Child Care in General Practice

To all our sons and daughters

Child Care in General Practice

Edited by

Cyril Hart MA, MB, DLitt, FRCGP

SECOND EDITION

CHURCHILL LIVINGSTONE
EDINBURGH LONDON MELBOURNE AND NEW YORK 1982

CHURCHILL LIVINGSTONE
Medical Division of Longman Group Limited

Distributed in the United States of America by Churchill Livingstone Inc., 19 West 44th Street, New York, N.Y. 10036, and by associated companies, branches and representatives throughout the world.

First edition 1977
Second edition 1982

ISBN 0 443 02591 6

British Library Cataloguing in Publication Data
Child care in general practice. – 2nd ed.
1. Children – Diseases
I. Hart, C.R.
618.92 RJ45

Library of Congress Catalog Card Number 81-69242

Printed in Singapore by Huntsmen Offset Printing Pte Ltd

Preface to the Second Edition

It is gratifying to receive a request from the publisher for a second edition of this book. Most of the original team of authors have been retained, but all except two of the original chapters have been revised, some radically. In an attempt to rectify omissions in the first edition, the number of chapters has been increased from 40 to 51. As before, contributors have been sought from among the ranks of general practitioners in active practice, though this rule has not been followed quite as strictly as in the first edition. There is greater emphasis on the preventive and social aspects of care, but clinical care has also received more coverage. The amount of progress in the theory and practice of child care in the past five years is surprising, and we are all faced with the formidable responsibility of keeping up to date. A series of multichoice questions has been added as an appendix to help established practitioners with this task. It is hoped that this innovation will find favour also with vocational trainees in general practice.

The editor is grateful to his partners, contributors, and other colleagues for constructive criticism, to his secretary, Mrs Janet Jaggard, for her patient and efficient help with retyping and in other directions too numerous to mention, and to his son, Dr Nicholas Hart, and daughter, Penelope Hart, for assisting with the index.

Peterborough, 1982 Cyril Hart

Preface to the First Edition

Child care is one quarter of all general practice. Of the wide spectrum of childhood disease and disorder presenting to the primary care team, only a small selection is referred for management elsewhere. The rest, the team members cope with themselves. Over the years they have evolved their own expertise in organisation, their own techniques of diagnosis and treatment, and their own philosophy of care. Our book is concerned with the quality of this service, and seeks therefore to supplement standard paediatric textbooks rather than to supplant them. We have tried to produce a balanced picture of our daily work with children. The book does not claim to be definitive or comprehensive; we have aimed rather at producing a practical manual for workers in the field.

Books on general practice are best written by general practitioners, but because we are generalists we have sometimes leaned heavily on colleagues from other disciplines for advice on specific topics. This has been readily forthcoming from helpers too numerous to mention individually; we are deeply indebted to them all. The editor is especially grateful to Dr Frederick Brimblecombe and to Dr John Horder for assistance in the early stages of planning, and to Dr Michael Webster for reading through the bulk of the typescript and contributing suggestions which improved the text substantially. Nicholas Hart, the editor's son, assisted with the index. Finally, thanks are due to Dr Paul Hooper for his generous and sustained support of this project. Few have done more for the improvement of child care in general practice.

Peterborough, 1977 Cyril Hart

Contributors

E. Alexander SRN, OND, HV
Health Visitor, Newport, Isle of Wight

W.W. Anderson BSc, MB, FRCGP, DObstRCOG
General Practitioner, Scarborough, Yorkshire

D.J. Bain MD, FRCGP, DCH, DObstRCOG
Professor of Primary Medical Care, University of Southampton

D.G. Barton MA, MB, FRCS, FRCGP, DCH, DObstRCOG
General Practitioner, Herne Bay; Clinical Assistant in Surgery, Queen Victoria Memorial Hospital, Herne Bay, Kent

K.J. Bolden MA, MB, FRCGP, DObstRCOG
General Practitioner, Exeter; Senior Lecturer in General Practice, University of Exeter

J.H. Briscoe MA, MB, MRCGP, DObstRCOG
General Practitioner, Eton, Berkshire; Medical Officer, Eton College and St George's School, Windsor Castle

N.J. Cook MB, ChB, DCH
General Practitioner, Bristol

G.H. Curtis Jenkins MA, MB, MRCGP, DObstRCOG
General Practitioner, Ashford, Middlesex

T.M. Davies MB, MRCGP
General Practitioner, Yaxley, Peterborough

D. Dean MB, MRCP, FRCGP, DCH
General Practitioner, West Bromwich

M.A. Downham BA, BM, MRCP, DCH
Senior Lecturer in Child Health, University of Newcastle

C.P. Elliott Binns MD, FRCGP, DCH, DObstRCOG
General Practitioner, Cogenhoe, Northampton

I. Gregg MA, MB, MRCP, FRCGP, DObstRCOG
General Practitioner, Kingston upon Thames, Surrey; Director, Department of Clinical Epidemiology, Cardiothoracic Institute

C.R. Hart MA, MB, DLitt, FRCGP
General Practitioner, Yaxley, Peterborough

A. Holden JP, BSc, ARCS
Principal Officer, Department of Social Services, Coventry

R. Holt PhD, MSc, BChD
Lecturer, Department of Children's Dentistry, Eastman Dental Hospital, London

P.D. Hooper MB, FRCGP, DObstRCOG
General Practitioner, Newport, Isle of Wight; Clinical Assistant in Surgery, Isle of Wight Hospital Group

Y. Horsfall Turner Cert Social Studies, Dip Social Work; Social Worker, Lewisham, London

D. Jenkinson MB, MRCGP, DCH, DObstRCOG
General Practitioner, Keyworth, Nottingham; Lecturer in General Practice, University of Nottingham

C. Josephs MD, FRCGP, DCH
General Practitioner, Stockwell Park, London

J.V. Lewis MB, MRCGP, DCH, DObstRCOG
General Practitioner, Stratford upon Avon, Warwickshire; Clinical Assistant, Casualty Department, Stratford upon Avon General Hospital

P. McWilliam MB, ChB, DCH
General Practitioner, Pontefract, Yorkshire; Hospital Practitioner in Paediatrics, Pontefract General Infirmary

T.M. Moore MB, FRCS
General Practitioner, Wickford, Essex

D.J. Pereira Gray MA, MB, FRCGP
General Practitioner, Exeter; Senior Lecturer in General Practice, University of Exeter

M. Pollak MD, MRCGP, DObstRCOG
Senior Lecturer in Social Paediatrics, King's College Hospital, London

M. Rogers MB, ChB, DObstRCOG
General Practitioner, Yaxley, Peterborough

R.G. Russell MB, ChB
General Practitioner, Stourbridge, Worcestershire

N. Silverston MB, FRCGP
General Practitioner, Bottisham, Cambridge

G.H. Smerdon MB, FRCGP, DCH, DObstRCOG
General Practitioner, Liskeard, Cornwall

I.M. Stanley MB, MRCP, MRCGP
General Practitioner, Leeds; Lecturer in General Practice, University of Leeds

T.I. Stewart MB, FRCGP, DCH
General Practitioner, Sonning Common, Berkshire

C.G. Sykes MB, FRCGP, DCH, DObstRCOG
General Practitioner, Huddersfield; Clinical Assistant in Paediatrics, Huddersfield Hospital Group

B. Tanner MD, FRCGP
General Practitioner, Lancaster Medical Centre, London

M. Thirlwall MB, MRCGP, DObstRCOG
General Practitioner, Aylesbury, Buckinghamshire

E. Tuckman MD, MRCGP, DCH, DTM&H
General Practitioner, Orpington, Kent

J.W. Tuke MB, MRCGP, DCH
Senior Clinical Medical Officer, Child Health, Northumberland

C. Waine MB, FRCGP
General Practitioner, Bishop Auckland, Durham; Hospital Practitioner in Paediatrics, Bishop Auckland General Hospital

J.H. Walker MD, FFCM, FRCGP, DCH
Professor of Family and Community Medicine, University of Newcastle

M.J. Whitfield MA, MB, MRCGP, DPH, DCH, DObstRCOG
General Practitioner, Bristol

P.G. Whitfield MB, MRCGP, DCH
Specialist in Community Medicine (Child Health), Hampshire

R.H. Wilkins (Ben-Dov), MD, MRCGP, DCH, DIH, DObstRCOG
Practitioner, Jerusalem, Israel

T. Wilkinson MB, BS
General Practitioner, Shepherd's Bush, London

G.B. Winter MB, BDS, FDSRCS, DCH
Professor of Children's Dentistry, Institute of Dental Surgery, London

Contents

1. THE ORGANISATION OF CHILD CARE

1. **The quality of child care** *C.R. Hart* 3
2. **Primary and secondary care** *M. Downham* 22
3. **Child care legislation** *A. Holden* 29
4. **Education in child care** *I. Stanley* 41
5. **Research in child care** *D.J.G. Bain* 45
6. **Child care and the computer** *K.J. Bolden* 53
7. **The practice health visitor** *E. Alexander* 57
8. **The social services and the practice** *Y. Horsfall Turner* 63

2. CHILD CARE AND PREVENTIVE MEDICINE

9. **The fetus at risk** *M. Rogers* 72
10. **Birth trauma** *M. Thirlwall* 86
11. **Immunisation** *D. Jenkinson* 91
12. **The child health clinic** *J.W. Tuke* 101
13. **Surveillance in the first year of life** *G. Curtis Jenkins* 105
14. **Surveillance in the pre-school years** *P.D. Hooper* 111
15. **The school health service** *J.H. Walker* 115
16. **Ill-treated children** *D.J. Pereira Gray* 120
17. **Health education** *C.R. Hart* 127

3. CLINICAL CARE IN ACUTE ILLNESS

18. **Acute disorders of the ear, nose and throat** *W.V. Anderson* 132
19. **Acute infections of the respiratory tract** *I. Gregg* 138
20. **Influenza in childhood** *J.D.H. Briscoe* 146
21. **The acute exanthemata** *E. Tuckman* 151
22. **Some common viral infections** *C.R. Hart* 157
23. **The acute abdomen in childhood** *P.D. Hooper* 174
24. **Accidents and poisoning in childhood** *J.V.V. Lewis* 181

4. CONTINUITY IN CLINICAL CARE

25. **Care of the newborn** *C. Waine* 194
26. **Problems of maturity** *P.D. Hooper* 202
27. **Nutrition in infancy and childhood** *M.J. Whitfield* 205
28. **Infestation with worms and insects** *N. Silverston* 211
29. **Some common skin disorders** *D. Dean* 218
30. **Some common orthopaedic disorders** *T.M.C. Moore* 224

31. Urinary infection in childhood
D.G. Barton 230

32. Blood disorders in childhood
C. Josephs 236

33. The teeth in childhood
G.B. Winter and R. Holt 250

34. Prescribing for infants and children
T.M. Davies 258

5. CLINICAL CARE IN LONG-TERM DISORDERS

35. Congenital heart disease
C.G.W. Sykes 267

36. Rheumatism and allied disorders
T.I. Stewart 278

37. Asthma and bronchitis
I. Gregg 283

38. Diabetes in childhood
R.G. Russell 299

39. Epilepsy in infancy and childhood
P. McWilliam 308

40. Deafness in childhood
J.W. Tuke 322

41. Visual disorders in childhood
P.G. Whitfield 327

42. The clinical care of handicapped children
D.J. Pereira Gray 333

6. ESSAYS IN FAMILY CARE

43. The sick family
G.H. Smerdon 343

44. Poverty and child health
B. Tanner 346

45. Behaviour problems in childhood
N. Cook 354

46. The spoilt child
C. Josephs 362

47. Communication and learning disorders in childhood
E. Tuckman 365

48. The care of immigrant children
M. Pollak 369

49. Children with alcoholic parents
R.H. Wilkins (Ben-Dov) 380

50. The handicapped child at home
T. Wilkinson 384

51. Death in childhood
C. Elliott Binns 386

Appendix: Voluntary organisations for child care
C.R. Hart 393

MCQs
I. Stanley 401

Index 409

PART ONE

The organisation of child care

1

The quality of child care

Cyril Hart

'In many crucial respects our findings have given us profound anxiety about the present state of child health in this country, about the shortcomings of the services and those working in them, and about the prospects for new generations if they are to grow up in the same deprived physical and emotional circumstances as many children today contend with.'

Court Report, 1976

The pattern of medical care available for children in the United Kingdom is governed almost entirely by the National Health Service, which was brought into being in 1948, reorganised radically in 1975, and is now (1982) undergoing a further administrative upheaval. The Health Service attempts to provide all necessary care for all children at all times, an ideal which is of course unattainable but which nevertheless forms a valuable template against which our success and our failures can be measured.

Within this framework, we are concerned in our book with the range and quality of services for children provided by the general practitioner and the primary care team. The first edition was published on the eve of the *Report of the Committee on Child Health Services,* which had been set up by the government under the chairmanship of Professor Donald Court. Such an authoritative review had not been carried out in this country before, and so great is its merit that ever since its appearance the report has rightly dominated every discussion on the future of child care, defining our objectives and guiding our efforts to achieve them (Curtis Jenkins *et al*, 1979). It is in response to the challenge of the opening statement of the Court report, which I have placed at the head of this chapter, that this review of the quality of child care in general practice has been undertaken.

In assessing quality we need a yardstick, and it was natural that the Court committee should begin by analysing such statistical information as was available to them. Infant mortality, the death rate per thousand live births in the first year of life, has been the traditional and most easily accessible index of child health in a country, and the committee began by plotting the rate for England and Wales against those of selected countries on a logarithmic scale for the years 1954 to 1974. The countries selected for comparison were Japan, France, Sweden and Finland. The famous graph that resulted is reproduced here (by kind permission) as

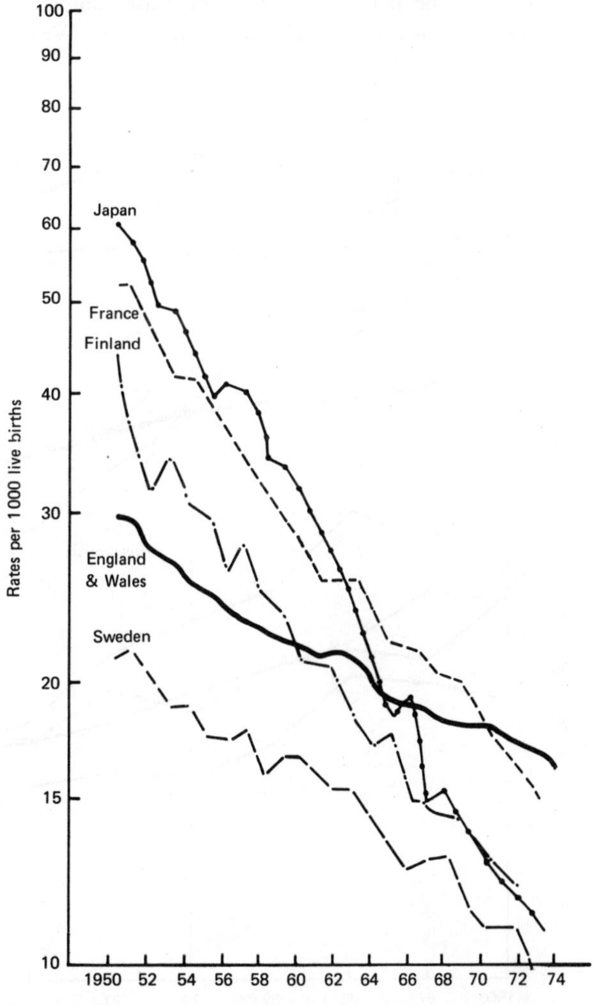

Fig. 1.1 Infant mortality rates in selected countries 1950–1974. Source: Court report, 1976

Figure 1.1. In 1950 only Sweden could show a better figure than England and Wales in this grim league table; by 1970 we were lying bottom (according to the committee's graph France was then still behind us, but revised figures now available show that this was not in fact the case). Nor were the countries selected for comparison just isolated examples; among others, Australia and New Zealand, Switzerland, Holland, Iceland, Norway and Denmark have all retained their early lead over us; by 1970 Canada and West Germany had overtaken us, to be joined later by such countries as Hong Kong and Singapore.

In Figure 1.2 I have sought to enlarge the scope of the graph in the Court report, and bring it up to date, as far as the published statistics will allow. It seems to me that the most valid comparison must be with Europe. To balance the account some East European countries have been included, and the figures for the United Kingdom as a whole replace those for England and Wales. The poor showing of the East compared with the West at once becomes apparent; in the West, only Portugal did worse than Eastern Europe. Hungary and Romania have made progress in recent years, but still have rates too high to be included on our graph, and the infant mortality rate in Byelorussian USSR actually increased between 1971 and 1974, the last available figures. (A request for later figures from the Soviet Embassy has been unsuccessful.) Within the western group, the United Kingdom is now shown to have maintained an average rate of improvement since 1970, the slope of its graph being very similar to those of the Scandinavian countries, Holland and West Germany. France has done better than Britain, but not remarkably so over the last seven years. The provisional figures for 1979–80 for the United Kingdom show a further substantial improvement.

The consistency of the improvement shown on the United Kingdom graph compares well with the more erratic graphs of Belgium, Ireland and West Germany. The picture for the United Kingdom today is therefore rather more favourable than that presented in the Court report; in Western Europe we are now just about holding

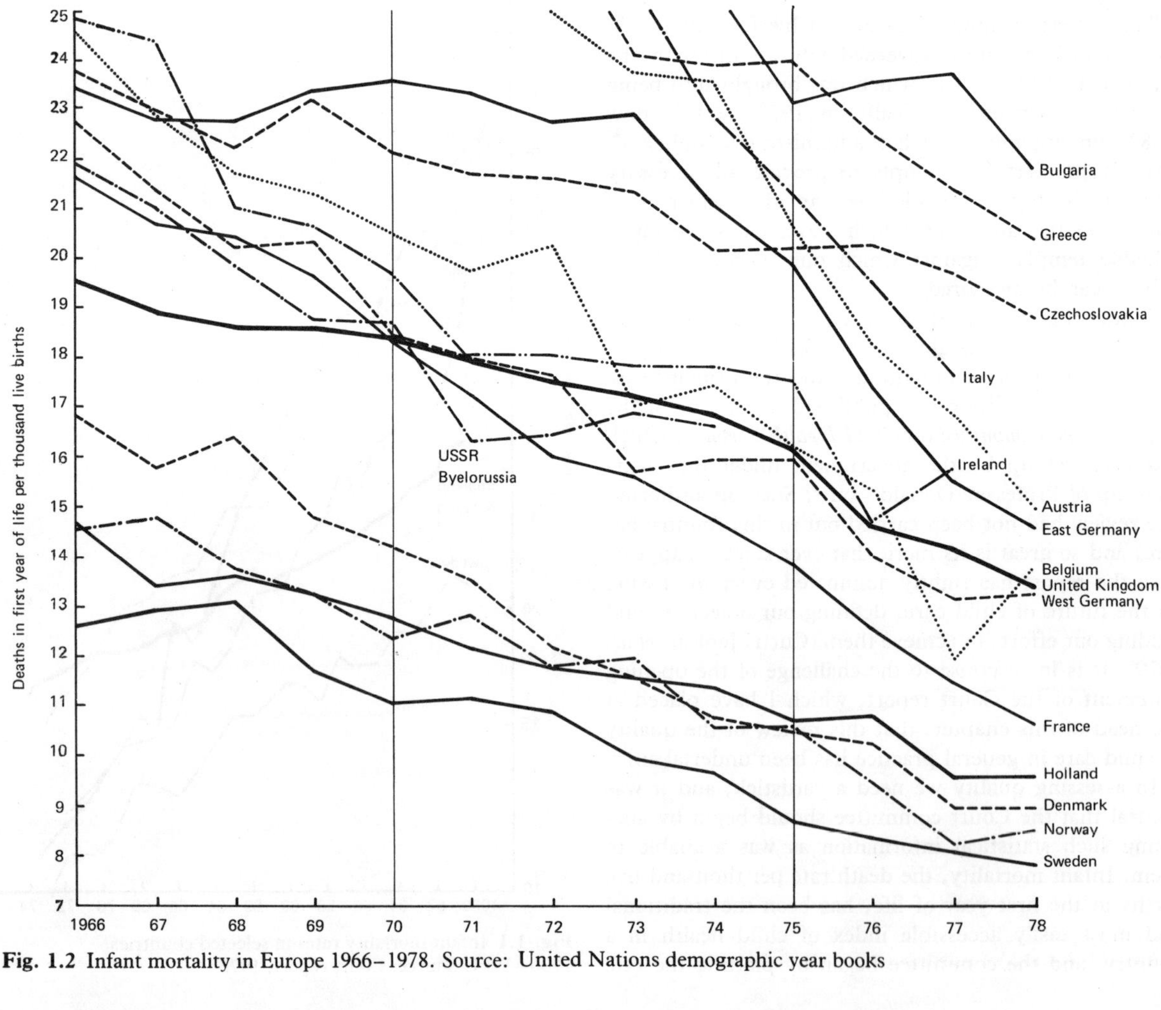

Fig. 1.2 Infant mortality in Europe 1966–1978. Source: United Nations demographic year books

our own as far as improvement of infant mortality is concerned, though we remain some ten years behind the figures of the Scandinavian countries, Holland and Switzerland.

Not that this gives us any reason for complacency, for infant mortality rates are but a blunderbuss method of assessment. As soon as the overall figures are broken down, enormous scope for further improvement is revealed. The more advanced countries of the West subject their mortality figures to minute scrutiny, and publish annual reports of which those for Holland and Denmark are fine examples. It is a pleasure to record that our own reports, published annually by HMSO for the Office of Population Censuses and Surveys, are as good as any to be found. We in general practice need to pay more attention to them.

Of the many permutations and combinations in this process of scrutiny, a vertical division into the days and weeks after birth when death occurs is one of the most useful. Thus the neonatal mortality rate measures the deaths per 1000 live births in the first month of life, and this can be further broken down into deaths occurring within 24 hours of birth, those from one to seven days after birth, and those from one to four weeks after birth. A histogram for infant mortality in the UK from 1967 to 1977 showing this breakdown appears as Figure 1.3. As is commonly the case world wide, there are more deaths in the first week of life than in the whole of the subsequent year.

The process of analysis can be extended by bringing the stillbirth rate into the picture, and by further breaking down the post neonatal mortality into deaths occurring between one and three months, between three and six months, and between six and twelve months, so revealing the total infant wastage step by step for the first year of life. The histogram of infant wastage for England and Wales from 1975 to 1978 is shown in Figure 1.4. We find there that the greater part of the improvement in recent years has been concentrated on that section of the wastage comprising the stillbirths together with the deaths within 24 hours of birth, and this is termed the crude perinatal mortality rate (in Fig. 1.4 this wastage is calculated per 1000 live births, but the true perinatal mortality rate (PMR) is usually calculated per 1000 live and stillbirths combined).

Let us pause here a moment to get things in perspective, for every integer in our statistics represents a human life. We have to remember that the improvement of perinatal mortality in Britain started well over a century ago. One might reasonably attribute its beginnings

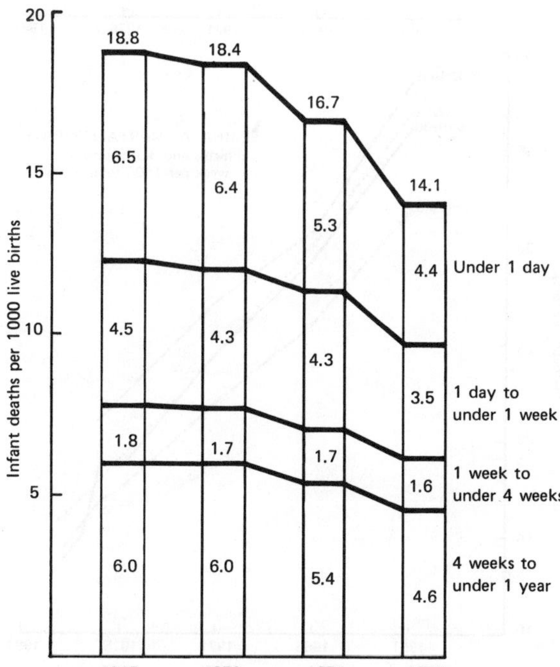

Fig. 1.3 United Kingdom infant mortality 1967–1977. Source: CSO annual abstract of statistics, 1979

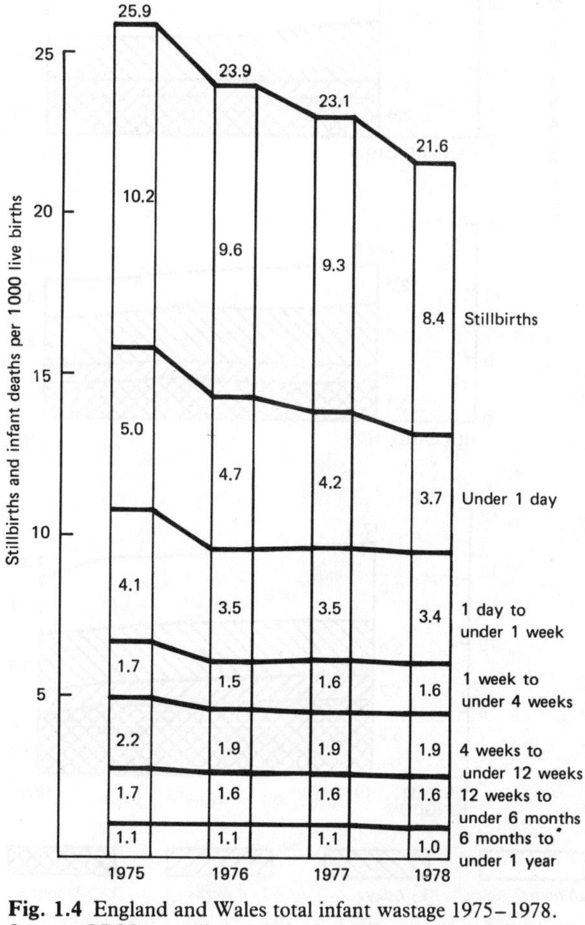

Fig. 1.4 England and Wales total infant wastage 1975–1978. Source: OPCS mortality statistics – childhood and maternity. HMSO, 1980

to Charles Dickens, who awakened the conscience of the nation to the plight of the poor in childbirth. Here is his description, written in 1837, of the birth of Oliver Twist in a workhouse:

'For a long time after it was ushered into this world of sorrow and trouble by the parish surgeon, it remained a matter of considerable doubt whether the child would survive to bear any name at all ... The fact is, that there was considerable difficulty in inducing Oliver to take upon himself the office of respiration ... and for some time he lay gasping on a little flock mattress, rather unequally poised between this world and the next ... There was nobody but a pauper old woman, who was rendered rather misty by an unwonted allowance of beer ... Oliver and Nature fought the point between them.'

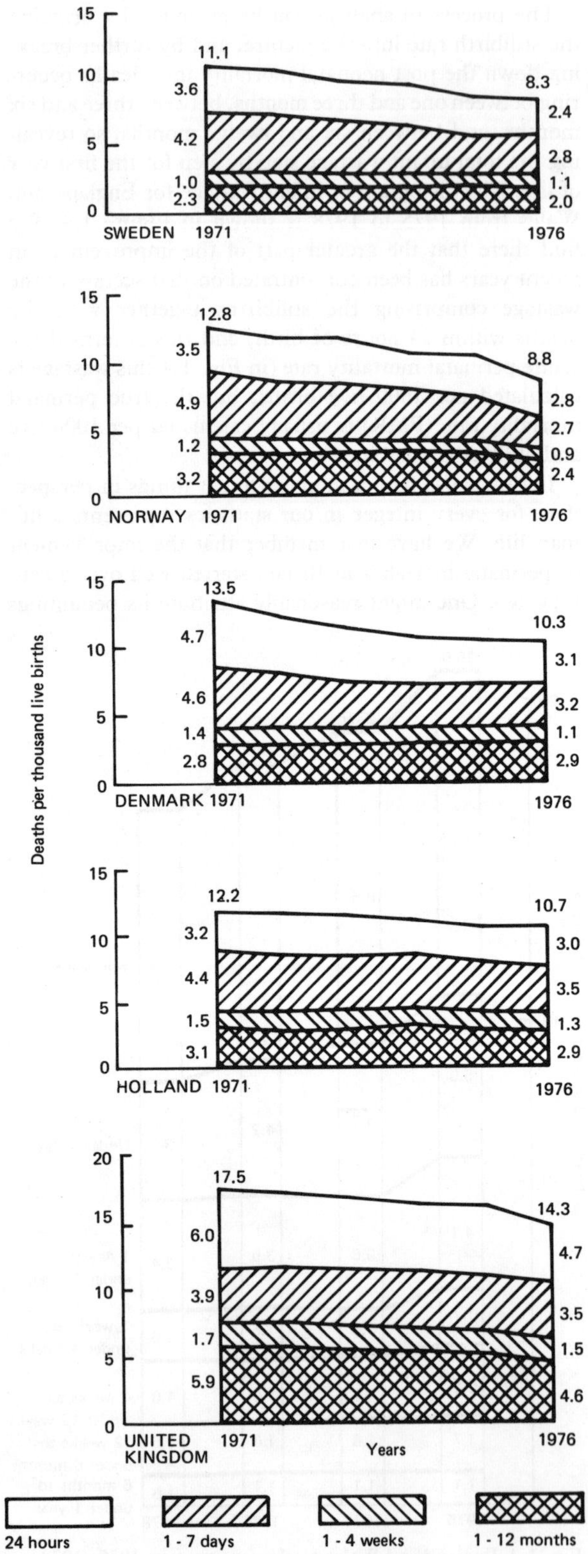

Fig. 1.5 Infant mortality in Northern Europe 1971–1976. Source: United Nations demographic year books

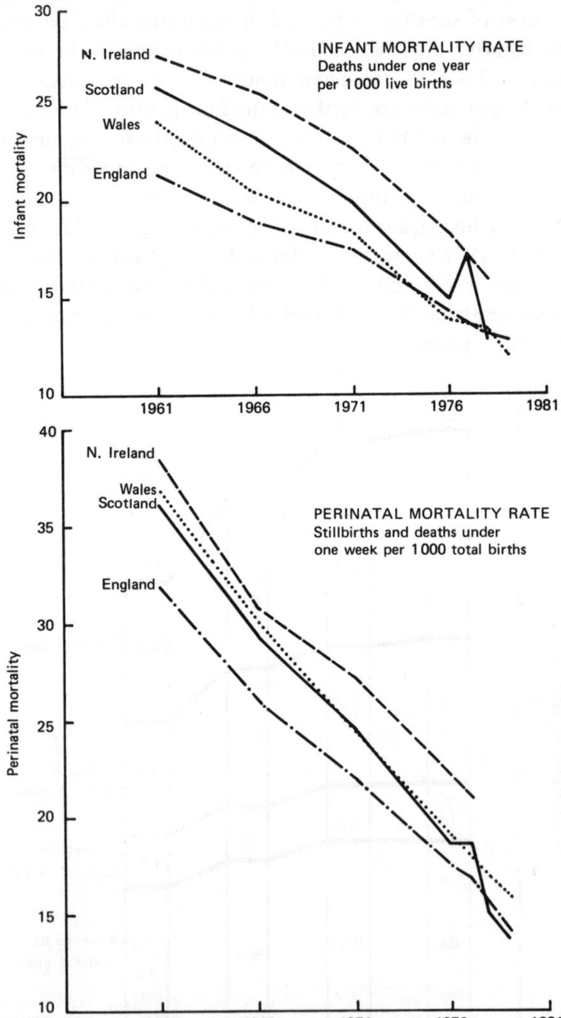

Fig. 1.6 Perinatal and infant mortality in England, Wales, Scotland and Northern Ireland 1961–1978. Source: CSO regional statistics 14, 1979

To return to modern times, this relatively greater improvement of perinatal mortality compared with post neonatal mortality is a common feature of statistics from advanced countries. Setting the stillbirths on one side, it is worthwhile to compare the United Kingdom infant mortality performance in detail with those of the Scandinavian countries and Holland, whose marvellous figures compel our respect and admiration. Those who still think our Health Service is the envy of the world would do well to examine Figure 1.5 carefully. Our neonatal and post neonatal figures both need to be halved before they compare well with the best, and a similar reduction is needed in our stillbirths.

Carrying the analysis of our own figures still further on a national basis, the first point of interest to emerge is that Scotland and Wales, which two decades ago had perinatal mortality rates close to those of Northern Ireland, have now dropped their figures to England's level, leaving Northern Ireland trailing behind. The same is true of the infant mortality rate, though less markedly so (Fig. 1.6). Yet Southern Ireland, starting from a much higher level, has managed to reduce its infant mortality to a figure near to that of England (Fig. 1.2). It could be argued that the troubles in Northern Ireland have caused more deaths of babies than of adults.

At a regional level, in England and Wales earlier disparities have been greatly reduced, yet remarkable anomalies persist. Perinatal mortality in 1978 was half as much again in the North West as in Wessex, and the death rate of babies between one and four weeks after birth for the period 1975 to 1977 was running nearly twice as high in Yorkshire and Humberside as in the West Midlands (Figs 1.7; 9.6).

We have now to consider to what extent these variations are ascribable to social, economic, biological and environmental causes, and to what extent they may arise from differences in the quality of care. In recent years it has been suggested that the crude perinatal mortality should be modified regionally to take into account the high loss due to babies born with very low birth weight; this latter component has been thought to be an index of socio-economic variation, rather than the quality of obstetric, paediatric, or nursing care. By applying regression analysis to eliminate the effect of babies born of 2000 g or less birth weight, a set of adjusted perinatal mortality rates has been produced for administrative areas in England and Wales (Chalmers *et al*, 1978). Yet even if we suppose the rationale of such an adjustment to be valid, we are still left with very large differences in rates, both regionally and at area level. This is shown for example in Figure 1.8, where the crude and adjusted PMRs for the Oxford and Yorkshire regions in 1976 are compared. The differences between the north and south of the country are well understood, but how can one account for the fact that the adjusted figure for Buckinghamshire was nearly twice that for neighbouring Oxfordshire?

So far, little firm evidence has emerged to support the naive assumption that the proportion of low birth weight babies born in a region or area reflects socio-economic variations in the population, rather than variation in the quality of overall care given by the health professionals. Many more factors than this are at play, some of them subtle and elusive, and further analysis is needed (Mutch *et al*, 1981). Effective care has a large preventive component, and greater attention to the early

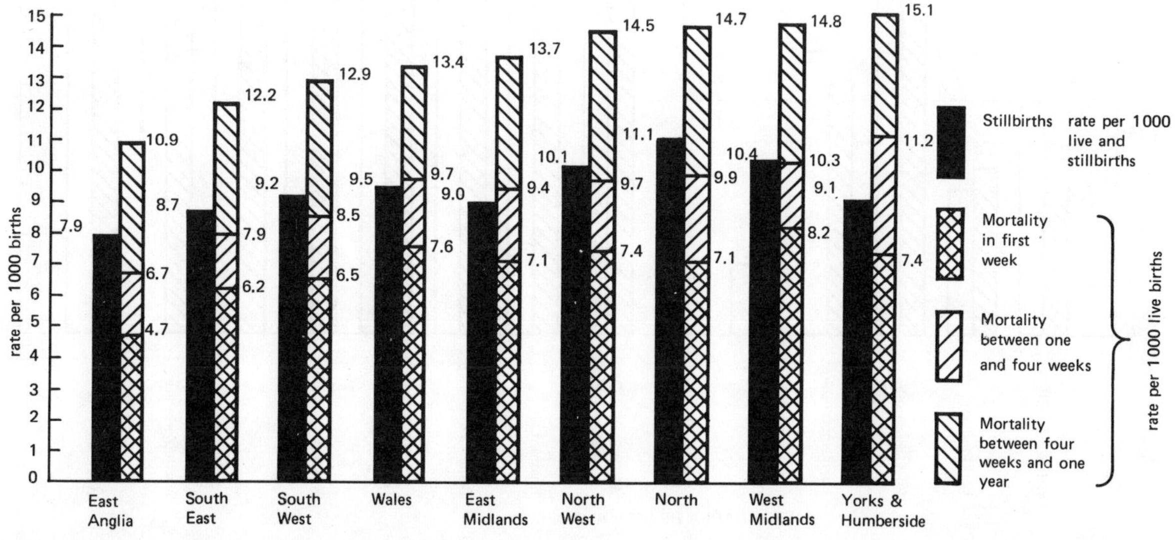

Fig. 1.7 England and Wales stillbirth and mortality rates in the first year of life for legitimate births in 1975–1977, by regions. Source: Studies in medical and population subjects, 41. HMSO, 1980

identification and detailed antenatal management of high risk groups would undoubtedly result in a corresponding reduction in births of premature and light-for-date babies. We are led to postulate that variations in the crude PMR may depend in part on the quality of antenatal care, whereas variations in the adjusted PMR are more likely to reflect the quality of intrapartum or post partum care. While there may be an element of truth in this proposition, it must be conceded that both rates are still influenced profoundly by social and economic factors, many of which are outside the reach of doctors and other health care professionals, whether working in hospitals or in primary care teams. We can only hope to influence this stubborn and unyielding component of perinatal death rates by patient education of our politicians, and of the general public who vote them into office, for an important part of the remedy lies in informed political decisions.

Some of these social and economic factors are discussed further in Chapters 44 and 48, and the professional aspects of perinatal care are pursued further in Chapters 9, 10 and 35. There is no doubt that the substantial general practitioner involvement in antenatal and perinatal care has received insufficient scrutiny in our efforts to improve the PMR. For example, the report on perinatal and neonatal mortality by a parliamentary committee under the chairmanship of Mrs Renee Short fails notably to appreciate the importance of the general practitioner services (Short, 1980; Davies, 1980). As another recent instance, one might quote a discussion document on the reduction of perinatal mortality and morbidity produced by the Children's Committee (*Children's Committee Report, 1979*). This was prepared by a working party which included two obstetricians, a paediatrician, a midwife, and a social worker, but not a single general practitioner or health visitor. As a result,

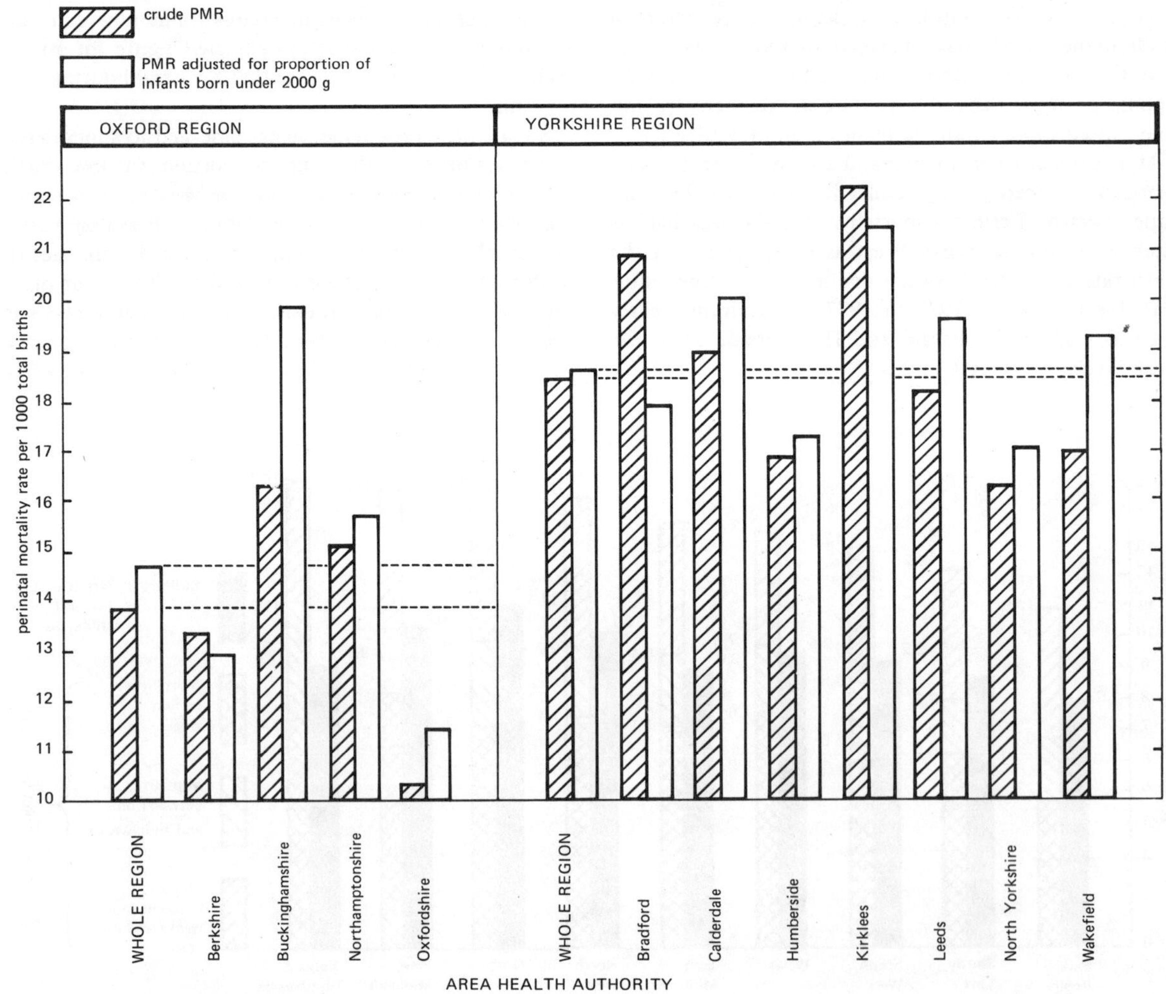

Fig. 1.8 Crude and adjusted perinatal mortality rates: Oxford and Yorkshire regions compared 1976. Source: Chalmers *et al*, 1978

whilst the report made many wise suggestions on the management of antenatal and postnatal care and of the delivery, the sections devoted to primary care in general, and to general practice in particular, were vague and superficial. The report's suggestion for 'a randomised controlled trial of home delivery' would appear to be quite impractical in view of present trends. In Holland, so often quoted as an example of what can be done, home delivery is now disappearing fast. Any increase in British home delivery rates now would require a radical and costly reorganisation of our maternity services, if safety for mother and baby is to be secured. The future for general practice participation in delivery must surely lie with GP obstetric units based on maternity hospitals where consultant help and advice is at hand.

I wish to turn now to consideration of the post-neonatal component of infant mortality, which has not changed very greatly in the last two decades (Fig. 1.9). The post-neonatal mortality has evened out in all the advanced countries over this period, but in Scandinavia the rates have levelled at about half those in the United Kingdom. We have much to learn from Sweden, where routine surveillance of babies is highly developed, and there is excellent parental compliance with immunisation and other forms of preventive care (Rooth, 1979; Harker, 1980). Can we hope to approach the Scandinavian level in the foreseeable future? I believe we can, but only if we make a tremendous effort, and only if there is more financial support for child care from central government.

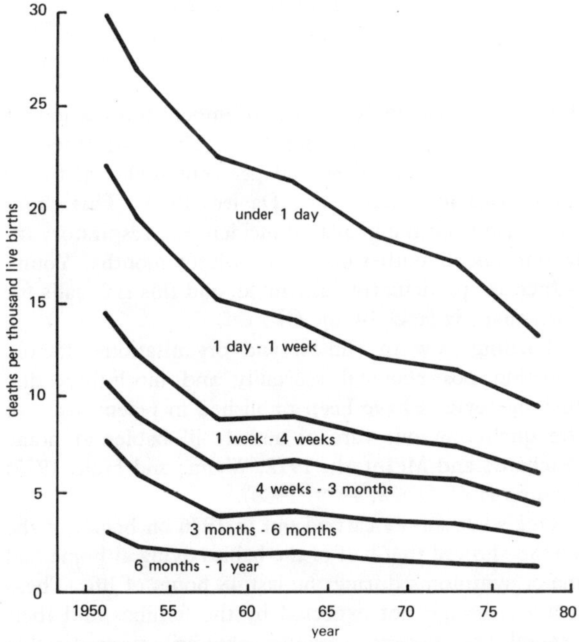

Fig. 1.9 Infant mortality by age groups, England and Wales, 1951–1978. Source: OPCS

Figures 1.10 to 1.12 show that a number of key social factors affect the baby's chance of survival almost as much in the post-neonatal as in the neonatal period. These are the social class, age and parity of the mother, and the legitimacy of the baby. The class factor is of course well known and is discussed elsewhere (Ch. 44). The considerable variation of post-neonatal mortality with age and parity of the mother is perhaps less well appreciated. The low late mortality of babies born to mothers under 16 years old is doubtless due to their adoption. But the increased risk to both legitimate and illegitimate babies of mothers in the 16 to 20 age group compounds with the greater vulnerability of third and later babies in a family, so that the post-neonatal mortality rate becomes substantially increased when a young mother has a large family quickly. The very high risk for the illegitimate babies of young mothers must also give cause for concern, because of the steep rise in illegitimacy (Fig. 9.8), which is now reverting in incidence to Victorian levels. At the time of writing, the provisional figures for 1979 show that 14 per cent of all births in England and Wales were illegitimate. It can be argued that a substantial proportion of these births are to couples having a stable relationship, but the hard statistical facts are that illegitimate babies do less well than legitimate babies in the mortality stakes. The class factor compounds these risks.

Once again we need only to turn to Dickens to remind ourselves that the bearing of these social factors on mortality has been well understood for many years. Here is Oliver Twist's slatternly midwife trying to revive his ailing mother after his delivery:

> 'Lor bless her dear heart, when she has lived as long as I have, and had thirteen children of her own, and all of them dead except two, and them in the workus with me, she'll know better to take on that way . . . Think what it is to be a mother, there's a dear young lamb, do.'

But Oliver's mother was too exhausted to respond:

> 'It's all over, Mrs Thingummy,' said the surgeon at last . . . 'She was a good looking girl too, where did she come from?'
>
> 'She was brought here last night,' replied the old woman, 'by the overseer's order. She was found lying on the street. She had walked some distance, for her shoes were worn to pieces; but where she came from, or where she was going to, nobody knows.'
>
> The surgeon leaned over the body, and raised the left hand. 'The same old story,' he said, shaking his head: 'no wedding ring, I see. Ah! Goodnight!'

Thanks to the parish surgeon's efforts, Oliver survived, but the problems of high parity, illegitimacy,

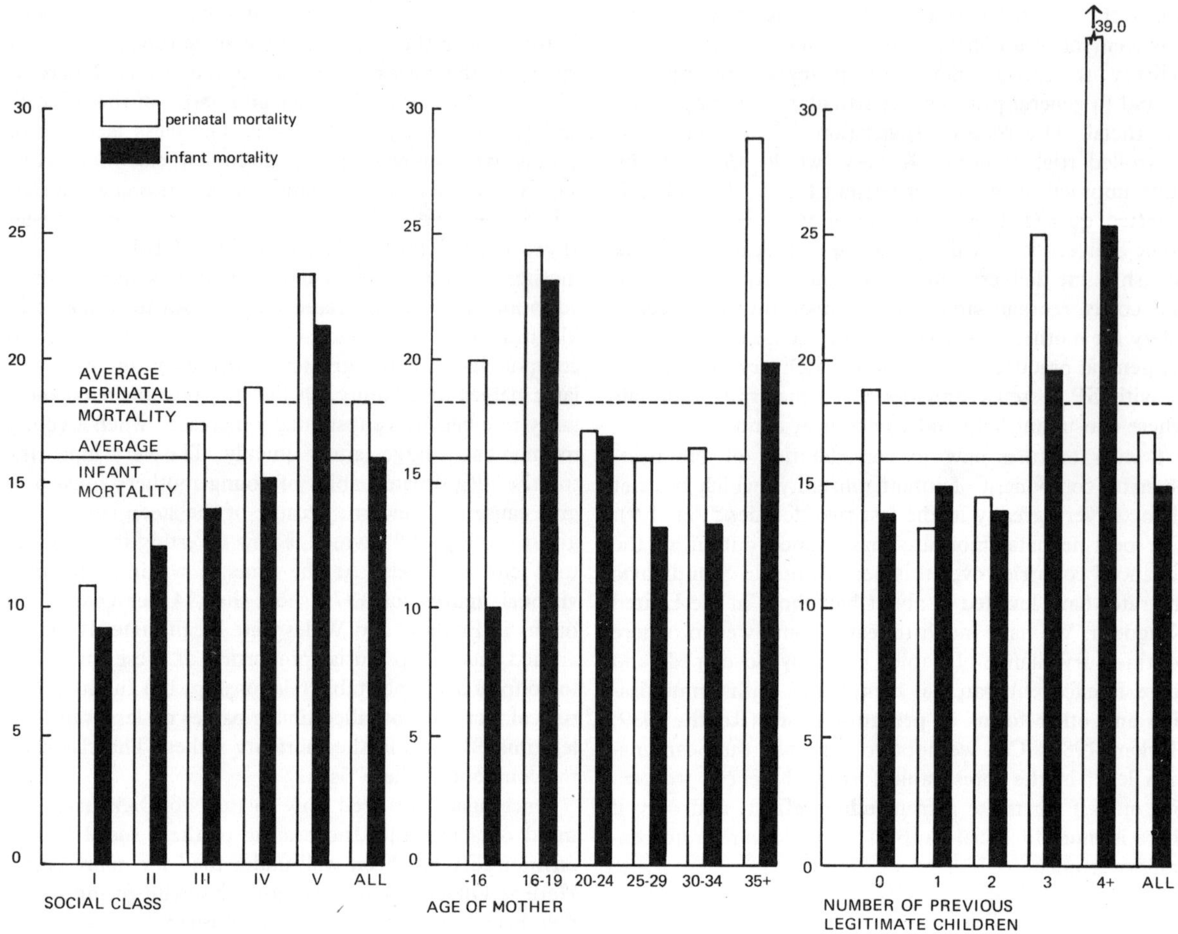

Fig. 1.10 Scottish perinatal and infant mortality in 1977. Source: *BMJ*, 1979

teenage pregnancy, poverty, and those who move frequently from place to place, all remain with us to the present day. We are still not doing nearly enough to combat them. The social differences between now and Victorian times are merely those of degree.

I believe that present day statistics point decisively to the need for a much more vigorous drive to educate young mothers, particularly those in social classes 4 and 5, to plan their families and space their babies by using the pill; at the same time, young fathers should be invited to consider vasectomy as soon as their families are complete. There is nothing new in these ideas, but we have not been active enough in pursuing them. The responsiblity for success in this field lies largely with general practitioners and health visitors, who are best placed to achieve it. When every baby is a wanted baby, the post-neonatal mortality will fall.

Another important factor affecting survival in the post-neonatal period is the season in which the baby is born. The highest post-neonatal death rates occur in children born between July and November, and the lowest in those born in March and April. The death rates for those born in August are 50 per cent higher than for those born in March (I.M. Davies, 1980). This could well arise from the increased incidence of respiratory infection and hypothermia in the winter months. Young babies are particularly vulnerable, and this risk calls for particular vigilance by the GP.

Turning now to clinical and organisational factors affecting post-neonatal mortality and morbidity, disturbing reviews have been published in recent years of the quality of our care of acutely ill babies at home (Richards and McIntosh, 1972; Wynne and Hull, 1977; Stanton *et al* , 1978, 1979, 1980).

One such survey carried out in 1976 on behalf of the DHSS showed that half of the babies dying at home had major symptoms during the last 48 hours of life. These deaths, though not expected by the families and their general practitioners, were not necessarily unpredictable from the symptoms described. It was concluded that some

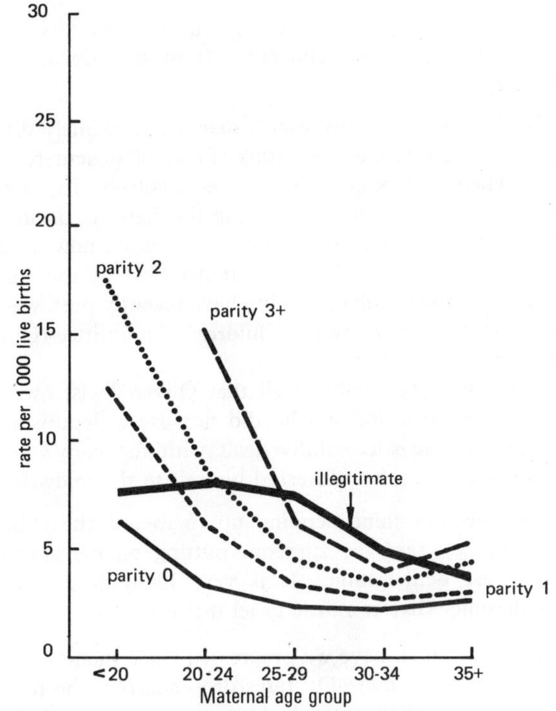

Fig. 1.11 Postneonatal mortality, England and Wales, 1977. Source: Studies in medical and population subjects, 41. HMSO, 1980

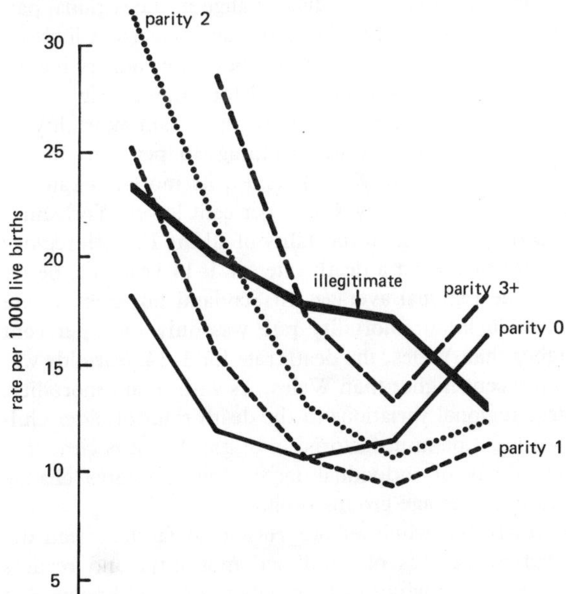

Fig. 1.12 Infant mortality 1977, England and Wales. Source: Studies in medical and population subjects, 41. HMSO, 1980

of these babies might have survived had the importance of their symptoms been recognised, and appropriate medical aid had been sought and provided. A second study undertaken in the winter of 1977-8 by Dr A.N. Stanton and his colleagues concerned the home management of acutely ill infants prior to their admission to hospital. Retrospective enquiries were made about 150 babies admitted to hospitals in Sheffield and Gateshead, who survived their illnesses. Of those admitted, more than two-thirds when first assessed by their family doctor had not been considered to require admission. Follow-up was arranged in only 14 of these cases. For the remaining 94 ill babies the initiative for recall of the GP was left to the parents. 33 cases (nearly one quarter of all acute admissions) were admitted from casualty without referral by the family doctor. Of these, 14 (nearly one in ten of all acute admissions) were taken direct to hospital without having seen a family doctor. It was found that babies aged between four and twelve weeks had over twice the admission rate of older babies, an index of their greater vulnerability (Fig. 1.13).

It is unfortunate that these reviews result from investigations carried out by hospital doctors rather than general practitioners. As a result, one could easily find fault with their methodology, and hence question their conclusions. Nevertheless, I believe that there is a substantial element of truth in their criticism, which we cannot afford to ignore. Instead, we should try to identify the underlying weaknesses in our day-to-day practice, and strive to overcome them.

The common early symptoms of serious illness in babies were listed by Dr Stanton as irritability, missed

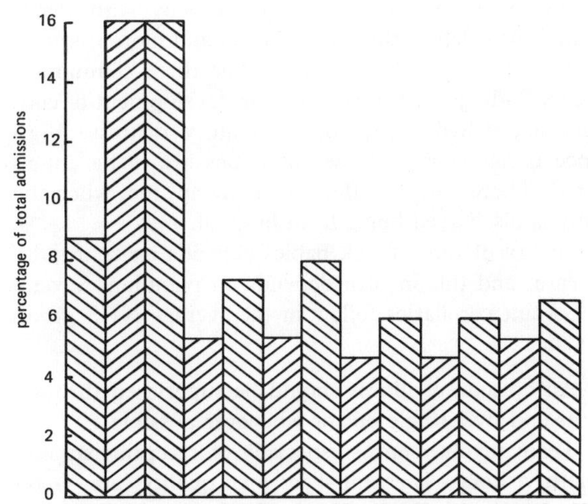

Fig. 1.13 Ages of babies admitted to hospital: 150 acute admissions, winter 1977–1978. Source: Stanton *et al*, *BMJ* 1980, 1, 897

feeds, vomiting, drowsiness, altered breathing, diarrhoea, altered cry, fever, wheeze, and shortness of breath, in that order of frequency. Often there are no objective clinical signs to be elicited in the early stages, so one has to depend on these symptoms for arousal of suspicion. Unfortunately they are all non-specific, and in fact they all occur far more frequently in babies with minor upsets than in those heading for severe illness. The great majority of babies in the former category are going to get better with the simplest of nursing care. However, as everyone knows, the condition of a mildly ill baby can change for the worse with alarming rapidity, and more often than not it is the suddenness of the change that leads to loss of confidence, and later to criticism, by parents and others. It is so easy to be wise after the event.

For the most part, therefore, the deficiencies in home care that have been revealed by these surveys are organisational, rather than clinical. What can we do about them? Dr Stanton has suggested that three criteria should be taken into account in the initial assessment of a sick baby:

1. Symptoms are more important than signs.
2. Behavioural changes are frequently the only warning signals before death.
3. Parents are in the best position to judge changes in their baby's behaviour, though they may not be able to interpret their importance.

If it is decided not to admit an ill baby to hospital, then effective follow-up must be considered. We should keep the initiative for this in our own hands, and be less ready to place the onus for further consultation on the parent. Daily reassessment by doctor or health visitor should be normal practice when a baby with major symptoms is left in the parents' care, and more frequent visiting may often be indicated. The three commonest events leading to admission are the development of convulsions, dehydration, and respiratory distress. Vigilance is necessary if these conditions are to be anticipated. There must be effective follow-up, too, when the baby is discharged home from hospital.

Quality of care of sick babies depends on continuity of care, and this in turn depends on planning. Several important corollaries follow in the average NHS group practice:

1. An episode of illness should be supervised through to its end by a single doctor whenever possible.
2. Team involvement – especially of receptionists and health visitors – is essential for high quality care. Good communication within the team is vital.
3. When the doctor concerned goes off duty at night or of a weekend, he should hand over the case formally to his partner on duty, with an up-to-date account of the baby's condition.
4. Good note taking is necessary if responsibility for care is to be passed efficiently from one doctor to another.

All this means, to my mind, that it is extremely difficult to ensure proper continuity of care of an acutely ill baby when a deputising service is involved. In such cases, surely, the safest thing for the baby is usually admission to hospital. Deputising services are now used by nearly half the general practitioners in England and Wales, and the problems arising have recently been well reviewed in a report by the Children's Committee (Out of Hours Care, 1980).

In passing, we might recall that Oliver Twist owed his survival to a doctor who did not use a deputising service. Having successfully dealt with the baby's respiratory distress, he addressed himself to the midwife:

> 'You needn't mind sending up to me, if the child cries, nurse,' said the surgeon, putting on his gloves with great deliberation. 'It is very likely it *will* be troublesome. Give it a little gruel if it is.'

Just how much have we progressed since then?

After infancy, mortality rates drop sharply, the total deaths for the whole of the 1–14 age group being only 30 per cent of the deaths in the first year of life. Rates continue to be related closely to social class and housing density, but there is a radical change in the regional pattern, which no longer shows the same clear-cut increase in death rates from south to north of the country for the 1–14 age group as is evidenced for infants (Fig. 1.14). For example, whereas in 1977 the infant mortality in the Northern region was running 30 per cent higher than that of South West Thames, its mortality rate for the 1–14 age group was nine per cent lower. Yorkshire, with the worst infant mortality of all the English regions in 1977, achieved a death rate for 1–14 year olds better than the regional average. In Scotland however, where the 1976 infant mortality rate was only nine per cent higher than Wales, the death rate for 1–14 year olds was 25 per cent higher than Wales. As with infant mortality, these regional variations in the death rates of older children must be multifactorial in origin, but it is clear that the effects of individual factors on the rates change greatly as the age groups progress.

Nearly the whole of our review so far has been devoted to analysis of childhood mortality, and readers will be asking why this is so, when it is well known that the overwhelming bulk of the GP's work with children is concerned with non-fatal conditions. There are two main reasons for this approach: firstly, mortality statistics enable the outcome of incidence and management of disease to be quantified more precisely than any other yardstick, and secondly in the United Kingdom as elsewhere, childhood morbidity as opposed to mortality has been ill recorded in statistical terms.

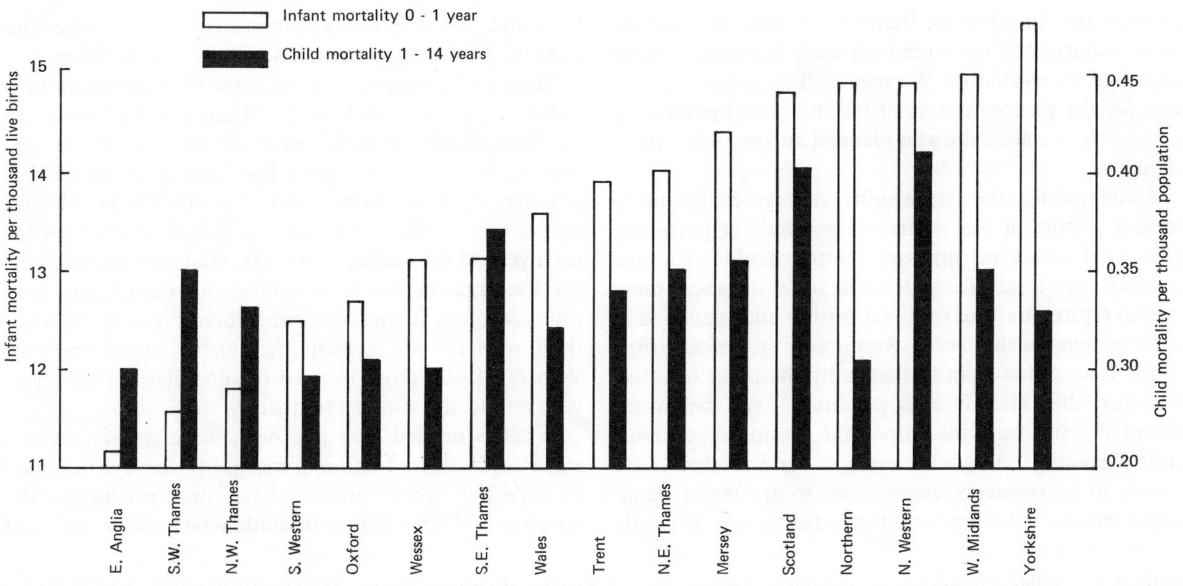

Fig. 1.14 Regional mortality rates by age group Great Britain, 1976–1977. Source: OPCS mortality statistics DH5

Our fundamental source of information is the now rather dated second *National Morbidity Survey* for the years 1970–1 and 1971–2 by selected general practitioners in England and Wales, published by the Stationery Office in 1974 and 1979. Unfortunately the scheme of disease classification adopted for this study is not well suited for extracting useful statistics concerning the younger section of the practice population. There is no provision for measuring the parts played in the identification and management of episodic illness by individual members of the primary care team other than the family doctor, so the work of the nurse and health visitor goes unrecorded. There are few disease categories reserved specifically for children (for example, there is no code number for wheezy bronchitis) and this together with the division of reporting into only two age groups, of 0–4 and 5–14 years, prevents any close analysis of childhood morbidity. Moreover, there is only the crudest regional breakdown by age groups (Table 1.1), and no breakdown at all by social class. There is no record of seasonal variations in morbidity. The time lag between the surveys and their publication further limits their usefulness, as patterns of morbidity in childhood appear to be changing rapidly. However, these

Table 1.1 Childhood morbidity in England and Wales 1971–2: crude regional breakdown. Source: HMSO (1979) OPCS, DHSS, RCGP studies in medical and population subjects No. 36

	Males			Females		
	All ages	0–4 years	5–14 years	All ages	0–4 years	5–14 years
Consultation rates per 100 population in selected practices						
All practices	267.3	396.1	189.3	360.1	357.7	192.2
North	286.3	405.5	174.7	373.6	372.4	176.6
Midlands and Wales	275.9	370.7	189.5	336.9	327.6	176.6
South	252.6	401.9	198.2	362.2	362.3	208.2
Patients consulting per 100 population in selected practices						
All practices	62.2	89.1	61.2	70.0	87.5	61.6
North	63.7	90.6	60.3	71.3	89.1	60.7
Midlands and Wales	61.4	85.1	59.5	67.8	83.0	58.9
South	61.8	91.1	63.0	70.6	89.6	64.0

surveys are considerably better than nothing, and no other country has yet attempted such a comprehensive review of its morbidity. We may well be grateful therefore for the pioneer efforts of the individual practitioners and their colleagues who planned and recorded these statistics.

Aetiologically, these morbidity surveys enable us to form a picture of the relative importance of particular groups of childhood illnesses for the workload of the primary care team (Table 1.2). In some instances these overall figures are broken down further and tabulated in later sections of this book. Respiratory infections come to the fore, followed in incidence by the other infective illnesses, then allergy, skin conditions, and behaviour disorders, and next the important group of accidents and poisoning. Anaemia, epilepsy and diabetes are shown to be relatively uncommon, so are major handicaps; cancer and congenital heart disease are distinctly rare, and tuberculosis and rheumatism are fast following rickets, diptheria, polio and smallpox into oblivion.

Measured by consulting rates, the 0–4 age group provided 10 per cent, and the 5–14 age group a further 15 per cent, of all the workload of the practices in the survey. Child care is therefore one quarter of all general practice. Roughly 90 per cent of the 0–4 year olds and 60 per cent of the 5–14 year olds consulted their doctor each year of the survey. This has important implications for the organisation of screening and surveillance programmes, but it must be remembered that of the children who do not consult the doctor, some are very vulnerable and more in need of surveillance than those who attend the surgery frequently.

What is needed now is a new, more specialised and more sophisticated national morbidity survey, designed to reveal in much greater detail than previously the spectrum of morbidity in childhood, the social and

Table 1.2 Childhood morbidity in England and Wales 1971–2. Selected disorders. Source: HMSO (1979) OPCS, DHSS, RCGP studies in medical and population subjects No. 36

Cause of consultation	*Episode rates per 1000 population*			*Consultation rates per 1000 population*		
	All ages	*0–4 years*	*5–14 years*	*All ages*	*0–4 years*	*5–14 years*
All conditions	1835.8	2909.2	1453.8	3156.8	3773.9	1907.1
Diseases of respiratory system	402.1	1025.2	491.1	590.1	1299.4	673.5
Acute nasopharyngitis – non febrile	69.5	325.0	78.4	80.8	375.8	88.1
Acute nasopharyngitis – febrile	40.5	126.9	42.6	55.5	169.5	52.9
Acute pharyngitis and tonsillitis	94.7	213.7	191.5	120.5	272.6	235.9
Acute bronchitis and bronchiolitis	70.7	194.9	62.1	117.7	274.7	94.6
Pneumonia	3.4	5.8	1.9	10.2	14.0	4.9
Asthma	11.9	13.5	18.4	31.9	24.9	43.3
Hay Fever	11.7	4.8	18.8	17.1	6.6	26.4
Diseases of CNS and sense organs	142.2	326.9	163.8	220.6	487.4	235.8
Epilepsy	3.3	2.8	2.5	9.1	7.3	5.4
Migraine	8.9	0.2	5.0	14.6	0.2	7.8
Conjunctivitis and ophthalmia	20.1	73.3	19.6	26.2	87.4	23.3
Acute otitis media	34.9	198.1	82.9	56.7	330.1	132.7
Skin Disorders	133.1	229.9	140.7	195.0	294.9	179.0
Impetigo	8.6	29.1	23.9	10.6	34.3	28.3
Eczema and dermatitis	37.2	113.2	30.6	53.9	149.3	40.4
Infective and Parasitic Diseases	93.7	267.4	180.2	132.4	337.1	234.3
Intestinal infections	78.8	101.6	26.2	37.8	131.3	30.4
Viral warts	12.9	4.7	45.2	19.7	5.9	71.0
Digestive System	97.3	153.1	55.9	160.4	182.4	67.1
Teeth	9.1	17.9	8.0	11.2	16.3	9.0
Acute vomiting and diarrhoea	23.7	84.0	20.6	31.4	103.4	23.2
Constipation	9.0	15.4	5.3	12.7	18.4	6.3
Genito urinary System	98.4	39.6	28.3	161.4	62.1	43.5
Mental Disorders	147.5	64.4	42.8	325.2	91.7	68.6
Accidents, poisonings & violence	105.2	84.3	103.1	165.3	108.4	126.7
Congenital anomalies	3.0	16.1	4.5	4.9	23.9	6.8
Symptoms + ill defined conditions	151.6	261.5	136.6	221.8	312.5	169.1

biological factors of greatest significance in its causation, and the effectiveness of its management at primary care level. The unique structure of the NHS would enable us to plan and implement such a survey more easily and more efficiently than any other country. The rewards would be immense. Armed with the results of the survey, we would have much more clear-cut objectives when planning the child care component of vocational training; we could identify the most pressing problems in child care, and restructure our practices to meet them; we could assess the quality of child care and its outcome with more precision than ever before. A new form of morbidity classification would be needed. As a start, the BPA classification should be considered (BPA, 1979). Suggested guidelines for a national child morbidity survey are outlined in the appendix to this chapter.

In the absence of a widespread organisation of screening and surveillance, the incidence of ill-health recorded in morbidity surveys is limited to those conditions leading to consultation with members of the primary care team. It has long been realised that much ill-health does not reach medical attention, and the term 'illness iceberg' has been used to describe this phenomenon (Last, 1963; Hart, 1975). The extent of chronic illness in children as seen through the eyes of their parents is surprisingly high. *The General Household Survey* carried out in 1973 revealed that parents considered over three per cent of children aged under five years to be suffering from a severe chronic illness, and a further two per cent from chronic illness of a minor degree of severity. The corresponding figures for the five to fourteen age group were over 5 per cent (boys) and 3.5 per cent (girls) considered to have severe chronic illness, and a further 4 per cent of boys and 3 per cent of girls thought to have minor chronic illness (Fig. 1.15). Nor is this perceived ill health limited to chronic illness. The *General Household Survey* of 1976 recorded that about 9 per cent of the 0–4 age group and 8 per cent of the 5–14 age group had episodes of restricted activity due to illness during the two weeks prior to the survey. The average number of days of restricted activity due to illness during the previous year was reported as 12.5 for boys and (surprisingly) 10.4 for girls. There was a social class variation for boys, but not for girls (Fig. 1.16).

These figures may seem impossibly high to primary health care professionals, but a recent survey in

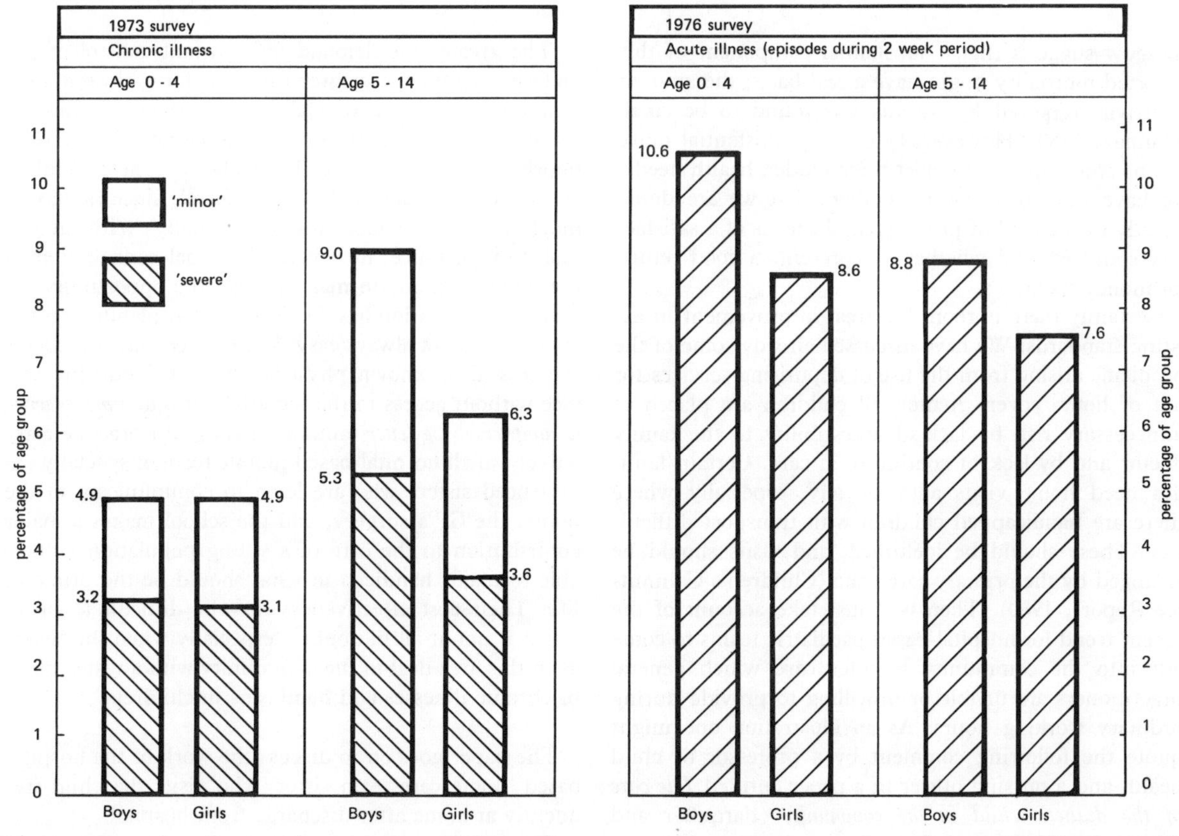

Fig. 1.15 Chronic and acute illness in children as perceived by parents. Source: OPCS General household surveys, 1976 and 1978

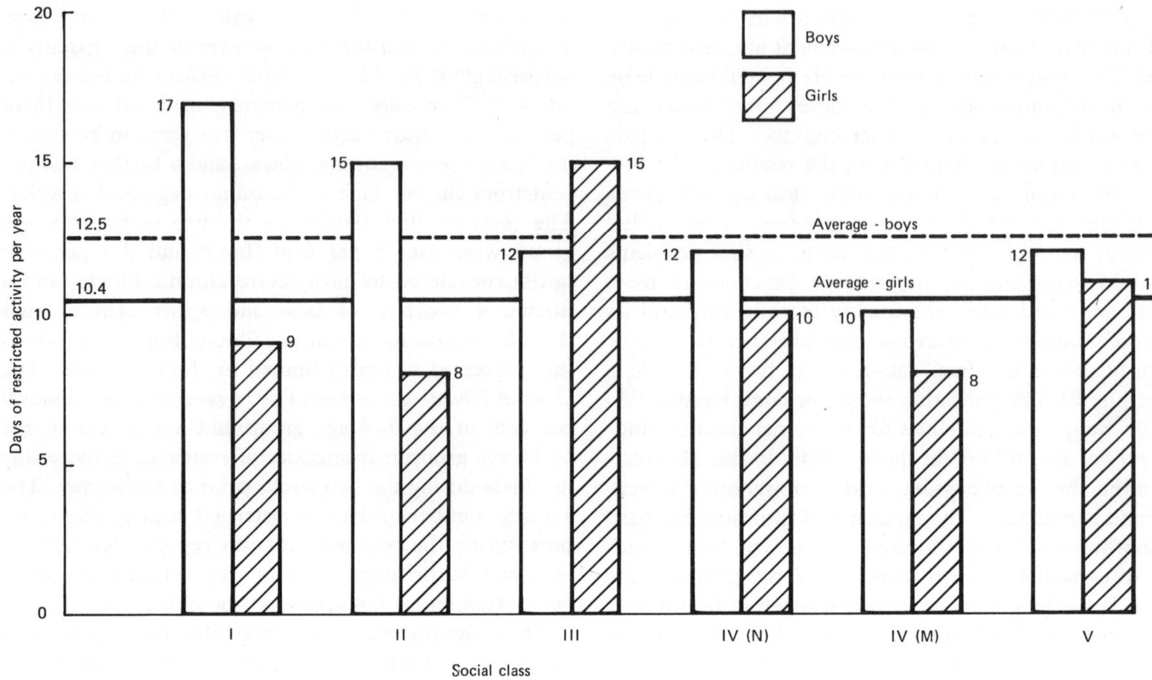

Fig. 1.16 Acute childhood illness by social class. Days of restricted activity in 1976. Source: OPCS General household survey, 1978

Glasgow suggests that a substantial component of this reported morbidity might have a real basis; the amount of 'trivia' reported by parents was found to be small (Hannay, 1980). However, before any substantial move can be contemplated to meet these hidden health needs, we have first to discover whether what we are doing already in the field of primary child care is of a satisfactory standard, and whether it represents a good return for money spent.

Certainly there is room for great improvement in existing standards. We have discussed already some of the problems arising from the use of deputising services for out of hours cover. Acutely ill children are placed at unnecessary risk by lack of accessibility to the family doctor and by lack of continuity in care. Certain families need home visits automatically, especially where there are handicapped children with transport difficulties. These should be identified, and visits should be arranged by the primary care team (Children's Committee Report, 1980). Then we must take account of the recent trend for hospital-based paediatric teams to come out into the community to offer care which general practitioners are unable or unwilling to provide during ordinary working hours. As an illustration one might quote the following comment by a professor of child health and a nursing officer in a paper entitled *The care of the diabetic child in the community* (Farquhar and Campbell, 1980):

'The greater the demand for constant control of the highest quality, the greater the need for a close understanding of the psychosocial factors concerned, and for clinical skill. The nature of the home and family relationships should in theory be available from the child's general practitioner at the first referral, since he has so much information about the whole family. With the virtual disappearance, however, of mutual consultation in the patient's home in many places, the opportunity for oral communication has declined, and availability on the telephone is not always easy. *The busy general practitioner* (far less an unknown physician from a deputising service without access to the records) *has little time to write a comprehensive letter* (author's italics). In practice a relatively small hospital-based mobile team of specially experienced sisters who are keen to communicate in the home, the GP's surgery, and the school makes a major contribution to the care of a young population vulnerable to major handicap in what should be the prime of life. Their cost effectiveness may be difficult to prove but it is not at all in doubt – especially when the sisters as in this area deal in the community with a wider range of chronic illnesses and handicaps in children.'

The paper goes on to discuss the work of the hospital based 'home care team sister' who visits the child frequently at home after discharge from hospital.

The case is argued persuasively, but do we in general

practice really wish to hand over to others our responsibility for an essential component of the primary care of children? Do we really have too little time to write comprehensive letters?

Or take this recent comment by a practising paediatrician (Pratt, 1980):

'It appears to be the exception rather than the rule for family doctors to see their young patients between attacks of asthma: few visit them in hospital as used to be the case ...without some such follow-up there is certainly an inadequancy of ambulatory care, and if the family doctor's commitments are such that he cannot provide it (or if this tiresome illness does not inspire his interest; we are not all "hooked" on asthma) then it seems preferable that a policy of informed care is provided by the hospital.'

Do general practitioners really find childhood asthma too tiresome an illness to be bothered with? If so, whatever are they doing in general practice?

These activities, be it noted, do not arise from an agreed policy of shared care between hospital and general practice, but from hospital staff moving in to offer service to the community for important areas of care which they feel general practitioners are not providing. They are not isolated examples, but representative of a growing trend, which if carried to its logical conclusion would leave the general practitioner with precious little responsibility for the care of ill children; no doubt the hospital based teams would willingly leave to us the care of the child with a running nose or a single loose motion, but when it comes to *real* illness our competence and our commitment is being increasingly called to question.

If the interests of our child patients would be better served by such a policy, then the argument in its favour would be irresistable. But few general practitioners with a real interest in their job would concede this to be the case. What then is the answer?

I believe that we must all of us go back and study the Court report again, because in the few years since its publication event after event has validated its conclusions. In the report we will find a comprehensive analysis of the problems still besetting the child care services, and a series of sensible and practical solutions are put forward. We in general practice were scared off by the suggestions in the report for the creation of General Practitioner Paediatricians (GPPs); many GPs who could not see themselves becoming GPPs were frightened that they would lose all contact with their child patients. The government harkened to these criticisms with relief (for the report would undoubtedly be expen-

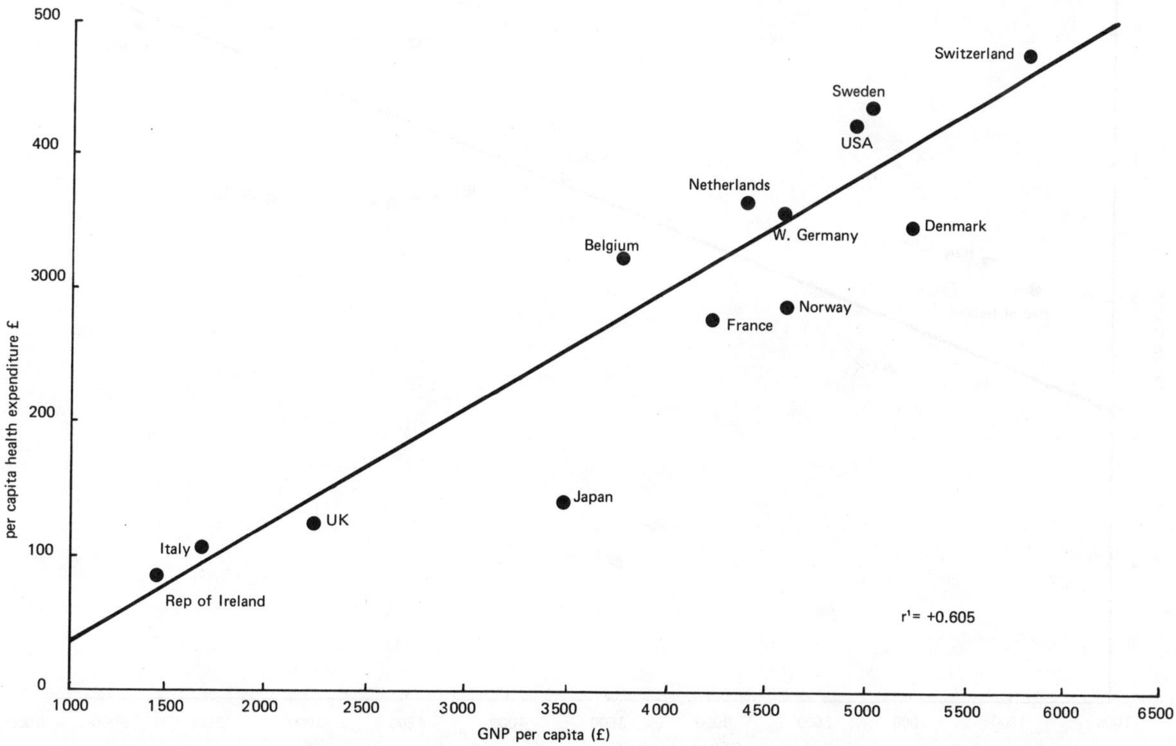

Fig. 1.17 Regression of 'per capita health expenditure' on 'GNP per capita', by selected OECD countries in 1977 (£). Source: Compendium of health statistics. Office of health economics, 1979

sive to implement) and the report was pigeonholed in the hope that it would soon be forgotten. But like Banquo's ghost the report keeps resurrecting itself, for the issues at stake are too fundamental to be disposed of in this fashion.

Much of the strength of the report lies in the real compassion running through the whole of its recommendations; something that appears to be lacking in important sections of our government and administration, and even (dare one say it) in some members of our profession today. Are we really not bothered about the inadequacy of our present standards of child care? Are we really content to drop further and further behind our European neighbours?

Let us forget the title GPP and look at the report's proposals once again. With a little amendment to make it clear that *all* GPs would continue to be heavily involved in child care, the Court proposals are far and away the best solution yet offered for our difficulties. They are just as valid today as when they were first written, and we in general practice would do well to insist on their full implementation.

It may be argued that our country cannot or will not afford to spend fresh money on its child health services, and indeed in Chapter 2 Dr Downham puts forward the case for a policy of 'positive discrimination' as the only practicable alternative. If new money cannot be found, he argues, then we must reallocate our existing resources, taking some away from those areas at present better provided for, to hand over to the deprived areas of the inner cities and other black spots. He may well be right. But before abandoning ourselves to this policy of despair, we would do well to examine once again the case for the injection of new money.

We may usher in the conclusion of this review with one final quotation from *Oliver Twist*:

He rose from the table; and advancing to the master, basin and spoon in hand, said, somewhat alarmed at his own temerity:
'Please, Sir, I want some more.'

Figures 1.17 and 1.18 show that our Health Service expenditure, whether measured per capita or as a percentage of the Gross National Product, lies among the

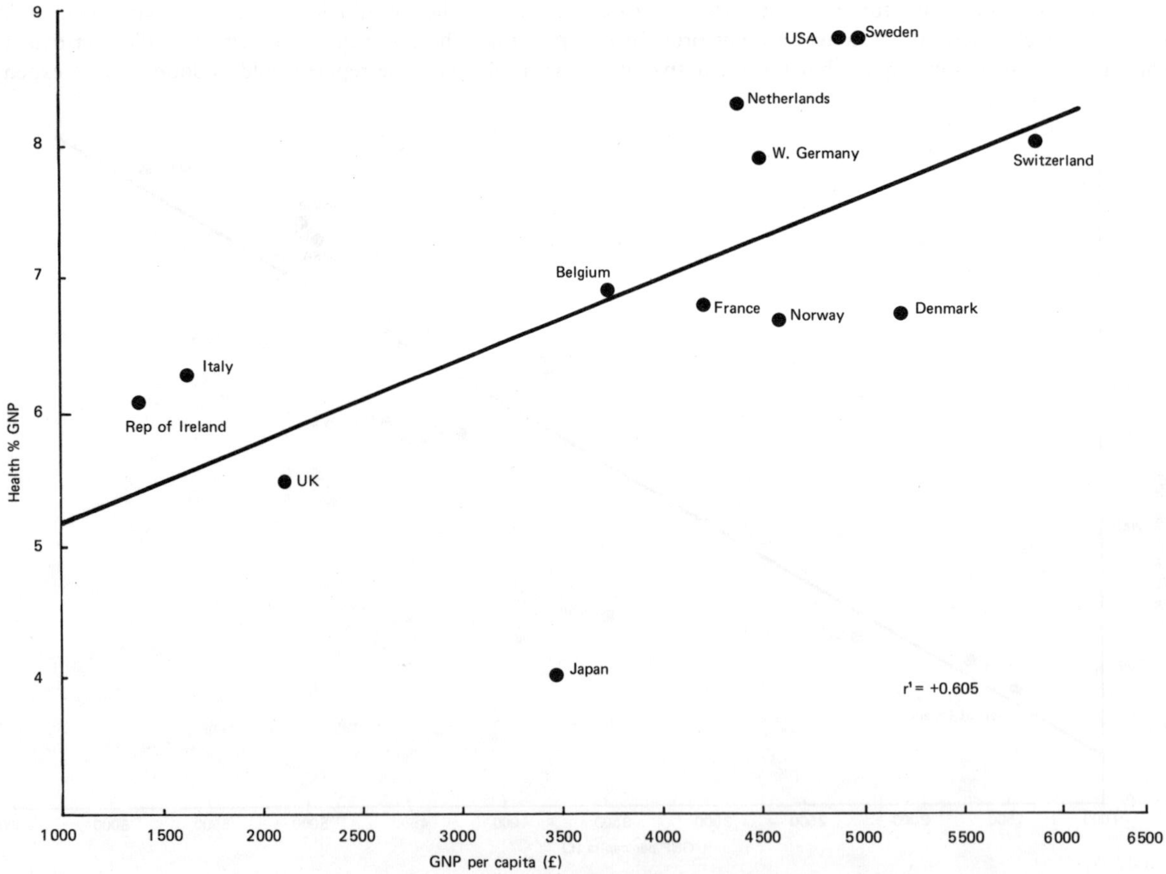

Fig. 1.18 Regression of 'health service expenditure as % of GNP' on 'GNP per capita' by selected OECD countries, 1977 (£). Source: Compendium of health statistics. Office of health economics, 1979

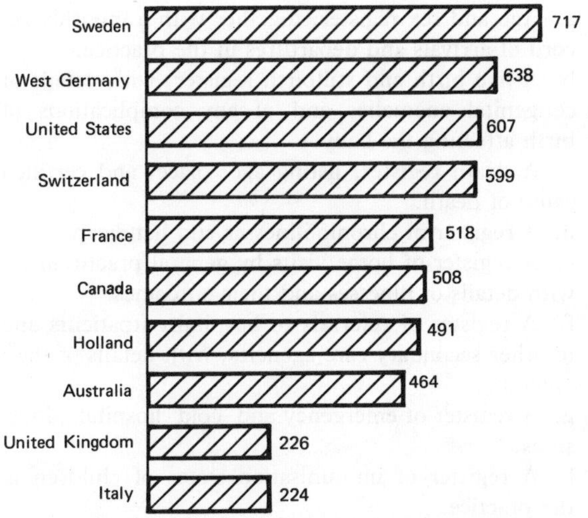

Fig. 1.19 Total health expenditure in 1975. US $ per head of population (public and private, capital and current). Source: Maxwell, 1980

lowest in Western Europe. Figures 1.19 and 1.20, if they can be substantiated, show that these generalisations are also true of our total health expenditure, both public and private, capital and current. Moreover this trend started with the inception of the NHS, and (what is not shown on the graphs) due to cuts in expenditure in recent years, the disparity between us and the rest of Western Europe is widening. Indeed the trend in our expenditure resembles the pattern of Eastern Europe far more than the West, and we have nothing to congratulate ourselves about in that.

Still more remarkable is the graph showing breakdown of our NHS current expenditure into components representing the cost of primary and secondary care, where we discover that the amount spent in the United Kingdom on the primary care of children represents a minute fraction of the total NHS expenditure of the country (Fig. 1.21). We are running our primary child care services on a shoestring.

Viewed in this light, and taking full account of the fact that we are now one of the poorest countries in Western Europe, we may well be grateful that our infant mortality, and indeed the general standard of primary child care in this country, is as respectable as it is. Certainly the country is getting excellent value for the little money it chooses to spend in this field, and we in the NHS have much to be proud of, for managing as well as we have done.

No one however can afford to be satisfied with the present position. In too many areas the provision of adequate primary care is crumbling and the health of the nation's children is increasingly at risk. We in general practice need first to put our own house in order. We need to remind ourselves of our vocation,

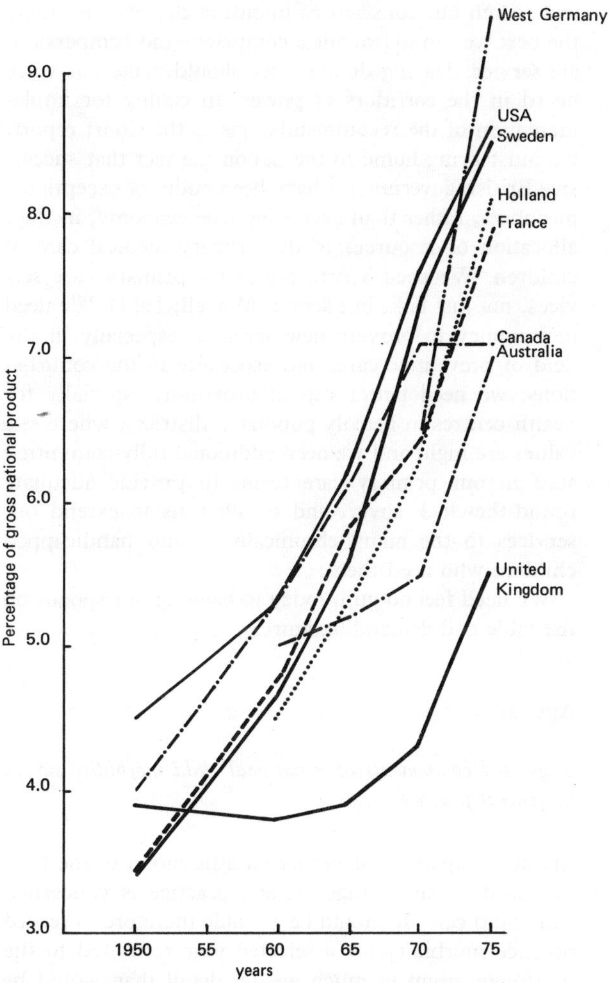

Fig. 1.20 Health care expenditure as a percentage of GNP (public and private, capital and current). Source: Maxwell, 1980

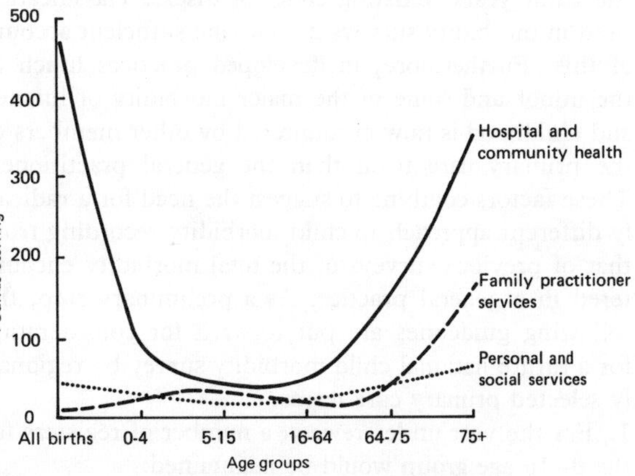

Fig. 1.21 Estimated current expenditure per capita 1975–1976, Great Britain. Source: Maxwell, 1980

and search our consciences to ensure that we are doing the best we can to provide a competent and compassionate service. Having done so, we should make our voice heard in the corridors of power. In calling for implementation of the recommendations of the Court report, we must bring home to the nation the fact that successive British governments have been guilty of exceptional meanness, rather than exercising true economy, in their allocation of resources to the primary medical care of children. We need a firm policy for primary care services, not just talk, but action (Morrell, 1981). We need new money to provide new services, especially in the field of preventive care, and especially in the conurbations; we need better capital provision, especially for health centres in heavily populated districts, where site values are high; and we need additional fully committed staff in our primary care teams to provide adequate round-the-clock cover, and to allow us to extend our services to the many chronically ill and handicapped children who need them.

We need feel no guilt today in banging our spoons on the table and demanding more.

Appendix

Suggested components of a national child morbidity survey in general practice

About one quarter, or perhaps a little more, of the total workload of an average general practice is concerned with child care. It should be possible therefore to record practice morbidity for a selected year restricted to the 0–16 age group in much greater detail than would be practicable for a complete morbidity survey of all age groups. The spectrum of disease and disorder in the first year of life differs greatly from that of the subsequent years of childhood, and it changes once again for the adult years. Existing codes of disease classification used in morbidity surveys do not take sufficient account of this. Furthermore, in developed practices much of the minor and some of the major morbidity of infancy and childhood is now encountered by other members of the primary care team than the general practitioner. These factors combine to suggest the need for a radically different approach to child morbidity recording from that of previous surveys of the total morbidity encountered in a general practice. As a preliminary step, the following guidelines are put forward for consideration for a future national child morbidity survey by regionally selected primary care teams.

1. For the year under review, a number of registers for the 0–16 age group would be maintained:
   a. Age and sex register, together with a monthly record of arrivals and departures in the practice.
   b. A live birth and stillbirth register, with details of congenital anomalies and of any complications of birth affecting the baby.
   c. A death register, listing age, place, and certified cause of death.
   d. A register of chronic illnesses and handicap.
   e. A register of home visits by general practitioners, with details of illnesses and their outcomes.
   f. A register of referrals to hospital outpatients and to other secondary care agencies, with details of their outcomes.
   g. A register of emergency and 'cold' hospital admissions.
   h. A register of immunisation states of children in the practice.
2. Separate records of encounters would be kept by the following members of the primary care team:
   a. the practice nurse
   b. the district nurse
   c. the midwife
   d. the health visitor.
3. The general practitioner morbidity recording would have the following features:
   a. Two schemes of classification, one for the first year of life, and one for the 1–16 age group. These would be designed specifically to cover the spectrum of disease and disorder appropriate for the age group. Each classification would have diagnostic and problem-orientated components.
   b. Entries for the first year of life would be broken down by age as follows: age in weeks for the first month, then age in months.
   c. Entries for the 1–16 age group would record the age in years.
   d. separate recording of episode and consultation rates, as in previous morbidity surveys.
   e. Recording of encounters by date, to enable a seasonal breakdown of morbidity.
   f. Recording of four social factors for each encounter: legitimacy, social class of parent, number of siblings, and age and sex of accompanying parent or adult.
4. To secure full national coverage, special arrangements might be necessary for inner city areas and for single handed practices.
5. It might be desirable to include some record of the preventive aspects of child care undertaken by each practice, particularly health education and developmental surveillance.
6. It is desirable to institute such a survey quite soon, as its findings could radically affect the design of computer programmes for general practice.

REFERENCES

BPA (1979) British Paediatric Association Classification of Diseases. London: BPA.

Chalmers *et al* (1978) Adjusted perinatal mortality rates in administrative areas in England and Wales. *Health Trends*, **10**, 24–28.

Children's Committee Report (1979) The Reduction of Perinatal Mortality and Morbidity. A discussion document. London: Children's Committee. Brook House.

Children's Committee Report (1980) The Needs of the under fives in the Family.

Court Report (1976) Fit for the Future. The Report of the Committee on Child Health Services. Chairman. S.D.M. Court, London: HMSO.

Curtis Jenkins, G.H.*et al* (1979) Child care in general practice. Report of the Developmental Paediatric Research Group. *Journal of the Royal College of General Practitioners*,**29**, 644–646.

Davies, I.M. (1980) Perinatal and infant deaths: social and biological factors. *Population Trends*, **19**, 19–21.

Davies, P. (1980) Perinatal mortality. *Archives of Disease in Childhood*, **35**, 833–837.

Farquhar, J.W. & Campbell, M. (1980) Care of the diabetic child in the community. *British Medical Journal*, **2**, 1538–1541.

Hannay, D.R. (1980) The iceberg of illness and trivial consultations. *Journal of the Royal College of General Practitioners*, **30**, 551–554.

Harker, P. (1980) Child health services in Sweden. *Public Health*, **94**, 144–148.

Hart, C.R. (1975) The History of Screening. In Hart, C.R. (ed.) *Screening in General Practice*, London: Churchill Livingstone.

Last, J.M. (1963) The clinical iceberg in England and Wales. *Lancet*, **2**, 28–31.

Maxwell, R. (1980) *International Comparisons of Health Needs and Services. A working paper for the Royal Commission on the NHS*. London: King's Fund Centre.

Morbidity Statistics (1974) *Morbidity Statistics from General Practice 1970–1971. Second National Study. OPCS, DHSS, RCGP*. London: HMSO, Studies in Medical and Population Subjects No. 26.

Morbidity Statistics (1979) *Morbidity Statistics from General Practice 1971–1972. Second National Study. OPCS, DHSS, RCGP*. London: HMSO, Studies in Medical and Population Subjects No. 36.

Morrell, D. (1981) Inner London general practice – is there a solution? *British Medical Journal*, **1**, 162–163.

Mutch, L. *et al* (1981) Perinatal mortality and neonatal survival in Avon: 1976–9. *British Medical Journal*, **1**, 119 122.

Out of Hours Care(1980) *Out of Hours Social and Health Care. Report of a working group the Children's Committee*. London: Mary Ward House.

Pratt, H. (1980) Trends in the care of acute childhood asthma. *British Medical Journal*, **2**, 1560–1561

Richards, I.D.G. & McIntosh, H.J.(1972) Confidential enquiry into 226 consecutive infant deaths. *Archives of Disease in Childhood*,**47**, 697–706.

Rooth, G. (1979) Sweden. *Lancet*, **2**, 1170–1172

Short, Renee (1980) *Perinatal and neonatal mortality. Second report from the Social Service Committee, 1979–1980*. Short, R. (chairman) London: HMSO.

Stanton, A.N. *et al* (1978) Terminal symptoms in children dying suddenly and unexpectedly at home. *British Medical Journal*, **2**, 1249–1251.

Stanton, A.N. *et al* (1980) Management of acute illness in infants before admission to hospital. *British Medical Journal*, **1**, 897–899.

Stanton, A.N. & Oakley, J.R. (1979) Meningococcal infections during infancy: confidential enquiries into 10 deaths. *British Medical Journal*, **2**, 468–469.

Wynne, J. & Hull, D. (1977) Why are children admitted to hospital? *British Medical Journal*, **2**, 1140–1142.

2

Primary and secondary care

Michael Downham

THE INTERFACE BETWEEN GENERAL PRACTICE, HOSPITAL AND COMMUNITY HEALTH SERVICES, AND HOW COOPERATION CAN BE IMPROVED

Should general practice, supported by hospital paediatric services, absorb the work of clinical medical officers, and provide a comprehensive family-based service for children? There are few who seriously dispute the desirability of this development any longer. The needs of children are inseparable from the needs of their families; prevention and health advice are more effective if they come from the same source as cure; modern doctors and nurses are no longer satisfied with a fragmented role; and the economic sense of two services rather than three is manifest.

If there is little dispute about the long term objective, there is a great deal about how and when it can be reached. Many people, some of them deeply concerned with the needs of children, point to the difficulties for general practitioners in assuming a new comprehensive role: their work load, governed by a system of remuneration which does not differentiate between the healthy patient who needs little help from his doctor and the unhealthy who needs a great deal, is already heavy, and is heaviest in socially disadvantaged areas where preventive services for children are most needed; their training in child health has not always been adequate; their practice populations may not be concentrated round their surgeries, especially in cities; and their premises are often poorly designed for groups of young children.

This chapter is written in the belief that general practice is changing rapidly, and that these difficulties can be overcome in most areas during the next few years. This will happen only if all those concerned with health services for children are prepared to move towards the same goal by making innovations, whether small or large, in the way they work. Some suggestions for innovation are described.

Open sessions for children in general practice

A growing number of general practices are moving towards comprehensive care by offering special weekly or fortnightly sessions for the babies and young children on their lists. This pattern of service however remains the exception, especially in areas where social deprivation is common and the need for such sessions is greatest. The pressures on practices in these areas make it extremely hard for them to commit time and energy to new initiatives, even if they can see likely long term benefits for both their patients and themselves.

If however the content of such sessions is kept simple, it may be possible for even the most stressed practices to make a start, and the benefits can become apparent in a very short time. A misconception which often discourages a start being made is that a formal programme of developmental screening is an essential feature of child health sessions from the outset. There is so far no evidence that such a programme benefits children more than a service which is readily accessible and attentive when parents perceive a problem. In disadvantaged communities the pressure of illness and problems may leave little room for screening the development of all children, and this should not be seen as the first priority.

The essential feature of the session is that it should be open, in the sense that parents should feel free to bring their child without an appointment if he is ill, if they are not sure whether he is ill, if they are worried about his development or his behaviour, or if they have family difficulties they want to discuss.

A limited programme of purely preventive procedures can be grafted on to this problem centered approach – immunisations, a hearing test at eight months, and perhaps an attempt to see all babies at the age of six weeks – using an age/sex register or the health visitor's birth notification list. The work of the session can be divided between the health visitor, one or more of the practice partners, and the practice nurse, in whatever way they choose. After the session there is an opportunity for health visitor, doctor, and practice nurse to review briefly their work together, and to plan the next approach for non-attenders or those causing special concern. This is also a good time for social workers and others (teachers, psychologists, speech therapists, paediatricians) to make contact with the health team, either on a regular basis or according to need.

If the practice premises are too cramped, it may be possible for the practice to use a nearby AHA clinic for the session. Many of these clinics are underused, and health authorities should welcome limited use by general practitioners, waiving rental charges in the interests of innovation.

Sessions of this kind can dramatically improve immunisation rates and are enjoyed by both the families and the professionals involved. General practice is a business as well as a service, and the extra work is balanced by immunisation fees, and by a reduction in the number of surgery appointments and home visits for young children, especially those perceived by the doctor as inappropriate.

General practitioners as school doctors

Most private schools continue to choose general practitioners as their school doctors, but it is unusual to find a general practitioner doing sessional work in local authority schools. The only viable explanation for this is that general practitioners as a rule are not invited to be school doctors by health authorities. The alternative explanations – that general practitioners do not like working in schools, or that they do not have the skills or attitudes to do the work well – are greatly over-stated. As in the case of developmental screening of pre-school children there has been a tendency to inflate the importance of technical skills required by the school doctor. What he needs much more than the uncertainly defined skills of 'educational medicine', is a close and regular relationship with the teachers, and also with the nurse, psychologist, educational welfare officer, and social workers relating to the school. These people can guide the doctor towards the children and families for whom they need his help, and towards clarification of his role within the school team, which will vary widely for different schools. The general practitioner is in a strong position to develop such individual relationships with one or more schools over a period of years, and to form a valuable extra bridge between school and home.

The content of the school doctor's work is not very different from that of general practice. First there are the physical problems which may present in school – asthma, petit mal, urinary frequency – and the school's need for advice about children with established handicaps. For these children the doctor in school can call as he needs on the hospital paediatrician, just as the doctor does in general practice. Then there are the children whose school attendance is persistently poor. Investigation by the school doctor of the medical reasons usually offered for school absence will reveal a minority with under-diagnosed genuine illnesses such as asthma and recurrent tonsillitis, and a majority with psychosocial difficulties which cannot be approached until the veil of physical excuses has been lifted. For these children, and for those presented to him with frank emotional and behavioural difficulties at school, the doctor will often want to turn to psychologist, social worker, or child psychiatrist.

The school doctor's contribution to health education in school needs clarification, but if as seems likely his major opportunities for influence are informal, in the private consultation and by personal example, the general practitioner should be as well or as poorly equipped as any doctor.

There are enough examples of general practitioners as school doctors to know that they can do school work well, and that it offers a challenging variation to their other work, and a valuable new perspective about the life of the community they serve.

Rationalising children's health records

The confused proliferation of children's health records reflects on the one hand a growing concern for childen on the part of health professionals, and on the other their difficulties in translating this concern into effective action.

Many children have eight separate health records! One for the events of birth, one in general practice, one with the health visitor, one in the child health clinic, one for school, one for hospital admissions or outpatient attendances (often duplicated if different hospital departments are visited), one for the health authority computer, and one held by the parents (generally restricted to weights and immunisations). It is not surprising that comparison of the information contained in these eight places reveals both incompleteness and inconsistency. None provides a reliable profile of the child's problems and management.

This chaos of thought springs first out of the lack of integration of our child health services. It also springs from our failure to think clearly about the three distinct purposes of health records – first as an aide memoire for an individual professional's care of an individual patient; second as a means of communication between different professionals, or between professionals and patient; and third as a means of providing epidemiological information about needs and service provision.

How could our records for children be rationalised, having recognised these three separate functions? The first function, that of aide memoire for continuing care, depends heavily on the integration of curative and preventive services, in the ways suggested earlier in this chapter. If the general practitioner is also responsible, along with the health visitor and the school nurse, for the child's health surveillance before and at school, then it is not difficult to conceive of a record which is used jointly and freely by doctor, health visitor, and school nurse; which is largely open ended in design, but also contains a proforma for a small number of age-related screening tests and for immunisations; and which includes a growth chart running from birth to eighteen years.

In this way four of the eight record systems could be reduced to one at a stroke, and the one greatly enriched as an aid to the care of the child. There is also a need, already met in some areas but inhibited in others by geographical splits in hospital services, for an integration of each child's hospital records, so that the perinatal and all subsequent hospital contacts, whatever the specialty involved, remain in a single folder.

The second function of child health records is communication between professionals, and between professionals and the child's parents. Written communication fails unless it is brief and simple. If the format is allowed to become long or complex, transmission will become delayed or be avoided because of the labour involved for the transmitting person, and reception will be incomplete because the receiving person cannot afford the time to read and decode the message. Letters from hospital paediatric departments to general practitioners are a notorious example. A rational solution is a summary list for each child of problems active and inactive, and of management decisions. Such a system would require two difficult conditions to be met – ready availability of the record to all health professionals sharing in the child's care; and a reliable method for up-dating it. The obvious solution is the regional computer; the less obvious, but one which carries with it many theoretical advantages, is to give the job of carrying and up-dating the record to parents. Both these methods need careful experimentation.

The third function of child health records – to provide epidemiological information about children's needs and service provision – is often allowed to dominate and compromise the clinical and communication functions, both in the design of the record and in making extra demands on the clinician's time in completing it. Worse still, a record which attempts to include all three functions, can exercise a drastic influence on the methods and standards of clinical care. The check list of 'defects' in the fossilised school health record (form 10M) is a factor which has prevented many school doctors from abandoning routine medical inspections for all children at set ages, which were appropriate when the school health service began in 1907 but have been increasingly inappropriate since 1948. Epidemiological objectives should, in a free and progressing society, vary considerably with time and place. These objectives should be kept under frequent review, and the information required to meet them should be carefully and economically defined. The process of gathering the information must always be seen as a service to patients and to the professionals caring for them, and not as an industry in itself. Those responsible for designing methods of gathering must beware in particular of compromising clinical care in the process. Usually this will involve a totally separate 'record' designed specifically for the epidemiological function, and completed and held by non-clinical personnel. These are great challenges to the new discipline of community medicine.

Suggested reform of record systems is always met with the full weight of reactionary resistance, because experiments with new systems must, if duplication is to be avoided, involve the risk of abandoning the old. But if it is the needs of children that concern us, rather than those of health service administration, almost any change is likely to be an improvement on the present shambles.

Setting standards through peer audit

One of the encouraging developments in general practice over recent years has been the gathering together of small groups of doctors to review their diagnosis and management of patients, and to set their own standards of care for common presenting conditions. It seems likely that standards derived internally in this way, provided the doctors involved have adequate information on which to base their conclusions, will be more effective in bringing about improvements in care, than standards imposed from outside by expert groups or individuals. (A large study to test this educational hypothesis, which could have far-reaching applications for influencing professional attitudes in general, is about to start in the North of England, focussing on the care of children in general practice).

The system of peer audit has so far naturally concentrated on the curative aspects of health care in the general practice setting. If it is to reach its full potential in improving the overall care of children, it needs to extend in three directions: towards the methods of *preventing* illness in children (such as immunisation, and screening tests); towards both the prevention and management of those problems which overlap the boundaries between health services and social and educational services (such as child abuse, and poor school attendance); and towards children whose care is partly in the hands of hospital services. This would necessarily involve the inclusion in the peer groups of health visitors, school nurses, school and clinic doctors (where integration remains incomplete), social workers, teachers, hospital paediatricians, and others. The essential smallness of the group would be lost if all these people were to attend all the audit meetings, but it should be possible to design a selective system according to the topic under discussion.

A further limitation of the existing peer group network, is that it operates almost exclusively in training practices. There are relatively few training practices in disadvantaged areas, and yet these are the areas where there is most need for general practitioners to examine their work within the security of small audit groups. One solution is to appoint more general practice trainers from practices in inner cities and other disadvantaged areas. Another is for university departments or divisions of general practice to catalyse the setting up of peer groups among non-trainers, and for the profession to negotiate financial recognition for this activity as it has for trainers.

The paediatrician's contribution

Does the paediatrician have a contribution to make to the health needs of children outside hospital? In health districts centered on small cities or towns, most paediatricians have long since established personal links with primary care teams, community clinics, and schools, so that their specialist skills are readily available to the wide range of professionals concerned with children. In the larger conurbations however the picture is generally different. Here the paediatrician tends to be tied more closely to his hospital base by a narrower special interest, regional responsibilities, and teaching commitments. At the same time his appointment is usually not specific to any single health district, so that the number of professionals and institutions outside hospital with whom he must relate is very large, and the opportunity for building specific relationships is correspondingly diminished.

Yet it is the children in conurbations whose health needs are greatest, and it is the primary care and preventive services in conurbations which most need support.

The conurbation paediatrician can move in three ways towards filling this gap: by forming direct personal links with some practices; by re-examining the contribution that his hospital department can make to emergency primary care for children; and by turning more of his academic attention in both teaching and research towards the common and the preventable.

A personal link between a paediatrician and a practice can be particularly fruitful at the time when a practice decides to develop a special session for children, along the lines described in a previous section. By making himself regularly available for the weekly or fortnightly session, the paediatrician can contribute towards the planning of the session, helping the practice to define its objectives and methodology. By sharing the clinical load of the session, working in an adjoining room alongside the general practitioner, he can contribute time, without which the practice might be unable to countenance the new initiative, and immediately available expertise if the general practitioner needs it. He will also learn a lot himself about the common problems of children, and about the opportunities and restrictions of primary care. Similarly if a general practitioner decides to take on a commitment as a school doctor, this is a time when he may welcome a direct link with a paediatrician, sharing time and expertise. In both these situations the hope is that the paediatrician can act as a pump-primer, gradually reducing his input as the general practitioner becomes established in his new role. Thereafter the relationship can be maintained, but on a less intensive level, the paediatrician acting as a resource which the practice feels able to call on for clinical problems with children in the practice, for advice about evaluation or changes in their service for children, or for discussion of problems thrown up at peer group sessions.

Emergency primary care is provided by many hospital casualty departments but few of them have adequate paediatric participation to deal appropriately with their child patients. If an analysis of the work of a casualty department shows a substantial number of child attenders, the paediatrician must seek ways of providing a regular paediatric presence or availability in casualty. In some cities casualty departments play little part in primary care, and the main cover for nights and weekends comes from a deputising service. The rapid progression of acute illnesses in young children, and the importance of the social context in the diagnosis and management of all childhood illness, makes the discontinuous and impersonal nature of deputising services especially unsuitable for children. Paediatricians should discuss with general practitioners alternative systems, such as encouraging parents to use the hospital casualty department for their children when their general practitioner is not personally available.

Increasingly, undergraduates and postgraduates from medicine and many other disciplines look upon the paediatrician as a teacher not only about paediatrics as a hospital specialty, but also about child health in its widest sense. He has a duty therefore to balance his knowledge of the rare and the technical with an understanding of the common and the preventable, and to reflect this balance in his teaching. His teaching needs to be securely based on research interests that include the problems that are more prevalent among children in his area. Sometimes this 'research' will be largely a matter of uncovering local misconceptions and clarifying existing knowledge (for example, the management of asthma, or the contraindications to immunisations). Sometimes there will be clear indications for experimental inquiry (for example, to establish the value or otherwise of screening tests for squint, or for delayed language development).

The contribution of other hospital specialists

The concept that the general paediatrician, especially in conurbations, should be turning more of his attention to the needs of children outside hospital, holds equally for many other hospital specialties – in particular obstetrics, child psychiatry, handicap, ENT, ophthalmology and dermatology. In all these disciplines there are under-explored opportunities for early diagnosis and prevention, and an inadequate understanding of the origins and management of the commoner problems, many of which never reach hospital. Direct links between consultants in these specialties and individual practices, in the way described for paediatricians in the previous section, is one model for approaching these opportunities.

The contribution of the specialist in community medicine

In 1974 the new post of specialist in community medicine (child health) was created and given a mixture of roles which were recognised to be incompatible but seen as a temporary necessity. On the one hand the SCM (CH) was expected to provide on-going epidemiological information to his AHA about health needs of children and the extent to which these needs were being met by services; on the other hand he was asked, pending the recommendations of the Court committee, to manage the child health clinic and school health service, and to be responsible to the LEA and the AHA for the actions of the doctors in clinics and schools. Even supposing such diverse skills could be acquired and practised by the same person, it is contrary to the concept of professional training and responsibility that any professional group should be 'managed' in the way that the SCM (CH) is expected to manage clinical medical officers.

The Court recommendations for resolving the anomalies of our tripartite system were blocked, at least temporarily, and so the contradictions remain. The worst of the sequelae from this chain of events is that in many areas the epidemiological skills are either not available or are not being applied, and there is a damaging and frustrating shortage of relevant, reliable, and up-to-date information about needs and services.

Those who provide preventive services often experience problems with motivation and professional satisfaction. The basic training of all doctors and nurses encourages their fundamental expectations as healers, in which they provide a requested service to sick people and are rewarded, in most instances, by their patients' gratitude. Preventive work is different; in the first place the service is often not requested and sometimes not welcomed; and secondly the reward is less tangible. Health workers can continue preventive work to a high standard and with personal satisfaction only if they are given the results of their activities, to measure against their own activities of the past and those of other workers.

It is just this sort of information that should be the priority of the SCM (CH)'s and the challenge of the new discipline of community medicine: information which is quickly available, and which can be broken down for individual health visitors, schools, practices, and small geographical areas. The dangers of a blanket approach to information, in which neither objectives nor methodology have been carefully considered, have been discussed in the section about child health records.

Two in the hand, or three in the bush?

The arguments so far rehearsed lead to an inescapable conclusion about the tripartite structure of our child health services. If general practice is to be encouraged to assume preventive as well as curative responsibilities for children, raising its standards through peer audit networks as well as vocational training, and supported more directly by paediatricians and other hospital specialists; and if community medicine addresses its whole attention to the information issues which are its only justification to stand as a specialist discipline; then it follows that the separate service of clinical medical officers will become superfluous, not immediately but over the next ten years.

Those who are, or who would have chosen to become, clinical medical officers will choose in future between family medicine and paediatrics. In-service training or retraining for both options must be made available for existing clinical medical officers, designed with imagination to strike a compromise between the ideal and the acceptable. New aspirants to the preventive service would be unwise to enter it without assurance of a training programme that is also recognised as a preparation for either general practice or paediatrics.

Most doctors are also parents. Full-time commitment to medicine is not compatible with a major commitment as a parent to the care and nurture of young children. Child health clinics and schools provide one of the few opportunities for combining medicine with family life. Unless more part-time work at convenient hours is made available within both paediatrics and general practice, the third service will be perpetuated by the needs of doctors rather than those of children.

All this was seen clearly by the Court committee in 1976. It is also seen clearly by the majority of practising doctors, whether clinical medical officers, general practitioners or paediatricians. When will government appreciate that it is only hierarchial jealousies and ambitions which are blocking progress, and that phasing out the third service is both logical for the needs of children and economically attractive?

Community nurses

The health visitor, school nurse, and community midwife are specialists in the care of children. Their experience spans the total population of children. They spend much of their time in homes, where needs can be more easily understood and help more readily accepted than in surgery, clinic or hospital. These are great advantages for the nurse over the doctor as a health advisor. They also bestow, especially on the health visitor, a tremendous potential for guiding the family doctor towards a better appreciation of the needs of children in his practice.

Yet somehow the best is not always made of these advantages. Many parents and more doctors do not recognise the health visitor for the expert she is, or if they do recognise her it is often with a sense of remoteness which lessens her influence on their behaviour.

There are perhaps two reasons for this. The first, mentioned earlier, is that advice about health is accepted more readily if it comes from someone who is also seen as a source of advice and help at times of illness. The intentional disintegration between curative and preventive community nursing is a fundamental mistake which was again identified by the Court committee. Until the health visitor is seen by parents as someone to turn to when their child is ill, and as a full partner preferably round the clock with their family doctor, her ability to help parents promote the health of their children will not be fully realised.The second reason is more difficult to express, for a doctor, because it involves serious criticism of the attitudes of nursing managers. In all our professions the weight of hierarchy threatens the success of the services offered, but in none more than nursing is this so devastatingly true at the present time. Policies and guidelines increasingly threaten the professional principle of individual responsibility based on training and continued support. Enforced vertical reference and deference cripple the natural development of horizontal relationships with doctors, social workers, and teachers. In many areas the health visitor or the school nurse can no longer choose to share (or not share) with the doctor the giving of immunisations, and the respect which goes with such practical procedures. And once child abuse is suspected the health visitor is caught up in a dilemma of loyalties which leaves all but the strongest paralysed.

Thankfully there are areas where these criticisms are largely unjustified, and where nursing managers feel secure enough in their own professional identity to allow initiative, professional responsibility, and the natural partnership between nurses and doctors to grow.

Positive discrimination

The principle of 'positive discrimination' was first spelt out by the Plowden Committee in 1967, in relation to primary schools. It means providing extra services where they are most needed *by withdrawing and reallocating services from areas where they are needed less*. The concept has been widely misunderstood in health service circles, where the idea has got about that it involves extra services for some areas *without* withdrawing them from others, and hence a net increase in total provision. Against a background of scarce resources, this misconception usually results in no change.

And yet there is surely even more justification in health than in education for scaling down services, especially preventive services, for some sub-populations and thereby encouraging a degree of self-reliance?

Positive discrimination can be operated at several levels. The principle underlines a number of regional policies which have attempted to redistribute health service provision across the country. Within the single district health area of Newcastle upon Tyne, childhood morbidity and mortality rates for different city wards have been used as an argument for the redistribution of child health services. But perhaps the most effective level is within the individual case loads of the health visitor and her primary care team. Health visitors invariably focus more of their time and attention on certain families, but more often at expense to themselves than by withdrawing their services from other families. There is a dangerous myth that *all* families with young children need regular home visiting, whereas the truth is that the majority can thrive without, as long as they know where to turn in need. The same is true for over-ambitious health surveillance programmes involving doctors. A great deal of valuable medical and nursing time can be wasted in this way.

The selection of families for extra help has been a subject of much research and debate. Risk-scoring systems have been advocated for the prevention of handicap, cot death, child abuse, and perinatal difficulties. They pose great problems for the epidemiologist in terms of specificity, sensitivity, and variability in time and place – but still greater problems at the clinical interface. A good health visitor or general practitioner will know which families need their extra help, and will also know that it can often be a problem to get that extra help accepted. A centralised anonymous system which on the one hand labels a family, and on the other tells a health visitor things she knows already, is likely to defeat its own object.

Deprofessionalising health care

We have a lot to learn about harnessing twentieth century technology for human benefit. In medicine the technology explosion has thrown up a proliferation of specialist health workers, welfare services, and health pedagogues which has steadily eroded the skills and responsibilities of self and family care. For children the dilemma is greatest: on the one hand we see the need for our society to increase its investment in the young; and yet by so doing we risk weakening parents, whose potential for influencing the health and attitudes of their children is pre-eminent.

One approach to this dilemma, already discussed in the context of 'positive discrimination', is that we should become better at accepting that some sub-populations of children need very little professional health care, and at identifying those who do need us. Another approach is to recognise that what many families with young children need is not so much highly skilled professional help, but more someone with whom they can communicate. The use of less highly trained personnel runs contrary to the trends towards increased periods of training and sharper demarcation of professional roles within our health service. And yet in countries where economic necessity has forced the use of such personnel, great gains have been realised in terms both of understanding health needs and of accepting health advice, especially where the health workers have been recruited locally. Are we, the highly trained professionals, prepared to take a step back, and see part of our role as the recruitment, training, and support of less skilled workers?

Finally, the great challenge in the practice of medicine and nursing, whether at primary care, preventive, or supporting care levels, is to strike a balance between technical skill and care. Many doctors, distracted or seduced by the new technology made available to them over the past thirty years, have lost this balance. Over the next thirty years we must strive to give prestige and priority to care, a sense of responsibility to our patients, listening to and seeking out their total needs, and helping them towards solutions which do not necessarily involve our technical intervention.

3

Child care legislation

Alan Holden

Ignorance of the law excuses no man — John Selden

There is more legislation surrounding the welfare of children than for any other group in society. Much of the legislation seeks to protect children from abuse, neglect or exploitation. This is surely a reflection of the ambivalent attitudes which, individually and collectively, we all hold regarding children. The emotions which children arouse are strong. Their dependency and vulnerability arouse concern and love, but at the same time also give rise to fear and anger. Children have need of both control and nurture. The law attempts to reconcile these needs, which sometimes sit together very uneasily.

Three main strands can be discerned in the legislation about children: the criminal law, family law, and the protection of children. These elements have evolved independently, and there are many examples of anomalies between different acts of parliament in their treatment of children.

WHO IS A CHILD?

Nowhere is this inconsistency more apparent than in the fundamental question of 'who is a child?' For some purposes (e.g. marriage without parental consent, the right to vote, inheritance) a child is a person aged less than 18. At 18 a child attains his 'majority'. The terms 'minor' and 'infant' are sometimes encountered, and these are synonymous with this definition of child. A person of 16 or over may legally have heterosexual relationships and may marry with parental consent. Homosexual relationships involving males aged under 21 are still illegal.

In the criminal law a child is aged less than 14, whilst a young person is aged 14 but less than 17. Someone aged 17, although still a minor, will, if he is accused of a criminal offence, be dealt with by the ordinary courts and not by the special juvenile court. The criminal law contains special provisions concerning the sentencing of people under 21. The term 'juvenile' is often used in criminal matters to encompass both children and young persons.

For many other purposes the seventeenth birthday is taken as the practical upper limit of childhood, e.g. in the provision of substitute family care. For still other purposes, the upper age limit for compulsory school attendance is the relevant milestone.

PARENT AND GUARDIAN

In the case of a legitimate child his mother and father have equal parental rights and duties. An illegitimate child has only one legal parent, his mother, although his natural father may have a responsibility to maintain him. A child may acquire new legal parents through the process of adoption. An adoption order severs all legal ties with the family of origin, and places the child in the same position within his new family as the legitimate child of his adopted parents. The status of illegitimacy was recently reviewed by the Law Commission, which has recommended its abolition in law.

Step-parents are a common feature of modern family life, but they have limited legal status. Under matrimonial law a step-parent has financial responsibilities towards his step-child who is a child of his family. His existence is often ignored by other facets of the law.

A guardian is a person with special responsibilities towards a child whose parents have died. A legal guardian is appointed either by the will of his deceased parent, or by a competent court. A person who looks after another person's child does not thereby become the child's guardian. Such a person may be a foster parent, concerning whom special legislation exists. Anyone who cares for a child in any way, even for a short period, and is therefore in loco parentis, has a duty to exercise due care towards the child's welfare, and can, in appropriate circumstances, be prosecuted for neglect, or for failing to send the child to school.

LOCAL AUTHORITY

Local authorities have many different powers and responsibilities towards children. The authorities involved with the greatest number of children are local education authorities. The authorities concerned in the widest range of legislation are local social services authorities. The councils of London boroughs, metropolitan districts and shire counties are social services authorities. Outside inner London these same councils are also the local education authorities. The Inner London Education Authority is the education authority for the central area of London.

Local social services authorities have a broad range of responsibilities affecting many different groups in the community. As part of those functions, their social work staff are responsible for the protection, care and supervision of children in many varied situations. They are also concerned in criminal procedures involving children.

THE CRIMINAL LAW – JUVENILE OFFENDERS

The Children and Young Persons Act 1969

The appropriate response to anti-social behaviour by children and young people has been a subject of controversy for many years. The level of offending by juveniles has been increasing for many years, and is rightly a matter for concern. But the increases have not been disproportionate to parallel trends in offending by adults, as is sometimes alleged, and there are signs that the rise in juvenile crime is beginning to abate, which cannot be said of offences by adults.

Controversy has focussed on the causes of juvenile crime and the best methods of dealing with children in trouble. All penal policy rests on a combination of punishment, deterrence and rehabilitation. The basis of current practice is the *Children and Young Persons Act 1969*, which is principally concerned with rehabilitation. The philosophy behind the act rests on the premise that anti-social behaviour by a juvenile is induced by a complex set of social factors, which involve the child, his family and the wider community. It is thus symptomatic of a social condition which could have equally become manifest as maladjustment or behavioural problems, or family breakdown, none of which would have been classified as criminal. As a consequence, juvenile offenders should be treated according to their needs, and children should be protected as far as possible from the stigma of criminality, as with other children with special problems.

The act has never attracted universal support. Certain provisions, notably those which would have curtailed the prosecution of juveniles, have not been brought into force. The law is therefore a very uneasy mixture of measures aimed at rehabilitation and punishment.

The juvenile court

Allegations of criminal behaviour against juveniles are usually heard in a juvenile court. The juvenile court is a special magistrates' court, established under the *Children and Young Persons Act 1933* to determine matters involving juveniles. The court deals mainly with criminal matters, but also hears other cases, notably care proceedings. The normal procedures of the magistrates' court are adapted to offer protection to the welfare of any child appearing before it. The times and places for juvenile courts to sit must be chosen so that children do not come into contact with adult offenders. The public are not admitted to the court. Newspaper and other reports of cases must not identify children appearing in the court. The terms used are modified: a juvenile is asked to admit or deny a charge, not to plead guilty or not guilty; he promises to tell the truth, he does not swear to do so. The magistrates who sit in a juvenile court are specially selected because of their particular experience or expertise.

Summary proceedings

For the adult offender criminal offences are divided into summary offences (always tried in a magistrates' court); indictable offences (always tried by judge and jury in the Crown Court); and offences triable either way. For the young offender this distinction does not exist. He will always be tried summarily in the juvenile court, unless:

1. he is charged jointly with an adult.
2. he is charged with a 'grave crime'.

When charged together with an adult a juvenile may be tried in the ordinary magistrates' court or, if the adult defendant wishes, and the charge is an indictable one, by the Crown Court. A juvenile found guilty of an offence by either of these courts will usually then be remitted to a juvenile court for that court to decide the appropriate action. A juvenile therefore has no right to a trial by jury.

The age of criminal responsibility

An act which, if committed by an adult, would be a crime, may be committed by a juvenile without its necessarily becoming a criminal act. In order to prove a criminal action it is necessary to prove that the person charged committed the alleged act, and that he was aware that the action was wrong. The law assumes that no child under the age of 10 can have sufficient knowledge of right and wrong to be guilty of an offence. Ten is the 'age of criminal responsibility', and no person under 10 can be prosecuted. A child under 10 who commits acts which would be crimes if committed by an older person, can be dealt with by the juvenile court as being in need of 'care or control' (see Care Proceedings).

A child aged between 10 and 14 can be guilty of an offence, but it must be shown in each case that the child involved had sufficient knowledge to be aware he was doing wrong. The prosecution must prove this to the satisfaction of the court. A boy under 14 can never be guilty of rape or attempted rape, although he could be guilty of indecent assault.

When the defendant is aged 14 to 16, it is assumed that he aware of the wrongness of his actions, unless the contrary can be proved. With increasing age the balance of proof has moved onto the defendant.

Grave crimes

In contrast to what has been said above, a child or young person may be tried and sentenced by the Crown Court on indictment, if he is charged with a grave crime. For a child the only grave crime is homicide: for a young person a grave crime is an offence which in the case of an adult offender would carry a maximum sentence of 14 years' imprisonment or more (which includes homicide). A juvenile found guilty of a grave crime may be sentenced to be detained for any period up to the maximum period of imprisonment available to the court for an adult convicted of the same offence. The Secretary of State is responsible for finding a suitable institution in which the juvenile can be detained, which cannot, whilst he is still a juvenile, be a prison.

Adjournments

Criminal proceedings against a juvenile may be adjourned for a number of different reasons, e.g. so that the defendant can seek legal advice or for social enquiry reports to be prepared. When a case is adjourned, the defendant is remanded. A juvenile defendant has the same rights as an adult to be remanded on bail. Under the *Bail Act 1976*, a person remanded must be released on bail unless the court is satisfied that the special reasons for not doing so, which are set out in the act, apply. The reasons for refusing bail are a substantial suspicion that the defendant would not surrender his bail at the next hearing, or that he would commit further offences whilst on bail. A juvenile may also be refused bail if the court believes he should be held in custody for his own welfare, or for the purposes of reports being prepared about him.

When a juvenile is refused bail he will usually be remanded to the care of an appropriate local authority. The authority will provide care for him as they would for any other child in care (see p. 35). The social workers caring for him may also prepare a report for consideration by the court at the resumed hearing. If the court is persuaded that the juvenile is 'of so unruly a character' that he cannot be safely entrusted to the care of a local authority, he may instead be placed in a remand centre. Such centres come under the jurisdiction of the Prison Department and are staffed by prison officers. A certificate of unruliness may only be granted if the juvenile is a boy; is aged 14 or over, and the local authority reports in writing that:

1a. he is charged with a very serious offence, or an offence of violence
 b. he cannot be safely accommodated in a local authority home.
2. he has persistently absconded from, or disrupted the running of, a home in which he has been living.

The intention of these conditions is to restrict the numbers of young people remanded to Prison Department establishments.

The court's decision

Before deciding what action to take in respect of a juvenile offender, the court will normally consider social enquiry reports describing the child, his family situation and background. These reports will be compiled by either a probation officer or a social worker from the local authority. Generally probation officers deal with older juveniles, and social workers with the younger, but this division is not a rigid one. The court will also receive a school report, and in many cases may also request a medical or psychiatric report.

Any court may defer passing sentence on a person found guilty of an offence: the deferment may be for a maximum of six months. This power is sometimes used by juvenile courts who wish, for example, to see the effects of changed home circumstances on a young person before deciding what action to take. At the end of the period of deferment the court may take any action it could have taken immediately (except sending him for Borstal training).

The options available to a juvenile court dealing with a juvenile offender are:

1. absolute or conditional discharge
2. binding over child or parent
3. imposing a fine
4. imposing supervision
5. making an attendance centre order
6. making a care order
7. sending a young person to a dention centre
8. seeking Borstal training for him

1. *Discharge*. An absolute discharge means that no action is taken concerning an offence, although it remains on his record. It is usually granted when the offence has occurred through circumstances over which the offender had no control, and is therefore used relatively rarely. A conditional discharge means that no action will be taken if the offender is not found guilty of another offence within a specified period, normally one or two years (maximum three years). If another offence is committed, the offender may have a penalty imposed on

him for the original offence as well as for the subsequent one.

2. *Binding over.* Any court may bind over a person found guilty of an offence, in a determined sum of money, to be of good behaviour or to keep the peace. If the conditions are not complied with, the court can order the offender to forfeit the specified sum of money. This power is little used in the juvenile courts. A parent may be ordered to enter into a recognisance to take proper care of, and exercise control over, a child or young person who has been found guilty of an offence. If the juvenile offends again, the parent can be ordered to forfeit all or part of the recognisance.

3. *Fine.* A fine can be imposed as a penalty for virtually all offences, and it is the most frequently used penalty in the courts. A juvenile may be fined; the court must have regard to the juvenile's means when deciding the size of the fine. A young person may not be fined more than £200 for one offence, or a child more than £50 (provided the offence carries a maximum penalty in excess of these limits). If the offender is a child the court will usually order the child's parents to pay the fine, and may do so if the offender is a young person. If a young person does not pay his fine it may be transferred to the parent at a later stage.

4. *Supervision.* Supervision is the juvenile equivalent of probation for adult offenders. A supervision order may last for a maximum of three years. Supervision will be by either a probation officer or a social worker. Again, social workers tend to be responsible for younger offenders, with probation officers taking the older, but the division is not rigidly applied, and will vary from place to place. The task of the supervisor is to 'advise, assist and befriend the supervised person'. The supervisor will attempt to resolve social problems and interpersonal difficulties affecting the juvenile and his family, with the aim of reducing tendencies to re-offend. Methods used by supervisors vary: many will rely on individual counselling or informal discussion with child and family members. On other occasions group work methods or approaches based on behaviour modification techniques will be adopted.

The court may include in a supervision order conditions which it considers appropriate for the purpose of preventing the commission of further offences. In particular, the order can impose 'intermediate treatment' on the supervised person. Intermediate treatment (or IT) is so called because it is intermediate between ordinary supervision and an order resulting in the child's long-term removal from home. Children following IT programmes can be required to take part in a wide variety of activities; sometimes activities available in the general community, sometimes specialised activities exclusively for children in trouble. An IT programme can include short periods of residential care. The aim of IT is to foster in the young person a sense of achievement and a positive self-image, the lack of which is often a precipitating factor in juvenile offending, and to introduce the young person to constructive ways of using leisure time.

5. *Attendance centres.* Attendance centres are run by the police. They are activity centres which children and young persons can be ordered to attend for a specified number of hours, usually 12 or 24. The young person will attend on a number of occasions, generally for two hours at a time, until the specified hours have been completed. Often the centres function on Saturday afternoons. Originally conceived as mainly punitive, they are now constructive in their approach and share in a modest way the same goals as intermediate treatment.

6. *Care.* The care order is the order available to the court when it decides that a juvenile offender should be removed from home. The order places the juvenile in the care of the relevant local authority, generally the authority in whose area he lives. The order will last until the age of 18 (19 in some cases) but may be discharged early. Under the order the local authority has the powers and duties of a parent, and may decide where the child shall live. Any of the authority's child care facilities may be used to accommodate the child, and he can be allowed to live at home. The time at which the child returns home is within the discretion of the local authority, but the child and his parents may at any time apply to the court for the order to be discharged.

7. *Detention.* A detention centre is an establishment run by the Prison Department, to which young offenders (over 14) can be sent for periods of three months. With remission, six weeks is the normal length of stay for a person under 17. The principle behind detention centres was one of deterrence, and they were almost wholly punitive in intent when first set up, with a firm regime. This approach has been modified to some degree, and educational classes are now provided, for example. The regime is still strenuous, with emphasis on physical activity and strict discipline. The success rate of detention centres, measured in terms of the proportion of those discharged who do not re-offend, is poor. Following the change of Government in 1979, one junior detention centre is to adopt an even tougher regime, although it is difficult to see how this can be easily done. It remains to be seen what effect this will have on the boys sent there. There are no detention centres for girls.

8. *Borstal training.* Borstals are named after the first special prison institution set up for young offenders at Borstal, a village near Rochester. A sentence of Borstal training is an indeterminate sentence, with a maximum of three years. A magistrates' court cannot impose Borstal training directly: the offender must be remitted to the Crown Court for sentence, with a recommendation

for Borstal training. The Crown Court is not bound to follow the recommendation, but may instead impose any other order which the lower court could have made. Borstal training cannot be imposed on a person under 15 years old.

The average length of stay in a Borstal is about nine months. On release, an offender will be subject to supervision, and can be recalled to the Borstal. The regime followed within a Borstal varies, although all attempt some degree of training, both in the sense of trade training, and in social skills and personal relationships. Borstals also have varying degrees of security. As with detention centres, the success rate of Borstals is low.

Compensation. In addition to the above orders, the juvenile court can order a juvenile offender to pay compensation to the victims of his offences. It is exceptional to make a compensation order in conjunction with an order which results in custodial treatment.

Proposed changes

The Goverment has published a White Paper on Young Offenders (HMSO, October 1980) outlining proposed changes in the powers available to courts when dealing with young offenders, including juveniles. The minimum period of detention centre orders is to be reduced to three weeks. Borstal training is to be replaced by determinate sentences of youth custody, with a minimum sentence of four months. Remission of sentence will be possible, but recall will not. The establishments which now accommodate young adults imprisoned or sent to Borstal will be used for youth custody. Training is to remain an important element in the new sentence, at least for those subject to medium-term sentences (up to 18 months). A residential care order will be introduced for young people who re-offend after being committed to care. The order will limit the local authority's discretion to allow the juvenile concerned to live at home. Community service, under which offenders do unpaid work in the community to help people in need, is to be extended to 16-year-olds. At present only adults (over 17) are eligible. All these changes require amendments to legislation, and no guide can be given to the date of their introduction.

Scotland

A different legal system operates in Scotland. There are no juvenile courts, and decisions on guilt and innocence are separated from the selection of appropriate treatment. The former is reserved for the sheriff court, whilst the latter is decided by a children's hearing. The children's hearing is an informal tribunal, which is not a court. Its decisions are, however, binding. The Hearing can impose supervision, or supervision with a condition of residence. Fines cannot be imposed, and Borstal and detention centres are not available for juveniles in Scotland.

Protection of children

Child destruction

This offence was created by the *Infant Life (Preservation) Act 1929*, which provides that any child of 28 weeks gestation is considered as capable of being born alive, and must not be caused to die before it has an existence independent of its mother, unless in good faith for the purpose only of preserving the mother's life.

Infanticide

This concerns a child once it is born. A mother is guilty of infanticide if by any wilful act or omission she causes the death of her child before it reaches the age of one year, in cases where it can be shown that the balance of her mind has been disturbed by giving birth or by lactation.

Neglect and ill-treatment

The common law requires that every parent, and any person acting in loco parentis, exercise reasonable care of his child. *The Children and Young Persons Act 1933* creates a number of criminal offences to strengthen parental obligations. The most important of these is contained in Section 1. A person having custody, charge or care of a child commits an offence if he 'wilfully assaults, ill-treats, neglects, abandons or exposes him (the child) . . . in a manner likely to cause him unnecessary suffering or injury to health'. The act specifies that anyone with a legal liability to maintain a child will be guilty of neglect if he fails to provide 'adequate food, clothing, medical aid or lodging for him'. A lack of means is no defence, for failure to make appropriate use of welfare facilities is also deemed to be neglect. The offence carries a maximum penalty of a £400 fine and six months imprisonment, if dealt with by a magistrates' court, or an unlimited fine and two years' imprisonment when heard in the Crown Court.

A parent who refuses, or fails to obtain, medical treatment for a child may render himself liable to prosecution for neglect under the *Children and Young Persons Act 1933*. At one time the use of care proceedings as a means of overcoming parental objections to blood transfusions and other life-saving treatment was favoured. It has since been recognised that such proceedings may not offer any additional protection to a doctor who operates without parental consent. Advice from the Ministry of Health (Circular F/P9/1B) suggests that as long as a second opinion has been sought to confirm the risks to life if treatment is withheld, there is little risk of subsequent action in the courts if treatment is given in an emergency in the face of parental opposition. In cases of chronic resistance to treatment the matter should be brought to the attention of the local authority as if it were a case of child abuse.

More than one person may have an obligation towards the child at the relevant time, and all involved could be charged under Section 1. For example, if a baby-sitter assaults or neglects the child in his charge, the parent who placed the child under his care could also be guilty of an offence under Section 1. It is not essential for actual injury or suffering to have been inflicted on the child. This may have been prevented by the intervention of a third party. If actual injury or suffering has not occurred, evidence will be required that this could have been the likely consequence. Such evidence may have a strong medical component.

An assault may be committed without physical ill-treatment being inflicted. Placing a child in fear of physical abuse can constitute assault. Sustained verbal abuse, or prolonged 'mental cruelty' can also be an adequate basis for proceedings against the parent. Placing the child in a situation of risk may also constitute an offence, depending on the circumstances. There is, for example, no absolute rule concerning children being left alone without adult supervision. Proceedings could be taken if the child's being left places him at risk. The child's age, his capabilities and the nature of the surroundings will all affect the likelihood of his being caused unnecessary suffering or injury. A very young child clearly cannot be left alone without substantial risk. Many children in their early teens can be left safely for a short period. There is no absolute point at which parental responsibility ceases – it is a matter of degree. This is sometimes very confusing for parents.

In addition to the major offence in Section 1, the 1933 act also creates a number of subsidiary offences. It is, for instance, an offence to give alcohol to a child under five, to expose a child under 12 to a risk of burning, to sell tobacco to a child under 16 or to allow a child under 16 to be used for begging. Separate acts dated 1937 and 1968 govern child protection in Scotland and Northern Ireland respectively.

Specific risks to children

A number of specific risks to children are covered by individual acts. The *Explosives (Age of Purchasing) Act 1976* raised the age for purchase of fireworks from 13 to 16, and increased the penalties for selling them to under-aged children. *The Consumer Protection Act 1961* provided *inter alia* that nightdresses for children should be made of material which meets a prescribed standard of low flammability. Since 1977 it has been mandatory for all drugs containing aspirin and paracetamol sold 'over the counter' to be supplied in child resistent containers. *The Tatooing of Minors Act 1969* establishes the practice of tatooing of minors as an offence. The *Hypnotism Act 1952* prohibits demonstrations of hypnotism for the purpose of public entertainment on young persons aged under 18.

Vaccine damage

The *Vaccine Damage Payments Act 1979* provides for the payment of £10 000 to a person of any age who is severely damaged by vaccination against diphtheria, tetanus, pertussis, poliomyelitis, measles, rubella, tuberculosis, or smallpox.

Treatment of minors

Under the *Family Law Reform Act 1969* a person aged 16 is considered capable of giving consent for medical or surgical treatment. For children under that age, consent by a parent or guardian is required, but in the case of life-saving treatment it is unlikely that parental objection would be upheld in the courts. There is no legislation concerning medical confidentiality for children under 16, but most doctors would respect the wishes of older children.

Sexual offences against children

The Law offers protection against rape and indecent assault to children and adults alike. In addition, the *Sexual Offences Act 1956* and the *Indecency with Children Act 1960* create offences specifically concerned with children. Sections 5 and 6 of the 1956 act make it illegal for a man to have intercourse with a girl under the age of 16. No offence will be committed if the girl is at least 13, the male is aged less than 24, and he can show that he had reasonable cause to believe the girl was 16 or more. Many occurrences of unlawful sexual intercourse with girls under 16 which come to light involve boys of similar ages. In such circumstances it is unusual for a prosecution to result, although action to protect the girl may well be taken as care proceedings. A doctor who becomes aware of such an offence may feel himself to be in a difficult position.

Although criminal proceedings are unlikely, if the matter is not reported to the police and the local social services authority any person having knowledge of the offence would himself be in breach of the law. Feelings of loyalty to a patient and her family should not obscure this fact. Similar conflicts may be experienced if a case of incest arises. Incest between father and daughter, or indecent assaults by fathers on their daughters, occur much more frequently than is generally supposed. It is likely that it will be a doctor who discovers that an offence has occurred.

Incest is an offence whatever the ages of the parties concerned. Incest with a child is not a special offence, although it is viewed most seriously by the courts. The man involved will almost invariably be sent to prison and care proceedings taken in respect of the girl.

Care proceedings
The law provides for the protection of children 'in need of care or control'. Care proceedings may be brought by the police, the NSPCC or a local authority. The proceedings take place before the juvenile court, under Section 1 of the *Children and Young Persons Act 1969*. The court may make an order to secure that the child receives adequate care or control if it is satisfied that:

a. one of the primary grounds is made out
b. the child is in need of care or control which he is unlikely to receive unless the court makes an order.

The primary grounds for care proceedings are:

a. his (the child's) proper development is being avoidably prevented or neglected, or his health is being avoidably impaired or neglected or he is being ill-treated;
b. it is probable that (a) will be satisfied because a court has found that it has been satisfied in the case of another child in the same household;
c. it is probable that (a) would be satisfied because a person who has been convicted of an offence set out in Schedule 1 to the *Children and Young Persons Act 1933* is or may become a member of the same household as the child;
d. he is exposed to moral danger;
e. he is beyond the care and control of his parent;
f. he is of compulsory school age and he is not receiving efficient full-time education suitable to his age, ability and aptitude;
g. he is guilty of an offence excluding homicide.

Paragraph (a) permits proceedings when the child has been neglected or ill-treated. It is written in the present tense, and so appears to exclude action to protect children in potentially harmful situations. It is not essential for criminal proceedings to have been taken against a parent for this ground to be used. Paragraph (b) extends protection to other children in the family. Paragraph (c) offers some protection where the previously assaulted child was not a member of the same family. (Schedule 1 offences are mainly offences of indecency or violence towards children.) Paragraph (g) was intended to provide an alternative to criminal prosecution for children, but is used very little.

If the court accepts the need for an order to be made, it will consider social enquiry reports prepared by social workers or probation officers. The most commonly imposed orders are care orders and supervision orders, which are identical to the corresponding orders made in criminal proceedings against a juvenile. As an alternative, the court may choose to bind over the parent to exercise proper care or control, or make a hospital order or guardianship order under the *Mental Health Act 1959*. The other powers available in criminal proceedings cannot be used in care proceedings.

Emergency powers
The circumstances justifying care proceedings may indicate the child should be removed from home as a matter of urgency. If there are reasonable grounds for believing that one of the grounds for care proceedings would be satisfied, the police can arrange for a child to be held in 'a place of safety' (e.g. a hospital or a children's home) for a maximum of eight days. A local authority social worker, or an officer of the NSPCC, must apply to a magistrate for authority to take a child to a place of safety, but in this case the order may be for up to 28 days. Care proceedings will be started within the period of the place of safety order; the juvenile court will make interim orders if it cannot complete the proceedings in one sitting.

Children beyond control
A parent who believes his child to be beyond his own control cannot himself bring the matter before the courts. He can approach the local authority, with a request that court action be started. If the local authority does not accept the need for action the parent may then bring proceedings against the local authority.

Child abuse registers
Much attention has been focussed on child abuse in recent years, and complex machinery has been set up to detect and manage cases. All local authorities are now maintaining 'at risk' registers. Doctors may well find themselves involved in case conferences held under the auspices of an area review committee. These arrangements have no legal foundation, although they serve a very useful purpose. The practice of holding case conferences is endorsed by the DHSS. Decisions reached by a case conference have no standing in law, and the conference has no executive power. Responsibility still rests with the individual agencies represented at such a gathering.

Children in care
As well as children placed in care by courts, local social services authorities also care for many children living apart from their own families. Because of the absence of a court order, children received into care by a local authority are sometimes described as being in 'voluntary care'. A local authority has a duty to receive into care any child within its area who has no parent or guardian, who has been and remains abandoned, who is lost or whose parent or guardian is for the time being or permanently prevented by reason of mental or bodily dis-

ease or infirmity or other incapacity or any other circumstances from providing for his proper accommodation, maintenance and upbringing (*Child Care Act 1980*, s.2). The child must be under 17, and the intervention of the local authority must be necessary in the interests of the child's welfare.

During the first six months of the child's stay in care his parent has an unlimited right to take over his care again. In view of this, if the local authority is aware of the parent's whereabouts at the time the need for care becomes apparent, it would be pointless for the child to be received into care against his parent's wishes. Local authorities have no powers to take children away from home without recourse to the courts.

If the child stays in care for longer than six months, the parent's right to discharge from care is modified. The local authority can require him to give up to 28 days' notice of his intention to remove the child. The main purpose of this delay is to facilitate a smooth transfer for the child, so that any emotional impact on moving from one home to another will be minimised.

If the authority believes it is not in the child's interests to return home it can, at any time the child is in care, pass a resolution assuming the rights and duties of a parent. This can be done if:

1. the child's parents are dead and he has no guardian
2. the child has been in care throughout the preceding three years
3. a parent of the child:
   a. has abandoned him
   b. suffers from a permanent disability, or a mental disorder within the terms of the *Mental Health Act 1959*, which renders him incapable or unfit to have the care of the child
   c. has so consistently failed without reasonable cause to discharge the obligations of a parent as to be unfit to have the care of the child.

The parent (if there is one) can agree to the assumption of parental rights by the authority. If he objects, the authority must go to the juvenile court for the resolution to be upheld.

Unless parental rights have been assumed, the local authority has a duty to encourage the return home of children in care. Advice, guidance, material help and financial aid may be given to assist discharge, or to prevent the need for children to be received into care.

However they come to be in care, whether as a result of a court order or a voluntary reception, all children are to be treated equally. In reaching any decision about a child in care the caring authority must take account of all the circumstances, 'first consideration being given to the need to safeguard and promote the welfare of the child throughout his childhood'. The authority must also take account of the child's own wishes and feelings. The majority of children in care live either with foster parents or in children's homes (sometimes called community homes). The supervision of children living with foster parents and the management of children's homes are both the subject of detailed regulations.

School attendance

The *Education Act 1944* requires that every child over 5 and under compulsory school leaving age must receive efficient, full-time education suited to his age, ability and aptitude. The end of compulsory schooling is currently fixed as the end of the spring or summer term next following the child's 16th birthday. Education does not have to be received in school, but it is very difficult for parents to satisfy the requirements of the act by educating children at home.

The duty to ensure that a child attends school regularly rests with the parent. If the child does not attend, the parent can be prosecuted. Care proceedings can be brought against the child in the juvenile court. Either or both courses may be followed. All local education authorities employ education welfare officers to investigate non-attendance and to counsel children who are truanting.

Employment of children

The employment of children is strictly controlled by the *Children and Young Persons Act 1933* and the *Employment of Children Act 1973*. Under these acts local education authorities have power to inspect and regulate the conditions in which children are working. Such an authority can require a parent and/or an employer to furnish particulars of how any child is employed. If it appears to the authority that the child is lawfully employed, but that, for reasons of health or other reasons, he is unsuited to that employment, the authority may serve notice on the employer prohibiting the child's employment, or specifying conditions of employment which must be observed if the child is to remain at work.

In general no child may be lawfully employed:

1. so long as he is under 13 years of age
2. before the close of school hours on any day on which he is required to attend school
3. before 7 a.m. or after 7 p.m. on any day
4. for more than two hours on any day on which he is required to attend school
5. for more than two hours on a Sunday
6. to lift, carry or move anything so heavy as to be likely to cause injury to him.

Special arrangements apply to children taking part in entertainments on stage, television, etc. Children may only perform if they have a licence to do so from the local education authority. Exceptions are made for very occasional performances and entertainments organised by schools and similar bodies. A licence to perform may specify conditions about the child's hours of work, provision of education, etc. Children under 13 can be granted licences in special circumstances.

Privately arranged fostering

Children may be placed in the care of foster parents without the intervention of a statutory agency, the arrangements being concluded directly between the child's family and the foster parents. Such placements must be notified to, and supervised by, the local social services authority. Any person proposing to receive a foster child into his home must give a minimum of 14 days' notice to the local social services department of his intention, unless the arrangements are made in an emergency. The department will investigate, and if the prospective foster parents are thought to be unsuitable, action can be taken in the courts to prohibit the placement.

Arrangements of less than six days' duration are excluded, although if the child is under five, and payment is involved, a short placement may come within the terms of the *Nurseries and Child Minders Act 1948* (see below). If the placement is for less than 28 days, and the persons proposing to look after the child are not regular foster parents, then the arrangement does not become one of formal fostering. A regular foster parent is someone who has cared for a child (or children), not his own, for at least three months or on at least three separate occasions. A child cared for by *close* relatives (grandparent, uncle, aunt) does not become a foster child within the terms of the act.

Although payment will usually be made to the foster parents by the child's family, it is not an essential requirement before the child may enjoy the protection offered by the act. All such arrangements must be notified to the authorities, even if no payment of any kind is made.

Whilst living in a foster home, the child is under the supervision of the local authority. Visits to the home will be made by social workers from the authority. If there are grounds to suspect that the care given to the child is inadequate or potentially harmful, the authority has the power to intervene and remove the child to a place of safety. The foster parent has no legal rights over his foster child. He does have the same duty as a parent to give adequate care and protection.

Daily minding

The care of young children of working parents presents a constant problem. Day nursery facilities are provided by some local authorities but these are inadequate to meet the demand, and most day care of young children is provided by private individuals. Such arrangements are again under the supervision of the local social services authority. Two registers are maintained by social services departments: one of persons who offer day care to children under five in their own homes, and the second of premises not being private homes (or schools) in which children are received to be looked after for all or part of the day. Offences are committed if unregistered premises are used to receive children for more than two hours per day, or if an unregistered person receives children under five into his home for more than two hours per day.

The act (*The Nurseries and Child-Minders Regulation Act 1948*) therefore covers daily minding, playgroups and private day nurseries, whether held in private homes or in other premises, such as church halls, etc. The authority with whom a person, or premises, is registered, will supervise its activities, give advice and guidance where appropriate, and may impose conditions, e.g. regarding the numbers of children who may be looked after at any one time. The supervising authority has power to refuse or withdraw registration. Note that arrangements for daily minding in private homes come under the act only if the child is under compulsory school age, and some payment is made.

Family law

Adoption

Adoption is a process whereby the legal bonds between a child and his family of origin are severed, and he becomes a full member of an alternative family. The purpose of adoption is to provide substitute families for children who require them, not to provide children for childless couples. Throughout, the law lays emphasis on the child's welfare. 'In reaching any decision relating to the adoption of a child, a court or adoption agency shall have regard to all the circumstances, first consideration being given to the need to safeguard and promote the welfare of the child throughout his childhood' (*Children Act 1975*, s.3). In some circumstances prospective adopters with children may be preferred to childless persons.

The majority of adoptions of children by strangers are arranged by registered voluntary adoption societies or by local authorities. It is still possible for a parent to make her own arrangements for the adoption of her own child, or for a private individual to act as an intermediary in private adoption arrangements, but such adoptions are fraught with difficulties. Anyone who does act as an intermediary must take responsibility for assessing the suitability of the prospective adopters, and must comply with a complex legal procedure. A general practitioner who is consulted by a patient seeking adoption for her child would be well advised to refer her to a recognised agency. When implemented, s.28(1) of the

Children Act 1975 will prohibit private placements for adoption.

Adoption may be by a married couple or a single person, but in practice adoptions by one person alone are very rare. The selection of suitable adopters is the responsibility of the placing agency, which must comply with the detailed requirements of the Adoption Agency Regulations. The child must live with the prospective adopters for at least three months before the adoption order can be made, during which time the placement will be supervised by the relevant local authority.

Adoption applications can be made to the High Court, the local county court or the local magistrates' court. The court will appoint a social worker (who will not be connected in any way with the agencies concerned in the placement) to be the *guardian ad litem*, with responsibility to protect the child's interests. The guardian ad litem will investigate the circumstances, interview all the parties, and make a report for the guidance of the court. Medical certificates confirming that the prospective adopters are in good health are required. A report on the child's medical history and state of health will also be required. The court will wish to be reassured that the adopters are fully informed of the child's history and of any abnormality found on examination.

An adoption order normally requires the agreement of the child's natural parents. In the case of an illegitimate child only the mother's agreement is usually needed. The court may dispense with a parent's agreement on certain grounds, i.e. if the parent:

1. cannot be found or is incapable of giving agreement
2. is withholding agreement unreasonably
3. has persistently failed without reasonable cause to discharge his parental duties towards the child
4. has abandoned or neglected the child
5. has persistently ill-treated the child, and (for whatever reason) the rehabilitation of the child within the parent's household is unlikely.

As the law now stands parental agreement to adoption only becomes final when the adoption order is made. Similarly, a court may only be asked to dispense with agreement when considering an application to adopt. This can cause much anxiety for adopters, and many natural parents also find the drawn-out procedure distressing. The *Children Act 1975* contains provisions, not yet implemented, which would permit a child to be declared 'free for adoption'. It is probable that these provisions will come into effect in 1981 or 1982.

Once made, an adoption order is irrevocable. The child is invested with the same legal status which he would have had if he had been the legitimate child of the adopters. The original parents lose all rights and duties towards the child. It is probable that the original parents will not know the child's new identity. The court procedure has been devised to keep the adopters' identities confidential. Every adopted person, on reaching the age of 18, is entitled to apply for a copy of his original birth certificate, which will reveal the identity of his first parents. Anyone adopted before 12th November, 1975 must be offered counselling about the possible consequences of attempting to find his first parents, before he may have access to his original birth records.

Illegitimacy

A child born to a married woman is presumed to be the legitimate child of her husband unless they are judicially separated, or evidence can be produced showing without a doubt that the husband cound not have been the child's father. Guardianship proceedings for custody or access may be brought by either parent of an illegitimate child under the *Legitimacy Act 1959*, in England and Wales. Rights of illegitimate children to share in the parents' estates are governed by the *Family Law Reform Act 1969*, for England and Wales, or for Scotland the *Law Reform (Miscellaneous Provisions) (Scotland) Act* 1968. A short form of birth certificate which does not disclose illegitimacy or the parents' names may be obtained.

Affiliation

Under an affiliation order a man judged by the court to be the putative father of an illegitimate child may be required to pay maintenance to the mother for the child. Application for an affiliation order is made to the mother's local magistrates' court. The application must be made within three years of the child's birth, unless the man had, within that time, voluntarily paid maintenance in respect of the child. The order lasts until the child reaches 16 or completes full-time education.

Questions of proof in affiliation proceedings can be very difficult, and medical evidence may be a vital component of both application and defence. Generally a court will not find an allegation of paternity proved on the unsubstantiated evidence of the mother alone. Some form of corroboration will be required. Affiliation is defined in the *Affiliation Proceedings Act 1957*.

Custodianship

The Houghton Committee, which reviewed adoption law in 1968/70, recognised that for some purposes adoption was too final. Their recommendations led to the passing of Part II of the *Children Act 1975*, which provides for custodianship. This part of the act is not yet in force, but is likely to be implemented by the end of 1982. A custodianship order will permit the legal custody of a child to be vested in the people actually looking after him if they are not his parents. They may be step-parents, relatives or foster parents. In the case of a step-parent who is the spouse of a parent having legal custody of the child, that legal custody will be shared between actual parent and step-parent. In other cases the caretakers will be given legal custody, to the exclusion of the patents. The parents' rights will be suspended, but not terminated. The parents may retain a right of access, and have a continuing duty to maintain the child. Custodians (other than step-parents) may be eligible to receive special allowances from the local authority.

Guardianship
The term 'legal guardian' is very specific. It means a person appointed by deed or will, or by a court of competent jurisdiction, to be the child's guardian. A child will have a guardian only if at least one of his parents is dead. A parent may nominate a guardian for his children in a will. After his death the guardian assumes responsibility for the child. If there is a surviving parent the guardianship is exercised jointly by the guardian and the surviving parent. In the case of a child with no parents, the court may appoint a guardian. A guardian has responsibilities towards his ward's property (if any) as well as towards his person. The *Guardianship Acts 1971 to 1973* also provide a framework within which disputes between parents or guardians can be resolved. In any such dispute the court is required to give first and paramount consideration to the child's welfare.

Marriage of children
Persons under 16 cannot legally marry in the United Kingdom. A marriage, one party to which was under 16, would be void. The invalidity of a marriage because the girl is under age does not necessarily make the male guilty of an offence under the *Sexual Offences Act,* if he reasonably believed the marriage valid. The courts will generally recognise as valid a marriage solemnized abroad where one party is under 16, if the marriage was lawful in the country where it was performed. Again, no sexual offence would have been committed.

Between 16 and 18 marriage normally requires the consent of both parents. If the young person intending to marry is the subject of a custody order, only the consent of the parent having custody is required. If parental consent cannot be obtained (as distinct from the parent refusing consent), the Registrar General may dispense with consent and permit the marriage to proceed. Where a parent refuses consent, the person intending marriage may apply to a county court or a magistrates' court for permission to marry. If, by some oversight, a couple were married in circumstances in which parental consent was required for one or both, without that consent being given or dispensed with, the marriage would probably still be valid, although the couple would be well advised to seek guidance from the Registrar General.

Matrimonial proceedings
Marital disputes are the most frequently occurring family proceedings in the courts. By their very nature, these proceedings affect many thousands of children. Divorce can take place only in the High Court and the county courts. The magistrates' courts can grant legal separations. In both types of proceedings, the court may make orders for the custody and maintenance of, and access to, 'children of the family'. This phrase includes a child of the marriage, and also any child of one party, towards whom the other party has accepted some responsiblity as a step-parent. The powers of courts in divorce cases are defined by the *Matrimonial Causes Act 1973;* those of the magistrates' courts by the *Domestic Proceedings and Magistrates' Courts Act 1978*. Both acts make it possible for the court, in exceptional cases, to place a child under the supervision of a local social services authority, or to commit a child to the care of such an authority.

Registration of births
Every birth must be registered within 42 days. The primary obligation falls on the parents, but any person present at the birth is a qualified informant. In the case of the death or inability of both father and mother, a statutory liability falls on every qualified informant to give the necessary particulars to the registrar.

If the child is that of a married woman, the particulars of her husband will normally be entered as the father. If the mother is single, widowed, divorced or separated no entry will be made in the Register of Births for the father's identity. The father's particulars will usually be entered only if he and the mother make a joint request for this to be done. A father's name can be added to a birth registration after the expiration of the 42 days' time limit, again on the joint application of father and mother.

Stillbirths also require registration. A stillbirth is 'a child which has issued forth from its mother after the 28th week of pregnancy, which did not, at any time after being completely expelled from its mother, breathe or show any other signs of life' (*Births and Deaths Registration Act 1926*, s.12). The certificate has to be signed by the midwife or medical practitioner who attended the birth or examined the body. The certificate must state that the child was not born alive, and include details of weight, duration of pregnancy and cause of death. Books of these certificates are obtainable from the Registrar of Births and Deaths.

Wardship
The High Court has an inherent power to interest itself

in the well-being of individual children, and to exercise its authority on their behalf. The power of the Court to make a child a 'ward of court' does not rest on statute law, but in the very nature of the English legal system. Wardship is amongst the oldest of legal remedies for disputes involving children, and remains a powerful tool. Because it is not constrained by the words of an Act of Parliament, the Court has maximum discretion to ensure that paramount consideration is given to the child's welfare. In modern times wardship is finding an increasing role in resolving the many anomalies which occur between different parts of the statute law regarding children.

Anyone with a valid interest can apply for a child to be made a ward of court. The initial process is rapid; after which the child's circumstances cannot be altered until the Court has investigated and made a decision about the child's future. If the Court confirms the status of wardship, the child then remains a ward of court until 18, and the Court will continue to interest itself in the major decisions in the child's life.

FURTHER READING

A more detailed description of aspects of child care law can be found in the following:

Holden, A.S. (1980) *Children in Care*. Leamington Spa: Comyn Books.

Harris, B. *et al* (1977) *Clarke Hall and Morrison on Children*, 9th edn, supplement 1980. London: Butterworths.

Bevan, H.K. (1973) The Law Relating to Children. London: Butterworths.

To consult published acts of parliament can be very misleading. Acts are published by Her Majesty's Stationery Office as enacted, and do not show amendments, repeals or sections not yet in force.

4

Education in child care

Ian Stanley

How important is child care in general practice? In terms of consultation rate the average general practitioner will see about 250 patients under 15 years of age per month i.e. approximately 12 per working day. What is more, since about two-thirds will be under 5 years of age, usually at least one parent will be seen at the same time. There is evidence that the consultation rate for the 0–4 age group is increasing (GHS, 1978). Much of this work will be for self-limiting minor illness when considered only in physical terms. The importance of the event lies in other dimensions of the continuing care of families.

The presence of serious or life-threatening illness is a small but significant risk. Consider for example deaths from respiratory disease in children. In 1974 in this country about 1000 children under five years old died at home from respiratory disease (Jenkins and Newton, 1981). It is difficult to escape the conclusion that some at least of these children were poorly assessed in respect of physical disease or the capacity of the home environment to provide care and vigilance.

The Court report (1976) documents the social inequities of childhood in the United Kingdom, with respect to health and life expectancy.

'A child born into the family of a semi-skilled or unskilled worker is twice as likely to die between the end of the first month and the end of the first year of life . . . as a child born to parents in social classes I and II'.

A very natural reaction to this sort of statistic is to suggest that social causes imply social rather than medical solutions. However a preventive approach by the medical profession implies concern, even prime responsibility, for raising the standard of care received by the disadvantaged. How then should education prepare doctors for the care of children in the community? Perhaps first by looking back.

Childhood is a universal experience; part of it consists of illness and resulting contact with the doctor. Those students entering medical school from a United Kingdom background bring with them impressions of the role of the general practitioner from first hand experience. The Court report documents this for 5th and 6th form school children. An early aim of medical education might be to explore this experience of the individual student and his peers. Two consequences are likely. Firstly, we might learn more of the origins of the medical vocation and, hopefully, how to nurture it more successfully than we do at present. Secondly, when the experience is looked at in terms of national morbidity (physical, psychological and social) in childhood, the limitations of our viewpoint as professional recruits should be obvious. It follows that medical education must provide a great deal more than knowledge of a system of disease.

The undergraduate curriculum in medicine is not lacking in relevant sociological and psychological content. What is missing is a continuing context in which to apply it and thereby to appreciate and define its limitations in the understanding of individuals and families. The appropriate context is the community, in which at present only a small proportion of undergraduate experience is obtained.

A shift in emphasis from the teaching hospital to the community need not result in more pressure on curriculum time, since it should focus the teaching of factual knowledge on relevant concerns, and encourage the acquisition of skills common to the consultation whatever its setting (Wright and MacAdam, 1979).

It is not surprising then that the experience provided by teaching in general practice should be such a cultural shock to undergraduates who have spent the preceding years in professional isolation from the community. In many medical schools this takes place at a time when, in terms of pay-off for final MB, the experience is seen by the student as limited. Nevertheless it exerts a substantial influence on the undergraduate in the long term. For many it is the first experience of a more balanced relationship with the patient, of coping with uncertainty, of practical preventive care, of selectivity, of team work and of continuity. Above all, while general practitioners in the United Kingdom continue to visit patients it remains the only widely available contact between the student and the patient's home environment. Without an understanding of the latter, a good deal of present knowledge cannot be translated into improved standards of family care. To give an example, students are likely to know what constitutes good ante-natal care; they are less likely to know why women fail to attend ante-natal clinics or appreciate the health implications for the offspring of non-attenders, extending beyond pregnancy into the early days and weeks of life (Court, 1976).

Specialist training and continuing education for general practice cannot be considered in isolation from what has gone before.

To quote from a recent article (Evered and Williams, 1980):

'Training a doctor is expensive and time-consuming. Substantial public funds (about £100 000 000 a year in the United Kingdom) are invested in this process and yet little has been done to ensure that the community obtains the maximum return on its investment. The Medical Schools accept only the most gifted students and then expose them to an educational process so rigid in its structure and limited in its horizons that at graduation the medical student is the best informed but most poorly educated of all graduates. This system, which is designed to eliminate the incompetent, also often succeeds in stifling the inventiveness and the imagination of the most competent and signally fails to develop those intellectual attitudes necessary for continuing self-education. These errors are subsequently compounded by the creation of systems of continuing medical education that have rarely been subjected to objective evaluation and often seem inappropriate to the needs of the medical graduate'

This statement is perhaps more symptomatic of present disatisfaction with the profession than strictly true. For example, I am not sure that the system of selecting medical students is capable of finding the most gifted, rather than the most knowledgeable. This is an important distinction, which may have greater implications for general practice than for any other branch of medicine. The importance of the statement resides in its implication that continuing self-education is vital to the profession. The acceptance and implementation of this principle is the yardstick against which we should measure the quality of education provided by vocational training.

For those who wish to undertake a career in general practice as a principal, vocational training is now mandatory. Although some variations occur, it usually consists of two years hospital experience followed by one year in general practice.

At the present time there seems to be little enthusiasm for extending the training period to five years as originally envisaged. This probably arises from doubts about the quality of much of the present three year programme. These reservations concern both the hospital based training and that taking place in training practices.

The content and methods of paediatric training required for general practice are the subject of a report by the British Paediatric Association and the Royal College of General Practitioners (1978). This document suggests, and the Court report recommends, that all trainees should undertake a hospital post in paediatrics. The contribution of such a post to the objectives of training will vary with its setting, but is likely to be limited in the main to acute conditions threatening life and to familiarity with the normal and abnormal neonate.

The vexed question of how long such a post should last, i.e. 3, 4 or 6 months, reflects organisational rather more than educational concerns. At present there seems to be no satisfactory alternative to a period of paediatric residence in an acute unit based in a district general hospital. Two reservations remain, however.

The first concerns the educational value of acute paediatrics managed under supervision and on cases selected for admission by a GP. This is a far cry from management in the home including consideration of the pros and cons of hospital admission. My second reservation concerns an attitude engendered by hospital posts, i.e. that the trainee has 'done paediatrics'. It is difficult to convince trainees that the majority of the objectives of paediatric training can only be achieved in the community (Franklin, 1976).

Although there is some evidence that paediatrics does not loom large in the curricula of day-release courses, this should not be taken at face value since many of the skills of general practice are relevant to the consultation involving a child. The nature of day-release courses provides opportunities for tutorial learning, project work, and the exploration of resources for the normal and abnormal child.

There seems little doubt that these courses are often stimulating and valuable in defining patterns of learning for the future principal. What is not clear is whether course organisers see themselves as responsible for imparting the basic or core knowledge of paediatrics needed for work in the community. Examples of this would be developmental assessment routines, immunisation schedules and contraindications. From personal experience of candidates presenting for assessment by the MRCGP examination, it is evident that some trainees have not absorbed this essential knowledge. Given the uneven quantity of hospital and practice teaching, and the educational efficiency of the day-release course, they would seem to be the setting in which this learning should occur. In the 'heady' atmosphere engendered by shared experience and heuristic methods much that is educationally valuable occurs.

The penalty may be that it is more difficult to define and cover a curriculum of study which is comprehensive, in respect of essential knowledge.

For many, the present limitations of vocational training reside principally in the uneven nature of teaching practices. To an extent this is inevitable. The complexity and uncertainty of much of general practice make it a difficult subject to impart. Unlike other branches of medicine there is no tradition of teaching junior staff. Nevertheless, there is now considerable collective experience of training and wide acknowledgement that the rewards for the practice are substantial, financially and professionally. As we have seen, the present structure of vocational training and the nature of its educational objectives for paediatrics make the one year spent in practice all-important.

For the year (or two periods of six months) in practice, the trainee is appointed to a principal rather than a partnership. The principal, his trainer, will have been appointed on the basis of education and experience rather more than on the setting in which he works. This one-to-one approach to training, whilst it may have been inevitable in the early days, needs to be reconsidered. It is the practice which reaps the rewards of training; it should be prepared to provide an appropriate working and educational environment. Considerable influence would be exerted on standards of 'structure' and 'process' in training practices if the criteria for selection were based rather more on the practice than on one, perhaps outstanding, principal. The involvement of more GPs, within a suitable practice, in the training process is likely to help the trainee and at the same time serve to define the educational needs of the established principal.

Throughout this brief review I have been at pains to emphasize 'the continuum of education' (Aims for Training, 1978). The training practice should exemplify this in providing an educational environment suitable for the needs of trainee and principal. What does this consist of? In essence, the sharing of experience and its translation into learning. In practical terms, the provision of opportunities for the exchange of information at a number of levels, administrative and professional. Such information will comprise that derived from outside sources (journals, books, people) and that arising from observation of the performance of the practice in a number of areas. These elements, the updating of knowledge and the monitoring of performance are essential attributes of a profession (Greenwood, 1966).

There is substantial overlap in the educational needs of the trainee and principal. In addition they almost certainly learn from one another given opportunity and appropriate attitudes. I want to give two examples. Initially the trainee will almost certainly find the time constraints of general practice difficult. While he must develop skills of selectivity which enable him to operate efficiently within these constraints, the practice might usefully evaluate those factors (for example, follow-up policy) which are contributing to the pressure on consulting time.

As a second example, a regular meeting to review journals (including book reviews) provides an important forum for the acquisition and exchange of knowledge. The contribution of the trainee will reflect his more recent education and hospital experience, that of the principal the knowledge derived from, and reinforced by, experience in general practice. This leads not only to an exchange of information but to a critical evaluation of publised articles from differing aspects. In the process, many basic assumptions will be examined. If conflict arises between the published findings of research and the lessons of experience, the importance of evaluative skills in assessing the quality of research (and the limitations of experience) will be evident. These skills are important not just to the doctor who wishes to conduct research but to all those who read journals or the 'literature' of the pharmaceutical industry.

It may well be that at the level of the practice these skills are not available. The regional advisor and his course organisers should be capable of responding by appropriate educational provision for the trainee and practice.

Paediatric educational objectives for training necessarily include a number of aspects of practice organisation. A preventive approach involves not just the provision of appropriate clinics and the fostering of a team, but flexibility of access in the event of illness. In the dialogue within the practice between the administration and the partners, there is much for the trainee to learn. Direct experience of the role of the receptionist is desirable. He should appreciate the responsibility the practice has to their education and the influence they exert upon his style of practice, his attitudes and his knowledge of the community.

The greatest contribution of the training year should be to the trainees depth of understanding of human behaviour. He will gain most of this from direct experience supplemented by well-directed reading. The necessary catalyst seems to be that those around him exhibit appropriate attitudes (Charvat *et al*, 1968). In this respect he should experience the role of other team members at first hand. In this way he will come to see them not merely as resources but as colleagues with differing priorities and distinct skills. It has been proposed that undergraduate teaching and vocational training should include combined sessions for the education of future members of the primary health care team. Even if this becomes a reality for students of medicine, health visiting, midwifery etc., the team concept in general practice is likely to extend to encompass clinical psychologists, physiotherapists and others, whose education remains distinct.

In paediatrics the trainee should be absorbing a substantial knowledge of common disease and its management; he should be acquiring skills needed in the consultation involving parent and child. In monitoring his progress two assessment methods are particularly appropriate. They are the use of audio-recordings of consultations and random case-analysis based on the patients' notes. These techniques are appropriate to the education of all the doctors in the practice. It is likely that habits of consultation acquired early persist into independent practice (Maguire and Rutter, 1976). Retrospective random case-analysis based on the patients' notes and conducted some weeks after the chosen consultation reveals the accuracy of hypothesis formation and the appropriateness of management. This evaluation is not possible without adequate patient records. Thus the first pay-off is likely to be an improved standard of record keeping.

The majority of paediatric training is then, rightly, inseparable from general professional training.

The Court report indicated deficiencies in the care of children in the community; its recommendations, however, have not all proved acceptable to the profession. Mandatory vocational training is only likely to influence professional standards in the long-term if continuing education is seen as an essential complement to the process. In the training practice, as I suggest, they should overlap to a great extent. Elsewhere much will depend on the influence that a vocationally-trained GP can exert on the practice to which he moves as a principal. Too little attention is given during training to the skills needed by a young principal if he is to cultivate and propagate his education once he is translated to the atmosphere of friendly inertia which pervades many practices.

There is at present no mandatory assessment of postgraduate training for general practice. 'Satisfactory completion' is little more than an acknowledgement of the physical presence of the trainee in a scheme for three years. So far as the paediatric content is concerned there are two relevant public examinations.

The Diploma in Child Health (DCH) requires the candidate to have spent six months in a resident paediatric hospital post. It is unlikely therefore to be available to all trainees in the immediate future.

The examination for Membership of the Royal College of General Practitioners aims to assess competence for independent practice (RCGP, 1981). There is a substantial paediatric content, examined in the context of family practice. Since the assessment is of basic competence at the end of vocational training, the failure of a trainee should lead to a review of methods by all those involved. Unfortunately this is often too late for the failed candidate who will be close to the completion of training by the time the result is known. Some form of external assessment at a mid-point in training would appear to be needed.

The paediatric knowledge, skills and attitudes appropriate to the established GP are not as yet clear. Voluntary reassessment is likely to be available to Members of the Royal College of General Practitioners within the near future. This may make possible a concensus view of standards of paediatric practice appropriate to the established principal.

The urgent need in general practice, now that vocational training is firmly established, is the transformation of continuing education from a hobby to an acknowledged professional responsibility.

REFERENCES

Aims for Training (1978) *Some Aims for Training for General Practice*, Occasional paper 6. London: Royal College of General Practitioners.

Charvat, J., McGuire, C. & Parsons, V. (1968) *A Review of the Nature and Uses of Examinations in Medical Education*. World Health Organisation: Geneva

Court report (1976) *Fit for the Future*. Report of the Committee on Child Health Services, Vol. 2, pp. 6, 416. London: H.M.S.O.

Curtis Jenkins, G. & Newton, R.S.F. (1981) *The First Year of Life*. Library of General Practice, Vol. 2. Edinburgh: Churchill Livingstone.

Evered, D.C. & Williams, H.D (1980) Postgraduate Education and the Doctor. *British Medical Journal*, **1**, 626–7.

Franklin, A.W. (1976) *Widening Horizons of Child Health*, p 124. Lancaster: M.T.P. Press.

G.H.S. (1978) *General Household Survey*, p 119. London: H.M.S.O.

Greenwood, E. (1966) The Elements of Professionalisation. Vollmer, H.M., & Mill, D.L. (eds) *Professionalisation*. London: Prentice Hall.

Maguire, P. & Rutter, D. (1976) Training Medical Students to Communicate. In Bennett, A.E. (ed.) *Communication Between Doctors and Patients*. Oxford University Press.

RCGP (1981) Obtaining and maintaining membership: a Council discussion paper. *Journal of the Royal College of General Practitioners*, 31, 521–524.

Wright, H.J. & MacAdam, D.B. (1979) *Clinical Thinking and Practice*, Ch. 8. Edinburgh: Churchill Livingstone.

5

Research in child care

John Bain

1970-1979: A REVIEW

The period 1970–1979 saw a series of reports concerned with the organisation of child care in the United Kingdom (*Paediatrics in the Seventies 1972, Towards an integrated Child Health Service 1973*, and *Fit for the future 1976*) and the decade ended with the International Year of the Child in 1979.

The past decade also included advances in academic general practice with the majority of medical schools in the United Kingdom setting up Departments of General Practice, with vocational training flourishing during this period of time, and by 1981 mandatory for all new entrants to general practice. Richardson (1975) stated that any specialty must meet four criteria in order to develop and maintain itself as an academic discipline. These are a distinctive cross-section of illness, the possession of special skills, the application of a characteristic philosophy, and the production of original research. While Richardson's principles referred to the whole of general practice, the same criteria can be applied to the content of child care in general practice.

The principles of research in child care in general practice are no different from the principles of research in any other field of medicine. It is not the purpose of this chapter to outline research methods or discuss the organisation of clinical trials. Ethical problems are discussed in a recent report (Working Party on Ethics, 1980). There are few books on research in general practice, but two in particular are worth mentioning. Eimerl and Laidlaw (1969) provided details of the methods of collecting data by means of the age sex register, the E book, the F book, and the W book, systems which have formed the basis of many reports produced by the Royal College of General Practitioners. More recently, Howie (1979) has provided a personal account of his approach to original work. Both these books can be commended for their attention to detail and their emphasis on research method. That method starts with the asking of questions and the proposing of hypotheses, progresses through the design of studies, the analysis and interpretation of results, and culminates finally in the presentation and discussion of findings.

The following review is based on studies reported by general practitioners which have included measurement of child care in the setting of general practice during the period 1970–1979. It has not been possible to refer to all articles pertaining to children published by general practitioners in the last 10 years, and review articles and opinion pieces have been largely excluded. Articles on subjects similar to the studies from general practice have also been quoted, in addition to a number of reports from paediatricians which have direct application to child care in general practice. The research work conducted by general practitioners can be considered under four main headings : 1-the natural history of illness and patient management, 2-preventive and social medicine, 3-organisation of services, 4-clinical trials.

Natural history of illness and patient management

Respiratory illness

Respiratory tract infections and disorders of the respiratory tract are the most common conditions in children seen in general practice. Fry's original work (1961) on the catarrhal child remains an excellent account of the natural history of a common condition and his methods are a model of simplicity. More recently Stott (1979) studied the prescribing behaviour of general practitioners in relation to upper respiratory tract infections in children. He found that the different management plans by general practitioners did not correlate with clinical outcome as judged by complications, recall rates, and demand for treatment of similar episodes in the future. General practitioners who prescribed antibiotics for 20 per cent of upper respiratory tract infections had similar complication rates to those who gave antibiotics to sixty per cent of such cases. On the same theme Howie (1971) and Howie and Hutchison (1978) have shown that contrary to popular belief the prescribing of antibiotics on a large scale neither lessens the number of return consultations nor saves work.

While doctors' beliefs and behaviour will be important factors in determining prescribing habits, the outcome in respiratory disorders in children will also be affected by patient behaviour. Millac (1975) showed that there was an increase in adenotonsillectomy in children of mothers referred to hospital with gynaecological symptoms and suggested that the outcome for children with apparently frequent respiratory tract infections is often determined by the consulting habits of the parents. It will never be possible to have absolute rules for prescribing and referral, but the measurement of the determinants and associations of prescribing and referral behaviour is crucial to an understanding of the discipline of general practice.

Despite the fact that otitis media remains a common problem seen in children in general practice there have been few original reports from general practice since Hazzard's paper (1970) describing the presenting symptoms of children with presumed middle ear infection. Price (1976) showed that the commonest cause of earache in his practice was otitis externa, and five new cases of otitis externa were seen for every case of otitis media. He rightly recommended that each case of earache should be scrutinised with a more critical approach.

The natural history of asthma has been admirably reviewed by Blair (1979). He commenced with 267 asthmatics registered in an East London practice between 1948 and 1952 and twenty years later was able to review 237 of these patients when 48 per cent of childhood asthmatics were found to be still asthmatic. The factors which adversely affected long term prognosis were the degree of inheritance as indicated by family history, the absence or limitation of breast feeding, and the history or presence of other atopic disease in the patient. In a similar long term follow-up study of asthmatic children Blair (1977) found that the final prognosis was further influenced by the severity of asthma at onset. Any discussion of asthma is beset by difficulties in definition, but Blair's work in asthma is an excellent example of the one man, one subject piece of research conducted over many years in general practice.

The aetiology of respiratory infections and in particular the role of viruses in wheezy bronchitis has been studied by Horn et al (1973, 1975, 1979) and Gregg (1975, 1977) has also reported original work on the management of asthma in general practice. Horn (1975) described her asthma/bronchitis clinic in general practice where regular follow-up using peak flow meters and the use of a physiotherapist led to a reduction in hospital admissions. Horn's conclusions are difficult to assess when the skill and enthusiasm of the individual doctor may have a notable effect on the outcome of the condition being studied. Guille and Clark (1977) stressed the need to perform objective tests of respiratory function in children, and found that those with exercise-induced bronchospasm measured by lung function tests had a higher consultation rate for respiratory symptoms while their consultation rates for non respiratory symptoms were the same as the remainder of the samples studied. This result raises the question of whether children with raised bronchial lability are at risk to respiratory problems later in life.

Other work in respiratory infection worth noting included Cullen's finding (1972) that, contrary to expectations, the warmer the climate the greater the prevalence of bronchitis, asthma and hay fever. Ross (1972) reported on the causation and incidence of sore throat in children but his suggestion that all children with sore throat should have a throat swab is unlikely to get much support in general practice circles.

Among epidemiological studies in respiratory illness Colley (1975) showed that the incidence of pneumonia and bronchitis in the first year of life was associated with parents' smoking habits, and that the child vulnerable to respiratory illness should be sought for, particularly in families where parents have chest symptoms and smoke.

Urinary tract infection

This subject has attracted a lot of attention from both general practitioners and paediatricians in the last few years. Mond et al (1970) calculated that the incidence of urinary tract infection in children in general practice was 1.4 per cent per annum in children under thirteen years of age and 4.9 per cent per annum in children under the age of five years. Mond also found that there was little or no relationship between upper respiratory tract infection and the finding of bacteriuria. Brooks and Houston (1977) reported on the presentation of urinary tract infection during a four year study; they found an incidence of 7.7 per thousand girls at risk per year and 3.8 per thousand boys at risk per year, while Dickinson (1979) who used three consecutive specimens exceeding 100 000 organisms per ml as an indication of definite infection found an incidence of 3.1 per thousand girls at risk per year and 1.7 per thousand boys at risk per year, and out of fourteen children investigated three were found to have radiological abnormalities. On the basis of small studies both Brooks and Dickinson suggested radiological investigation of children at the time of the *first* urinary tract infection, a policy supported from a hospital study (Saxena, 1975). While this may be a reasonable approach in boys, this counsel of perfection would lead to many thousands of girls undergoing additional and costly investigations. Robson et al (1979) over a ten year period, showed that dip slide cultures for children were practicable, a fact previously shown in a hospital study by Baum et al

(1972). Unfortunately Robson made no comment on what savings there may have been for the local laboratory in terms of time and money during the period of the study. The reasons why dip slides are not so popular as might have been expected are largely unknown, and with the advent of health centre practice and the growth of treatment room facilities dip slide investigations require further study.

Outwith general practice the main focus of attention has been on asymptomatic bacteriuria and a number of studies have looked at covert bacteriuria in children and concluded that there was not sufficient evidence to warrant the prescriptive screening of children for urinary tract infection (Savage et al, 1973; Davies et al, 1974; Boothman et al, 1974; Saxena et al, 1975; Report of the Newcastle Research Group, 1975).

Infant feeding

The main focus of research work in this field has been on the relationship between early feeding practices and subsequent obesity. Hodgson (1978) and Thorogood et al (1979) in studies from general practice found no relationship between the age of introduction of solids and obesity at one year of age, which was a similar finding to that of paediatricians (Davies et al, 1977) who found no evidence that the introduction of solids to bottle fed infants at any time in the first few months of life had a significant effect on growth. While these results may be reassuring to mothers, the possibility of hypernatraemia in young babies given thickened feeds cannot be ignored (Oates, 1973). Sunderland et al (1979) from Sheffield attributed much of the reduction in deaths due to hypernatraemia to intensive local campaigns to encourage breast feeding and to instruct mothers in the correct dilution of milk feeds. Although the importance of health visitors and health education must not be minimised, to what extent this reduction in hypernatraemia was also related to the withdrawal of national dried milk is difficult to determine.

Psychological illness

While psychological illness in adults has been studied widely in general practice, psychological problems in children have attracted much less attention. Bailey et al (1978) reported on the psychological and social factors in 1127 consecutive attendances in children and adolescents in four London practices. The proportion of pure psychological problems was low (3.5 per cent) but in 25.7 per cent of attendances a psychological component existed in the presenting problem. There was also a significantly higher proportion of the children with psychological problems who had mothers with concurrent psychological difficulties.

Common conditions with a possible psychological component are sleep problems and enuresis, the incidence of which have been reported by Seiler (1972) and Hodes (1973). In a study of psychotropic drug prescribing in children Bain (1975) found that in a group practice in a new town 13 per cent of all psychotropic drug prescriptions were for children under the age of 12 years and six per cent of the child population had received one or more psychotropic drugs in one year. Bain's study also showed that the majority of psychotropic prescriptions were for children with sleep difficulties and enuresis, two problems where there are few specific guidelines for the GP to follow. Studies by psychologists (McAllister and Philip, 1975; Davis et al, 1977; Ives, 1979) showed that one area where the psychologist may have an important part to play in primary care is in the management of developmental and behaviour problems in children. Further research is required to determine if problems such as hyperactivity, sleep problems, enuresis, and encopresis might be more appropriately dealt with by psychologists than by referral to paediatricians.

While on the subject of psychological problems and the prescribing of psychotropic drugs mention might be made of the controversy over the use of tricyclic antidepressants in children. Poisoning by tricyclic antidepressants has attracted some recent comment because they are the commonest cause of fatal poisoning of children under five years of age. Cronin (1979) recommended that no child with nocturnal enuresis should be treated with tricyclic drugs. While studying the use of psychotropic drugs in general practice Bain (1973) expressed caution about the use of tricyclic antidepressants in enuresis, but found that the large majority of children who died from tricyclic poisoning had accidently ingested parents' or relatives' drugs and not medicines prescribed for enuresis.

Only about seven per cent of children with recurrent abdominal pain will have an organic cause for their complaint (BMJ, 1975). In a study from his own practice Turner (1978) concluded that recurrent abdominal pain in childhood is often a reflection of family disorder. He found that relations between mothers and children with recurrent pain were often unstable and inconsistent. He went on to suggest that the longer term management of these families might be handled better by health visitors and social workers but produced no evidence to support these proposals.

Psychological problems in families can often be related to the incidence of accidents in children, and the 'accident prone family' can be readily identified (Husband and Hinton, 1975; Julyan and Kuzemko, 1975).

Parents and children

Although parents are constantly sharing their concerns with their family doctors, little is known about how parents decide on the course of action to be taken when treating their own children's illnesses.

Bassett and Bain (1976) used a multiple choice questionnaire in measuring mothers' knowledge of child health and produced some evidence to show that low scoring mothers do have higher consultation rates with their doctor.

A paediatrician and a general practitioner (Rutter and Metcalfe, 1978) found that parental management of febrile convulsions was often inappropriate and suggested that simply written instructions on how to handle febrile illnesses might help.

An outstanding example of general practice research in this field was Pereira Gray's study (1970) of handicapped children and one of his main conclusions was that sustained abnormal emotional tension was the commonest single finding in families of handicapped children. The family doctor is in an ideal position to report on patients' concern for and management of their children, yet this is a sadly neglected area of research in primary care.

Preventive services and social problems

Three topics dominated this area of child care in the 1970s: 1-developmental screening, 2-whooping cough vaccination, 3-child abuse.

Developmental screening. A number of general practitioners have reported on the organisation and outcome of developmental screening in clinics and general practice (Hooper, 1971; Starte, 1974; Bain, 1974; Rowlands, 1975; Curtis-Jenkins, 1978). On average, ten per cent of children examined at these clinics will have problems requiring further follow-up and three per cent will be referred for specialist opinion. Starte (1974) Barber (1976) and Curtis-Jenkins (1978) have made important contributions to the design of developmental screening forms and methods of examination. However, it is remarkable that after decades of routine pre-school surveillance so little is known about the general application of suggested methods of examination of the pre-school child.

Curtis-Jenkins (1975) has shown that the existence of a child development clinic in a group practice can lead to a reduction in consulting rates for illness in pre-school children. If this finding were to be confirmed in other settings, this would have considerable implications for the provision of primary care for children. Freer (1977) has highlighted the problem of non-attendance at screening clinics, and in a Glasgow study found a default rate of 41 per cent and raised the question of whether selective screening should be a more realistic alternative to comprehensive screening. There are also considerable variations in the standards applied by different general practitioners when examining children and in screening clinics in general practice over 60 per cent of children will be examined by health visitors alone, or health visitors in combination with general practitioners (Bain, 1977). From an analysis of school-entry examinations Wintle (1972) suggested that a suitably trained nurse could conduct the pre-school examination, but there have been no meaningful comparisons between general practitioners' and health visitors' performances in the developmental examination of children.

Bolden (1976) expressed doubt about the value of screening and found that 81 per cent of developmental abnormalities in his practice were identified outwith the screening clinic. The study was not entirely without bias in that he looked at a selected and uncontrolled sample, but it would be equally fair to say that those in favour of screening can be faulted for overstating their case. A number of questions remain unanswered about routine surveillance, and there is a need for more controlled studies of outcome and cost of screening programmes.

Starte's interest in child development has also resulted in two interesting findings (1975, 1978). He found that the poorly communicating two-year-old was a sensitive index of possible high risk families in terms of psychosocial impairment (1975), and also reported on a study (1978) which showed that the degree of influence of illness in children under two years of age on developmental progress was for the most part small. Child development has been at the centre of Pollak's work (1972, 1974) on the differences between various ethnic groups, and Pollak (1979) has also shown that the adequacy of maternal care was highly significant in relationship to satisfactory child development, while quality of housing was not found to affect children's developmental needs. Curtis Jenkins (1978) reported on the identification of children with learning problems in general practice but this study will only have relevance to doctors with special training and interest in children.

Immunisation. Two reports from outwith general practice stimulated considerable debate on the value of whooping cough vaccination. Bassili and Stewart (1976) argued that the persistence of whooping cough in some areas was more strongly correlated with adverse socio-economic conditions than with lack of immunisation, and Stewart (1977) claimed that there was evidence to show a strong relationship between pertussis vaccination and the development of neurological abnormalities in children. The correspondence generated by this latter article would require a chapter on its own, but the majority of doctors seem to approve of the retention of whooping cough vaccination.

Two general practitioners reported on outbreaks of whooping cough in their practices. Jenkinson (1978) found that one in five children at risk under the age of five years got the infection; of those who had been immunised within one year of the outbreak none got whooping cough. He relied mainly on clinical diagnosis of whooping cough, being able to confirm the diagnosis in only 40 per cent of 50 patients who had swabs taken. Ditchburn (1979) reported on his findings during an epidemic in his practice in the Shetland Isles. The practice policy had been to discontinue whooping cough immunisation after 1974 and he found that the incidence of infection was similar in those who had been immunised and those who had not, and concluded his article by questioning the value of whooping cough vaccination. His study could be criticised on a number of grounds: firstly the diagnosis of whooping cough was on clinical presentation only; secondly the two groups of children were not strictly comparable; thirdly the efficacy of whooping cough vaccines used in the late 1960s and early 1970s have been questioned (Abbot et al, 1971; Public Health Laboratory, 1973). As a result the older children in Ditchburn's study probably received less effective vaccines.

It would have been of interest to know if the workload of health visitors and general practitioners increased at the peak of the whooping cough debate but there were no reports to indicate that this was any more than a subjective impression.

Other immunisation procedures were studied by Watson and his colleagues (1975) who followed-up children after measles vaccination and raised questions about revaccination. Gringras et al (1977) showed that women at risk to rubella could be readily identified and vaccinated in general practice without much addition to workload.

Child abuse. Beswick et al (1976) and Roberts et al (1977) described a joint project which had been set up between their practice and a child abuse research team to provide help for families with child rearing problems which could lead to abuse. Hardy et al (1979) concluded that their policy of regular team meetings, active developmental screening programmes, and open discussion with mothers about their fears were the reasons for the low incidence of child abuse in their practice compared to the surrounding area. It is difficult to be critical of well motivated colleagues in general practice, but this latter study did not take into sufficient account the many differences that may have existed between the two populations compared. However, attempts to reduce the number of child abuse cases are to be applauded and it was encouraging to read of the efforts of practices which had adopted a positive approach to preventive care.

Organisation

While the Scottish Home and Health Department report *Towards an integrated child health service* (1973) and the Court report *Fit for the future* (1976) have put forward proposals for children's care, and the Royal College of General Practitioners (1978) has recommended that every child receive a comprehensive curative and preventive service through general practice, there are few studies which have looked at how these services can be organised. The only report which has described a comprehensive child care service based in general practice is that from Livingston New Town where integration of services and an element of specialisation in general practice has been fostered (Stark et al, 1975).

A survey of attitudes of vocational trainees in general practice submitted to the Court report revealed that the trainee practitioners agreed that curative and preventive services were both necessary and desirable in general practice but only three out of 53 trainees had any experience of preventive care for children (Report of an Independent Working Party, 1977). If the aims of the Royal College of General Practitioners are to be met the content of vocational training has to be constantly reviewed. The outcome of the experimental scheme in the Lothian region in Scotland where trainees have an extended course in community paediatrics will be watched with interest (Donald et al, 1979). Experiments in primary care for children have often been thwarted by lack of investment and by the absence of meaningful attempts to evaluate alternative systems of care. When this occurs visions of change are too often circumscribed by tradition. The inequalities in paediatric care in different practices have been shown by Wright (1973), and the problem of providing primary care to children in inner cities, new towns, and large housing estates is well known. What is lacking are well designed studies to examine whether general practice as presently constituted is the most appropriate means of providing for those at the centre of the problem – namely the children who require our care and attention.

Clinical trials

The only well controlled trial including children and conducted by a general practitioner was that of Everett (1973) who found that there was no significant difference in the duration of diarrhoea between patients treated with kaolin and neomycin and those treated with kaolin alone. He concluded that antibiotics had no place in the treatment of acute gastro-enteritis general practice. It might be well worth while repeating this study to find out if drugs have any place at all in the treatment of acute gastro-intestinal upsets in children.

Gordon et al (1974) and Taylor et al (1977), from Australia and New Zealand respectively, have conducted trials on the use of antibiotics in upper respiratory tract infection in children. In a controlled trial of 89 patients Gordon found that for the ordinary run of upper respiratory tract illness in children, antibiotics neither shortened the course of the illness nor prevented bacterial complications. Taylor and his colleagues in a double blind trial conducted on 197 children with upper respiratory tract infections found that any benefits of antibiotics which were noted were marginal, and that they should not be routinely prescribed. It will never be possible to have absolute rules for prescribing, but while there is a lack of controlled studies many apparently mild disorders will continue to be managed as though they were serious diseases.

Other controlled trials with relevance to general practice were Stansfield's finding (1975) that there was no difference in outcome in terms of recurrence of UTI in a two week treatment period compared with a six month treatment period, and the investigation of Cooper et al (1976) who found that co-trimoxazole and amoxycillin were equally effective in the treatment of acute otitis media in children.

Clinical trials outwith the setting of general practice have not been reported in this review.

Conclusions

If there is to be one major criticism of the studies reported, there were probably too few adequately controlled reports of patient management, prevention, and organisation of services. This is not surprising when general practice has no long-standing tradition of research. Few of us have the rare ability to pool the multitude of random facts in child care into coherent and enlightening theories but I see no reason why the general practitioner cannot be an experimental thinker.

It is now ten years since Porter (1971) complained that much of general practice research was too concerned with medical and practice organisation. There are signs in the field of child care research that the more recent studies from general practice have concentrated more on clinical problems and their management. There has been less emphasis on multi-doctor studies and more concentration on the research of individual doctors working with their own patients, a trend firmly supported by Howie (1979). It would be a mistake to think that research always requires sophisticated record systems and access to computers – indeed these may be a hindrance when the research worker gets diverted from his original hypothesis and becomes more concerned with the collection of data. 'Problems exist which can be defined, if not solved, by using only the five senses and a notebook' (Watson, 1972).

While the fleeting hour remains the constant enemy of the general practitioner there are very real difficulties in maintaining a disciplined approach with an adherence to the scientific sequence of idea, hypothesis, test, and evaluation, which will produce the true reward of a sense of creative satisfaction. The time contraints of practice workload may be the reason for the relatively few meaningful investigative efforts from general practice. Yet similar problems concerning available time exist in other clinical specialties, and they have collectively organised themselves in their fields of interest.

The dominant values in the specialty of paediatrics are still to do with rare conditions and complex pathology not perceived as directly applicable to the work of the family doctor. It may well be that we are more concerned in general practice with what we believe to be true rather than the 'sterile' truths of scientific fact but research can only be ignored at the risk of allowing one's work to slip into a complacent repetition of sloppy habits. If general practice is to retain the privilege of being the main provider of primary care for children, the achievement of better medical care can be reached only by transforming commonplace experiences into matters of scientific enquiry, and as a result practice can become more stimulating.

REFERENCES

Abbott, J.D., Preston, N.W. & MacKay, R.I. (1971) Agglutinin response to pertussis vaccination in the child *British Medical Journal*, **1**, 86–88.

Bailey, V., Graham, P. & Boniface, D. (1978) How much child psychiatry does a general practitioner do? *Journal of the Royal College of General Practitioners*, **28**, 621–626.

Bain, D.J.G. (1973) Tricyclic antidepressant drugs in the treatment of childhood enuresis. *Journal of the Royal College of General Practitioners*, **23**, 222–224.

Bain, D.J.G. (1974) The results of developmental screening in general practice. *Health Bulletin*, **32**, 189–193.

Bain, D.J.G. (1975) Prescribing psychotropic drugs for children. *Journal of the Royal College of General Practitioners*, **25**, 49–53.

Bain, D.J.G. (1977) Methods used by general practitioners in developmental screening of pre-school children. *British Medical Journal*, **2**, 363–365.

Barber, J.H., Boothman, R. & Stanfield, J.P. (1976) A new visual chart for pre-school developmental screening. *Health Bulletin*, **34**, 80–91

Bassett, W.J. & Bain, D.J.G. (1976) The use of a multiple choice questionnaire in measuring maternal child health knowledge. *Health Bulletin*, **34**, 335–341.

Bassili, W.R. & Stewart, G.T. (1976) Epidemiological evaluation of immunisation and other factors in the control of whooping cough. *Lancet*, **1**, 471–473.

Baum, J.D., Darrell, J.H. & Lambert, R.A. (1972) Evaluation of dipinnoculum urine culture. *Archives of Disease in Childhood*, **47**, 977–978.

Beswick, K., Lynch, M.A., Roberts, J. (1976) Child abuse and general practice. *British Medical Journal*, **2**, 800–802.

Blair, H. (1977) Natural history of childhood asthma. *Archives of Diseases in Childhood*, **52**, 613–619.

Blair, H. (1979) Childhood asthma. *Proceedings of the Royal Society of Medicine*, **72**, 42–48.

Bolden, K.J. (1976) Developmental screening in general practice. *Proceedings of the Royal Society of Medicine*, **69**, 385–388.

Boothman, R., Laidlaw, M. & Richards, I.D.E (1974) Prevalence of urinary tract infection in children of pre-school

age. *Archives of Disease in Childhood*, **49**, 917–922.
British Medical Journal Leading Article (1975) Recurrent abdominal pain in children. *British Medical Journal*, **2**, 459.
Brooks, D. & Houston, I.B. (1977) Symptomatic urinary infection in childhood. *Journal of the Royal College of General Practitioners*, **27**, 678–683.
Colley, J.R.T. (1975) The vulnerable child *Journal of the Royal College of General Practitioners*, **25**, 257–262.
Cooper, J., Inman, J.S. & Dawson, A.F. (1976) A comparison between co-trimoxazole and amoxycillin in the treatment of acute otitis media in general practice. *The Practitioner*, **217**, 804–809.
Court, D. & Jackson, A. (1972) Paediatrics in the seventies: Developing the child health services. Nuffield Provincial Hospitals Trust: Oxford University Press.
Cronin, A.J., Chalil, R. & Little, T.M. (1979) Poisoning with trycyclic antidepressants; an avoidable cause of childhood deaths. *British Medical Journal*, **1**, 722.
Cullen, K.J. (1972) Climate and chest disorders in school children. *British Medical Journal*, **4**, 65–67.
Curtis Jenkins, G.H. (1975) The pre-school child. In Hart, C.R. (ed.) *Screening in General Practice* Chapter 9, 91–99. Edinburgh: Churchill Livingstone.
Curtis Jenkins, G.H. (1979) The identification of children with learning problems in general practice. *Journal of the Royal College of General Practitioners*, **29**, 647–650.
Curtis Jenkins, G.H., Collins, S. & Andren, S. (1978) Developmental surveillance in general practice. *British Medical Journal*, **1**, 1537–1540.
Davies, D.P., Gray, O.P. & Elwood, P.C. (1977) Effects of solid foods on growth of bottle fed infants in the first three months of life. *British Medical Journal*, **2**, 7–8.
Dickinson, J.A. (1979) Incidence and outcome of symptomatic urinary tract infection in children. *British Medical Journal*, **1**, 1330–1332.
Ditchburn, R.K. (1979) Whooping cough after stopping pertussis immunisation. *British Medical Journal*, **1**, 1601–1603.
Donald A.G., Farquhar, J.W. & Gilleghan, J.D. (1979) An experiment in training in child care for general practitioners. *Journal of the Royal College of General Practitioners*, **29**, 641–643.
Eimerl, T.S. & Laidlaw, A.J. (1969) *A handbook for research in general practice*. Edinburgh: E. & S. Livingstone.
Everett, M.T. (1973) The place of antibiotics in the treatment of acute gastroenteritis in general practice: a controlled clinical trial. *Journal of the Royal College of General Practitioners*, **23**, 183–193.
Freer, C.B. & Ogunmuyiwa, T.A. (1977) Pre-school developmental screening in a health centre – the problem of non attendance. *Journal of the Royal College of General Practitioners*, **27**, 482–430.
Fry, J. (1961) The catarrhal child. London, Butterworth.
Gordon, M., Lovel, S. & Dugdale, A.E. (1974) The value of antibiotics in minor respiratory tract and illness in children. *Medical Journal of Australia*, **1**, 304–306.
Gregg, I. (1975) The place of beclomethasone dipropionate aerosol in the treatment of asthma. *Drugs*, **10**, 161.
Gregg, I. (1977) The difficult asthmatic. *Drugs*, **13**, 35–45.
Gringras, M., Reisler, R. & Caisley, J. et al (1977) Vaccination of rubella susceptible women during oral contraceptive care in general practice. *British Medical Journal*, **2**, 245–246.
Guille, S. & Clark, E.M. (1979) Respiratory morbidity and exercise induced bronchoconstriction in children. *Journal of the Royal College of General Practitioners*, **29**, 652–654.
Hardy, M., McElroy, E. & Patchett, D.R. (1979) Prevention of baby battering. *The Practitioner*, **222**, 243–247.
Hazzard, A.J. (1970) Symptoms associated with acute otitis media in children. *The Practitioner*, **205**, 683–686.
Hodes, C. (1973) Enuresis – a study in general practice. *Journal of the Royal College of General Practitioners*, **23**, 520–524.
Horn, M.E.C. (1975) The asthma and bronchitis clinic for children in general practice. *Update*, **10**, 759–767.
Horn, M.E.C. & Gregg, I. (1973). The role of viral infection and host factors in asthma and chronic bronchitis. *Chest*, **63**, Supp, 4, 44.
Horn, M.E.C., Brain, A.E. & Gregg, I. et al (1979a) Respiratory viral infection in childhood. A survey in general practice. *Journal of Hygiene*, **74**, 157–168.
Horn, M.E.C., Brain, A.E. & Gregg, I. et al (1979b) Respiratory viral infection and wheezy bronchitis in childhood. *Thorax*, **34**, 23–28.
Hodgson, S.V. (1978) Early infant feeding and weight gain. *Journal of the Royal College of General Practitioners*, **28**, 280–281.
Hooper, P.D. & Alexander, E.L. (1971) Developmental assessment in general practice. *The Practitioner*, **207**, 371–376.
Howie, J.G.R. (1971) A new look at respiratory illness in general practice. *Journal of the Royal College of General Practitioners*, **23**, 895–904.
Howie, J.G.R. (1979) Research in general practice. London: Croom Helm.
Howie, J.G.R. & Hutchison, K.R. (1978) Antibiotics and respiratory illness in general practice – prescribing policy and work-load. *British Medical Journal*, **2**, 1342.
Husband, P. (1975) The child with repeated injuries – a family problem. *Journal of the Royal College of General Practitioners*, **25**, 419–423.
Ives, G (1979) Psychological treatment in general practice. *Journal of the Royal College of General Practitioners*, **29**, 343–351.
Jenkinson, D. (1978) Outbreak of Whooping Cough in General Practice. *British Medical Journal*, **2**, 577–578.
Julyan, M. & Kuzemko, J.A. (1975) Accidental poisoning in children: the sick family. *The Practitioner*, **214**, 813–815.
Millac, J (1975) Incidence of adeno-tonsilleotomy in children of women referred with gynaecological symptoms. *The Practitioner*, **215**, 220–222.
Mond, N.C., Gruneberg, R.N. & Smellie, J.M. (1970) Study of childhood urinary tract infection in general practice. *British Medical Journal*, **1**, 602–605.
McAllister, T.A. & Philip, A.E. (1975) The clinical psychologist in a health centre: one year's work. *British Medical Journal*, **4**, 513–514.
Oates, R.K. (1973) Infant feeding practices. *British Medical Journal*, **2**, 762–764.
Pereira Gray, D.J. (1970) *Transactions of the Hunterian Society*, **28**, 121–175. This essay is reproduced as Chapter 16 of the present book (p. 120).
Pollak, M. (1972). The development of three-year old children in a south London practice. *Update*, **5**, 445–452.
Pollak, M. (1979) Housing and mothering. *Archives of Disease in Childhood*, **54**, 54–58.
Pollak, M. & Mitchell, S. (1974) Early development of negro and white babies. *Archives of Disease in Childhood*, **49**, 40–45.
Porter, A.M.W (1971) Clinical research in general practice. *British Medical Journal*, **1**, 600–602.
Price, J. (1976) Otitis externa in children. *Journal of the Royal College of General Practitioners*, **26**, 610–615.
Public Health Laboratory Service (1973) Efficacy of

Whooping Cough Vaccines in the United Kingdom before 1968. Whooping Cough Committee and Working Party. *British Medical Journal*, **1**, 259–262.
Report of the Committee on Child Health Services (1977) *Fit for the Future*. CMND 6684 London: HMSO.
Report of an independent working group in Newcastle-Upon-Tyne (1977) *British Medical Journal*, **2**, 811–813.
Research Group on Asymptomatic Bacteriuria (1975) Asymptomatic bacteriuria in school children in Newcastle-upon-Tyne. *Archives of Disease in Childhood*, **50**, 90–101.
Richardson, I.M. (1975) The value of a university department of general practice. *British Medical Journal*, **4**, 740–742.
Roberts, J., Beswick, K., Leverton, B. & Lynch, M.A. (1977) Prevention of child abuse: group therapy for mothers and children. *The Practitioner*, **219**, 111–115.
Robson, J., Lurie, N. & Hart, J.T. (1979) Ten years experience in general practice of dip-slide urine culture in children under five years old. *Journal of the Royal College of General Practitioners*, **29**, 658–661.
Ross, P.W., Chisty, S.M.K. & Knox, J.D.E. (1971) Sore throat in children: its causation and incidence. *British Medical Journal*, **2**, 624–626.
Royal College of General Practitioners (1978) College Policy – the care of children. *Journal of the Royal College of General Practitioners*, **28**, 553–556.
Rowlands, P. (1975) Developmental assessment in general practice. *Update*, **10**, 379–388.
Rutter, N. & Metcalfe, D.H. (1978) Febrile convulsions – what do parents do? *British Medical Journal*, **2**, 1345–1346.
Savage, D.C.L., Wilson, M.I. & McHardy, M. et al (1973) Covert bacteriuria of childhood. *Archives of Disease in Childhood*, **48**, 8–20.
Saxena, S.R. Collis, A. & Laurance, B.M. (1975a) Prevalance of asymptomatic urinary tract infection in pre-school children. *The Practitioner*, **214**, 257–260.
Saxena, S.R., Laurance, B.M. & Shaw, D.G. (1975b) The justification for early radiological investigation of urinary tract infection in children. *Lancet*, **2**, 403–405.
Scottish Home and Health Department (1973) *Towards an integrated child health service*. Edinburgh: HMSO.
Seiler, E.R. (1972) Sleep problems in children. *The Practitioner*, **208**, 271–276.
Stansfield, J.M. (1975) Duration of treatment for urinary tract infection in children. *British Medical Journal*, **3**, 65.
Stark, G.D., Bassett, W.J. & Stewart, F.I., Bain, D.J.G. (1975) Paediatrics in Livingston New Town: evolution of a child health service. *British Medical Journal*, **4**, 387–390.
Starte, G.D. (1974) Developmental assessment of the young child in general practice. The Practitioner, **213**, 823–828.
Starte, G.D. (1975) The poor-communicating two-year-old and his family. *Journal of the Royal College of General Practitioners*, **25**, 880–887.
Starte, G.D. (1978) Influence of illness in developmental progress in children under two. *Journal of the Royal College of General Practitioners*, **28**, 273–277.
Stewart, G.T. (1977) Vaccination against whooping cough. *Lancet*, **1**, 234–237.
Stott, N.C.H. (1979) Management and outcome of upper respiratory tract infections in children aged 0–9 years. *British Medical Journal*, **1**, 29–31.
Sunderland, R. & Emery, J.L. (1979) Apparent disappearance of hypernatraemic dehydration from infant deaths in Sheffield. *British Medical Journal*, **2**, 575–576.
Taylor, B., Abbot, G.D., McKerr, M. & Fergusson, D.M. (1977) Amoxycillin and co-trimoxazole in presumed viral respiratory tract infection of childhood: placebo controlled trial. *British Medical Journal*, **2**, 552–554.
Thorogood, M., Clark, R., Harker, P. & Mann, J.I. (1979) Infant feeding and overweight in two Oxfordshire towns. *Journal of the Royal College of General Practitioners*, **29**, 427–430.
Turner, R.M. (1978) Recurrent abdominal pain in childhood. *Journal of the Royal College of General Practitioners*, **28**, 729–734.
Watson, G.I. (1972) General practitioners and medical research. *Journal of the Royal College of General Practitioners*, **22**, 789–798.
Watson, G.I., Nichols, J.A. & Robshaw, I. (1975) Revaccintation against measles – a pilot study. *Journal of the Royal College of General Practitioners*, **25**, 863–873.
Wintle, C.J., Clay, J.S. & Davis, R.H. (1972). The school medical examination in an integrated group practice. *Journal of the Royal College of General Practitioners*, **22**, 327–329.
Working Party On Ethics (1980) guidelines to aid ethical committees concerning research involving children. *British Medical Journal* **1**, 229–231.
Wright, H.J. (1973) Primary paediatric practice in industrial and rural Britain. *Journal of the Royal College of General Practitioners*, **23**, 815–820.

6

Child care and the computer

Keith Bolden

Computers have become a household word over the past few years and are rapidly making great changes in established ways of life. In no sphere have they had greater impact than in the field of medicine, and within this field child care is no exception.

The use of computers in child care is not new as immunisation programmes using computers have been in operation since the mid 1960s.

Some general practices have used manual record systems to identify their children via the age/sex index and in this way to arrange supervision of developmental surveillance and immunisation procedures. However, there is a limit to the number of activities, especially in the field of recall and cross indexing, which can be done on a manual system. For these reasons plus the rapidly advancing technology combined with a fall in costs there has been an increasing awareness over the last few years of the possible role of computers within the framework of general practice.

Before one can appreciate the possibilities of the situation it would be appropriate to pose the question 'what is a computer?'

WHAT ARE COMPUTERS?

A computer is essentially a calculating machine; information is fed in at one end and the required calculation carried out on this information. The answers are then printed out and between time the information is stored within the computer or in a separate storage device.

There is some jargon which is unfortunately inevitable in this field.

1. *Input*. This is the act of feeding information into the computer and can be done in various ways. In early computers use was made of coding and punched cards. Using this method of input facts are coded by punching a card in the appropriate places and the card then inserted into a machine called a *card reader*. This converts the holes into electrical impulses which are in turn accepted by the computer. This way of entering data is called batch processing because the cards can be collected together and fed in as a batch.

Most modern computers use an ordinary typewriter keyboard in direct communication with the computer so that the information is just typed in.

2. *Memory*. The information is stored within the computer in that area devoted to memory. If there is a lot of information to be stored it may be held separately as *external or additional* memory and only fed into the machine when calculations are being carried out. This external memory may be in the form of cassettes, tapes or discs.

3. *Processor*. The calculations carried out on the stored information are performed by the processor. There may be a number of different calculations which have to be carried out and each calculation is presented as a set of instructions called a *programme*.

Individual programmes may also be held on cassettes, tape or disc and fed into the machine when required. Programmes are called *software* and the computer and other machinery is known as the *hardware*.

4. *Output*. The answers to the various calculations are presented on a small television screen, on tapes or as printed material on paper.

Computers come in all shapes and sizes:

A *mainframe computer* is vast with almost unlimited storage capacity, requires a building to itself and is highly expensive to set up and run. It is only suitable for very large businesses or a region such as a health authority or for national projects.

A *mini computer* is smaller, will easily fit into one small room, and has a moderate degree of storage capacity.

A *micro computer* is the smallest, cheapest version and the one that is most likely to be readily accessible to all general practitioners in the near future. It looks like a television with a typewriter keyboard.

Nevertheless all these types of computer have the same basic principles and their differences are really related only to the quantity of information which can be stored and processed. Equally they all need a way of presenting their processed data and this invariably requires a printer.

CONFIDENTIALITY

One of the main problems of storing vast quantities of information about individuals is the difficulty of preserving the confidentiality of the material for the individual concerned. The Exeter Computer Project has been developing a combined hospital/GP computerised record system for over ten years and has been most concerned to preserve this confidentiality. In the project all information e.g. name and address, marital status, social history, medical history and current history is protected by built in safeguards such as user access with passcodes and strict ethical standards about the handling of records and the release of data.

It was on just this issue of confidentiality that the National Child Health Computer System foundered. Attempts by the National Child Health Computing Committee to introduce pilot trials in various regions were abandoned when they failed to meet adequate safeguards agreed within the profession. The problem is that any individual questions may look innocuous and it is only when they are stored and collated with data about a patient collected from other sources that features and conclusions about the patient or his parents can be drawn which are a breach of confidentiality.

Examples of questions on the child health computer form to which doctors objected are:

1. Has this examination revealed any delay or defect not previously identified by anyone?
2. Did the previous examination result in any action which benefited the child?
3. Has any diagnosable condition previously been missed that could have been to the detriment of the child?

The Health Visitors Association also objected strongly to the last question and it has now been dropped. There have also been occasions in various regions where information about children has gone directly on to computer without the permission of either parents or the general practitioner of the child concerned. In some cases information was taken directly off letters from consultants to general practitioners.

In 1978 as a result of increasing disquiet the Child Health Computing Committee took heed of the advice of the BMA ethical committee and agreed that its system would be based on the following principles:

1. Identifiable information should be regarded as held for the specific purpose of the continuing care of the patient and should not be used without appropriate authorisation or the consent of the patient, or guardian in the case of a child, for any other purpose.

2. Access to identifiable information should be confined to those persons clinically responsible for the patient during the episode from which the data has been collected (or their successors) for the purpose for which it was supplied. The author has the discretion to release the information in the best interests of the patient.

3. An individual should not be identifiable from data supplied for statistical or research purposes except when follow-up of the individual patient is a necessary part of the research.

For those not clear about the function of the Child Health Computing Committee it was set up in 1977 to consider proposals for the development of a computer based child health system for England and Wales, and to advise the centre responsible for the development accordingly.

The committee comprises members representing all National Health Service regions, the General Medical Services Council, British Paediatric Association, Royal College of Obstetricians and Gynaecologists, The Department of Health and Social Security as well as observers from Scotland and Northern Ireland.

To date very little progress has been made on the original proposals of the Child Health Computer System and it might be more profitable to look at the ways in which the computer might help the progress of child care when operated from within the practice.

A COMPUTER IN THE PRACTICE

Until recently the idea of the general practitioner having his own computer would have appeared ludicrous. However there have been some rapid developments in this area which make this situation almost a certainty during the decade of the eighties.

As already mentioned hardware is dropping rapidly in price as a result of the so called silicon chip revolution and within a very short time now (say three to five years) the cost of using a computer will be well within the means of the average practice.

Already (1980) systems are being advertised for less than £1000 but enthusiastic general practitioners must beware of rushing too quickly into this arena which is fraught with commercial pitfalls. For example, although systems are advertised for less then £1000 these advertisements take care not to mention that even at the simplest level of usage a printer will be required, which will double the cost of the equipment. In any case the programmes and equipment at this level of cost are still most unsatisfactory for all but the most simple tasks and at present a satisfactory system producing useful information from various recall methods would cost between £10 000 and £20 000 for a four man practice.

The Exeter Computer Project was started in the late 1960s and the original concept was to integrate a computerised record system between hospital and general practice. At this time the only possible system available was the large main frame computer and over the past ten years the development of the general practice aspects of the project have resulted in an approximate cost per patient of £1.70 if the capital costs were being written off over seven years and about 80p if capital costs are ignored. These costs are per patient per year and take into account full maintenance and running costs.

However, the Exeter Project also supported a computerised record system for the consultation and this is certainly the most expensive part of the system and at the present time probably the least valuable because technology has not yet advanced sufficiently to enable information to be entered easily at the time of the consultation. A modified version of the project omitting the recording of the consultation would cost much less than that stated here and indeed the project is moving into a new phase in which micro computers will be used in the practices rather than the cumbersome and expensive main frame computer.

The purpose of this discussion has been to emphasise that while computers are still expensive they are not prohibitively so and prices will continue to fall dramatically. In addition negotiations are going on between the GMSC and DHSS to explore other ways in which some costs may be defrayed.

The Royal College of General Practitioners formed a working party to consider the question of the place of computers in practice two years ago, and if has produced (1980) a comprehensive document suggesting guidelines to any general practitioner contemplating entering this field. In their interim report the working party produced a series of questions which general practitioners should ask themselves if they are contemplating having a computer. This report will undoubtedly be of great value to prospective users for several years during the difficult times when commercialisation, conflicting needs and abortive experiments add to the confusion of this exciting development.

HOW WILL THE COMPUTER HELP CHILD HEALTH?

Having discussed the very real possibility of general practitioners having their own computer it is now time to examine the ways in which it may be used in the practice.

The computer is capable of storing, comparing and reproducing data in an infinite variety of ways but the data produced is only as reliable as the data inserted and this, therefore, places a great responsibility upon those who input the data in the first place.

Within the field of child health two examples of areas where computer facilities are of particular value are in immunisation and in identifying at risk categories such as handicap and both these will be discussed in detail.

Immunisation

Keeping track of all the immunisation procedures which each child requires and making sure that they are done at the appropriate time has been a major problem for general practitioners ever since regular preventive procedures were started.

In the 1960s a number of local authorities started to collate the data required on computer and since then it has become common place for children to be called for immunisation in the first five years of life using local authority computer systems.

However, within the practice this could be extended to all immunisation procedures by using a practice computer.

Putting all patients records on to computer automatically provides an age/sex register within the practice. From this patients can easily be identified at the appropriate age for routine triple and booster immunisation, rubella, or, indeed, any other prophylactive procedure, at any age rather than specifically for the under fives.

The computer can print out a list of, for example, all the girls in the practice aged eleven years so that they can be called for their rubella immunisation. Not only will the computer print out the list, but also print out sticky labels with the patients' name and address to be fixed on a pre-typed recall card which is sent to the patient.

Attendances for rubella immunisation will be recorded as the girls get their injection and then those defaulting can easily be identified and chased up using the practice health visitor or school medical services.

The great advantage of using a practice based computer for this type of activity is that the numbers of patients involved are relatively small (say several hundred in any one year) and, therefore, the risk of patients being overlooked is slight. Indeed there is no risk of omission at all provided the data – in this case the date of birth, and whether the patient has had a rubella immunisation – have been entered correctly. This emphasises again what was stated earlier, namely that the data produced is only as reliable as the data inserted. In addition to the reliability of the information within the practice system there is plenty of evidence that patients are more likely to attend their general practitioner for routine procedures than go to a local authority or school clinic.

Those general practitioners who are financially orientated will have realised by now that a great deal of extra income can be made by tightening up on items of service charges within the practice and using the computer will help to formalise and improve the efficiency of what were previously almost random prophylactic procedures. Some of the cost of the computer system can be offset by extra practice income earned in this way.

It is probable that the general immune status of the population would improve considerably if general practitioners had the facilities to operate efficient supervisory and recall systems within their practice for all routine prophylactic immunisations.

At risk groups

If sensitive data such as adverse birth factors, possible battering or a family history of mental subnormality is to be entered on a computer then it is immediately apparent why this system has to be secure and confidential with data being totally under the control of the general practitioner. However, having this type of information available to him will enable him to compile a list of children who have adverse physical or social factors in their history. There is then no problem from time to time in printing out a list of, say, the under fives who have been queried as possibly belonging to a 'battering' family, or children between the ages of five and ten who have been noted to have had reduced hearing at a routine audiometry check.

These lists can then be used within the practice by the team to follow up the children concerned at intervals considered appropriate.

The potential of this type of approach is unlimited. For example, if a drug has been taken by a pregnant mother during the past x years (depending on how far back efficient recording goes), this can be identified immediately. Her children can likewise be identified and checked for the suspected abnormality.

As can be seen, if computerised systems were widely adopted the problem would not be 'what shall we do with the computer?' but 'where do we stop?'

CONCLUSION

This chapter has tried very briefly to introduce what to many general practitioners may seem an irrelevant topic.

However general practice, along with all other branches of medicine, has to move with the times and the future lies with computers where record systems are concerned.

It is hoped that the reader now has a clearer idea of what a computerised system has to offer him, particularly in the field of child health. Equally important is the realisation of all the possible pitfalls and particularly the enormous risk to our patients if the ethics of strict confidentiality are not observed.

REFERENCES

Bolden, K.J. (1976) Developmental assessment: luxury or necessity? *Proceedings of the Royal Society of Medicine*, **69**, 385–6.

DHSS Statement (1978) *Child Health Computing System*, 78/135. London: DHSS.

RCGP (1980) Computers in primary care. *Journal of the Royal College of General Practitioners*, Occasional Paper no. 13.

7

The practice health visitor

Eugenie Alexander

Health visiting has its origins in the Ladies Sanitary Reform Association of 1861. Florence Nightingale also saw the need of such a service, and helped to develop it in Buckinghamshire in 1891, since when it has been continuously changing and enlarging its scope.

The Council for the Education and Training of Health Visitors (1973) lists five main aspects in its description of the health visitor's work:

1. The prevention of mental, physical and emotional ill health.
2. Early detection of ill health and the surveillance of high risk groups.
3. Recognition and identification of need and mobilisation of the appropriate resources when necessary.
4. Health teaching.
5. Provision of care; this will include support during periods of stress, and advice and guidance in cases of illness as well as in the management of children.

An investigation into the principles of health visiting by the Council for the Education and Training of Health Visitors (1977) formulated the following four main principles:

1. The search for health needs.
2. The stimulation of the awareness of health needs.
3. The influence on policies affecting health.
4. The facilitation of health-enhancing activities.

The health visitor needs to ensure that the general practitioner has an understanding of the above in order that he may fully appreciate her function and make proper use of her as a team member.

The health visitor is a State Registered Nurse who has had midwifery experience, before commencing her health visitor training. The Briggs Report will, when implemented, make alterations in the nurse education programme, but at present the course is of one academic year at a university or polytechnic during which health visiting, social administration, psychology, sociology, health education, child development, medicine, human behaviour, psychiatry, geriatrics and social services are among the subjects studied.

In the first nine months, two thirds of the time is spent on theory and one third on practical experience. Much of the practical experience is spent in an area where the student is attached to a field work teacher who may be working with a practice. Here the student sees health visiting procedures and has the opportunity to practise and develop her skills by doing accompanied and unaccompanied visits; she learns the importance of record keeping and report writing. During this period she visits and studies in depth six families, usually including one primipara, one larger family, one family with a problem, possibly a handicapped child, and an elderly or handicapped person. Case histories on three of these she selects to present as part of her final examination, as well as a project and neighbourhood study.

After the written examination comes a three month supervised period with a case load of 100 families for whom she is responsible. This assessment period is followed by an oral examination and determines finally if she is awarded her certificate.

ATTACHMENT

The relationship between general practitioners and health visitors was poor for many years, but the 1960s and 70s have seen a great increase in attachment schemes. The Department of Health and Social Security (1973) figure was 79 per cent. This closer co-operation appears to have improved the understanding of each other's role, functions and limitations.

The use of the same premises is an advantage. The closer the proximity the better the opportunity that exists for frequent and regular meetings for discussion of cases, policy, and exchange of information between all members of staff. Such meetings are essential if attachment is to be of real benefit. The use of the same premises by the primary health care team also demonstrates to the families a more unified service than was once the case.

The traditional division between the GP's curative and the HV's preventive role has become less significant as general practitioners become more interested in preventive medicine and endeavour to find time to give to this matter.

The successful development of attachment depends a great deal on the goodwill and tolerance of both the GP and the HV in the early stages, but once initiated should bring a better service to the families by providing a more cohesive form of care, with both seeking to reinforce the advice and providing better follow-up care. It is up to the HV to demonstrate the areas in which she in particular may be of best use.

It is unfortunate that in some cases neither the GP nor the HV have the opportunity to partake in the decision about placement of the HV in a particular primary care team; sometimes attachments have been jeopardised by mutual incompatibility, or a reluctance to change the status quo.

Two disadvantages to attachment of the HV are sometimes quoted: (a) the larger geographical area to be covered, and (b) the fact that in the past the HV knew that all families in her area were under her care. With attachment this is not so, and co-operation with the practice secretarial staff is necessary to ensure that families transferring in are brought to her notice. The success of attachment can depend greatly upon the attitude of the secretarial and reception staff. Information about new patients, access to records, the age/sex register, hospital letters, admission information and clinic bookings can be of great assistance, as can willingness to type letters or reports.

The desirability of attachment to group practices and geographical allocation of health visitors was again raised in the Court report (1976). One's opinion in regard to this must depend upon the success of the schemes one has known. A successful attachment brings to the family far more advantages than a geographical allocation.

From the HV's point of view, attachment has increased her work load by increasing its scope and, if there is good communication, by making her aware of situations which have arisen earlier than might otherwise have been possible. It would be fallacious to imagine that attachment is a means of saving the GP's time. In some respects this may be so, but in her case-finding capacity the HV is equally likely to bring to the GP's notice situations of which he was previously unaware.

The HV has a responsibility to all age groups, but it is still the case that by far the largest proportion of her time is given to families with young children. Clark found in her study of health visiting in Berkshire that 70.6 per cent of visits were made to families where there were young children (Clark, 1973).

The HV has no right of entry to a home. She has a statutory duty to visit children from 0–5 years, but cannot insist upon entry. The fact that she has been unable to gain access would be reported to the nursing officer. If concern was felt about the family a discussion about the case with the GP, Social Services Department or NSPCC inspector would be appropriate. Fortunately this is not a common occurrence, but it underlines the importance of the HV developing a good relationship with 'her' families.

THE ANTENATAL PERIOD

Paediatric care for the HV should start in the antenatal clinic, where, particularly in the case of a primigravida, a relationship can be developed. The expectant mother can there see the GP, midwife and HV as a team, interested in her and her baby from the beginning. The HV is able to introduce herself and explain her future role. The mother can be invited to attend the parentcraft and relaxation classes, and the opportunity can be taken to enquire in a friendly way into the domestic arrangements postnatally, whether she hopes to breast feed, her previous experience and her anticipation of the coming event. Knowledge of the family background and circumstances may be important in helping to determine families where extra support may be required.

Early contact with unmarried mothers is very valuable, as they often need assistance and support, and may need advice about help which is available from social services or other agencies.

Parentcraft and relaxation classes are held in most areas; they vary somewhat from place to place. The relaxation exercises may be given by physiotherapist, midwife or HV and the mothercraft shared between midwife and HV. The subjects usually include breast feeding, preparation and sterilisation techniques for bottle feeding, nappy changing (particularly important since the advent of prepacked, sterilised, disposable bottles and disposable nappies in hospitals), mechanics of labour, the types of analgesia available, home safety, infant development, speech development, diet, care of teeth and the special dangers of smoking during pregnancy. If possible a film of a delivery is shown; the fathers may be invited in an attempt to involve them from the beginning. The first few weeks of the postnatal period, and common difficulties which may arise, are discussed. Many young mothers expect their babies to be always contented, and feel very anxious and sometimes guilty if they are not. The simple caring routines which we tend to take for granted may be a source of great anxiety to the mother, and interfere with the development of a good mother – baby relationship.

If a visit to the maternity unit can be arranged, to see the wards and nurseries and meet some of the staff, this may serve to allay some of the natural fears present at this time.

After the mothers have attended the class for a while,

they begin to gain the confidence to discuss their fears within the group. They may also develop friendships which can be supportive in an often stressful period after the baby is born.

THE NEONATAL PERIOD

The primary visit to a new baby, especially a first child, is probably the most important home visit the HV makes. It is at this time the mother is most receptive, and the relationship between the mother and HV can be developed to serve its purpose in the ensuing years. The HV can observe the degree of bonding, the interrelationship of the parents, baby and any other siblings, the quality of care, attitudes and standards without asking more than essential questions. The mother needs to feel that the HV is as interested in her as in her baby, and that she has someone available to answer her queries later. Mothers often ring up to ask for advice about what may be a minor ailment which they do not feel justifies calling their doctor.

Most young mothers will happily wake the baby to be examined and weighed if necessary, as they like to be reassured about weight and the umbilicus. This gives the opportunity to see the baby unclothed and look for abnormalities, but there are times when it is better to arrange to call again at a feeding time, or have the baby brought down to the surgery for an examination possibly by the GP, rather than waken a baby who has just fallen asleep after a long disturbed period.

Practical advice can be given about both mother and child. If she is breast feeding, she may need encouragement to continue, and information on care of breasts, rest and diet; if the baby is artifically fed, advice may be needed on the strength, quantity and frequency suitable for the baby. The presence of normal stools can be ascertained. The dangers of prop feeding, pillows and hypothermia are still insufficiently recognised and these matters could be mentioned. The mother's emotional state needs to be assessed, the necessity of a postnatal examination emphasised and family planning discussed. Information is given about the HV's availability and clinics. It is not helpful to give too much information at once.

Subsequent visits may then be arranged. Some mothers, particularly anxious, inexperienced ones, may need frequent visits, especially if breast feeding for the first time or if feeding difficulties arise, when a visit to watch the baby fed may be useful to observe feeding techniques or if artifically fed, to watch the feed being mixed, as the problem may be due to inaccurate mixing.

It is very important to give advice in a manner which does not undermine the mother's confidence in her own ability.

THE FIRST YEAR OF LIFE

During the first year visits should be at least monthly, or a visit to the clinic may suffice. However, the most useful contacts are usually in the home, where the mother is aware that she is the only one demanding attention, and may feel more free to express herself with the support of her own surroundings.

It is important during the early weeks to select the families who will need extra support. Those who are happy and coping well do not need much visiting, but unless they are seen occasionally one is unaware of changes in circumstances and may have lost the opportunity of building up a relationship which may be of use should a stress situation occur.

The topics discussed in the first year are mainly feeding, general care, the mother's physical and emotional condition, development, immunisation, home safety, care of teeth, other aspects of health education, play and the importance of the mother communicating both verbally and physically with her child. Many other topics may arise, sometimes relating to an older child in the family. These matters are discussed in a manner to suit that particular family.

A Guthrie test is performed by the midwife in the first few days and a hearing test between the ages of six and nine months.

INFANT FEEDING

This usually arouses the most anxiety in the early stages. Health education continues from the mothercraft classes onwards about the undesirability of obese children. Mothers do appear to be more accepting of this advice recently, probably largely due to the increasing publicity which has been given to this subject.

Mothers often appear to desire to start mixed feeding from about two weeks. Four months may be the best time for the introduction of solids (DHSS, 1974) but it is frequently hard to delay it for as long as three months! One cannot be too uncompromising; some babies do appear to require some additional food earlier than others, and it is better to have a contented mother and baby than to adhere rigidly to a principle. A few years ago it became fashionable to banish scales from child health clinics, but it is easier to weigh a baby monthly, and check an excessive gain, than wait until it is an obvious 'Michelin Man' and start a stringent slimming campaign. If caught early all that is required is to cut the calories by weakening the milk slightly and cutting down on unnecessary cereals and sugar. If the baby is fed on prepared baby foods it is more difficult to control the diet; it is also cheaper if the mother can prepare her own food for the baby by the use of a liquidiser, mouli or sieve. The convenience of prepared foods should not be undervalued, however, especially at first when only a small amount is needed.

The HV is in a strong position to encourage breast feeding. We have not been too successful in recent years –71 per cent initially, but only 18 per cent continuing to six months (Hide and Guyer, 1980). It may be that the increasing cost of living will do much to promote an increase. A higher rate could reduce the incidence of allergic manifestations in infancy. Vitamin drops need to be started at about one month, and these can be bought cheaply at the Health Authority clinics. Although one may feel strongly that it better to breast feed, if a mother or father finds it distasteful it is unwise to persist, but one can encourage the uncommitted and help those who wish to succeed.

Weaning a breast fed baby at about six months is another period where a young mother often needs support.

CHILD HEALTH CLINICS

These provide an opportunity for the mother to bring her child along to check its progress and seek advice if she wishes. The HV can take the opportunity to assess if a home visit is required. Mothers, especially those with their first babies, use these facilities frequently, particularly in the first year. It gives them a chance to meet other young mothers, discuss mutual problems and thus reduce the feeling of isolation which sometimes occurs when a previously working woman suddenly finds herself housebound. A mother and baby group, if this can be arranged, often proves very supportive in the post-natal period.

Where the clinic is held in the surgery, with immunisation and developmental screening as part of the routine, the mother feels that her doctor is not just interested in her child when ill, he has the opportunity to know the family better, and decisions about treatment can be implemented directly (Jones, 1975).

A policy regarding the immunisation programme and developmental screening must be arranged between the GP and HV in order that a suitable programme can be implemented and follow-up ensured where necessary. A register of immunisations needs to be kept and defaulters encouraged to attend.

THE TODDLER

The HV continues to visit the child until he starts school; there is observation and discussion of development, toilet training, diet, management, play, speech and behaviour. Mothers may be anxious about what are normal behaviour, speech and development patterns for a child of that age and need to talk about their anxiety. Advice can be given regarding the prevention and handling of behaviour problems especially when a new baby is expected, or if a domestic crisis occurs. It is very useful if the GP makes the HV aware of illness in the family which might reflect upon the child, so that she may visit and counsel where necessary.

Physical observations are made and the mother advised to see her doctor if, for instance, anaemia, squints or urinary infections are suspected. The child may need referral for child guidance advice, audiology, speech therapy, or the educational psychologist's assessment. The GP and HV should be kept informed of action to be taken, and personal contact with other departments is helpful.

HANDICAPPED CHILDREN

A family with a handicapped child requires more frequent visits to give support and advice about the appropriate care and available facilities. Information and encouragement to use toy libraries and associations such as the Spastic Society and Spina Bifida Association should be given. In some cases holiday arrangements can be made to enable the family to have a rest.

Interpretation may be needed regarding decisions made at a hospital appointment as many mothers are diffident about questioning the consultant or they may think up questions later which need an answer. Some hospitals have a HV at the paediatric clinic who informs her colleagues of decisions made, and this enables them to reinforce the advice given and report back if required. At the age of two years it is necessary to check that the parents have applied for an attendance allowance if eligible; the question of education may also arise.

PREMATURE BABIES

It may be necessary to visit the home of a premature baby before discharge, either to assess home conditions or to discuss the situation with the mother. It has been found that one group of children subject to non-accidental injury are those who have for some reason been separated from their parents in the early months. Thus the above groups are worthy of special attention to develop a good relationship. The mother may need encouragement to keep outpatient appointments and to continue the vitamin and iron supplements which have been prescribed.

THE SCHOOL CHILD

In some areas the HV is also the school nurse, but the pattern is changing and separate school nurses are now appointed in many places. However, it is still necessary for the HV to maintain contact with the local schools, as the staff can co-operate in discussion about a child who may have problems at home or at school. The HV has no statutory duty to visit children over the age of five, but mothers who have known her in the past will sometimes ask her advice, or the GP may refer a child. The problem may or may not fall within the HV's province, but often a visit to the school helps to clarify the situation and determine whether she, or for instance the school welfare officer, should continue with the matter. The mother then knows to whom she should turn with her problem.

In cases of scabies, head lice, and impetigo, especially close co-operation of the GP, school nurse, teacher, and HV is essential if an outbreak is to be contained and cleared as speedily as possible.

SELECTION OF VISITS

The HV must select her priorities herself, by her knowledge of the families and of her role. Many families who have psychological and social problems demand extra visiting; with attachment it is easier for the HV and GP to keep each other informed of current developments. The father and/or mother may be of low mental capacity, but may cope fairly adequately, provided encouragement and support are readily available. It is for this sort of family that frequent reiteration of advice may be needed, and often readily accepted. Mothers who are chronically over-anxious require more support to build up their self confidence.

Unfortunately, some families within these groups are either unwilling or unable to put into practice simple child care or home safety, and all one can do is to try to maintain a working relationship, in the hope of eventually promoting an improvement.

LIAISON

Liaison and referrals are an important facet of the work of the HV. It may be necessary, especially if ill treatment or neglect is suspected, to refer a family to the Social Services Department. In this event it is important for the social worker, GP and HV to work together. This should be facilitated if there is social worker attachment. The HV needs to continue visiting the family as well as the social worker, as the latter generally visits for a more limited period, and it would be unwise for the HV to lose the continuity of her work. With close liaison it should be possible to prevent the danger of conflicting advice, and arrange for visits to be spaced out to allow for better observation of the situation.

Hospitals frequently contact HVs about missed appointments and it is often possible if she visits and explains the necessity, to persuade the mother to keep subsequent appointments. It may be necessary for her to take the mother and child to the hospital or arrange care for other children in the family. If a journey to a hospital outside the area is necessary, the HV can arrange travel vouchers for the children and one accompanying adult. Red Cross escort can be arranged where this is required.

In some areas the HV is supplied with information on all child casualties by the hospitals in the district. This is a useful way of ensuring that non-accidental injuries are noted and the HV and GP can use their knowledge of the family to decide what follow-up care is advisable, or where home safety guidance is needed.

The HV is also in contact with the environmental health officer, housing department and probation department where this is necessary for the wellbeing of the family. Liaison is also maintained with the play groups and nurseries in her area, although the Social Services departments now have responsibility for these. Much useful information can be gathered from such visits. The nursery matrons and play group organisers have an excellent opportunity to observe the behaviour of a child away from the family, and with its peers. It is useful if one is concerned about the behaviour or development of a child to see him in these surroundings, and it may help to give a better overall picture.

It is essential that close liaison be maintained between the members of the primary health care team. The GP, midwife, district nurse and health visitor all have a part to play in child care in general practice.

HEALTH EDUCATION

Health education is a continuing part of the HV's work from the antenatal period onwards. This may be in a one to one situation as in the home visit, or in a small group as when a subject arises in the baby clinic, or more formally as in the mothercraft and relaxation classes or organisations. Health education is given in the schools by arrangement with the teaching staff. This may be for any age group from the primary school to the technical college, and provides an important opportunity to promote better health at a receptive age.

CONCLUSION

The problems arising in the course of work may vary from area to area but the basic objectives remain the same: the promotion of physical, mental and emotional health by the recognition of need and the provision or mobilisation of such advice, support and health education as may be necessary to achieve these ends.

The HV cannot be an expert in every field. She needs to know when and to whom she should refer those who are beyond her terms of reference.

REFERENCES

Clark, J. (1973) *A family Visitor*. Royal College of Nursing.
Council for the Education and Training of Health Visitors (1977) *An Investigation into the Principles of Health Visiting*.
DHSS (1973) *The Health Visitor. Functions and Implications for Training* Annual Report, Department of Health and Social Security. London: HMSO.
DHSS (1974) *Present Day Practice in Infant Feeding*.London: HMSO.
Hide & Guyer (1980) *Archives of Disease in Childhood*.
Jones, M. (1975) Paediatric liaison and the general practice team. *Update*, **11**, 25–31.

8

The social services and the practice

Yvonne Horsfall Turner

The provision of good child care is one of the many functions to be fulfilled by the primary health care team, for the babies of today are the adults of tomorrow and the investment in their physical and emotional well-being will pay dividends for future generations.

'Taking care of their children, seeing them grow and develop into fine people, gives most parents – despite the hard work – their greatest satisfaction in life' (Dr B. Spock). Yet there is little preparation of young couples for their roles as parents. They come to parenthood with little experience of their own, having been brought up in small nuclear family settings with little opportunity to experience how their own or other parents go about raising small brothers and sisters.

Parents need help in providing good child care and it is to the primary health care team that they often come for guidance. On its part the team will seek out those who may need guidance yet who, for whatever reason, are unable to ask for help. For such guidance to be effective there must be cooperation between team members and an understanding of child care practice and each individual's role in promoting child care. It is the intention of this chapter to discuss the team, its role in relation to child care with emphasis on the social work involvement, and how the service can best be delivered to the consumer with full cooperation between team members.

THE TEAM

The primary health care team usually comprises GPs, district nurses, health visitors and, under ideal circumstances, social workers. It is important to acknowledge each individual member's unique training and expertise, including any overlap within their professional knowledge. An understanding of each other's role and skill is vitally important so that appropriate referrals can be made. The view that some doctors express, 'the health visitor is my social worker', is not acceptable and health visitors should not collude with doctors in being put into the social work role.

The report of the Committee on Local Authority and Allied Personal Social Services (1968) acknowledged the importance of team work amongst general practitioners and recommended that 'as soon as doctors in a health centre or sizeable group practice feel that they want a worker of the social services department to be attached to them to become a member of their team, the department should do all they can to meet their request'. More easily said than done, for eight years later, a survey showed that only one half of the local authorities in Britain had some formal link with group practice (Gilchrist et al, 1978). This involved only 220 social workers. Two thirds of them described their work in the setting of group practice as a rewarding professional experience. The mean time they spent in group practice work was just under five hours per week, and in only 12 schemes throughout the country were social workers working solely in group practice. In 99 schemes social workers were working part-time in general practice, with their main work elsewhere; and in 82 schemes, social workers were involved in liaison work only. This gives some indication of the size of the problem, with very few practices having formalised links with social workers, in spite of the advantages having been well documented (Goldberg and Neill, 1972; Ratoff, 1973), and in spite of it being shown that the use made of the social services by the GP improves as the result of attachment of a social worker.

THE ROLE OF THE PRIMARY HEALTH CARE TEAM

The primary care team has a vital role to play in identifying those children and their families in whom for medical, social or economic reasons the wellbeing of the family unit is threatened or there is concern that the proper development of a child in all aspects is adversely affected. Each member should be aware that social and economic problems frequently manifest themselves in physical symptoms or lead to varying degrees of ill health, both in children and their parents, which can result in the eventual breakdown of the family unit if appropriate help is not given. So often one hears of the single parent who has 'had enough', who can no longer cope with the demands of a growing family, coupled with financial difficulties, and who turns to her GP for 'something to help me sleep'. The degree of care the depressed parent can give must affect the family and it is often in circumstances like these that the child resorts to petty theft in order to help his mother, and their relationship with the social services begins.

Although the GP may be the first person that the patient will go to see, and who will learn of the family difficulties at a consultation, often masked with the 'respectability' of a stomach ache or headache, the other members of the team through routine visiting of families often pick up the signs and symptoms of stress and can then refer appropriately. For instance, referral by the health visitor to the social worker of a young unmarried mother with depression revealed that the mother was in fact lesbian, and in trying to conform she had taken a lover, fallen pregnant, then realised she could not marry and was living with her girlfriend. The health visitor had visited routinely as the patient had newly registered with the practice; she had referred her to the social worker because she felt she was not getting 'through' to the patient, and the social worker's revelation that the patient was lesbian helped to increase the health visitor's understanding of the mother's needs. After a few counselling sessions with the social worker there was no need for continued contact with the social services and subsequent contact was with the health visitor on routine child care and development matters.

Different members of the team will have different interests and different skills, resulting from their training and experience. Their concern for the wellbeing of the child in the family applies not only to those who are disadvantaged because of social/economic reasons, but also to those who are disadvantaged through handicap, both physical and mental. One must also be aware that the handicapped child's siblings could equally be at risk as prime attention is given to the handicapped child to the exclusion of the siblings.

Who are at risk, and what are the main reasons for children coming into care?

The National Children's Bureau study *Born to Fail* showed that only 64 per cent of children in the study could be described as having 'ordinary family backgrounds'. The others were members of families in whom, for reasons such as low income, poor housing or an absent parent, there was disharmony or stress in their physical environment. These figures only took into account poverty in the physical environment and did not include children who were disadvantaged physically, educationally or emotionally. In every local authority the number of children in care is small compared with the number still in the community who lack an 'ordinary' stable background and have special problems to face. Children who could be deemed to be at risk include those for whom any of the following circumstances apply:

1. material standards in the home are poor
2. one or both parents are of low intelligence
3. one or both parents suffer from chronic ill health
4. the parent is single-handed through separation or bereavement, or is unmarried
5. there is marital disharmony
6. there is lack of understanding between parent and child
7. the child is unwanted or unplanned
8. the parents themselves have had an unhappy childhood and are as a result unable to adjust positively to parenthood themselves.

Such parents perpetuate their own experiences with their own children – in their desperate search for love they abuse their child when their needs fail to be satisfied.

Although some people who have had a poor mothering experience may learn from this and make a determined effort not to let their own children suffer as they did, they often do not have the degree of maturity or insight to mould their parenting into a better kind of experience for their child – they have often been in care themselves and carry a chip on their shoulder, for 'once a child has lost his own home he is in danger of feeling a lodger in the world all his life' (Stroud, 1973).

In 1977 in England and Wales 101 000 children were in local authority care – many of whom will be 'lodgers' in the world for the rest of their lives. The handing down of behaviour from one generation to the next has been called 'intergenerational continuity' and the primary health care team must have a vested interest to break this cycle down and this can best be achieved by identifying those who are potentially at risk and by giving them necessary support.

Ways of ensuring good child care

Child care starts in the womb and ante-natal care is the forerunner of good child care later on. The health visitor, through ante-natal classes, is able to get to know the 'parents to be' prior to the baby's arrival and early contact may highlight potential areas of worry which she can relieve at an early stage. The health visitor will be able to keep a special eye on those expectant mothers who she feels may have difficulties in adjusting to motherhood. Some women feel ambivalent about their pregnancy and may refuse to attend ante-natal classes – a form of 'denying' the fact they are pregnant. Young unmarried mothers may refuse to attend because of embarrassment about their condition or because they are working and they cannot afford to take time off.

Fortunately the more enlightened employers are sympathetic to the needs of their pregnant workers, allowing them time off to attend classes. It has been shown that workers receiving full ante-natal care are less likely to have days off during pregnancy than those who don't, for they take greater care of themselves and thereby keep in better health during pregnancy.

Ante-natal classes for the mother who is pregnant for the second or subsequent time are just as important and everything should be done to encourage her attendance through the provision of creche facilities for her children or provision of a baby-sitting service. Here is an area where health visitor and social worker can cooperate, for the latter may know of a willing volunteer or elderly person who is only too eager to be a substitute granny.

The health visitor is able to visit the home prior to the birth of the baby and establish relationships with the parents through fathers' evenings. Frank discussion at the ante-natal classes of the impact of the new addition to the family – in physical and emotional terms – should be common sense based, enabling positive and negative feelings to be expressed. So often parents have expectations of parenthood that are quite unrealistic, resulting in disappointments and frustrations after the birth, and this can be a factor in the battered baby syndrome.

Prematurity can also affect the bonding between mother and child and mothers of premature babies will need extra support and help. Often they have to leave the baby in hospital to look after the other members in the family and it is not always easy for them to organise visiting times to the baby. This may create tension and anger at times in the hospital staff; and mothers may take longer in bonding with their child. Cooperation between the health visitor and social worker in discussing availability of resources can do much to help and support a mother at such a time.

The child care task for the social worker and her role in the team

Most social workers in general practice are employed by local authority social service departments and consequently their work brief is wider than the traditional concept of providing support and guidance to people in need. The social worker has certain specific obligations to fulfil in relation to children which derive from the powers and duties imposed on local authorities through statutory legislation. There are three main elements in the many legal enactments relating to children, namely:

1. Prevention
2. Protection
3. Care

In order to fulfil their duties in these areas, social services departments, to a greater or lesser degree, provide practical resources such as day nurseries, children's homes, intermediate treatment centres and a counselling and advisory service from social workers.

In the majority of cases the main emphasis in child care work is on the preventive elements. This means not just the prevention of children coming into local authority care but the 'positive promotion of the welfare of children by meeting their social needs . . . so that only when there is no alternative will long term care or treatment be provided' (Leeding, 1980). A social worker in the general practice setting is in a prime position to do preventive work, for many people present their problem to their GP in the first instance long before crisis point is reached. An unfortunate stigma is attached to most local authority social service departments and the referral to the attached social worker may be much more acceptable to the patient when suggested by the doctor. Nor is this an anonymous, 'I'll refer you to the social service department' (who may or may not take the case on), but the doctor can refer to a named social worker, his colleague, and often will make the introduction personally. The patient does not see this as being fobbed off but an extension of the doctor's care for him.

For their part, social workers acknowledge that the primary responsibility for welfare and upbringing of children is with the parents but the social worker can and must provide help to enable those parents who are in need to carry out their responsibilities and enrich their children's lives. The social workers main concern is to promote the child's best interests and at the same time keep within the precepts of the law. If the family does break down then protection must be afforded to the child within a substitute family. The social worker would then work towards returning the child to the care of his original family when this became possible, though recently child care experts have suggested that if family ties have proved to be too weak they should be severed in favour of adoption or long term fostering.

Such considerations of prevention, protection and care form the background to the social worker's role in relation to child care and to her involvement as a member of the primary care team. Her expertise in child care matters reflects the back-up of services provided by her local authority department. She needs also to be informed about the contribution made in the voluntary sector, where much exciting, innovating work is being carried out.

The social worker's position is not always an easy one, particularly when she is required to exercise the more authoritative aspects of her duties, such as removing a child at risk from home against the parents' wishes. At such times the involvement and cooperation of the other team members can be invaluable in ensuring the continuing care of the remaining members of the family. Too often social workers are criticized for dallying over important decision making, especially in removing a child into care or returning a child home following a period in care. The other members of the team can often provide useful information which will facilitate the decision making, and often they will provide backup to the patient once the decision is made.

A fundamental difference exists between GP and social worker in that the GP is used to making decisions quickly and he expects the social worker to do the same. This is not always appropriate as facts have to be gathered together and it may take some time before all members of the family can be interviewed and a total assessment can be made. It is important for the doctor to recognize the social worker's different method of working — a five minute consultation is not enough for her to decide whether a parent is a fit person to look after a child. Although most social workers in general practice are qualified they usually have to refer to a senior when decisions about reception into care are being made. Doctors often feel frustrated at this for they do not consult with their colleagues to the same extent – for example when deciding to admit a patient to hospital. A patient either has or has not a specific ailment and treatment is prescribed accordingly. Referral to a social worker for assessment can be equated with referral of a patient to another doctor for a series of tests for a complaint which the GP has otherwise failed to diagnose.

Although social workers may use the medical model of assessment, diagnosis and treatment, they do not usually come to a conclusion on the basis of one interview. They are as far as possible involved in attempting to help the patient define, assess, and eventually find a solution to the problems with which he is faced. This can often be a painful process as negative feelings are handled. The mother who comes in desperation saying she will kill her child unless something is done to take him off her hands may have to come face to face with painful insights about herself and what makes her have murderous feelings towards her child. She may equally have to cope with the anger when she is not given what she has asked for, and yet in the long term she may well be thankful for having had an opportunity to work through her feelings. Ultimately she may feel that she has grown as a person as a result of the counselling she has received. However doctors are not mind readers and it is important that the GP is kept in the picture while the assessment is being made and the social worker should at the earliest possibility inform him as to what action is being taken.

The role of the social worker within the primary health care team may be enumerated as follows: she is accountable to (1) the practice/health service for the general provision of a social work service and confidentiality concerning patients' records and interests; (2) the social services district office for casework, maintenance of professional standards and implementation of departmental policy.

Her duties involve:

1. Casework of patients, including those with severe emotional and relationship problems, the physically and mentally ill and the aged and children at risk.
2. Statutory work – representing the council in court in child care and other cases as required.
3. Advice and consultation – as a member of the primary care team she contributes to the diagnosis and treatment plans, reporting direct to all team members and giving advice on the social and emotional aspects of patient care.
4. Development of service – she has a responsibility for developing social work in the practice by
   a. establishing the social worker's role
   b. demonstrating a high standard of casework practice
   c. extending the range of casework referrals
   d. contributing towards the planning of similar projects.

Instances of her other duties include an involvement in training, liaison and administration.

Achieving cooperation

Understanding comes from working together and sharing not just tasks but also ideas. Ways of doing this are:

1. By *discussion of cases* and explanation of the individual member of the team's involvement. What is the role of the team in helping a family where a young mother with two children is nursing her terminally ill husband who is suffering from a brain tumour? Should all members of the team be personally involved from the outset, or should the case be handled by one or two members with advice from the rest? The GP and district nurse may decide they can cope but without discussion involving the health visitor and social worker, aspects such as play group facilities, attendance allowance may be overlooked. While being 'strong' in the presence of the GP and district nurse the mother may need to break down with someone else and express her fears and feelings etc. Nor should any member of the team think it a sign of weakness or inadequacy on his professional part in referring to his colleague.

2. *Identification of those at risk*. Given the knowledge that certain factors within a particular family situation may be more likely to lead to breakdown than others it would be beneficial for GPs, health visitors and social workers to go through their caseloads in an attempt to identify those at risk and a decision can then be made as

to who should keep an overall eye on a particular family.

3. *Joint visiting* by different members of the team would benefit certain classes of patients at risk. In the case of a handicapped child the health visitor and social worker could visit the family at the onset of diagnosis of a handicap and explain their role. So often the social worker is introduced at a very late stage, when the affairs of the family have reached a crisis, and she is seen as the person who will 'put the child into a home'. Ideally a register should be kept of all handicapped children in the practice indicating whether they live at home, or attend residential school, and what their needs are both in the long and short term. Families need to know what resources and services are available to them and cooperation between professionals is most important in achieving the dissemination of knowledge about local facilities.

4. *Post-natal support.* Mention has been made of the need for good antenatal care. Increasingly attention is being paid to post-natal care in the form of post-natal support groups. Some people are natural parents, others need to be encouraged to interact with their child. Discussion evenings, led by the GP, and involving other team members on topical subjects such as bed wetting, temper tantrums in the toddler etc, can do much to educate the parents and to increase their confidence in their abilities as parents. Encouragement is most important and many mothers need to be told that they are doing a good job in bringing up their children, hence the importance of well-run baby clinics and regular developmental check-ups.

The use of volunteer groups can greatly help and stimulate those families who for one reason or another are disadvantaged. Time is often the most important thing one can give and yet because of high caseloads and increasing clerical duties the individual professional may not be able to give the amount of time required, for example to show a mother how to play and relate with her child. A volunteer with the necessary understanding could do this most successfully and the parent may not feel she is being undermined to the same extent or that she is taking up the professional's time.

5. *Field conferences.* So often seen by doctors as decision-deferring meetings as opposed to decision-taking ones, case conferences conjure up protracted discussions amongst professionals, often involving the upper hierarchy of the social services department who have no personal knowledge of the patient/client, and whose main function would appear to be that of holding the social worker's hand – a situation which doctors find it difficult to accept when trying to work with a professional as an equal. Such formal conferences may be necessary in situations such as non-accidental injury where one tries to pool knowledge about the family and where it is appropriate to contact agencies such as the police and the education department. However, their size often makes them unwieldly and ineffective.

It is to be hoped that the present trend of 'field' conferences, i.e. meetings involving only those actually working with the family, will render many of the more formal case conferences unnecessary. The group practice setting is an ideal place for these field conferences to be convened, often at short notice, to discuss the family situation and the team's involvement in it. Every opportunity should be given for the patient/client to participate in these discussions, and here again the group practice setting will facilitate such participation, and help the child and his parents to realise that the primary health care team are working together with his interest foremost in mind.

Voluntary organisations

The role of voluntary organisations is historic for often they set the pace in providing care for all conditions of men, establishing the need and getting to grips with it in terms of provision. Many began as services for the deprived and under-privileged and have gradually become incorporated in present day health education and welfare services for all.

Voluntary services are often able to offer a flexibility which escapes local authority provision, all too often tied down by rules of petty bureaucracy. Voluntary bodies are often able to initiate new methods of working with children and can function in an experimental manner. The social worker has a responsibility to take into account the resources available through the auspices of voluntary organisations and use them where appropriate to the individual's need. It is important for the social worker to liaise with her colleagues in voluntary organisations lest there be duplication of services. This frequently occurs when working with handicapped children – for example an application for help to the Family Fund may be submitted simultaneously both by the attached social worker and by the social worker of the voluntary agency.

The voluntary society is often more flexible and willing to cater for the individual patient. In these days of financial restraint there is the possibility of greater use being made of voluntary bodies resulting in a greater call on their resources and services by the individual social worker feeling the pinch of local authority cutbacks. Voluntary organisations however will themselves feel the pinch in a reduced income from local authority funding which regretably will affect the service they offer.

One must not forget the small local voluntary organizations which serve the needs of a particular area. A volunteer group attached to a south east London practice has provided valuable service to the health care team and patients alike for several years. Referrals are made by a member of the team to the coordinator, a practice patient herself, and she then matches the need to a volunteer, most of whom are also practice patients. Tasks include escorting people to the surgery for consultation – this is not intended to 'save' the GPs from a home visit but is therapeutic for the patient, often housebound from one consultation to the next, to make the effort and to get out of the house; sitting with the frail elderly to give a caring relative time to do her shopping regularly; baby sitting for a couple with a young family to enable them to have an evening together. The social worker takes a special interest in the group, often introducing volunteers when appropriate, as part of their therapy.

The problems of child care in immigrant families

When working with immigrant families it is important for the team to appreciate that ethnic minorities are not homogenous but consist of several different groups, and even communities within these groups. Different races have different attitudes and morals with regard to child care and religious beliefs also influence the pattern of care.

A community development project in Batley, Yorkshire, examined various approaches to working with immigrants (CDP, 1974). It concluded that there are few studies of the contribution of community work to race relations. Particular problems expressed by the Asian organisation in this study included the religious needs of the community such as special additional classes after school for children in religious matters, a desire for Muslim marriages to be recognised as legal and the availability of circumcision as a regular service in local hospitals. The need for play groups was apparent and recognized not only for the children's benefit but also was offering their mothers the opportunity to mix and learn English. The study also highlighted the general lack of knowledge about the social services and the individual's eligibility for them.

There is an increasing awareness of the need to understand the cultures or particular beliefs of the differing groups in the ethnic minorities. Hoggarth (1979) has commented, 'The new attitudes (arising from young blacks born and growing up in Britain) are causing an important rift in many West Indian families. Social workers will often be involved in problems where tensions between a young black and his family play a major part.' Many of the young people are experiencing a crisis of identity for whereas their parents sought acceptance by becoming as English as possible, their children are expressing a great pride in blackness, and there has been a resurgence of traditional customs, often expressed in hair styles and dress.

A study of West Indian one-year-olds compared the use made of the health services by West Indians in Paddington with a control group of non West Indians. This showed that lack of effective communication between medical workers and the immigrant group had a great bearing on the use made of the services. Problems highlighted amongst this group included poor housing conditions, a high number of children with both parents working, and a need for health education particularly in relation to feeding as there was a tendency for the children to suffer from nutritional deficiency diseases. Studies such as these serve to inform the members of the primary care team, for there are few teams comprising coloured members, which in itself is a drawback to providing a comprehensive service for the immigrants, and the ratio of coloured social workers and health visitors to GPs is also small.

CONCLUSION

It is acknowledged that 'general practice is in touch with a higher proportion of those who are in difficulties than any of the social services and it needs the full support of them all' (Report of the Committee on Local Authority and Allied Personal Social Services, 1968).

The general practitioner is often the first person people approach when they have a problem, be it physical or emotional, and they consult him seeking 'something' to make it better. Often the problem may be alleviated by 'someone', not necessarily the GP himself but another member of the primary care team, who can meet the patient's need in an appropriate way.

Two main themes run through the professional tenets of GP, nurse, health visitor and social worker: (1) interest in and care for the patient and his family and (2) acknowledgement that help may best be given by other workers. No profession is an island and the key to exploding some of the myths held by professional members about each other is inter-professional cooperation and training with a view to providing all aspects of good patient care, including the promotion of good child care.

In these days of financial restraint we have an incentive to look at opportunities for pooling resources, both of finance and teaching equipment for their most effective use at both pre- and post professional levels of training. Each profession shares common areas of knowledge, albeit at different levels. But, it should not be without the bounds of possibility for various student groups on professional courses to share lectures on subjects such as sociology, psychology and psychiatry. A start has already been made at a recent sympossium held by training groups of the four professions (RCGP

1980). As Dr G Beales commented at a conference on inter-professional collaboration 'somehow, somebody has to try to teach an approach which looks at all patients' needs and which poses the questions: What can't I do for this patient? What can other people do?'

An atmosphere of trust must exist between team members if they are going to be able to discuss individual cases and to look at their mistakes and to learn by them. So often it is assumed that the health visitor, social worker or GP is going to be responsible for this or that and nothing is done because each member of the team thought that another member was involved.

Inter-professional cooperation is often hindered by ignorance of one another's skills, differences in case load numbers and methods of working, and petty resentments often as a result of individual preoccupation with power and status within the team.

Teaching should be combined with humility so that students of all professions can recognise their own limitations and the necessity of and advantages from working with other people with complementary skills and training. The standard of care provided by the team is a reflection of the team's understanding of each member's role and function within the team – 'whole patient' care can only be achieved when team members have that understanding of each other's function and are mature enough to refer to their colleague when appropriate – so often a patient/client is kept on a list/caseload because of the worker's needs and involvement.

It is hoped that primary health care teams will develop and the attachment of social workers to them will continue and enhance the provision of an effective and efficient health and social service to the public whom they strive to help.

ACKNOWLEDGEMENTS

My experience in this field derives from an attachment as social worker to the group practice of Drs Meyrick, Cox and Grabinar and their patients at Catford, London SE6.

I am grateful to Dr M Johnson, of the Research Unit on Ethnic Relations, and to Mrs P Oliver, District Officer, London Borough of Lewisham Social Services, for help in preparing this chapter.

REFERENCES

CDP (1974) Community work with immigrants. *British Journal of Social Work*, **42**.

Gilchrist, I. *et al* (1978) Social work in general practice. *Journal of the Royal College of General Practitioners*, **28**, 675–686.

Goldberg, M. & Neil, J. (1972) *Social Work in General Practice.* National Institue of Social Services Library, 24. London: George Allen & Unwin.

Hicks, D. (1976) *Primary Health Care – a review.* DHSS. London: HMSO.

Hoggarth, E. (1979) *Social Work Today*, **II**, 13.

Leeding, A.M. (1980) *Child Care Manual for Social Workers*, 4th edn. London.

Marsh, D. (1965) *An Introduction to the Study of Social Administration.* London: Routledge & Kegan Paul.

Paine, T. (1976) The role of part-time workers in general practice. *Journal of the Royal College of General Practitioners*, **26**, 695–6.

Ratoff, L. (1973) *Journal of the Royal College of General Practitioners*, **23**, 736–742.

RCGP (1980) *Education for Cooperation in Health and Social Work.* RCGP Occasional Paper, 14.

Stroud, J. (1973) *Services for children and their families. Aspects of Child Care for Social Workers.* The Commonwealth and International Library. London: Pergammon Press.

PART TWO

Child care and preventive medicine

9

The fetus at risk

Michael Rogers

The quality of human life can now be improved by good antenatal care. Preventive obstetrics has become increasingly important over the years and is now a well recognised part of any good antenatal clinic (Elstein *et al*, 1975; Lloyd, 1975; Crocker and Clements, 1976). The GP involvement is substantial. In 1978 in England and Wales, 9609 births (1.6 per cent of all confinements) were at home. In many practices up to 20 per cent of mothers are confined at GP obstetric units. It is probable that well over 50 per cent of the medical care in antenatal clinics in the United Kingdom is by GPs.

It has become customary to judge the effectiveness of our antenatal care by the perinatal mortality rate (PMR). The PMR is the sum of stillbirths and first week deaths per 1000 total births. This has been halved since 1939 and now stands at around 15 per 1000 in England and Wales. Comparison with the rates for other European countries shows that this could and should be halved again (Ch. 1). It is our responsibility as GPs to ensure that we play our full part in achieving this as quickly as possible.

CAUSES OF PERINATAL DEATHS

The major causes of perinatal death in this country are shown in Table 9.1. It will be seen that the neonatal mortality, the number of deaths in the first week of life, is almost equal to the number of stillbirths. The largest single factor is congenital anomaly, which is the cause of just over 20 per cent of all stillbirths and neonatal deaths. This is broken down into individual systems in Table 9.2, where the pre-eminence of CNS defects as a cause of death is well illustrated. Circulatory defects (mostly congenital heart disease) form an important runner up. These are discussed further in Chapter 35. It is important to appreciate that the total incidence (as opposed to mortality) of congenital malformations shows a wide annual variation, as a recent review from Northern Ireland demonstrates (Fig. 9.1).

Open neural tube defects can now be prevented, and this is discussed later in this chapter. A start has already been made, as Figures 9.2 and 9.3 show, but we still have a long way to go before the incidence of these horrible disorders is reduced to an acceptable minimum.

Neural tube defects form the most important group of those mid-trimster abnormalities that can be detected by amniocentesis. Selective abortion can then be performed when indicated. The general practitioner, in his role as primary physician, can contribute greatly to the detection of such abnormalities. He has an intimate knowledge of the family unit and will be aware of any previous fetal abnormality. His vigilance during early pregnancy may be the key factor in suspecting fetal abnormality, and it is to be hoped that more emphasis will be placed on prenatal diagnosis in the future.

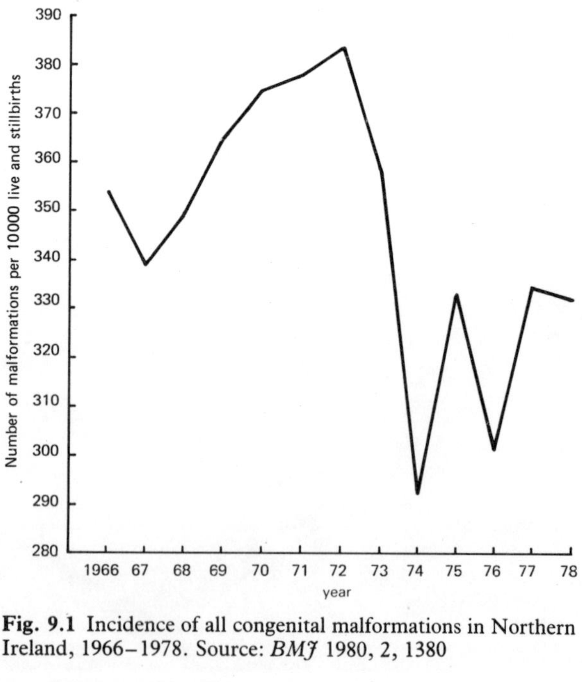

Fig. 9.1 Incidence of all congenital malformations in Northern Ireland, 1966–1978. Source: *BMJ* 1980, 2, 1380

Table 9.1 Some causes of perinatal deaths, England and Wales, 1978. Source: OPCS Infant mortality Statistics, series DH3 no. 5

Cause	*Stillbirths*		*Death under one week*	
	Number	*Percentage*	*Number*	*Percentage*
Maternal				
Unrelated to pregnancy				
Hypertension	114	2.23	1	
Diabetes mellitus	61	1.19	10	
Other	97		8	
Related to pregnancy				
Toxaemia	438	8.57	30	
Ante and intrapartum infection	16		10	
Difficult labour				
Pelvic abnormality	7		0	
Disproportion	19		12	
Malpresentation	80	1.57	35	
Abnormality of forces of labour	11		9	
Unspecified	22		16	
Complications of pregnancy and labour				
Multiple pregnancy	139	2.72	253	5.05
Premature rupture of membranes	32		19	
Hydramnios	14		1	
Other	156		47	
Conditions of placenta				
Premature separation	509	9.96	32	
Infarction	96	1.72	0	
Placenta praevia	42		7	
Insufficiency (unspecified)	700	13.70	6	
Conditions of umbilical cord	400	7.83	39	
Conditions of fetus and newborn				
Anoxia and Hypoxia	337	6.60	1344	26.78
Maceration	217	4.25	0	
Birth injury	33		319	6.38
Immaturity	31		500	9.99
Haemolytic disease	85	1.66	33	
Haemorrhagic disease	4		75	1.50
Congenital abnormalities (see Table 9.2)	1050	20.6	1035	20.7
Other	344	6.73	72	1.44
Total	5108	100	5003	100

Table 9.2 Perinatal mortality from congenital defects, England and Wales, 1978. Source: OPCS Infant Mortality Statistics, series DH3 no. 5

Abnormality	Stillbirths	Deaths in first week
Anencephalus	553	68
Spina bifida	130	153
Hydrocephalus	137	28
Other CNS and eye	27	50
Circulatory	22	303
Respiratory	3	85
Digestive	43	47
Genitourinary	11	77
Musculoskeletal	15	41
Down's Syndrome	7	6
Multiple systems	74	154
Other unspecified	28	23
Total	1050	1035

FACTORS AFFECTING THE FETUS

1. Social and environmental

Even the best obstetric care can, to some extent, be offset by poor social and environmental conditions. This can be shown by the wide variation of perinatal mortality rates throughout the country. The rate is worse in Northern Ireland than in the other components of the United Kingdom. Within England there is a big regional variation; the rates are worse in the north than in the south, and worse in conurbations than in rural areas. However, this variation is reducing steadily as the years go by (Fig. 9.4).

The PMR also varies enormously, as one would expect, between the five social classes. The rate for social class V is still nearly double that of social class I despite improved housing, education, and medical care in all

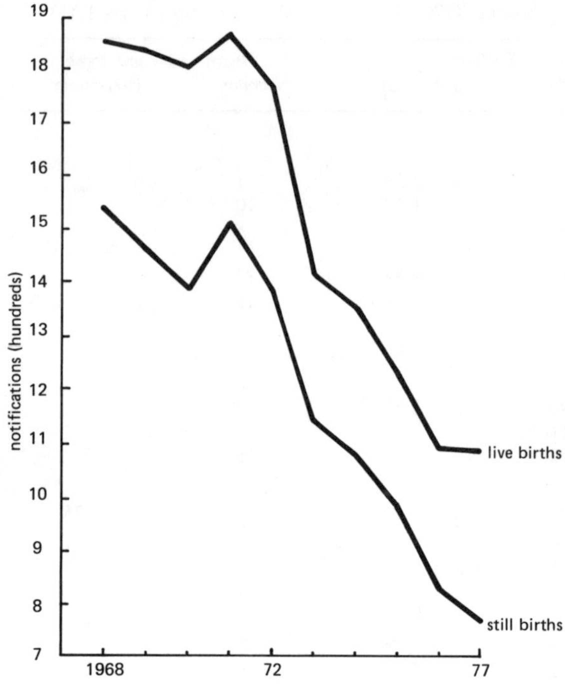

Fig. 9.2 Notifications of live and still births with CNS malformations, England and Wales 1968–1977. Source: OPCS Population trends 19, 1980

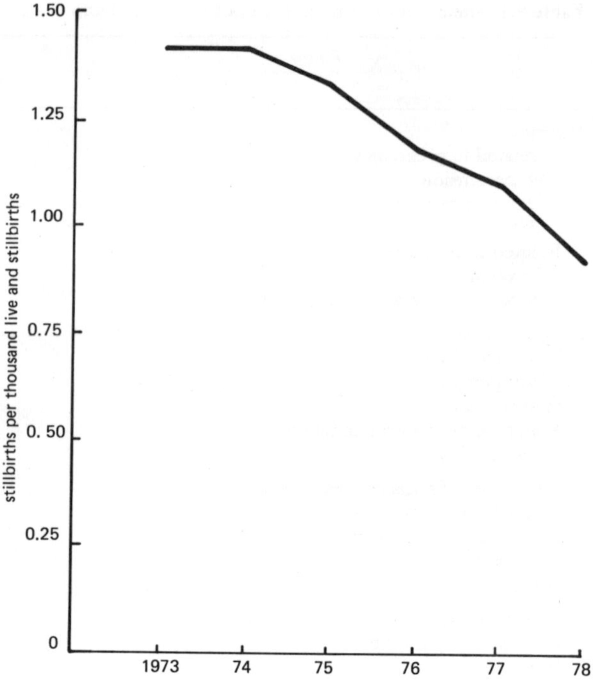

Fig. 9.3 Stillbirths from anencephaly England and Wales 1973–1978. Source: OPCS

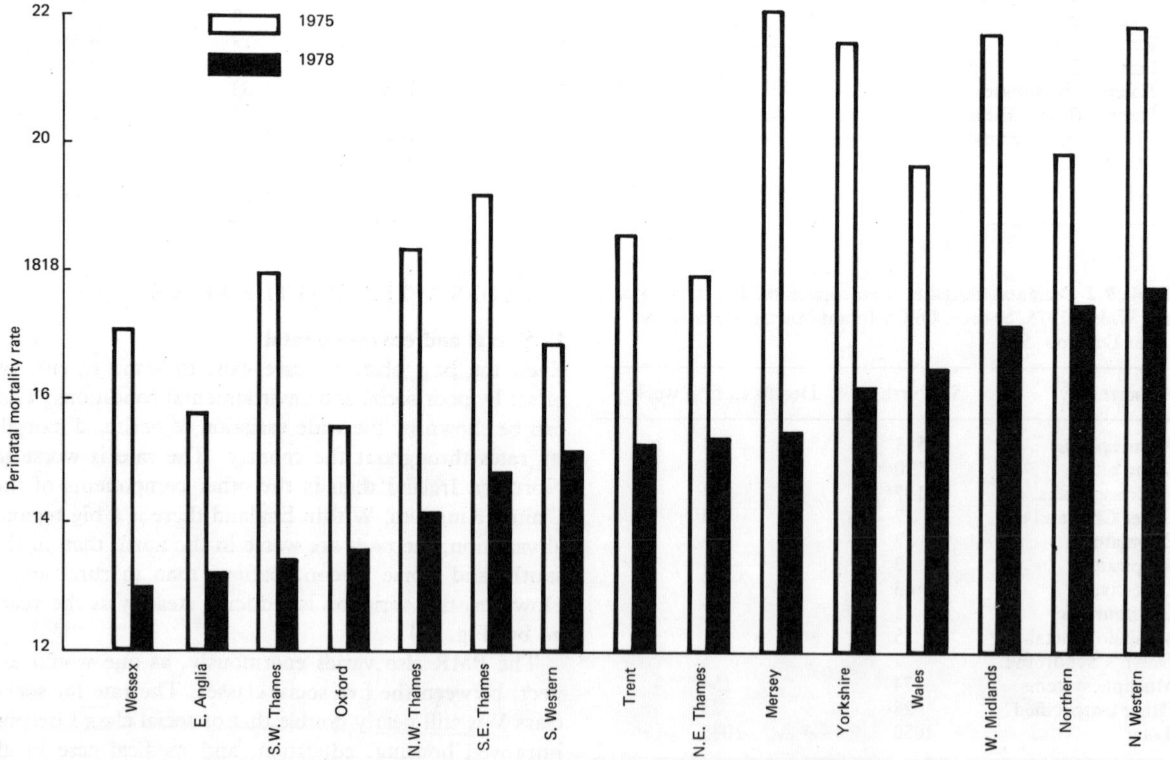

Fig. 9.4 Regional variations in perinatal mortality 1975–1978 England and Wales. Source: OPCS

classes. Figures released in a parliamentary written answer show that the United Kingdom PMR was 10.9 per 1000 among professional classes in 1977 and 20.6 per 1000 among unskilled workers (Fig. 9.6). This variation is common knowledge among GPs, but all too often we fail to do much about it. In a memorable paper read at the spring meeting of the RCGP in 1980, Dr Geoffrey Marsh of Stockton outlined the measures taken in his own practice to reduce this great disparity. In his antenatal clinic, he reserves the examination of mothers in social classes IV and V for his own personal attention, leaving those in social classes I to III to be supervised in the main by the practice midwife. This simple measure must surely contribute to the outstanding PMR statistics obtained in his practice.

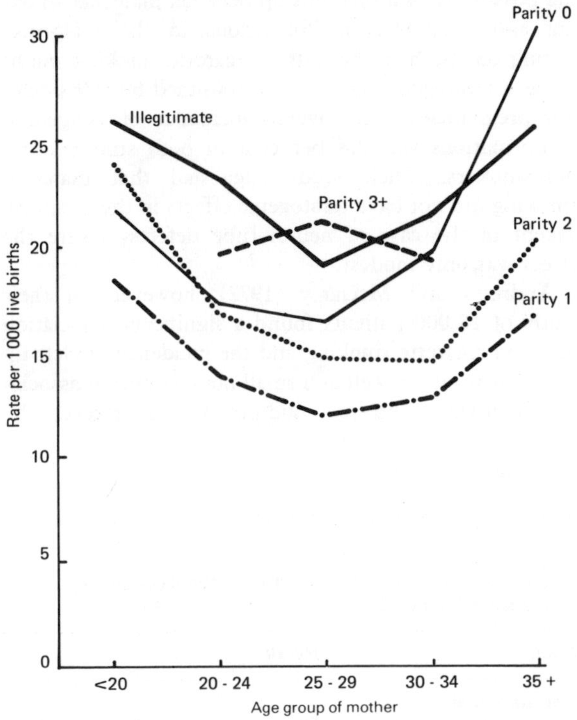

Fig. 9.5 Perinatal mortality 1977 England and Wales. Source: OPCS Studies in medical and population subjects, 41. HMSO, 1980

Another important social factor affecting the PMR is illegitimacy, the incidence of which has doubled in the last two decades. In 1978 11.32 per cent of live births and 15.85 per cent of stillbirths in England and Wales were illegitimate (Fig. 9.7). Perinatal mortality is particularly high for illegitimate children of teenage mothers (SBF, 1980). The PMR of legitimate children is also affected by the age and parity of their mothers, as is well known. The biggest risks to the baby are for those with mothers under 20 or over 35 years, and those whose mothers already have four or more children (Fig. 9.5). Another important consideration is the ethnic origin of the mother; the PMR is high for children whose mothers are immigrants from Pakistan and the New Commonwealth (Fig. 48.3). Moreover, these social and environmental risks often compound themselves. The risk of death in the perinatal period for the fifth child of a Northern Irish mother aged 35 in social class V is perhaps six times as great as that of the second child of an English mother aged 25 in social class I.

Clearly, expectant mothers in all risk groups should be identified as early as possible in pregnancy. They should be encouraged to attend the antenatal clinic as

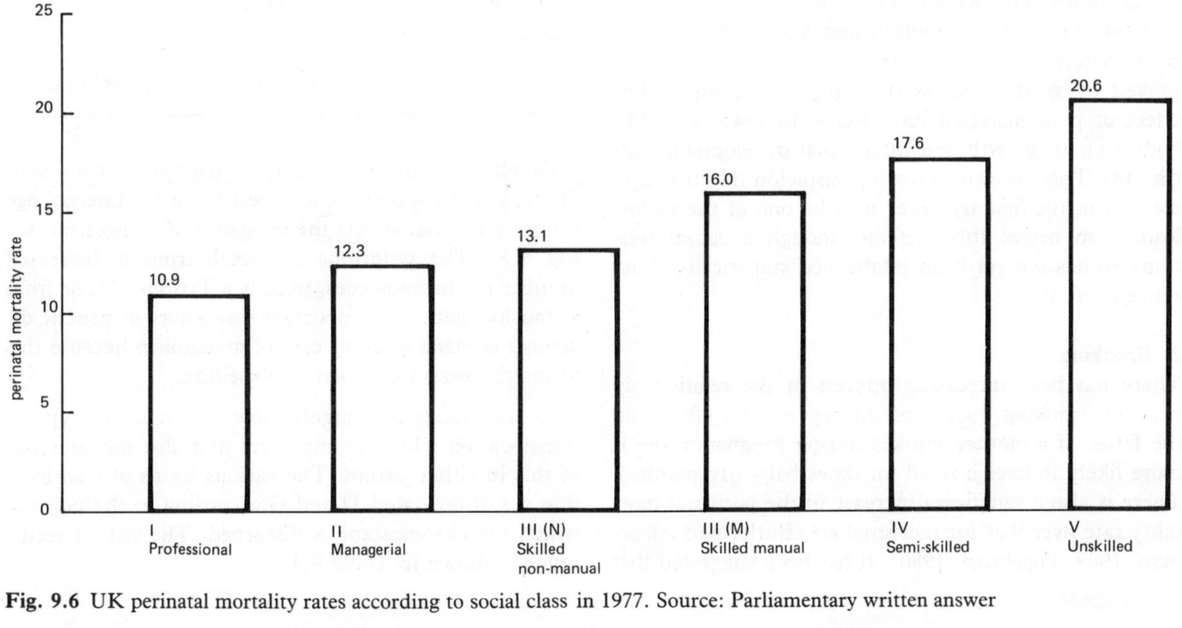

Fig. 9.6 UK perinatal mortality rates according to social class in 1977. Source: Parliamentary written answer

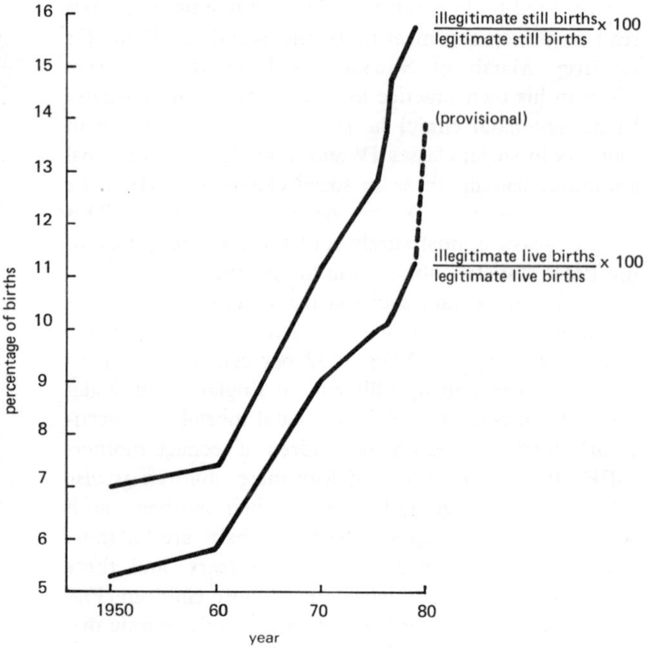

Fig. 9.7 Percentage of illegitimate live and still births England and Wales, 1950–1978. Source: OPCS mortality statistics childhood and maternity, 1978. HMSO, 1980, and Population trends, September 1980

soon as pregnancy is established, and they should receive special care and attention in the clinic. To achieve this is one of the most important tasks of the practice health visitors.

Diet

It was shown in the Rhondda experiment in South Wales in 1934, and later by Yudkin and Yudkin (1968) that both maternal and infant mortality rates can be improved by good nutrition throughout pregnancy. The effect of poor maternal nutrition is to lower a child's body weight, growth and intellectual development (see Ch. 43). There is also a growing suspicion that inadequate diet in the first trimester may be one of the factors leading to neural tube defects, though a causal relationship has not yet been established statistically (Laurence *et al*, 1980).

2. Smoking

There has been increasing interest in the relationship between smoking during pregnancy and its effects on the fetus. If a mother smokes during pregnancy she is more likely to have a small for dates baby (dysmature). There is also a significant increase in the perinatal mortality rate over that for non-smokers (Butler and Alberman, 1969; Fogelman, 1980). It has been suggested that this is due to a reduction in the potential supply of oxygen to the fetus by an increased maternal carboxyhaemoglobin level (Cole, Hawkins and Roberts, 1972).

Recently it was noted by Evans, Newcombe and Cambell (1979) that little attention had been focused on the possibility of a relationship between maternal smoking and congenital malformations in the offspring. Acting on the hypothesis that cigarette smoking might act as a teratogenic agent, they examined 69 609 singleton pregnancies. The overall incidence of congenital malformations was 2.8 per cent in both smokers and non-smokers. Their study suggested that maternal smoking did not have teratogenic effects in the offspring except in the case of neural tube defects, where the effect was only modest.

Andrews and McGarry (1972), however, in their study of 18 000 patients found a significant association between cigarette smoking and the incidence of cleft lip and cleft palate as well as a small non-significant association with gastro intestinal and neural tube defects.

3. Genetic factors

a. Chromosomal abnormalities (see Table 9.3)

Table 9.3 Examples of genetic risks to the fetus due to chromosomal abnormality

Fault	*Result*
Chromosomal	
a. Anomaly of number	Down's Syndrome (Trisomy 21) Turner's Syndrome (XO) Klinefelter's Syndrome (XXY)
b. Anomaly of structure	Translocation mongol
Gene mutations	Achondroplasia
Combination of factors	Spina bifida Anencephaly Talipes equino varus (club foot)

Of all the chromosomal abnormalities Down's syndrome is the commonest and best known. Maternal age is one factor that affects the incidence of mongolism (see Fig. 9.8). The syndrome can result from an increased number of chromosomes, usually a Trisomy 21, or from a translocation. It is important that a correct genetic diagnosis is made in every case of mongolism because this forms the basis for genetic counselling.

In translocation mongols, however, it is the type of translocation which is important and also the presence of this in either parent. The various forms of translocation are abbreviated D and G according to the point at which the chromosome is disturbed. The risk of recurrence is shown in Table 9.4.

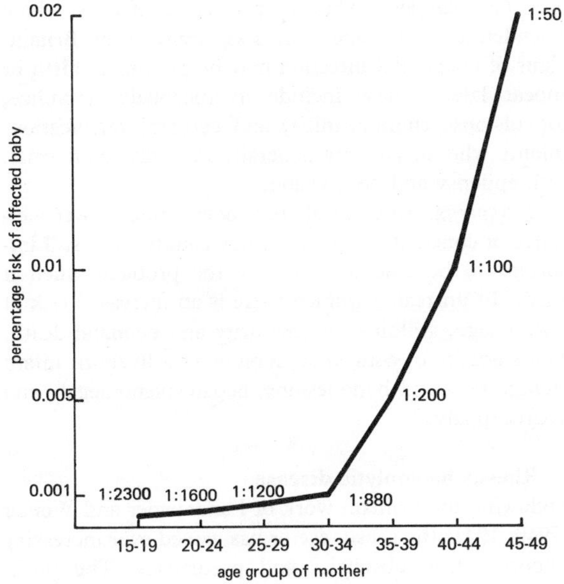

Fig. 9.8 Risk of occurrence of Down's syndrome according to maternal age (adapted from Crandon, 1979)

Table 9.4 Risk of recurrence of Down's Syndrome due to different chromosome abnormalities (reproduced by kind permission of Dr Rosalind Skinner)

Patient	*Carrier parent*	*Risk of recurrence (per cent)*
Translocation:		
D/G (Chromosomes 13 or 14/21)	Mother	10–15
	Father	5
21/22	Mother	10–15
	Father	5
21/22	Mother	100
	Father	100
Trisomy 21		1

b. Metabolic disorders

These are relatively uncommon but several can now be detected in early pregnancy by examination of the amniotic fluid. See Table 9.5.

Table 9.5 Enzyme defects of various metabolic disorders detectable by examination of amniotic fluid

Disorder detectable	*Enzyme defect*
Tay Sach's disease	Hexosaminidase A
Niemann Pick's disease	Sphingomyelinase
Galactosaemia	Galactose–1–phosphate uridylyl transferase

In phenylketonuria there is a deficiency of phenylalanine hydroxylase, and this can be detected by the Guthrie test using maternal blood (Guthrie and Susi, 1963). If the test is positive a special diet can be used during pregnancy, with benefit to the fetus. It was suggested by Raine (1974) that it is extremely doubtful if mass population screening for any inherited metabolic disease, other than phenylketonuria, should be established beyond the few pilot studies at present in progress.

4. Drugs and radiation

Since the thalidomide disaster women have become wary of taking any drugs during pregnancy and frequently consult the general practitioner for his advice. The recent ill-founded scare with regard to Debendox has brought this to the forefront again (Harron *et al.*, 1980). It is, therefore, important to be aware of the effects of various common drugs on the fetus. Drugs reach the fetus by transport across the placenta and if given in the first trimester can affect organogenesis. Cytotoxic drugs should never be given to a pregnant woman.

Other drugs may still affect the fetus even though they do not cause teratogenesis. Androgenic steroids can masculinise a female fetus. Hormones cross the placenta and thereby affect the fetus (King, 1975). Hormone pregnancy tests were therefore discontinued in 1979.

Stilboestrol and diethylstilboestrol are unique in their manner of damaging the fetus. If given in large doses to prevent habitual abortion there is a risk that a female child will develop a clear-cell adenocarcinoma of her vagina after puberty.

Antithyroid agents may lead to a fetal goitre. Radioactive iodine will destroy fetal thyroid tissue if given to the mother during pregnancy. Oral hypoglycaemic agents will cause prolonged hypoglycaemia in the newborn infant.

Of the antibiotics, tetracyclines are known to chelate with calcium ions and are thus deposited in bones, including teeth. This gives rise to a yellow discoloration of primary teeth (Ch. 33). Streptomycin can be ototoxic to the fetus, as well as the mother. Long acting sulphonamides can cause jaundice and kernicterus in the fetus if given in late pregnancy. This is because they displace bilirubin from the plasma albumin in the circulating blood.

Coumarin anticoagulants can alter fetal clotting mechanisms, but heparin, with its large molecule, has very little effect on the fetus because of its inability to be transported across the placenta.

Maternal ingestion of alcohol, even as little as one double whisky per day may cause the fetal alcohol syndrome. This is discussed in Chapter 49.

Maternal addiction to narcotics, such as heroin, can cause neonatal addiction and lead to serious withdrawal symptoms. All narcotics, and pethidine is a narcotic, given during labour can cause serious depression of neonatal respiration. The use of pethidine and other drugs in labour is discussed in Chapter 10.

With an ever increasing number of the population being referred for X-rays, the fetus must be protected from the hazard of leukaemia in later childhood. It is now recommended that X-ray investigation of the abdomen or pelvis in women of childbearing age should be restricted to the first ten days of the menstrual cycle (the Ten Day Rule).

5. Maternal infection

a. *Maternal rubella syndrome*. It was Gregg (1941) who first established a relationship between congenital cataracts and rubella in early pregnancy. Many of his cases had also congenital cardiac lesions. During the first 16 weeks of pregnancy rubella can cause death, multiple congenital abnormalities, or continuing disease of the fetus.

The common congenital abnormalities are patent ductus arteriosus, septal defects, cataracts, retinopathy, deafness and microcephaly. Signs of active rubella infection at birth include hepatosplenomegaly, thrombocytopenic purpura, myocarditis, skin rash, and lymphadenopathy.

The problem of rubella in pregnancy is well reviewed by Brimblecombe (1979).

b. *Other viral diseases*. Siegel (1973) has studied the incidence of congenital malformations following infection of the mother during pregnancy with chickenpox, measles, mumps, and virus hepatitis. In general his results showed no apparent difference in the incidence of congenital defects between the virus and control groups. There was, however, a somewhat higher fetal death rate when maternal infection with these viruses occurred. There was also an increased incidence of premature labour, prematurity and low birth weight.

Cytomegalovirus infection is asymptomatic in the mother, but can give rise to chronic infection in the fetus, and congenital abnormalities. The commonest defects are neurological, and include mental retardation, microcephaly, and hydrocephaly. Maternal infection with poliovirus and variola has been associated with similar fetal damage.

Genital herpes in the mother at term can affect the fetus adversely after delivery (Ch. 22).

The subject of virus infections other than rubella during pregnancy was reviewed by Waterson (1979). He concluded that some viruses, especially rubella and cytomegalovirus, can have serious effects on the fetus but that most other viruses affect the fetus only exceptionally or not at all.

c. *Toxoplasmosis*. This is a protozoon infection which is endemic in Europe, but less common in Britain. Signs of congenital infection may be present at birth or appear later. These include hydrocephaly, jaundice, convulsions, chorioretinitis, and cerebral calcification. Infants who survive are generally mentally subnormal, with epilepsy and poor vision.

d. *Syphilis*. Although there is now a much lower incidence of congenital syphilis in this country it is still important to be able to recognise the problem when it arises. In untreated women there is an increased risk of miscarriage, stillbirth, prematurity and neonatal death. The stigmata of congenital syphilis in a liveborn infant include skin and bone lesions, hepatosplenomegaly and hydrocephaly.

6. Rhesus haemolytic disease

Following the brilliant work of Landsteiner and Weiner (1940, 1941) the rhesus factor has gained ever increasing importance in obstetrics and paediatrics. The initial confusion was eliminated by the CDE classification of Fisher. This postulates that the rhesus complex consists of three closely associated genes, C, D and E, with allelic forms c, d and e. In clinical practice it is the D/d antigen which is most important. There are three possible genotypes: D/D (rhesus positive – homozygous); D/d (rhesus positive – heterozygous); d/d (rhesus nega-

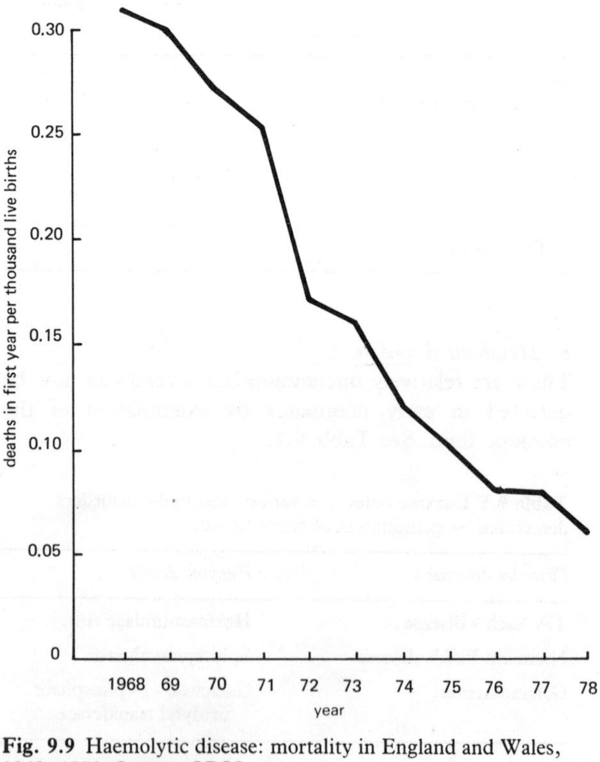

Fig. 9.9 Haemolytic disease: mortality in England and Wales, 1968–1978. Source: OPCS

tive). It is known that about 15 per cent of the British population are rhesus negative.

It is the rhesus negative mother who is at risk from isoimmunisation, if her husband is rhesus positive. If he has homozygous antigens (D/D) all children will be affected, but if he is heterozygous (D/d) only half will be affected. It is thus important that the rhesus genotype of each parent is established. The ABO groups should also be known, since isoimmunisation can occur rarely in differing incompatible ABO groups.

There are only two ways in which a rhesus negative woman can receive rhesus positive antigens: by mismatched blood transfusion, and by fetomaternal haemorrhage (FMH). This can occur at any stage of pregnancy and may be due to such factors as abortion, abruptio placentae, amniocentesis, external cephalic version, hypertension, Caesarian section, third stage of labour, retained placenta, and trauma. As a result of any of these factors, rhesus positive antigens (D antigens) can cross into the maternal circulation and stimulate Anti-D antibodies.

Unless action is taken, subsequent pregnancies can result in fetal damage by haemolysis of fetal red cells leading to anaemia. The three clinical forms are hydrops foetalis, icterus gravis neonatorum and congenital haemolytic anaemia. Hydrops foetalis is invariably fatal; icterus gravis neonatorum is the commonest and may lead to kernicterus; congenital haemolytic anaemia is the mildest.

The gratifying drop in mortality from haemolytic disease in England and Wales in the past decade is shown in Figure 9.9. This can only be maintained by meticulous monitoring of antibodies of susceptible women throughout pregnancy.

7. Obstetric problems

a. *Maternal.* Any mother, who is not entirely fit, may put the fetus at risk, but there are certain well recognised conditions which can lead to an at-risk pregnancy.

The grand multipara (five or more previous viable babies) is more susceptible to uterine rupture, antepartum haemorrhage, postpartum haemorrhage, prematurity, malpresentation and precipitate delivery. Maternal disease such as cardiac disease, diabetes mellitus (below), tuberculosis, thyrotoxicosis and anaemia can all put the fetus in a precarious state. Previous Caesarian section or hysterotomy can lead to uterine rupture. Hypertensive states can lead to intrauterine death, eclampsia, cerebral vascular accident or abruptio placentae. There were 114 stillbirths from this cause in England and Wales in 1978 (Table 9.1).

Diabetes mellitus can reduce the chance of pregnancy in affected women. Since the introduction of insulin, the fertility rate has risen to 20–30 per cent. Once pregnant, a diabetic woman is more likely to suffer from abortion, stillbirth, hydramnios, gross fetal abnormality, and pre-eclampsia. Babies of diabetic mothers are frequently large at birth. The fetal loss in diabetic mothers due to intrauterine and neonatal death still ranges between 40 and 50 per cent, but can be as low as 10 to 15 per cent in experienced centres. This disparity is a challenge to us all. The perinatal loss in England and Wales in 1978 was 61 stillbirths and 10 neonatal deaths (Table 9.1).

It is now common to induce labour in diabetic mothers at the end of the 38th week, because it is at this stage that the risk of intrauterine death overtakes that of neonatal death. Obviously one has to be absolutely sure of gestational age, because of the risk of a disastrous degree of prematurity. Here the use of ultrasonics, as mentioned later in this chapter, is an invaluable aid to predicting the optimum time for delivery.

The method of delivery of diabetic mothers depends on the obstetrician concerned, but vaginal delivery has been used increasingly recently, with a fall in the Caesarian section rate. The infant after delivery must be competently handled, since he may be oedematous, lethargic, premature, and prone to atelectasis and hypoglycaemia. The stomach is always full of swallowed liquor, and must be aspirated. During the first 48 hours the baby may develop a cyanotic attack, and die without warning.

It is for all these reasons that urine should be tested at every antenatal visit, and if sugar is present a low renal threshold must be confirmed by a glucose tolerance test (GTT). A previous history of large babies, or a family history of diabetes, is a mandatory indication for a GTT early on in the antenatal period.

b. *Fetal.* The obvious at-risk babies are those involved in a multiple pregnancy, breech and other malpresentations, disproportion and prematurity. The fetal and neonatal loss from these complications are listed in Table 9.1.

In this section on factors which may affect the fetus the problems facing us all in the antenatal clinic have been outlined. These are not to be regarded lightly, since we are responsible for the safe delivery of a fit healthy child to the mother. By an understanding of the above factors the general practitioner can really exert to the full his primary care role. Much of the early suspicion and detection will inevitably necessitate referral to specialist colleagues, and in this respect the team approach and shared care is paramount.

As standards improve, the criteria for selecting cases for domiciliary confinement grow increasingly strict. The risks are well documented (Fig. 9.10). Recently it has been strongly argued that increased efforts should be made to achieve 100 per cent hospital delivery (Cox *et al*, 1976). Provision of more GP obstetric units in maternity hospitals will inevitably encourage this trend.

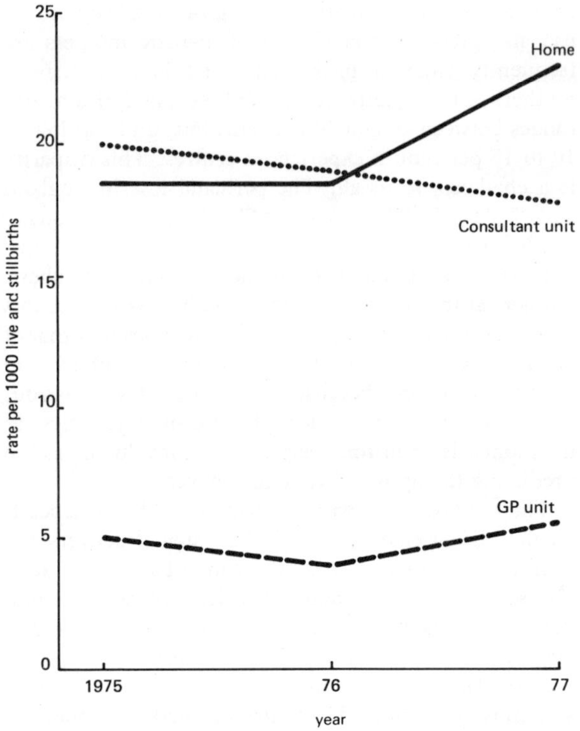

Fig. 9.10 Perinatal mortality by place of confinement 1975–1977 England and Wales. Source: OPCS perinatal and infant mortality: social and biological factors 1975–1977. Studies in medical and population subjects, 41. HMSO, 1980

More and more women are, however, asking for home confinements. In most cases these are being refused by the general practitioner and the burden then falls on the district midwife. Most general practitioners in rural areas realise that if home confinements do return then disasters may once more occur, especially from haemorrhage. The use of flying squads has inevitably fallen off in recent years and the efficiency of such a team must therefore be questioned. In some hospitals it is not always made clear who is on the squad. A paediatrician should be included in the team, as well as an obstetrician.

The most dangerous part of the whole pregnancy is labour and the few hours immediately afterwards. Probably the ideal compromise for women requesting home confinement would be delivery of the baby in a GP obstetric unit within the maternity hospital and *return home within six hours* if all is normal. The risks of home delivery should be sympathetically explained by the GP and midwife and this other alternative offered. The most vital danger time has then been spent in hospital with access for emergency resuscitation etc., but the mother is soon returned with her baby to her home environment.

Detection of the fetus at risk

Once the practitioner is aware of the many ways in which a fetus may be at risk during pregnancy, the problem becomes one of recognition and detection.

The general practitioner, with his knowledge of the family unit, will be able to classify pregnant women into their various social and environmental classes. He will also be aware of their smoking habits and exposure to drugs and radiation. Previous obstetric, medical and family history will be readily available.

More specialised tests are being used increasingly, and these are conveniently divided into tests of fetal maturity and tests of uteroplacental function.

1. Tests of fetal maturity

a. *Clinical.* By the addition of nine months and seven days to the first day of the last normal menstrual period an estimate of the date of delivery can be given. Palpation of the uterine fundus enables an estimate of the rate of growth to be obtained. The height of the fundus is usually related to the symphysis pubis, umbilicus and xiphisternum.

The date at which fetal movements are first felt is noted routinely on antenatal cards. A primigravida may not notice movements until as late as 22 weeks gestation, whereas a multigravida can usually detect movement as early as 16 weeks.

Any variation from the expected normal in the clinical findings should raise the first suspicions of a fetus at risk. The clinical methods of assessing fetal maturity are, however, so frequently unreliable that often other methods are now used to elucidate the problem.

b. *Amniotic fluid estimation.* An examination of a sample of amniotic fluid can be of considerable value, not only in estimating gestation, but for detecting chromosomal abnormalities, in monitoring rhesus isoimmunisation, and in predicting the respiratory distress syndrome (RDS).

Accurate location of the placenta by ultrasound reduces the risks, but amniocentesis is not a procedure to be undertaken lightly, nor will it normally fall within the competence of British general practitioners (Miskin, 1974; BMJ Editorial, 1975a). Amniocentesis should be fully explained to the parents and they must accept that if this procedure is to be carried out, any abnormalities uncovered should be acted upon by termination of pregnancy.

Amniocentesis is an invasive procedure and as such carries a risk. In early amniocentesis there is a risk of abortion in about two per cent of cases. This is twice the spontaneous incidence of abortion in normal pregnancies. Orthopaedic problems such as club foot are also increased slightly in infants whose mothers have had amniocentesis. In late amniocentesis the risks are of bleeding, both fetal and maternal. These can be reduced by the use of ultrasound before amniocentesis.

The problems of amniocentesis have been reviewed in recent articles (Valman, 1979; Scrimgeour, 1979, 1980; Bain, 1979; Bryan, 1979; Laurence, 1979; Gardner, 1979).

1. *For estimating gestation* Lind (1971) has produced a point scoring system for certain characteristics of the amniotic fluid. These are the cytological pattern, the amniotic fluid creatinine concentration and the difference between the urea concentrations of the amniotic fluid and maternal plasma.

2. If amniotic fluid is obtained at about 14–16 weeks gestation, its examination can detect chromosomal and metabolic abnormalities. The antenatal diagnosis of neural tube defects, such as spina bifida, can now be made by estimation of *amniotic alphafetoprotein* (AFP) (BMJ Editorial, 1975; Brock and Scrimgeour, 1974; Milinsky *et al*, 1974).
Because of the risks of amniocentesis it should only be performed in selected cases, and by staff experienced in the technique. The women who are usually offered amniocentesis are those who:
 (i) have previously had an anencephalic or spina bifida infant
 (ii) are over the age of 36 years
 (iii) have previously had a Mongol child
 (iv) have previously had a child with a rare metabolic disease such as mucopolysaccharidosis or galactosaemia.

3. In *monitoring rhesus haemolytic disease* the bilirubin concentration in amniotic fluid can be measured spectrophotometrically. Serial readings are taken in more severe cases, and intrauterine exchange transfusion may be carried out if the levels rise dangerously.

4. *In predicting RDS* it has been shown that the lecithin/sphingomyelin ratio of amniotic fluid can provide an indication of fetal lung maturity and thus a susceptibility to RDS (Gluck, 1971).
Amniocentesis is then done in later pregnancy if early induction of labour is being contemplated (Usually after 32 weeks gestation).

c. *Radiology*. The progressive change in ossification centres in the fetal skeleton has been used to determine fetal age. Thus, the distal femoral epiphyses appear at about 36 weeks gestation. On the whole, however, the method is not particularly reliable, especially if there is fetal growth retardation.

d. *Ultrasonic cephalometry*. Ultrasound can be used to measure the biparietal diameter of the fetal skull. Serial measurements of the biparietal diameter can be used to estimate fetal growth rate. If a reading is taken at about 14 week gestation (the fetal skull becomes visible at about 13 weeks) and then at a later stage, a fairly accurate estimate can be given of gestation. It is not possible, however, even in experienced centres, to assess gestation to within one week either way. Thus a single reading is of little value in predicting fetal growth retardation and serial readings are essential. Ultrasound is also a safe method of scanning the uterus to detect such things as missed abortion, twin pregnancies or breech. There is a theoretical risk that ultrasound might damage chromosomes and cell membranes, but reliable current opinion refutes this (Donald, 1974; Munro, 1976).

2. Tests of utero placental function (see Table 9.6)

Table 9.6 Some tests of uteroplacental function

Hormones	Urine	oestrogens
	Plasma	oestriol
	Serum	human placental lactogen (HPL)
Enzymes	Heat stable alkaline phosphatase	
	Transaminases	
Serial ultrasonic cephalometry		
Cardiotocography		
Acid-base balance of fetal blood		

Any single test of placental function can, at best, examine only a small fraction of placental activity. Many enzymes are produced by the placenta, but their estimation is not satisfactory for widespread use as an index of placental function.

In *acute placental failure* the effects are best looked for in changes of fetal heart rate; passage of meconium stained liquor, changes in cardiotocography (see p. 87) and changes in fetal blood pH.

Chronic failure of the placenta causing fetal growth retardation (FGR) can best be looked for with changes in maternal hormonal levels. As with ultrasonics it is the serial readings that are more useful than a single one. The two best known tests in current use are the urinary oestriol level and the serum oestriol level.

Serial oestriol assays are valuable in detecting FGR changes, because the level falls as placental function becomes impaired. In a series of 597 unselected pregnancies Beischer and his colleagues (1968) showed that oestriol excretion could be low in the absence of abnormal clinical signs and recommended that every pregnancy should be screened by at least two urinary oestriol levels. Klopper (1969) has suggested that fetal death is unlikely as long as urinary oestriol excretion exceeds 5 mg/24 hours. He regards an excretion of less than 8 mg/24 hours after 37 weeks of pregnancy as a signal for early delivery. Certain factors have to be taken into account, however, because lack of adrenal tissue in the fetus, as in anencephaly, can give low oestriol values. Drugs given to the mother such as ampicillin, meprobamate and stilboestrol can reduce urinary oestriol levels.

MANAGEMENT OF THE FETUS AT RISK

The management of the fetus at risk involves both general practitioner and specialist. The general practitioner, as the primary physician, will encounter or suspect some problems at an early stage and can refer to specialist colleagues for advice on future management.

Management can suitably be divided into preventive and active.

1. Preventive management

The best treatment of any medical condition is prevention, but in obstetrics, as with any other branch of medicine, the ideal state can never be achieved whereby all abnormalities are prevented. We have come a long way, however, over the last few years to diminish the risks, and as our knowledge of genetics increases so too perhaps will our powers of preventing genetically inherited conditions.

Any obstetric history should include previous genetic abnormalities and in suitable cases patients can be referred for genetic couselling. Ideally this should be done before pregnancy. Such an example would be Down's syndrome, the risk of which varies according to maternal age or translocation type. This has been referred to earlier in the chapter.

It is now more important than ever before to encourage our patients to attend for antenatal care at an early stage of pregnancy. Too many still do not contact us until 20 weeks gestation, and this is too late to give them the full advantage of the preventive care now available (Simpson and Walker, 1980). Moreover, those who arrive latest are usually those at greatest risk. It is a great challenge to the primary care team to improve this state of affairs.

The antenatal clinic is a hive of preventive activity in the form of screening procedures. It is important that we all maintain high standards, lest simple things are missed in the early stages of pregnancy and lead to disaster. Thus the first day of the last menstrual period must be established at the earliest opportunity, since patients will inevitably find it more difficult to remember it accurately as time goes on. A standard, routine, physical examination is obligatory at the outset. Urine should be tested at every antenatal visit for albumin and sugar. Urinary and serum oestriols need to be measured during the later stages of pregnancy.

It is most important to take blood specimens at an early stage in pregnancy. Ideally this should be done at the booking clinic by the primary care team, and there should be a regular collection service for transporting the specimens to the hospital laboratory. The delays still experienced all to commonly in securing early hospital appointments for antenatal care are quite indefensible.

Blood can be taken for estimation of haemoglobin, ABO group, rhesus type and antibodies, Wassermann, rubella, toxoplasmosis, cytomegalic inclusion disease, and Guthrie test. As pregnancy continues some of the above can be repeated to detect rising titres. The development of the serum AFP test is discussed below.

Ultrasonics, and occasionally radiology, should be used when indicated. The value of ultrasonics has been shown earlier in this chapter.

Amniocentesis may be performed at a suitable stage in pregnancy if there is any doubt about chromosomal or metabolic disease. As mentioned earlier amniotic fluid can also be used to estimate gestation, monitor rhesus haemolytic disease and predict the respiratory distress syndrome.

Serum alphafetoprotein and neural tube defects

The substantial drop in the number of children born with malformations of the central nervous system over the past decade must be due in part to improved genetic counselling and antenatal care (Figs 9.2, 9.3). There is no doubt that further large reductions are possible if we apply effectively our existing knowledge to the early detection of neural tube defects.

Alphafetoprotein (AFP) is a normal fetal protein capable of being passed into amniotic fluid. Its level rises to a peak at the end of the first trimester and then falls off rapidly. It is produced by the yolk sac and then the liver and is equivalent to the albumen of adult life.

A range for maternal serum alphafetoprotein (AFP) levels has now been established (Leighton *et al*, 1975). Figures above the normal range suggest the presence of a neural tube defect. Leighton and his colleagues were of the opinion that measurement of AFP in maternal blood should become a screening test in all pregnancies. They recommended that the finding of a raised maternal AFP in early pregnancy should lead to the following action:

1. repeat maternal serum AFP, plus review of clinical material to ascertain gestation. If the second AFP is also raised, the next steps should be:
2. ultrasonography to determine fetal number, gestation, and to locate the placenta, and:
3. amniocentesis to determine amniotic AFP; if this is raised then:
4. termination of pregnancy should be considered.

The serum AFP is now measured by radioimmuno assay, normally between the 16th and 18th weeks of pregnancy as recommended by the UK Collaborative Study (1977). Some centres take one serum sample and recommend amniocentesis if the level is raised. Others do two serum AFP before recommending amniocentesis.

The results of a year's screening by serum AFP were published by Woolfson and collaborators (1979). In their Health District of West Berkshire 17 per cent of deliveries and most of the antenatal care was undertaken by general practitioners. In the first year 4458 patients were screened and 43 (0.96 per cent) had raised serum AFP levels. Amniocentesis was performed on 31 patients (0.69 per cent). Ten fetuses with severe neural tube defects and one with exomphalos were detected and the pregnancies terminated. In six patients raised serum AFP was due to fetal death. No normal pregnancy was terminated. Patient acceptability was high. They concluded that maternal serum AFP estimation seemed to be a valuable screening test.

In a recent clinical review Bryan (1979) points out that more than 2000 babies are born each year with neural tube defects and over 90 per cent of these are born to women in whom there is no history of such deformities. Recent research is also showing that high AFP levels in normal pregnancies may be associated with low birth weight infants. The cost of a serum AFP test is currently (1980) about £3, but the cost to the State of an affected child missed during screening is extremely high. The emotional toll of a disabled child or a normal child aborted unnecessarily is incalculable.

In 1979 a working Group of the Standing Medical Advisory Committee, set up under the chairmanship of Sir Douglas Black, issued a report which recommended health authorities that mothers be invited to choose whether they wished to be screened, i.e. 'opting in' rather than 'opting out' (Black, 1979). This would involve GPs closely at the counselling stage.

The problem has been reviewed more recently by Harris (1980), and in a JRCGP editorial (1980).

2. Active management

Inevitably, preventive management fails in a large proportion of cases and a great deal of time is still spent managing such conditions as pre-eclampsia, rhesus isoimmunisation, diabetes mellitus and antepartum haemorrhage. Until we learn more of these conditions their total prevention remains impossible. With the advent of intramuscular Anti-D, however, given to mothers who have developed FMH it should become possible to reduce rhesus isoimmunisation to a minimum.

If a woman has been exposed to rubella in early pregnancy it is now possible to detect her immune status to the virus by a specific antibody titre. A rising titre would indicate clinical infection, whereas a stable titre indicates immunity due to infection in the past. The majority of women are immune to rubella because of past infection, but in the small number who are not, temporary passive immunity can be conferred by intramuscular gamma globulin. If the mother who is not immune to rubella develops a clinical infection, then the risks of fetal abnormality have to be considered. Termination of pregnancy might then be advised if the risk is considered great. The whole issue of management of mothers exposed to rubella in early pregnancy has been reviewed in the RCGP Journal (RCGP Journal Editorial, 1975).

Similarly, multiple pregnancy, malpresentation and unstable lie of the fetus still occur and call for active management by the obstetrician. Any at risk pregnancy should be referred by the general practitioner to a specialist colleague for delivery in hospital.

During pregnancy the active management will consist of serial readings of the various tests outlined, plus the specific treatment of any disease such as diabetes mellitus. Care of the fetus during labour is discussed in Chapter 10.

LOGISTICS OF FETAL CARE

Many of the newer tests available are costly, and their cost must be weighed against their value. In 1974 the figures were as follows: amniocentesis followed by chromosome studies or AFP level estimations cost up to £60 (Laurence, 1974); on the other hand the lifetime cost of an annual cohort of children, whose mental handicap might be attributed to perinatal causes, was estimated at £30 million (Chard, 1974). In England and Wales the initial capital cost for introducing routine maternal serum AFP screening has been estimated by Harris (1980) as £1.7 million, with a recurring revenue cost of £2.2 million.

Should we worry about the cost of amniocentesis, when it is theoretically possible to eliminate Down's syndrome completely by this relatively simple manouvre performed in every pregnancy? (Stein *et al*, 1973).

CONCLUSIONS

The fetus is at risk from conception until delivery, but with an ever increasing knowledge of the feto-maternal unit, and with increasing powers of prevention becoming available, the challenge of reducing the PMR to an acceptable minimum can be met with ever increasing confidence. This is a fast-moving subject, and GPs need to update themselves frequently in both the epidemiological and the clinical aspects of antenatal care, and apply existing knowledge vigorously in their everyday practice, if avoidable fetal damage is to be eliminated.

ACKNOWLEDGMENTS

I am grateful to Dr Marion McPherson for kindly reading through the revised chapter and suggesting many improvements, and to my secretary Mrs Barbara Munton for preparing the typescript with her usual efficiency.

REFERENCES

Andrews, J. & McGarry, J.M. (1972) A community study of smoking in pregnancy. *Journal of Obstetrics and Gynaecology of the British Commonwealth*, **79**, 1057–73.

Bain, D. (1979) Clinical Review – Amniocentesis – Nationwide Screening. *General Practitioner*, 2nd March 1979, 22.

Beischer, N.A., Bhargava, V.L., Brown, J.B. & Smith, M.A. (1968) The incidence and significance of low oestriol excretion in an obstetric population. *Journal of Obstetrics and Gynaecology of the British Commonwealth*, **75**, 1024.

Black, D. (1979) *Report of the Working Group on Screening for Neural Tube Defects*. London: DHSS.

BMJ Editorial (1975) Antenatal diagnosis of spina bifida. *British Medical Journal*, **1**, 44.

BMJ Editorial (1975a) Risks of amniocentesis. *British Medical Journal*, **4**, 485–486.

Brimblecombe, F.S.W. (1979) Rubella, *Update*, **19**, 9, 917–920.

Brock, D.J.H. & Scrimgeour, J.B. (1974) Alphafetoprotein in the prenatal diagnosis of CNS malformations. *Lancet*, **1**, 569.

Bryan J. (1979) Clinical Review – Amniocentesis – AFP screening: A need for great care, *General Practitioner*, 2nd March, 1979, 24.

Butler N. & Alberman, E.D. (1969) *Perinatal Mortality*. Edinburgh: Churchill Livingstone.

Chard, T. (1974) The fetus at risk. *Lancet*, **2**, 880.

Cole, P.V., Hawkins L.H. & Roberts, D. (1972) Smoking during pregnancy and its effects on the fetus. *Journal of Obstetrics and Gynaecology of the British Commonwealth*, **79**, 782.

Cox, C.A., Fox, J.S., Zinkin, P.M. & Matthews, A.E.B. (1976) Critical appraisal of domiciliary obstetrics and neonatal practice. *British Medical Journal*, **1**, 84–86.

Crandon, A.J. (1979) Antenatal diagnosis of fetal abnormality, *Medical News*, Vol. 11, No. 26, 14 and 18.

Crocker, S.G. & Clements, R.V. (1976) Early warning in obstetrics, *Update*, **12**, 831–848.

Donald, I. (1974) New problems in sonar diagnosis in obstetrics and gynaecology. *American Journal of Obstetrics and Gynaecology*, **118**, 299.

Elstein, M., Angus, W., Barker, I. & Dennis, K.J. (1975) The general practitioner-obstetrician – the evolution of his role in the next decade. *Journal of the Royal College of General Practitioners*, **25**, 373–376.

Evans, D.R., Newcombe, R.G., Campbell, H. (1979) Maternal Smoking Habits and congenital malformations: a population study, *British Medical Journal*, **2**, 171–173.

Fogelman, K. (1980) Smoking in pregnancy and subsequent development of the child, *Child Care, Health and Development*, **6**, 233–249.

Gardner, R. (1979) Clinical review – Amniocentesis – weigh up the ethical pros and cons, *General Practitioner*, 2nd March, 1979, 29.

Gluck, L. (1971) Diagnosis of the respiratory distress syndrome by amniocentesis. *American Journal of Obstetrics and Gynaecology*, **109**, 440.

Greenberg, G. & Inman, W.H.W. (1975) Hormonal pregnancy tests and congenital malformations. *British Medical Journal*, **2**, 191–192.

Gregg, H.M. (1941) Congenital cataract following German measles in the mother. *Transactions of the Ophthalmological Society of Australia*, **3**, 35.

Guthrie, R. & Susi, A, (1963) A simple phenylalanine method for detecting phenylketonuria in large populations of newborn infants. *Paediatrics*, **32**, 338.

Harris, R. (1980) Maternal serum alphafetoprotein in pregnancy and the prevention of birth defect, *British Medical Journal*, **280**, 1199–1202.

Harron, D.W.G., Griffiths, K. & Shanks, R.G. (1980) Debenox and congenital malformations in Northern Ireland. *British Medical Journal*, **2**, 1379–1381.

JRCGP Editorial (1980) Screening for Neural Tube Defects. *Journal of the Royal College of General Practitioners*, **30**, 581–2.

King, R.L. (1975) Exposure of girls to oestrogen during fetal development. *Journal of the Royal College of General Practitioners*, **25**, 252–254.

Klopper, A. (1969) *Foetus and Placenta*, p. 471. Oxford: Blackwell.

Landsteiner, K. & Weiner, A.S. (1940) An agglutinable factor in human blood recognised by immune sera for rhesus blood. *Proceedings of the Society for Experimental Biology* (New York), **43**, 223.

Landsteiner, K. & Weiner, A.S. (1941) Studies of an agglutinogen (Rh) in human blood reacting with anti-rhesus sera and with human isoantibodies. *Journal of Experimental Medicine*, **74**, 309.

Laurence, K.M. (1974) Fetal malformations and abnormalities. *Lancet*, **2**, 939.

Laurence, K.M. (1979) Clinical review – Amniocentesis – Prenatal help for at risk parents, *General Practitioner*, 2nd March, 1979, **27**.

Laurence, K.M. et al (1980) Increased risk of recurrence of pregnancies complicated by fetal neural tube defects in mothers receiving poor diets, and possible benefits of dietary counselling *British Medical Journal*, **2**, 1592–1594.

Leighton, P.C., Kitau, M.J. Goulon, Y.B., Leek, A.E. & Chard, T. (1975) Level of alphafetoprotein in maternal blood as a screening test for fetal neural tube defect. *Lancet*, **2**, 1012–1015.

Lind T. (1971) Composition of amniotic fluid and maternal blood through pregnancy. *Journal of Obstetrics and Gynaecology of the British Commonweath*, **78**, 505.

Lloyd. G. (1975) The general practitioner and changes in obstetric practice. *British Medical Journal*, **1**, 79–82.

Milinsky, A., Alpert, E. & Charles, D. (1974) Amniotic fluid alphafetoprotein in anencephaly. *Obstetrics and Gynaecology*, **43**, 592.

Miskin, M. (1974) Use of ultrasound for placental localisation in genetic amniocentesis. *Obstetrics and Gynaecology*, **43**, 872.

Munro, W.L. (1976) A guide to ultrasonics. *The Practitioner*, **216**, 191–208.

Raine, D.N. (1974) Inherited metabolic disease. *Lancet*, **2**, 996.

RCGP Journal Editorial (1975) Rubella in early pregnancy. *Journal of the Royal College of General Practitioners*, **25**, 783–784.

SBF (1980) Perinatal and infant mortality: social and biological factors 1975–1977. Studies in Medical and Population Subjects No. 41. HMSO.

Scrimgeour, J.B. (1979) The challenge of prospective obstetric care. *Mims Magazine*, **12**, 73.

Scrimgeour, J.B. (1980) Early screening for neural tube defects, *Pulse*, **40**, 18, 36–37.

Siegel, M. (1973) Congenital malformations following chickenpox, measles, mumps and hepatitis. *Journal of American Medical Association*, **226**, 1521.

Simpson, Hazel & Walker, G. (1980) When do pregnant women attend for antenatal care? *British Medical Journal* **2**, 104–107

Stein, Z., Susser, & Guterman, A.V. (1973) Screening programme for prevention of Down's syndrome. *Lancet*, **1**, 305.

U.K. Collaborative Study on Alphafetoprotein in relation to neural tube defects (1977), *Lancet*, **1**, 1323.

Valman, H.B. (1979) Amniotic fluid investigations, *British Medical Journal*, **2**, 1272–1273.

Waterson, A.P. (1979) Virus infections (other than rubella) during pregnancy, *British Medical Journal*, **2**, 564–566.

Woolfson, J., Holt, E.M. Whyman, A.E. & Mabbs, D.V. (1979) Maternal alphafetoprotein screening in a Provincial Health District, *British Journal of Obstetrics and Gynaecology*, **86**, 87–90.

Yudkin, S. & Yudkin, G. (1968) Poverty and child development. *Developmental Medicine and Child Neurology*, **10**, 569.

10

Birth trauma

Michael Thirlwall

Birth trauma may be defined as any condition that effects the fetus adversely during labour or delivery (Potter, 1961). It can be subdivided into trauma due to mechanical factors and trauma due to hypoxia.

MECHANICAL FACTORS

1. *Caput succedaneum*. A localised scalp oedema which is commonly seen – especially in prolonged labours and often in association with moulding of the skull bones. Although alarming in appearance it usually settles rapidly over 48 to 72 hours post partum with no need for intervention. It needs to be distinguished from cephalhaematoma.

2. *Cephalhaematoma*. This is due to subperiosteal bleeding in the fetal skull bones and its edges are demarcated by the periosteal attachments and therefore it does not cross suture lines (unlike caput succedaneum). It is seen more commonly after instrumental deliveries and also in larger babies. The incidence is said to be between 0.4 and 2.5 per cent of all deliveries. Usually the haematoma is small and occurs most frequently over the parietal bones. Most will settle spontaneously after a few days. A few are large enough to cause neonatal anaemia. They may become infected, particularly in the presence of scalp abrasions or lacerations. About 10 per cent are associated with underlying skull fractures and thus a skull X-ray is worthwhile (Gresham, 1975). Happily most of these fractures need no intervention either.

3. *Minor scalp lacerations*. These are commonly associated with artificial rupture of membranes, instrumental deliveries, fetal scalp electrode appliation or fetal scalp blood sampling, and require standard minor wound toilet only.

4. *Miscellaneous birth injuries*. Under this heading we include fractures of clavicle or humerus, brachial plexus or spinal cord damage, and even amputation of digits. The commonest of these was fracture of the clavicle in one series (Rubin, 1964) and at an incidence of one in 400 deliveries the average GP is very unlikely to encounter many of these rarer problems in his obstetric career. Most of them will become apparent during routine examination of the newborn and will require referral.

HYPOXIA

This is the most important subdivision of birth trauma and is implicated in the pathogenesis of fetal/neonatal brain damage leading to cerebral dysfunction in later life. The three commonest dysfunctions are cerebral palsy, mental retardation and epilepsy (some authors would also include psychopathy). The association between neonatal brain damage and the subsequent development of neurological problems has been recognised in scientific writings for over 100 years.

Towbin (1978), reporting a study of 50 000 pregnancies, outlined five basic concepts which emerged from this research:

1. Hypoxia is the commonest cause of cerebral damage in the fetus and neonate
2. There are two basic forms of perinatal brain damage
   a. *deep cerebral damage* – most commonly seen in the premature fetus
   b. *cortical cerebral damage* – occurring mainly in the mature fetus at term
3. The origin of brain damage is far more commonly due to prenatal factors than to damage occurring during delivery
4. Acute cerebral lesions found in hypoxia affecting the fetus/neonate correlate with the chronic lesions found in the brains of children or adults suffering from mental retardation, cerebral palsy and related cerebral dysfunctions
5. The severity of the brain damage is related to the severity and duration of the hypoxic 'insult'.

According to Whitelaw (1980), the sequence of events in hypoxic brain damage appears to be:

Partial hypoxia
↓
Cerebral oedema
↓
Raised intracranial pressure
↓
Reduced cerebral perfusion
↓
Prolonged cerebral ischaemia

The concept of birth trauma causing brain damage has been thoroughly reviewed by Illingworth (1979). In recent years publicity has been given to the idea that most cases of cerebral palsy and mental retardation have occurred by default – i.e. that lack of resources and consequent failure to apply obstetric/neonatal high technology have been responsible for many 'brain damaged' children (Spastics Society publications; Select Committee Report, 1980). According to Illingworth this would appear to be superficial thinking and he quotes several papers to support this argument. Penrose (1938) in a study of 1280 mentally defective patients found only 11 cases where their physical condition allied to their birth history warranted a diagnosis of birth injury as the main cause. Perlstein (1952) wrote that faulty obstetric practice was now considered by some authorities to account for only three to five per cent of 'birth injury'. Amiel-Tison (1969) followed up 41 children with clear histories of traumatic deliveries and found none with cerebral palsy.

From Illingworth's review it seems much more likely that prenatal factors such as prematurity, dysmaturity, congenital abnormalities, lower social class, and bleeding in pregnancy will adversely affect the subsequent physical and neurological development of the child. McBride et al (1979) concluded that, in the absence of other complicating events (e.g. poor antenatal history, prematurity, disorganised home environment), the method of delivery (comparing low cavity forceps to mid cavity forceps to manual rotation with forceps to elective Caesarian section to normal vaginal delivery) constituted an early risk factor which the young child was able to overcome.

It would seem then that the major contribution we can make to reduction in perinatal morbidity and subsequent cerebral dysfunction lies in vigilant and competent antenatal care – identifying the 'high risk pregnancy' and enlisting specialist help at an early stage. These factors have been dealt with in Chapter 9. However, there is still much to contribute during labour and delivery.

When the mother is admitted in labour the opportunity should be taken to review her antenatal record with the midwife. Evidence of prematurity or dysmaturity or any of the adverse prenatal factors outlined above should signal early transfer to specialist care where facilities for dealing with such high risk deliveries are concentrated. Her general condition should be assessed, including her mental state, state of hydration, temperature, pulse, blood pressure, and urinalysis (for sugar, protein and ketones). Her abdomen should be palpated to exclude malpresentation and a baseline fetal heart rate recorded. Pelvic examination will reveal the degree of cervical dilatation and the integrity or otherwise of the membranes. Where there is a history of ruptured membranes, cord prolapse should be excluded – a rare but potentially reversible cause of acute hypoxic stress to the fetus.

All being well, the labour will proceed and then the main task is to monitor the well being of the fetus and the progress of the labour. As yet we have no foolproof indices of fetal well being. We rely on three signs: the fetal heart rate (FHR – measured either intermittently or continuously), the state of the liquor (presence or absence of meconium), and fetal scalp blood sampling. Only the first two are commonly used by GPs.

FETAL HEART RATE

The FHR should normally be between 120 and 160 beats per minute. It is monitored in four main ways:

1. Intermittently
   a. traditional fetal stethoscope
   b. Sonicaid amplifier
2. Continuously
   a. cardiotocograph
   ±b. fetal scalp ECG.

The continuous methods are the province of the specialist units, though it is possible that with the rapid advance of microelectronics these machines may become cheaper and more available. Meanwhile, most GPs will rely on the intermittent methods.

The FHR can normally vary by 5 to 15 beats from minute to minute ('beat-to-beat' variation). Accelerations of FHR are sometimes heard during contractions and are probably a normal response to transient hypoxia. Decelerations of FHR are of more significance and are caused by (1) head compression – as it passes through the brim, (2) cord compression or (3) uteroplacental insufficiency. *Early* decelerations – occurring with the contraction and speeding up as the contraction goes – are of little significance unless the deceleration is marked (i.e. below 100 beats per minutes). *Late* decelerations – occurring towards the end of the contraction and only picking up between contractions – are thought to be of more significance and indicative of fetal myocardial depression. Late decelerations correlate with fetal hypoxia and acidosis. It is possible to recognise these changes with intermittent auscultation but they are much more accurately displayed on cardiotocographic traces. The early decelerations show up as 'Type I' dips in FHR and the later decelerations as 'Type II' dips. Also these continuous traces can show loss of normal 'beat-to-beat' variation associated with fetal hypoxia (and also with certain drugs, e.g. diazepam, given to mother).

THE STATE OF THE LIQUOR

Meconium staining of the liquor is a time honoured sign of probable fetal distress – 'no death without defaecation'. It is thought that when the fetus is subjected to hypoxic stress there is a reflex evacuation of the bowel. The weight given to this sign has varied over the years but a recent paper by Meis *et al* (1978) suggests a useful classification. They suggest that early, heavy meconium staining (likened to 'pea-soup') is associated with low Apgar scores (for the Apgar score, see Ch. 25). Late meconium staining of liquor is associated with prolonged labour. Clear liquor with only vernix mixed with it is a fairly reliable index of a healthy, unstressed fetus.

FETAL SCALP BLOOD SAMPLING

This is again a specialist technique used to measure arterial pH but worthy of brief mention. A pH of greater than 7.26 is normal. Between pH 7.20 and pH 7.26 close monitoring of labour is required, with further sampling at 30 or 60 minutes. A pH of less than 7.20 represents severe acidosis/hypoxia and signals the need for urgent delivery.

LENGTH OF LABOUR

Over the past 50 years thinking has changed over what constitutes unduly prolonged labour. In my own copy of Donald's *Practical Obstetric Problems*, published in 1969, a prolonged labour for a primigravida is defined as one exceeding 48 hours and for a multigravida one exceeding 24 hours. Four years later O'Driscoll proposed active management of labour with operative intervention if the labour was exceeding 12 hours. Plotting cervical dilatation against time, labour was accelerated if cervical dilatation failed to exceed one centimetre per hour. Such 'aggressive' management is not universally approved nor practised but it seems to me to offer reasonable guidelines for the GP in attempting to evaluate normal progress in established labour and to identify those labours which may need specialist intervention.

It is widely accepted that the second stage of labour should not exceed one hour for a primigravida and half an hour for a multigravida. It may well be that these figures can be cautiously exceeded if all parameters (e.g. maternal condition, FHR, liquor, etc.) are favourable. However, if they are being exceeded the situation should be reviewed and reasons sought for the delay (e.g. malpresentation, maternal exhaustion, full bladder/rectum, etc.). Specialist help should be sought unless delivery can be safely expedited by episiotomy or low cavity forceps delivery (if the latter is within one's competence).

Length of time in labour following rupture of membranes must also be monitored. It is well established that fetal morbidity and mortality increases with increase in the length of time the membranes have been ruptured. In our unit, transfer for acceleration of labour is advised if the mother is not in strong, established labour more than eight hours following rupture of membranes. It is as well to check that the liquor is coming from a forewater rupture rather than the less worrying hindwater leak. Maternal temperature should be checked regularly in labour as a rise might signify infection of the liquor.

USE OF DRUGS IN LABOUR

One likes to think that one prescribes with care at all times but this should be especially so in labour, as so many drugs in common use cross the placenta and have adverse effects on the fetus. In my experience there is little reason to administer any drugs other than analgesics in GP obstetrics.

Analgesics

Pethidine remains the drug of choice in labour analgesia. Some authorities recommend a test dose of 50 mg IM early in labour to assess maternal response. Routinely we would use 100 mg when the mother becomes distressed with contractions. However, the extent of cervical dilatation should always be assessed prior to the administration of pethidine. If delivery seems likely within the next four hours one should hold off using any further pethidine, because of the risk of neonatal respiratory depression – even though this can be mitigated by the use of naloxone given to the neonate post-delivery. It should rarely be necessary to exceed 200–300 mg of pethidine in a normal labour – if these figures are exceeded there is a need to review management and reassess the need for specialist help. Pethilorfan (a combination of pethidine and levallorphan – a narcotic antagonist) is used still in the belief that levallorphan reduces neonatal respiratory depression. There is little evidence that this is so.

Sedatives

Sparine (promazine) is commonly used to enhance the analgesic effect of pethidine. However, it is known to cause fetal/neonatal tachycardia and should be used as little as possible.

Valium (diazepam) is also used for its sedative action but is associated with neonatal hypotonia and impaired neonatal response to cold stress. Thus it has no place in GP managed labours.

Uterine stimulants

Syntocinon by nasal spray or intravenously may be used to accelerate labour in GP units. Intravenous Syntocinon should only be used where one can be confident that the standard of supervision of the drip will be high. Syntocinon should never be used in the presence of signs of fetal distress as it may worsen the hypoxic stress on the fetus.

Inhaled drugs

Turning the mother on her side and administering 100 per cent oxygen by mask has been advocated as a 'first aid' measure in first stage fetal distress. There is little evidence that it is effective.

Last but not least comes Entonox (nitrous oxide and oxygen in a 50/50 mixture) which is inhaled by mother from the Entonox apparatus. This provides valuable, safe 'topping up' analgesia in the late first stage and second stage of labour. It is wise to supervise intake, as excessive use is inclined to make mother rather intoxicated and less co-operative. However, there are no adverse fetal or neonatal effects.

Our conclusions so far, are summarised in Table 10.1.

Table 10.1 Summary of management of labour

1. *Early labour*
   check maternal factors:
   - general condition
   - urinalysis: sugar
     - protein
     - ketones
     - temperature/pulse/respirations (T/P/R)
     - blood pressure
     - integrity of membranes

   check fetal factors:
   - ? premature
   - ?dysmature
   - presentation (beware the undiagnosed breech)
   - FHR

2. *If abnormal*
   transfer to specialist care *early*

3. *If normal, monitor*
   maternal conditions: T/P/R, BP etc.
   contractions: frequency, duration, strength
   cervical dilatation (look for greater than 1 cm/hour)
   rate of descent of presenting part
   duration of labour following rupture of membranes (beware if more than 8 hours and still not in established labour)
   FHR:
   - 120–160 beats/min
   - pattern of response to contractions

   ? ± meconium – beware 'pea soup'
   length of 2nd stage:
   - 1 hour primigravida
   - ½ hour multigravida

   use drugs with care

4. *If normal*
   proceed to normal delivery

5. *If abnormal* (e.g. FHR ↑ or ↓, meconium stained liquor etc.)
   is delivery possible with aid of episiotomy or low cavity forceps (if within one's competence)?
   NO? → specialist care

The timing of and necessity for a request for specialist help depends on all the above factors. I believe GP obstetrics should be conducted in purpose-built units adjacent to specialist units. However, many units are geographically distant from specialist centres and the number of home confinements, though small at present, may well increase in coming years. Where the GP unit is adjacent to the specialist unit, one might reasonably 'hang on' in the presence of minor, transient abormalities (e.g. a prolonged second stage, or slight variations of the FHR outside normal range) if delivery seems imminent. In the home or a distant GP unit it is advisable to enlist specialist help *early* in labour even in the presence of minor abnormalities – far better to have a nice, normal delivery following early transfer than a nerve-wracking flying squad call after a failed forceps in the presence of mounting fetal distress.

Central to the safe, efficient management of labour is a sound working relationship with the practice midwife and the midwifery staff in the local GP unit. Decisions are far better taken in consultation – the relationship should be one of partnership rather than the traditional hierarchical doctor/nurse type. Time and again I have been grateful for the wise counsel of the midwives I have worked with. One should be realistic about what is within the competence of this partnership. For instance, are you prepared to perform forceps deliveries if necessary? If not, it is far better to be honest and have a clear policy for transfer if the need should arise for one.

In the fiscal year 1978–1979 approximately 25 per cent of the total paid in fees for the provision of maternity services were in respect of cases in which GPs provided complete care (Young, 1979). Taking into account those claims for partial care which included care during delivery, one surmises that GPs claimed for attendance at confinement in approximately one third of all booked cases. In a review by Barry (1980), the proportion of confinements attended by GPs in several repeated series varied from 18 to 92 per cent. In our own GP unit the figures are towards the lower end of this range (20 per cent). It would seem therefore that, as in other areas of medicine, GPs vary widely in their attitudes and behaviour towards the need for attending their booked cases in GP units and at home. It seems that other practice work often takes precedence over maternity work. I feel that this is a regrettable trend. I would suggest that it should be standard practice that GPs should be informed of the admission of their patients in labour and that the patient should be assessed early in labour. Ideally this should be by a visit, or at least by discussion with the attending midwife. The GP should again be informed when the patient is approaching full dilatation (it is usually possible to assess this stage) and he or she should then make every effort to be in attendance during the second and third stages of the confinement. It is likely that a completely normal delivery will be completed by the midwife and that all that will be required of the GP will be the repair of the episiotomy. However, we must be on hand to expedite delivery by forceps if necessary, to assess the need for specialist care in complicated labours, and to resuscitate the neonate if required.

It is apparent that we are letting our role in the management of labour wither away slowly by default. It is inadequate to await a request to attend only if problems arise – by that time it may well be too late to help. We should anticipate crises by being present during the confinement. If the Select Committee's recommendations are implemented, many GPs will have their responsibility for their pregnant patients severely restricted; we will have only ourselves to blame.

REFERENCES

Amiel-Tison C. (1969) *Biologia Neonatorum*, **14**, 234.

Barry C.N. (1980) Home versus hospital confinement. *Journal of RCGP* 105.

Donald, I. (1969) Practical obstetric problems, p. 504, 4th edn. London: Lloyd Luke.

Gresham, E.L. (1975) Birth trauma. *Paediatric Clinics of N. America*, **22**, 319.

Illingworth, R.S. (1979) Why blame the obstetrician? *British Medical Journal*, **1**, 797–801.

McBride W.G. et al (1979) Method of delivery and developmental outcome at first year of age. *The Medical Journal of Australia*. April 21, 301–304.

Meis et al (1978) Meconium passage. New classification for risk assessment during labour. *American Journal of Obstetrics Gynaecology* **131** 509–513.

O'Driscoll et al (1973) Active management of labour. *British Medical Journal*, **2**, 135–137.

Penrose L. (1938) A clinical and genetic study of 1280 cases of mental defect. Special report series of MRC (London) No. 229. HMSO.

Perlstein M. (1952) *Journal of American Medical Association*, **149**, 30.

Potter, E.L. (1961) *Pathology of the Fetus and Infant*, 2nd edn. Chicago: Year Book Medical Publishers.

Rubin, A. (1964) Birth injuries: incidence, mechanisms, and end results. *Obstetrics and Gynaecology*, **23**, 218.

Select Committee Report (1980) Report of House of Commons select committee on perinatal mortality. HMSO.

Towbin, A. (1978) Cerebral dysfunctions related to perinatal organic damage: clinical – Neuropathologic correlations. *Journal of Abnormal Psychology*, **87**, 617–635.

Whitelaw, A. (1980) Prevention of handicap by improved perinatal care. *Update*, **15** June, 1505–1520.

Young, Sir George (1979) (Junior Health Minister) Parliamentary Reply.

11

Immunisation

Douglas Jenkinson

Immunisation has always been controversial. For example, in 1853 smallpox vaccination was made compulsory, and although the smallpox prevention programme had considerable success, anti-vaccination groups created vociferous opposition. Now more than 120 years later there is still controversy. Considerable effort is still required to persuade the public of the need for immunisation.

Passive immunisation was practical against some diseases at the end of the last century, but the elements of our present programme involving active immunisation only came with the use of diphtheria toxoid between the wars, and tetanus toxoid during the last war. Tuberculosis, whooping cough, poliomyelitis, measles and rubella have now been added to the list and recommended as public policy. This policy underpins the reduced prevalence of these diseases, but it is presently threatened by changes in public attitudes which those involved in immunisation should understand.

When serious diseases such as smallpox, poliomyelitis and diphtheria were common, the advantage of immunity was quite clear. The threat to the individual or the community was great and seen to be so. Even moderate risks associated with immunisation could be accepted. Nevertheless, the balance has to weigh fairly heavily in favour of immunisation before people will trade the possible risk of getting the disease for the risks of deliberate immunisation.

The folk-memory of infectious diseases, which has provided the momentum for immunisation for previous generations, is fading also. The contemporary parent has heard of vaccine-damaged children but may never have heard a whoop. It is difficult for them to appreciate that the benefits of immunisation must be weighed against the risks they will run in an unimmunised population. They are living in a disease free community, where vaccine problems are conspicuous because of the large numbers involved, and the risks are less readily accepted because there is only a possibility of future disease. The advantages to patients of immunisation against relatively trivial diseases such as measles, or rarely encountered diseases such as congenital rubella, are even less obvious.

From the medical point of view, immunisation is one of the most successful measures. Doctors have received the accolades which have resulted from these successes and included more and more diseases within the vaccine repertoire. Past victories against smallpox and poliomyelitis have led to skirmishes with rubella and measles. The public has generally been ready to go along with these measures because of confidence in the profession, and the profession has accepted the innovations because the community benefits have been quite clear. Public attitudes to immunisation have, however, changed. There has been an erosion of the status of the profession and a greater readiness and ability of patients to question accepted procedures and make their own decisions. The benefits of some immunisations such as whooping cough, measles and BCG are being seriously questioned within the profession, and knowledge of this may reach the patient directly, or indirectly via the doctor's attitude. The realisation, however, that serious illness may occasionally result from immunisation has probably made the greatest impact.

Our present consumer-conscious society has allowed a critical airing by the media of some immunisation procedures, particularly those against whooping cough, to flourish, and immunisation against this disease has consequently fallen. It is clear that some sections of the public regard the media as the protector of the public interest, and it has probably had considerably greater effect on public attitudes to immunisation over the last few years than the medical profession. The revelation of possible brain damage associated with pertussis immunisation and doubts about its efficacy have led to a feeling amongst the public of being deceived, and the penalty has been a reduction in immunisations other than pertussis. The public has shown that it does not expect decisions to be taken on its behalf without frankness about the facts.

Another major public concern to emerge from the pertussis problem is that of compensation for vaccine damaged children. Natural justice would suggest that these children, immunised in the public interest, should be given some recompense from the public purse. Recent legislation has made this possible, but it is still far from satisfactory (Ch. 3). The rights of the individual have grown in relation to the rights of the community, a relationship that is of critical importance to many decisions about immunisation. The reluctance to subject a precious child to a slight risk for the public good is another reason for a low immunisation rate.

If immunisation rates are to be kept at an effective level, those involved with immunisation should try to meet the problems. The profession should be seen to be updating its recommendations with the changing pattern of infectious disease. Existing vaccines may be improved, the effects for good and ill monitored, and support given for adequate compensation for those damaged by vaccine.

It is reassuring for doctors to know that in spite of uncertainties patients still look to general practitioners for guidance on immunisation. Advice when given should be accurate, up to date and consistent. It is sad, but true, that many children are unimmunised because of imaginary contraindications. This denies them benefit and reduces in the parents' eyes the credibility of the doctors involved.

Advice about immunisation policy is the responsibility of the Chief Medical Officer of the DHSS, who is advised by the Joint Standing Committee on Vaccination and Immunisation. The committee is made up of experts from all branches of medicine related to infectious diseases and community health. The DHSS publishes a booklet describing immunisation policy, which is constantly updated by the issue of circulars to all involved personnel (DHSS, 1980). Doctors can be sure that information from this source provides a sound guide to current immunisation practice.

Immunisation is just as important now as it ever was. When the immunisation rate falls then the disease recurs. The seriousness of some diseases such as whooping cough may be diminished, and others such as tuberculosis may be declining, but the trend towards smaller families makes the occasional tragedy all the greater. Although the media have done much to exacerbate our present difficulties, we should be prepared to let the same techniques be used to advance the case of immunisation. We have a responsibility to 'sell' immunisation if we expect people to opt for it (Jones, 1980).

ORGANISATION FOR IMMUNISATION

The success of an immunisation programme can be judged by the immunisation rate, ideally 100 per cent, but rarely achieved. An immunisation service is offered by AHA child health clinics and school medical service, or by general practitioners. Health authority clinics are staffed by clinical medical officers who advise and immunise with the help of clinic nurses or health visitors. The records are derived from health visiting or school medical records and the organisation allows an efficient call-up and recall postal system to operate, either manually or by computer.

There is an increasing trend towards the incorporation of immunisation and developmental surveillance into practice-based child health clinics run by general practitioners. The increasing emphasis on primary prevention, with the GP taking on this role, coupled with the attitude of the Court report (1976), has given increased momentum to this trend. Immunisation thus becomes part of the whole person care that general practice seeks to achieve.

The advantages of immunisation by the family doctor are many. Provided the doctor is motivated and invests a little time, a far higher rate of immunisation can be achieved. It is probably easier for parents to discuss doubts about their child's immunisation with a familiar doctor and more difficult to default from him, as treatment may be needed in the future. The importance the general practitioner is seen to attach to immunisation also provides a useful lesson when he is seen as a preventer rather than a prescriber.

The average GP will have about 30 babies born into his practice each year. Five immunisation episodes per child are usually required in the first five years, which means about 150 procedures per year, per GP. Six special immunising sessions per year will cope with this number adequately, but a four-man practice with a high birth rate would need 12 to 15 sessions, efficiently organised, in order to keep the business civilised.

Most large practices find a special session necessary but may delegate the work to a suitably trained nurse or health visitor. Some doctors choose to do the first immunisation themselves, for the sake of public relations or to check for contraindications, and others may just be available in case of problems. It can be combined with a regular developmental surveillance clinic held more frequently, so that the number per session is less, the health visitor immunising while the doctor does the surveillance. Immunisation can be carried out during a regular surgery, and combined with developmental surveillance if appropriate ages are chosen. Single handed doctors may find this most appealing, especially if ancillary help is not available.

Parental motivation has to be high to achieve a satisfactory immunisation rate. Even when smallpox vaccination was compulsory, the rate was never higher than 76 per cent and 60 to 70 per cent seems to be the general level for polio or diphtheria and tetanus in many areas. The variability of the rate is striking, from 30 per cent in some areas to almost 100 per cent achieved by many practices for non-controversial immunisations.

To obtain a high immunisation rate the action must be continuous. This requires an attitude of expectation of immunisation in the practice, whose foundations are laid during the first pregnancy. Primagravid mothers are prevention minded, and immunisation should be discussed in the antenatal clinic with a health visitor if possible. Efforts to increase immunisation are most profitably directed towards the firstborn, as subsequent babies are likely to be immunised similarly.

The health visitor should discuss immunisation at the first home visit and obtain written consent. Doubts can be discussed and the practice policy explained. A specially prepared leaflet explaining the need for immunisation, the contraindications and reactions, given at the same time can be very useful, and can also be available at immunising sessions.

A GP organising his own sessions needs to use a recording system which is accurate and sensitive to default. There are several alternatives.

The health visiting record (HV1) can be used to record immunisation details and filed according to date of birth. A search then quickly reveals omissions.

An index card or FP73 record form can be filled out at the same time as the birth notification is received and filed according to the date the first immunisation is due. When the first is done it is refiled according to the date of the next, so that defaulters are brought to the front of the file automatically.

Standard MRE or alternative systems can be used but need to be checked against an accurate age-sex register to detect defaulters.

The simplest way is to keep a book of births and transfers-in, with a column for each immunisation or routine check. These can be marked off as each is done, either at the time, or from another recording system retrospectively. Each practice method will vary according to local needs and conditions. Appointment reminder cards are usually needed, either issued at clinics or posted. The latter is expensive but may be the best way of chasing up defaulters.

It is important that all pertinent information is available to the immuniser. The immunisation record should indicate which immunisations are consented to, any contradicting factors, the date given and the batch number. As soon as a contraindication is known, the parents should be told and the details recorded in the medical and immunisation record. It is inefficient and slow to enquire individually in the clinic, but this must be done if there is any doubt. A reliable recording system and a full explanation to parents using leaflets helps to avoid problems and eliminates the counterproductive practice of omitting an immunisation because there is uncertainty. There are a few real contraindications to immunisation, so it does not make great demands on organisation.

The health visitor plays a key role. On her falls the responsibility of enquiring after habitual defaulters, home-visiting if necessary to find the reason and when possible, to remedy it. It is essential that she and the doctor speak with one voice and pursue an agreed policy. The greater her and the doctor's enthusiasm the more difficult it is to default through apathy. The suggestion that the doctor will call at home to immunise the children if they are not brought to the clinic is often effective, and doesn't usually increase the number of such visits. The health visitor or nurse may occasionally immunise in the home when judged prudent. Special measures may be necessary in areas with a high immigrant population, such as multilingual information leaflets. The combination of language and cultural barriers may inhibit clinic attendance. A health visitor from a similar background speaking the same language might be an impossible luxury, but there is scope for local ingenuity to adapt to the community needs.

A simple audit is achieved by calculating the percentage immunised against a particular disease in any one year. This can be compared with the rate for the district, obtainable from the community physician.

Payment for GP immunisation is claimed on form FP73, which is also the record which is forwarded at present (1980) to the AHA. Courses should preferably be completed before claiming. A high rate is paid for the first two of a course and a low rate for third or reinforcing doses. Combined vaccines like DTP count as one, but polio is counted separately even though given simultaneously. Only public policy immunisations can be claimed for.

Vaccines will often be supplied by the AHA. Otherwise an FP10 should be made out for each person for the vaccine provided (the reverse should be left blank) and forwarded monthly with an FP34 claim form to the FPC. The cost of the vaccine plus a small percentage is refunded. Vaccines would normally then be obtained from a drug wholesaler or direct from a manufacturer.

Patients should be provided with a record of immunisation and encouraged to keep it. Immunisation records frequently go astray, especially when lying loose within an MRE. This information can often be retrieved from the AHA which keeps records for many years.

Immunisations during school years are usually done by the school health service. This would seem most appropriate since the immunisation rate should be high in a captive population. The GP should be notified of immunisations carried out at school so that defaulters can be followed up if desired.

Table 11.1 Basic immunisation

	Polio	*Tetanus*	*Diphtheria*	*Pertussis*	*Measles*	*Rubella*	*BCG*
Age	3 months	5 years (school entry) 15 years (or school leaving)	5 months	10 months	15 months	11 to 13 years	11 to 13 years
Specific Contra-indications	Immunological deficiency. First four months of pregnancy	None	None	Personal history of fits or neonatal cerebral irritation. Close family history of fits, C.N.S. disease. Untoward reaction to previous dose to this vaccine. Inter – current illness present or likely	Immunological deficiency. Hypersensitivity to antibiotics in vaccine	Immunological deficiency Pregnancy. Suspected pregnancy Thrombocytopaenia. Hypersensitivity to antibiotics in vaccine.	Immunological deficiency
Notes	May be ineffective in presence of diarrhoea or enterovirus infection. Small quantities of antibiotics present in vaccine, including penicillin. Take care in presence of severe hypersensitivity. History of penicillin rash alone is not a contraindication Consider IPV if OPV contra – indicated. Immunise unimmunised parents simultaneously	Nodule at injection site is of no significance	Nodule at injection site is of no significance	Nodule at injection site is of no significance Allergy is irrelevant.	Chronic debilitating illness, especially cardio-pulmonary or increased risk from reactions, requires simultaneous administration of human measles gamma globulin. Also consider delay and/or anticonvulsant prophylaxis if increased risk of fitting.	Subcutaneous only Females only. No need to establish immune status at this age.	Heaf test first. Immunise negative reactors only.

IMMUNISATION PROCEDURES

We are concerned in this chapter with basic immunisation. Procedures for those going overseas are not therefore discussed, nor is immunisation for influenza (Ch. 20) or mumps (Ch. 22).

A schedule of basic immunisation is shown in the Table 11.1. This is applicable to all children in the United Kingdom. The usual sites for injection are over or into the upper deltoid, the upper and outer quadrant of the buttock, or the lateral thigh. I prefer the deltoid in older children and the buttock in infants. Polio vaccine is given in syrup off a spoon or on a sugar lump. Cleansing the skin is traditional though probably ineffective. The skin must be dry before injecting live vaccine.

Mothers should be encouraged to hold their own babies, but some are squeamish and prefer somebody else to do it. In older children, parental trepidation is quickly mirrored by the child and one howl is infectious. The behaviour of parent and child in this situation often gives a valuable insight into the relationship. Polio vaccine can be given to infants when they open their mouth to yell after the injection. This saves time which is important, since the sooner the whole unpleasant procedure is over the better.

General precautions

It is important to understand the rationale for contraindications and precautions, so that balanced judgements can be made. There are few absolute contraindications, most are relative and the balance of risk must be evaluated. Some contraindications are theoretical and built into the product licence without scientific validation. Many precautions advised are in case of reactions that must be excessively rare or theoretical and are included more to protect the manufacturer from litigation than to guide the doctor. Advice urging caution where there is a history of allergy for example is singularly unhelpful. Immunisations are frequently omitted unnecessarily when there is the slightest history of hay fever, asthma, eczema, penicillin rash, or sometimes if there is a family history of these things. The correct response is to weigh the risks of immunising against the risks of not immunising and the latter is usually greater.

Specific contraindications to vaccines are discussed individually, but some general principles apply to all. Only well children should be immunised since any subsequent deterioration might be blamed on the vaccine, and a true reaction may be aggravated by an intercurrent illness. Snuffles that have been going on for some time in an otherwise well baby do not matter. If there is doubt postpone. A rectal temperature will solve some doubts. Live vaccine should not be given when there is immunological impairment as in leukaemia, Hodgkin's disease, immunosuppressive or cytotoxic therapy, or when therapeutic doses of corticosteroids are being used.

Many vaccines cause slight systemic or local upset which may be regarded as normal. Severe general reactions should be regarded as contraindicating further doses of that vaccine. If this occurred after DTP and polio, it would be reasonable to continue with DT and polio only.

Prematurity should be compensated for when timing immunisation.

Very rarely an immediate allergic reaction occurs after immunisation. Adrenalin 1 in 1000 should always be available for subcutaneous injection (taking care that it is not date expired) in a dose of 0.1 ml to 0.5 ml according to the size of the child.

Unusual, severe or unexpected reactions should be reported to the Committee on Safety of Medicines on a yellow card.

The correct potency of some vaccines depends on correct storage conditions, and some live vaccines are rapidly inactivated at normal temperatures, and by light when reconstituted. Manufacturers' instructions should be carefully observed.

Diphtheria

Between the wars diphtheria killed thousands of children every year in the UK. Widespread immunisation, commenced in 1941, has virtually eliminated the disease. The vaccine contains inactivated toxoid usually with a mineral adjuvant. It is usually combined with tetanus toxoid (DT) and pertussis (DTP). Three doses are required, with six to eight weeks between the first two and four to six months between the second two. A reinforcing dose at school entry is necessary, and this provides sufficient lasting immunity to protect the adult population amongst whom infectivity is low anyway.

Outbreaks nowadays usually occur in residential children's homes, so staff and children should always be immunised. Schick testing to determine immune status should always be done in children over the age of 10 years as pre-existing immunity can cause unpleasant reactions (Bainton *et al*, 1979). Plain vaccine is preferred for the same reason in this age group, for first and reinforcing doses.

There are no specific contraindications. Mild fever or malaise may occur in the first 24 hours. A nodule at the injection site due to the adjuvant is common and may persist for weeks. It has no significance.

There is some evidence of a recent drop in immunisation rates against diphtheria, concurrent with the much larger drop in pertussis immunisation (Fig. 11.1). However, overall between 70 per cent and 80 per cent of children are currently immunised. This is sufficient to keep the disease at bay because of herd immunity.

Tetanus

Immunisation is beneficial only to the individual. It provides a basic immunity which can be boosted as necessary throughout life, either in response to time lapse since previous immunisation or the occurrence of a wound suspected of being contaminated by tetanus. Three injections of adjuvenated toxoid at intervals of six to eight weeks and four to six months are required, usually in DT or DTP. Reinforcing doses are advised at school entry (usually as DT), at school leaving (alone or with polio), and every ten years thereafter.

There are no specific contraindications. Mild reactions as with diphtheria toxoid may occur as may some local tenderness. After repeated boosters, reactions become more common and occasionally a severe local (Arthus) reaction may occur or even frank serum sickness about ten days later. If a severe reaction has previously occurred and immunity is considered inadequate, intradermal plain vaccine should be used.

Whooping cough

Between the wars the case fatality rate from whooping cough was about one per cent and there was considerable permanent morbidity. Eighty to 150 thousand cases were notified each year. Vaccines were developed early in the century and were in use in the 1920s. There was considerable variation between vaccines, but in the main, controlled trials demonstrated considerable protection against the disease and reduced severity in the immunised.

Official approval for immunisation compaigns by local authorities came in 1942 with the start of the diphtheria programme, and by 1951 more than half the authorities were offering whooping cough immunisation in addition. By 1957, only ten of the 126 local authorities in England and Wales were not offering it. Financial support for whooping cough immunisation was promised by the Ministry of Health provided numbers were produced. Hence, official figures for whooping cough immunisation only start in 1957 although immunisation commenced, and notifications started to fall, before this time (Griffith, 1979).

The number of notified cases of whooping cough fell as 70 to 80 per cent of children accepted immunisation, and until the mid seventies varied between 2000 and 20 000 a year with peaks every three or four years (Fig. 11.1). The case fatality rate started to fall dramatically in the late forties, to reach the 0.1 per cent which has prevailed for two decades.

As a result of adverse publicity about the efficacy and safety of the vaccine in the early seventies, the immunisation rate started to fall, and by 1978 only 31 per cent of children were being immunised overall, dropping to 22 per cent or less in some conurbations (Fig. 11.2). The existence of a large number of unprotected children led to fears that the next outbreak would be more severe, and indeed, the outbreak that occurred in 1977–8 led to over 83 000 notifications, the highest for over 20 years, although the case fatality rate fell to 0.02 per cent. The effect of the outbreak on one large community has been well reported (RCGP, 1981; Roberts and Williams, 1981).

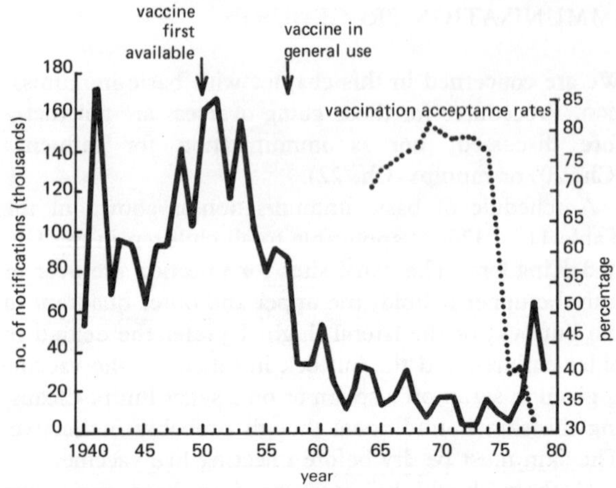

Fig. 11.1 Annual notification of whooping cough in England and Wales 1940–1979, and vaccination acceptance rates 1964–1979. Source: Galbraith *et al*, 1980

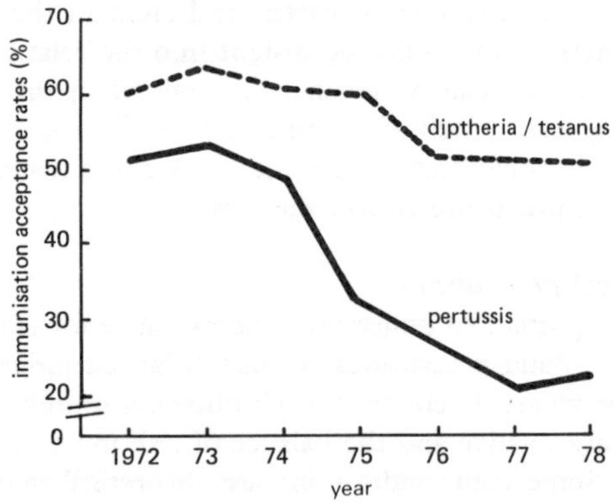

Fig. 11.2 Immunisation acceptance rates in Birmingham children during 1972–1978. Source: McKendrick *et al*, 1980

The controversy surrounding whooping cough immunisation involves three issues: 1. The efficacy of the vaccine; data collected during the 1977–8 outbreak has in general confirmed protection in the region of 80 per cent (Jenkinson, 1978; Church, 1979); 2. The inherent hazards of the disease, which are now much less than they were in the days when the vaccine was developed; 3. The safety of the vaccine; this is difficult to evaluate.

Reports of serious neurological sequelae following whooping cough immunisation have occurred with regularity. Many attempts have been made to determine the frequency of such reactions, but the difficulties are considerable. The supposed reactions are nonspecific in nature, taking the form of convulsions, an encephalopathy or infantile spasms. The former, convulsions, are relatively common, the latter are rare; all occur in the immunised and unimmunised. The important question is, do they occur more frequently after pertussis immunisation? Evidence from the National Childhood Encephalopathy Study suggests that they do (DHSS, 1981). Such reactions may occur once every 110 000 injections but most of the affected children recover completely. The risk works out at approximately one permanent brain injury for every 100 000 courses of immunisation.

In addition to nonspecific reactions, some seem specific to pertussis. These are characterised by shock, pallor, collapse, or persistent screaming, two to 12 hours after immunisation.

Since pertussis vaccine is prepared from whole bacteria it is likely to be more reactogenic since it contains a wide variety of materials. It is also possible that there are differences between various vaccines, since manufacturers use different techniques of preparation. The organisms may also differ, as fresh isolates of the prevailing organism have to be used.

Some of the older types of vaccine seem to have been more reactogenic, especially those of the quadruple type.

Since the cause of untoward reactions to pertussis vaccine is obscure, advice on contraindications and precautions is largely empirical. There have been reports of children who have had a mild reaction to the first dose and a more severe reaction with successive doses. For this reason further doses should be omitted following any abnormal reaction.

The evidence for increased risk where there is a history or family history of neurological disorder such as fits is scanty, and it is not regarded as a contraindication in the USA where one report describes its administration to thousands of such children without encountering unexpected reactions (Livingstone, 1972).

The DHSS advises the following contraindications:

'A history of siezures, convulsions or cerebral irritation in the neonatal period. A history or family history of epilepsy or other disease of the central nervous system. Children with neurological defects. Any febrile illness, particularly respiratory, until the patient is fully recovered.'

The climate of doubt about this immunisation is such that this broad view should be observed, but it is unnecessary to put an even broader interpretation on it, as some doctors do, and include migraine, prematurity, non-neurological neonatal illness and a variety of other irrelevant conditions as contraindications. Family history means first degree relatives or several family members with non traumatic seizures. Even so, the risks are greater from the disease than the immunisation and if the parents were keen for it, it could be carried out with considerable confidence.

It appears that whooping cough is a much milder disease than previously. The highest mortality is in very young infants, and they can only be protected effectively if older children from whom they catch the disease are immunised. The incidence of permanent injury from the vaccine is probably not a lot greater than from measles or polio vaccine, but the benefits are for the community and not the individual immunised. Even with limited knowledge of the incidence of vaccine damage, there can be little doubt that the community interests are best served by continued immunisation, while freedom of choice recognises that altruism is a variable individual quality.

The vaccine is given combined with tetanus and diphtheria toxoids (DTP) in three doses at six to eight week and four to six month intervals. A primary course only is given, commencing at about six months, but if the disease is prevalent it may be preferable to start at three months. The intervals are minimum only. If one is missed, the course is continued where it was left off, whatever the interval.

Poliomyelitis

The virtual elimination of poliomyelitis from this country is one of the great immunisation success stories. Inactivated polio vaccine was introduced in the late 1950s and was followed by a rapid decline in the incidence of the disease. Oral polio vaccine was introduced in 1962 and the trend continued. Cases are now rare.

There are three types of virus and immunity is specific in each. Vaccines therefore contain all three types. Oral vaccine (OPV) is recommended for routine use in this country, and has several advantages. Inactivated vaccine (IPV) is equally effective and may be indicated when OPV is not.

Oral vaccine is a mixture of all three types of attenuated virus. Being oral it imitates the natural portal of entry and replicates in the gut whence it may pass into the community and infect unimmunised individuals. In this way it can break the chain of transmission of the wild virus. Infection from one virus type may interfere with infection by the other two, so three separate doses with at least four week intervals are necessary. Immunity is thought to be lifelong. It is usually given with DT or DTP for convenience. Further doses are recommended at school entry and leaving. These can be regarded as fillers rather than boosters, to make up for any failure of take during primary immunisation. Other enterovirus infections or diarrhoea can cause such failure. Breast feeding need not be temporarily stopped.

One of the worries about OPV is that reversion to a paralytic type of virus after passage through the gut is suspected to occur occasionally, putting unimmunised contacts at risk. For this reason, unimmunised parents of children being immunised should be given OPV at the same time unless the mother is within the first four months of pregnancy, in which case both should be postponed.

The vaccine is remarkably free of reactions. Paralysis occurs about one in a million doses, but most of these have some pre-existing immunodeficiency.

OPV contains traces of several antibiotics, including penicillin. There is, therefore, a theoretical possibility of a reaction occuring in a sensitive individual. The quantity is so minute (0.004 IU penicillin) that this cannot be a consideration except in possibly the most exquisitely sensitive individual.

Measles

Before measles vaccine was available, most children acquired clinical infection between the ages of three and five years, with outbreaks every two years. Deaths from the disease are rare, about one in a million cases, but encephalitis occurs about once in 10 000 cases, and there is a small but serious morbidity from subacute sclerosing panencephalitis. Measles may be more serious in children debilitated by cardiac or pulmonary disease, and even in healthy children it leaves a trail of secondary infections such as otitis media, not to mention its unpleasantness and social disruption. In parts of the third world more than 10 per cent of children die of measles before the age of five.

Immunity is provided by a single injection of live attenuated virus of the Schwarz strain. When properly administered it produces a durable immunity in 95 per cent of cases. The object of the current programme is to eliminate measles from the community. This is feasible provided virtually 100 per cent of children are immunised. Since the vaccine came into wide use in 1968 the immunisation rate has been about 50 per cent. This has reduced the incidence so that it now takes longer for a sufficient number of susceptible people to build up for an outbreak to occur, and when it does so, many older children will be affected. A half-effective immunisation programme may simply postpone the disease for the unimmunised to an age when it may be more disrupting and possibly more severe (Roden, 1977).

The vaccine should not be administered under the age of fifteen months to avoid neutralisation by maternal antibodies. The second year of life after this age is the usual time but it should be offered to any child who has had neither the disease nor the immunisation. The incubation period of the vaccine virus is several days shorter than the wild virus, so that immunisation as an emergency measure soon after contact, should be preventative. Vaccine virus transmission does not occur.

Mild reactions consisting of fever, malaise and a mild rash on about the eighth day are common. Febrile convulsions may occasionally occur. Encephalitis occurs less than with the natural infection. The same holds for subacute sclerosing panencephalitis.

If there is a chronic debilitating illness, particularly cardio-pulmonary, when a reaction could have serious consequences, the injection of human measles immunoglobulin into the opposite arm is recommended. This can be obtained from public health laboratories, and given according to the vaccine manufacturer's instructions. If there is a history, or strong family history of convulsions, immunisation should be postponed until the age of three or four, and a prophylactic anticonvulsant such as phenytoin or sodium valproate given for about 16 days. If natural infection is likely, immunisation may be preferable with anticonvulsant cover. Gamma globulin will provide additional protection.

There are small quantities of polymyxin and neomycin in the vaccine so care should be taken if there is known hypersensitivity to these substances. Sensitivity to egg is a stated contraindication. This is theoretical. The vaccine is derived from tissue cultures of chick fibroblasts which are antigenically different from egg, and it has been given to children highly sensitive to egg without untoward effect (Kamin *et al*, 1965).

The incidence of measles in England and Wales in the past decade, since the introduction of vaccination, is shown in Figure 21.1 (p. 152).

The measles immunisation programme cannot be judged successful when only 50 per cent of children are immunised. If the rate cannot be improved considerably, it may be better to withdraw to a policy of selective immunisation in the future.

Rubella

Rubella acquired in the first month of pregnancy results in congenital abnormality in more than half the infants, and falls steadily to 5 per cent affected when it occurs in the fourth month. In addition, 10 to 15 per cent of affected pregnancies will abort spontaneously. The number of children affected varies widely from year to year, but from 1971 to 1978 over 500 children were affected in England, Scotland and Wales. It is also a reason for termination of pregnancy, and in the epidemic year of 1978 over 800 terminations were rubella-linked.

Natural rubella provides lasting immunity for practical purposes, but only serological confirmation should be taken as evidence. About 50 per cent of 15 year old girls are immune, and about 85 per cent of women of child-bearing age. Rubella vaccine is therefore advised for prepubertal girls aged 11 to 13 years. This avoids the risk of vaccine induced congenital defects, although the risk seems far less than with the natural disease. Seroconversion occurs in 95 per cent to 98 per cent of nonimmune subjects. The duration of immunity is not known for certain, but if given at this age it probably covers the main reproductive years (Gingram, 1980). If subsequent natural infection occurs, the viraemia required for fetal infection is thought not to occur. Subclinical natural infection is thought not to affect the fetus for the same reason.

The cohort of women which has now received immunisation will not reach their main reproductive years until the mid 1980's and only 70 per cent are currently accepting immunisation. The first pregnancy is most commonly affected, so those unimmunised are at risk unless deliberately sought out by their general practitioner.

In 1979, on the initiative of the newly formed Children's Committee, a campaign was started to increase the uptake of rubella vaccination in girls aged 11 to 14 years to at least 90 per cent, and to offer rubella vaccine to a larger number of seronegative women of child bearing age. It is important that the latter group should not include women already pregnant, and that contraception should be effective for three months after vaccination (Brimblecombe, 1979).

Two vaccine strains are available, Cendehill and RA27/3. The latter is thought to be marginally preferable as it induced a more rapid and higher antibody response, although the incidence of reaction is higher. A single subcutaneous dose is required.

Pregnancy or suspected pregnancy is an absolute contraindication. Minute amounts of polymyxin, neomycin or both may be present in the vaccine, so care should be taken when there is known hypersensitivity to these antibiotics.

Mild reactions similar to the natural illness but less severe are infrequent, but may occur on about the ninth day. Arthralgia is less common and mainly confined to mature adults. Thrombocytopaenia has been reported, but neurological reactions are probably extremely rare.

Tuberculosis

Immunisation against tuberculosis with the attenuated bacillus of Calmette and Guerin (BCG) has been available since the 1920s. The incidence of tuberculosis in the United Kingdom has been declining for many decades, but immunisation has only been partly responsible. Case finding, screening of contacts and effective treatment are some of the other factors responsible. High levels of immigration, from areas where tuberculosis is prevalent over recent years, has resulted in an incidence in this subgroup which is 30 times the national one.

The degree of effectiveness of BCG is open to some question, but evidence from this country suggests 80 per cent effectiveness, maximal at two-and-a-half to five years, with little immunity remaining after 10 to 15 years. Since tuberculosis is a prolonged serious illness, even a small degree of protection provides large benefit in terms of morbidity in areas of high prevalence. In many areas the prevalence is very low, and if the decline continues there may be little advantage in continuing BCG immunisation for everyone. However, in heavily populated areas, particularly those with a high proportion of immigrants, where future trends in the pattern of the disease are uncertain, immunisation may be of great importance.

BCG can be given at any age and repeated as necessary throughout life. At present it is recommended for children at 11 to 13 years and all others at special risk of developing the disease. It must be preceded by tuberculin testing in all but neonates, and only negative reactors immunised. Measles, measles vaccine, glandular fever and immunosuppression may cause a false negative reaction.

The vaccine is administered intradermally over the lower third of the deltoid. A papule develops which usually persists for several weeks. A small number ulcerate and cause parental anxiety. This is of no consequence and only needs a dry dressing. Axillary adenitis may occur, but no specific action is usually required. In the case of a rare severe reaction, specialist advice should be sought.

The procedure is usually followed by tuberculin testing after an interval of at least four weeks to ensure that seroconversion has occured. There are no specific contradications, but live vaccine precautions apply.

REFERENCES

Bainton, D. *et al* (1979) The immunity of children to diphtheria, tetanus and poliomyelitis. *British Medical Journal*, **1**, 854.

Brimblecombe, F.S.W. (1979) Rubella. *Update*, **19**, 917–926.

Church, M.A. (1979) Evidence of whooping cough vaccine efficacy from the 1978 whooping cough epidemic in Hertfordshire. *Lancet*, **2**, 188–190.

Court report (1976) *Fit for the Future*. Committee on Child Health Services. London: HMSO.

DHSS (1980) *Immunisation Against Infectious Disease*. London: HMSO.

DHSS (1981) Whooping cough: reports from the Committee on Safety of Medicines and the Joint Committee on Vaccination and Immunisation. London: HMSO.

Galbraith N.S., Forbes Pat & Mayon-White R.T. 1980 Changing patterns of communicable disease in England and Wales. Part III Increasing infectious disease. *British Medical Journal* **2**, 546–548

Gingram M. (1980) Follow up study of rubella vaccination in general practice. *British Medical Journal*, **2**, 18–19
Griffith A.H. (1979) Development of the pertussis vaccination programme in England and Wales and its effects on morbidity and mortality. International Symposium on Immunisation: Benefits versus Risk Factors. Brussels 1978. Developments in Biological Standardisation, **43**, 91–94. Basle: Karger.
Jenkinson D. (1978) Outbreak of whooping cough in general practice. *British Medical Journal*, **2**, 577.
Jones S.A.M. (1980) Health education to improve rubella immunisation. *British Medical Journal* **2**, 649–650.
Kamin P.B., Fein B.T. & Britton H.A. (1965) Use of live attenuated measles vaccine virus in children allergic to egg protein. *Journal of the American Medical Association*, **193**, 1125–1126.
Livingstone S. (1972) Comprehensive Management of Epilepsy in Infancy, Childhood and Adolescence, pp. 159–165. Thomas Springfield, Illinois.
McKendrick M.W., Gully P.R. & Geddes A.M. (1980) Protection against pertussis by immunisation. *British Medical Journal*, **2**, 1390–1391.
RCGP (1981) Swansea Research Unit, RCGP. Effect of low pertussis vaccination uptake on a large community. *British Medical Journal*, **1**, 23–26.
Roberts, A. & Williams, W.O. (1981) Whooping cough in nursery school children. *Journal of the Royal College of General Practitioners*, **31**, 470–472.
Roden A.T. (1977) Effects of vaccination against measles on the incidence of the disease and the immunity of the child population in England and Wales. *Health Trends*, **9**, 69–72.

12

The child health clinic

J.W. Tuke

Today's child health clinic involves the application of paediatrics in its broad sense and there can be no more rewarding investment in preventive medicine than the surveillance of our children from birth to school entry. This is an example of the shifting pattern of family medicine whereby patients are invited to attend. The primary purpose is the avoidance of the sequelae of conditions which will detrimentally affect the length or quality of life. The medical profession cannot claim a brilliant record for the early discovery of more disabling conditions such as metabolic disorders, mental handicap and deafness, much less the minor defects such as the 'clumsy child', speech delay, reading disabilities and intellectual retardation. In so many cases timely identification can vastly change the outlook for such a child.

DESIGN

Whilst the purposes of the child health clinic have changed since their initiation with the *Maternity and Child Welfare Act 1918*, more than sixty years experience has resulted in a structure with an organisation not to be lightly discarded. The need for the clinic is not in doubt and indeed the careful studies made by the committees of Sheldon (1967) and Court (1976) have confirmed this. Their place has been accepted by the Royal College of General Practitioners (1978) and by the Department of Health and Social Security (1978, 1980). Justification for their continuance into the next decade would include observation and discussion of nutrition and growth, reassurance and explanation of minor problems, screening for physical, neuro-psychiatric and metabolic disorders, immunisation against infectious disease and health education.

The ideal aim would be to examine every child and give time to question and listen to every mother at a series of appropriate times in the child's life. These ages have recently been officially recommended as birth, 6–10 days, 6 weeks, 7–8 months, 18 months, about 3 years and at school entry (DHSS, 1980), though some doctors advocate rather different programmes (Ch. 13). In many areas such routine surveillance is a realistic proposition where the great majority of infants attend when requested. In other districts, unfortunately the more densely populated with a higher proportion of socially under-privileged, the rate of default may be as high as 41 per cent (Freer and Ogunmuyiwa, 1977). In such a situation it is often those most in need who fail to attend. Possible solutions to this very unsatisfactory position would be the supply of transport for mother and child to the clinic, greatly increased establishment of health visitors in these areas enabling home visits to replace clinic visits when necessary, and more flexible timing of clinics. Freer (1977) suggests a reintroduction of the selective examination of 'high risk' children when resources are limited. Whilst the concept of the 'at risk' register has been disbanded with good evidence to do so (Richards and Roberts, 1967; Court, 1976), I believe that there is ample justification to re-consider the use of a modified system. Clearly there are many infants with a greater than average change of developing problems and many can be anticipated. It should be clearly indicated on the clinic record if a child has for example suffered a period of intra-uterine under-nourishment, hypoxia before or after birth, convulsions, hyperbilirubinaemia, hypoglycaemia or post-natal CNS infection. The well known extra risk run by these children surely deserves extra care in their surveillance. The fact that a very few highly specialised obstetric units have found as few as 10 per cent of their very low birth weight babies (less than 1500 g) to have subsequent handicap, does not yet justify the erasure of 'VLBW' on the record.

PREMISES AND STAFF

Some of the best medicine is carried out in the poorest premises but certain physical features are essential for developmental screening techniques. Both the health visitor's and the doctor's rooms must be warm and the consulting room should be carpeted. Part of the assessment of toddlers involves observation whilst playing on the floor, and vision testing may require the doctor to descend to the same level. At least one room should be insulated against noise in order to carry out hearing tests.

Informal attendance without appointment encourages busy mothers to seek help for minor problems but this may also lead to long and frustrating waiting times. Since many children will be attending for screening examination it should be possible to provide, in the words of Court, 'a judicious blend of appointments and open access'.

Originally staffed by health authority doctors and nurses, a transitional period occurred when some 10 to 20 per cent of clinics were run by general practitioners and health visitors for their own patients. We now appear to be entering a more rational phase where an increasing number of family doctors wish to carry out their own preventive services and this inclusion within the primary care base is strongly supported by the report of the Committee on Child Health Services (1976). Most of these clinics will be supervised by a doctor with a special interest and training in paediatrics and this concept will be nothing new. However, the acceptance by the Royal College of General Practitioners that all family doctors should receive a more adequate postgraduate paediatric training, and the new mandatory vocational training scheme for general practice, should provide a sufficient number of doctors with the necessary interest and expertise. The recommendations of Sheldon were backed up by a study on Tees-side where 502 mothers were questioned about their attitudes to clinics (Donaldson, 1974); information obtained included preference to seek the advice of their family doctor rather than the clinic medical officer. It seems clear that given a suitable organisation and premises, child health clinics would be better conducted by family doctors. It would be disappointing if those who possess the necessary training, interest and equanimity should be denied the opportunity to include this clinic in their services.

The present consultant paediatric service, being almost wholly hospital orientated, offers little help to the type of community service described. It has been pointed out with increasing clarity that the present number of consultants should be doubled to provide community paediatricians. These consultants would have extensive clinical paediatric training but also knowledge of social medicine and paediatric psychiatry (Court and Jackson, 1972). This topic is fully explored in the Court report. These physicians would have preventive and social expertise and would work in close association with group practices and with the School Health Service. They would also be responsible for the care of handicapped children in the community. This would provide the support for the general practitioner-based clinics and such a system is already operating in some areas. The better organised practice, whether in the doctor's own premises or a health centre with clerical staff and attached health visitors and nurses, will it is hoped, become the rule. The doctor responsible for the clinic will be the leader of a practice team and he should be fitted for this paediatric work by special interest and training because of the extent and character of children's needs. Whilst the natural urge to resist specialisation in family medicine is generally accepted, there is surely a place for a division of work (Ellis, 1974). There are also many doctors similarly equipped, previously employed by local authorities, who would perhaps be willing to run clinics in general practice centres. One anticipates that in due course most group practices will wish to provide their own child health clinics but a smaller practice and some busy groups, especially in urban areas, may prefer to call upon their health authority for assistance. The supply of facilities and personnel clearly needs to be balanced to the particular local needs and this may require an improvement in working relationships.

This refers to the need for personal contact. Community physicians should be frequent and welcome visitors in general practice (JRCGP, 1976). The proportion of women entering medical school is at present some 40 per cent and this is expected to increase. Woman doctors with paediatric training, together with personal experience of their own families, will provide an ideal source of suitable expertise to fill this need. Their help, perhaps on a part-time basis, will be especially welcome in the inner city areas where improved child care is most needed (DHSS, 1978). General practitioners and health visitors working in concentrated areas with moving population and immigrants and with large general practitioner lists, may look to their specialists in community medicine and area nurses to provide that extra help. Authority for meeting these provisions has been provided by the Department of Health and Social Security in their paper *Prevention in the Child Health Services* (1978).

THE CHILDREN

The need to continue to observe growth in weight and height remains. The use of centile charts proves most helpful to the doctor in early detection of failure to thrive reflecting in turn some underlying disorder. Any temptation to discard the clinic weighing machine should be resisted if only for the protection of the apparently contented breast fed baby who in fact fails to thrive. Another example of a common situation where centile charts can be helpful is where a mother of twins is worried about the increasing differential in weight and height between her twins. She is happy when shown the smaller is proceeding in his normal predicted manner adhering to his centile. Charts which allow for length of gestation are particularly useful in clinics (Tanner and Whitehouse, 1973). Adolescent and adult obesity is related to childhood obesity (Lloyd, Wolff and Whelan, 1961) and whilst results may not so far have been very encouraging, the child health clinic would seem to be the ideal situation to tackle this problem. Treatment, to be effective, requires constant surveillance, energy and continuity (Ch. 27).

Relatively minor problems such as feeding difficulties, sleep disturbance and breath holding attacks can worry a parent for a long time before seeking medical advice by appointment. The clinic provides an informal facility with easy access where fears can be allayed in an unhurried atmosphere. There are some who feel that a physician's time can be more effectively used than by reassurance on such matters (Anderson, 1970) but it is doubtful if these problems, which are of major importance to the parents, will be acceptably dispelled by ancilliary staff. At the same time it is realistic to accept that in some areas, for example new towns, health visitors will take a greater responsibility for screening and dealing with these problems (Freer, 1977). It is becoming increasingly clear that the organisation of child health clinics in the United Kingdom will require modification according to the particular needs of the locality. These differing needs offer an ideal opportunity for cooperation between the community medicine specialist, area nurse, general practitioner and health visitor.

The observations and comments of a parent should be carefully considered in an unhurried atmosphere. Experience and retrospective study shows that parents with an anxiety about their child's development or abilities are very frequently justified. Reassurance is only warranted after the appropriate examination reveals a normal child. Doubtful results may require re-examination or referral to a child development centre or specialist, the child health clinic not being primarily a place for diagnosis.

The absence of now unfamiliar, fatal and disabling infectious diseases results from efficient immunisation schemes, organised and carried out at a local level by the staff of the infant welfare clinic. The determination of these staffs is shown by attaining an immunisation rate of 100 per cent in some areas, while the problems of successfully protecting a moving population are shown by a rate as low as 25 per cent in some city areas. There were six cases of paralytic poliomyelitis notified in this country in 1979 none of whom had been previously vaccinated, three having contracted the infection abroad. The pre-existing Infant Welfare Clinic organisation is experienced in this important field and it is perhaps only the health visitors' determination to follow up defaulters which we have to thank for the present low mortality figures.

The child health clinic would seem the obvious place to promote health education for children. Accidents form the greatest single cause of death between the first birthday and the end of childhood and are the most important problem in social paediatrics today. Although a pictorial display of domestic dangers may be suggestive of the schoolroom, such attempts to modify the environment and the attitude of parents is surely part of preventive medicine. Safety devices built in as a constant feature of the environment are more effective than attempts to alter people's behaviour (Lancet, 1979).

CONCLUSION

There is much evidence to show that mothers and preschool children require observation by nurses and doctors with special paediatric skills. Mothers prefer to be seen by their own family doctor and there is an urgent need for general practitioners to find time to see their children regularly in addition to consultations for sickness. The organised regular contact between child, parent and family doctor in the practice itself, placed at appropriate points in the child's development, offers parents a unique opportunity to discuss with their family doctor individual problems and gives the doctor a chance to know the child and watch his or her progress (JRCGP, 1979).

REFERENCES

Anderson, F.P. (1970) Evaulation of the routine physical examination of infants in their first year of life. *Paediatrics*, **45**, 950–959.

Court, D (1976) *Report of the Committe on Child Health Services*.London: HMSO

Court, S.D.M. & Jackson, A.D.M. (1972) *Paediatrics in the seventies*. On behalf of the British Paediatric Association. Oxford University Press.

DHSS (1978) *Health Services Development: Court Report on Child Health Services*. Health Circular, HC(78)5. Department of Health and Social Security.

DHSS (1980) *Prevention in the Child Health Services*. Department of Health and Social Security.

Donaldson, R.J. (1974) *Child health clinics evaluated*. 81st Congress of the Royal Society of Health, Brighton.

Ellis, H.L. (1974) Britain's child health services. Some strengths and weaknesses. *American Journal of Diseases of Children*, **127**, 321–324

Freer, C.B. & Ogunmuyiwa, T.A. (1977) Pre-school development screening in a health centre – the problem of non-attendance. *Journal of the Royal College of General Practitioners*, **27**, 428

JRCGP Editorial (1976) Community Medicine and General Practice. *Journal of Royal College of General Practitioners*, **26**, 155

JRCGP Editorial (1979) The International Year of the Child. *Journal of Royal College of General Practitioners*. **29**, 635

Lloyd, J.K., Wolf, O.H. & Whelan, W.S. (1961) *British Medical Journal*, **2**, 145

RCGP (1978) Comments on the Report of the Child Health Services Committee. *Journal of the Royal College of General Practitioners*, **28**, 553

Richards, I.D.G., Roberts, C.J. (1967) *Lancet*, **2**, 711

Sheldon (1967) Report of a Sub-Committee of the Standing Medical Advisory Committee of the Central Health Services Council. Child Welfare Services. London: HMSO

Tanner, J.M. & Whitehouse, R.H. (1973) Growth charts. *Archives of Disease in Childhood*, **48**, 786–789. (Charts obtainable from: Creaseys, Bull Plain, Hertford, Herts. Ref. SHWB 28/29)

13

Surveillance in the first year of life

Graham Curtis Jenkins

Doctors working in general practice are becoming aware that, particularly in the case of the preschool child, the traditional posture of waiting for the sick to be brought to them for treatment is no longer acceptable (Tudor Hart, 1980).

The use of hospital accident and emergency departments by many parents wanting an instant service for their children both in and out of working hours (Jackson, 1980), and discoveries at the initial school medical examinations of children with what obviously have been long-standing disorders of growth and development undetected by both parents and the general practitioners to whom the children had been brought on average ten to fifteen times in the preschool period, are obvious examples that all is not well with the traditional style of curative primary paediatric care.

The numbers of unimmunized children, the problems of children being brought up in emotionally deprived environments undetected by the primary care team or anybody else (Pringle, 1974), the cases of child abuse that hit the national headlines, cause many thoughtful doctors twinges of anxiety.

Perceptive general practitioners working in those areas where the child health services are being run down or axed by district health departments short of funds are becoming worried about the inadequacy of preventive services and realize uneasily that they are going to have to do something about it.

Evidence from many parts of the country points to the widely differing rates of infant mortality and some figures from one provincial city show how the health, life and death of children is affected by the places in which they live even when these are only a few streets apart (Table 13.1).

What the doctors and fellow health professionals want to see in these two communities is something very different. Moreover it is obvious to all who work in communities with such divergencies that the two populations view the services provided in a totally different light.

Lack of contact with services *is* dangerous. A survey in Glasgow in 1972 which looked at child death showed which children were at risk and died. Just 60 per cent of all children attended a child health clinic in the first year of life but only 30 per cent of 146 infants that died from no known predisposing organic disease had done so. More revealing of parental attitude was that only 28 percent of the dead children who were old enough had received any immunization *at all* (Richards and McIntosh, 1972).

Table 13.1 Local variations in vital statistics of infancy in the U.K. (Bryant, 1979)

1970–1976	*Ward A*	*Ward B*
live births	2458	2945
still births	39	26
still birth rate/1000 total births	15.6	8.8
neonatal deaths	45	24
total wastage—still births and deaths in first 12 months of life	84	50
reported child abuse and neglect	50	7

Ward A: disadvantaged area, mainly rundown council housing
Ward B: well-to-do suburb with a small council housing estate

Lack of contact with services provided for them in Wandsworth in 1978–79 meant that eight per cent of children at school entry still had major previously undiagnosed disorders requiring urgent treatment. Many of these children had been seen frequently by their own general practitioner or at hospital accident and emergency departments, yet nobody had stopped to think of the whole child and his problems (Ismail, 1979).

Health visitors attached administratively (but not always emotionally) to general practice see their skills in child care diluted by other demands on their time. They are painfully aware that in a typical general practice without an age sex register, it is unlikely that they even know the names of all the children registered in the practice, let alone have visited them in the home or seen them all at preschool child health clinics run by 'their' GP or by the district health authority. The health visitor often finds 'her' general practitioner bemused by her activities and unappreciative of her efforts in promoting child health. Children she finds with squint or deafness and brings to the notice of the general practitioner are sometimes ignored and occasionally parents are assured, inaccurately, that the child 'will grow out of it'. The health visitor's advice on management of feeding and development, based in many cases on far more up to date information than that held by the doctor, is sometimes contradicted by the general practitioner, seemingly almost maliciously.

The involvement of the general practitioner in the care of children in the newborn period is sometimes haphazard and a 'collusion of anonymity' – a term coined by Balint that really means that each helper hopes the other will do the helping – ensures too often that the mother cannot get the help she needs without feeling that she is wasting somebody's time.

When the mother and her new baby reach home for the first time, the mother is ready to listen and act on practical advice and is very grateful for help. However, much advice given by friends, relatives and non-professional helpers at this time is inaccurate, and occasionally it may be dangerous. The midwife, sometimes regarded as the traditional foe of the health visitor, because 'she gets there first', normally stops visiting on the tenth postnatal day and in most cases the health visitor begins visiting at this time. Differing advice may be proffered on such basic matters as breast feeding, bathing of the baby and cracked nipples.

The family doctor usually visits routinely at this time too. All too often he resists the temptation to involve himself with the baby neatly wrapped in a crib at the foot of the bed, and reaches merely for the involuting uterus – repeating needlessly the daily examination already carried out by the midwife. A few doctors, however, do examine the newborn baby, repeating the physical examination already carried out in hospital by a paediatrician. In many practices that is the last time the baby is seen by the general practitioner for many months. The doctor vaguely hopes that the mother will attend a local child health clinic for immunizations and he hopes a hearing test will be done at eight months. The four or five contacts the mother and her baby make with the general practitioner in the first year will throw up a number of problems. Many general practitioners feel that some of them at least could have been handled by a health visitor or by the mother herself. Feeding and general management problems (usually concerned with sleep and its absence), snuffles and similar minor difficulties seem to characterise for many doctors the view they have of the infant in the first year of life. Contact with the mother is usually anxiety-ridden. Failure to cope, depression, sleeplessness, lack of libido and sheer exhaustion tax the therapeutic endeavours of most general practitioners. By the end of the first year, the pressure eases as the mother gains confidence and regains her strength and figure.

This is a bleak picture of child care in the first year of life in general practice, but for the 80 per cent of practices in the UK running no form of child care clinic and the 70 per cent not attempting any immunization other than on an unorganised haphazard basis, and for those practices (probably 40 per cent of the total) with a non-functioning primary care child health team, in which the health visitor, midwife and general practitioner rarely, if ever, meet together, the picture I have painted will often apply.

There is much discussion about what to put in its place. The Court report (1976) proposed the creation of a general practitioner paediatrician. Many doctors who fail to see the possibilities of this role argue that they are too busy to run clinics to see well children, adding as an aside that it is a pointless exercise and boring to boot.

Hidden within this set of attitudes is a basic misunderstanding of what constitutes child care, but how can an individual general practitioner make the transition to a more enlightened approach to his work?

I think the most important first step is to identify all the children of preschool age in your practice. The health centre staff in a certain midlands town thought they had. The 474 addresses supplied to a research team by the health centre could at best have been expected to tell them the whereabouts of 663 children. But the 1971 census for the town gave a figure of 847 children aged 0–4. Since there was no reason to suppose that the population had dropped substantially, then approximately 200 children had been 'lost' from health department records (Jackson and Jackson, 1979).

Ultimately 300 children under the age of five were found who had been 'lost' by the health department, more than a third of the total. The same research team also found that it was the most vulnerable children of single parents or of families on the move with poor communication skills and a low appreciation of their children's health needs who were most likely to slip through the net; another example of the inverse care law (Zinkin and Cox, 1976).

The example quoted is not an isolated one. Similar record discrepancies are reported for other areas (Heward and Clayton, 1980), and they must be widespread. This sad state of affairs needs our urgent attention.

Start by ensuring that the practice management structure is geared to identify all the children under five years old in the practice's care if you wish to introduce a comprehensive child care programme. An age/sex register (if you haven't one, the FPC can often be persuaded to provide one free) can be used initially, but from it 'year books' need to be built. These should be the sole responsibility of a named person, perhaps a health visitor or receptionist, but ideally a part-time clerk who can also serve the health visitors' clerical needs and physically run the proposed child health clinics. Into the books are entered new births and transfers in of children in month order for each year. Removals out are just as important a responsibility. From such books, one for each year, which will identify every child in the practice the likely clinic work load can be calculated. All members of the practice team should be instructed on the importance of maintaining these books accurately (Curtis Jenkins and Newton, 1981).

The second essential is a functioning health visitor, emotionally committed to such a programme. This is blindingly obvious to those of us already running such programmes but to general practitioners who never exchange a word with 'their' health visitor from one week to the next, this may be a revolutionary suggestion. Her co-operation and interest are vital. Divided loyalties caused by uncomprehending senior nursing management insisting that work outside the practice has equal if not greater priority, and inability to organise a satisfactory holiday rota can cause great harm. Some of the health visitors' teaching is unrealistic and inflexible and badly needs re-orientating. Moreover, many of the health visitors' skills may lie unused due to inefficient deployment and poor morale. This last can dramatically improve when a practice provides secretarial help for them (with 70 per cent of the secretary's salary reimbursed) and can identify all the pre-school children in the practice's care, and succeeds in drawing the health visitor into the antenatal period of care when their influence can be so profound.

For these reasons it is important to consult the managers at district health authority level. Senior nursing officers and community physicians can be very helpful when a clinic is proposed in providing, for instance, a clinic nurse to do the actual immunizations.

A demonstration to the community physician of a management system for identifying children (usually far more up to date than the best district health authorities' systems), physical provision of space suitable for clinic use, and skills in developmental paediatrics, will often persuade the community physician to pay the clinical medical officer sessional rates once the clinic is in operation.

At this point, it is important to calculate work load of the clinic. For instance, a 10 000 patient practice with a birth rate of 100 per annum will have around 500 children under five years old in its care. Two clinic sessions weekly, 46 weeks a year, of 2¼ hours with 7–8 booked appointments for routine surveillance examinations at 7 months, 12 months, 2½ years and 4½ years, and at other times requested by parent, health visitor or doctor, and 4–5 unbooked gaps will amply cover the well care needs of such a child population (with a 10 per cent first-time appointment failure rate).

To the clinic will come mothers bringing their children to be weighed, and to see friends including the health visitor who will, of course, be in attendance 'up front'. A steady stream of children will be guided to the health visitor's clerk who (as mentioned earlier) is responsible for their booking in, record retrieval, weighing and height measuring, prior to the doctor's consultation. A vacant consulting room suits admirably for this job and does not interfere with the running of the other activities in the clinic. Children whom the health visitor wants the doctor to see can be brought to the room and then wait for the next convenient moment to be seen. A health visitor confident in her skills and supported to the full by the doctor can reduce this sort of consultation to a minimum. The secret of success is the mix and the ability and willingness of the clerk to fit in unbooked patients around the booked ones. It is no good 'putting up the shutters' on mothers who present with a problem or whom the health visitor wants help with. This is no service and mothers quickly discover this and go elsewhere for help. I have visited towns where the general practitioners pride themselves on their developmental surveillance examination clinics and where the community health clinics are full of their patients wanting help and advice and unable to get it from their own general pracitioner. The clerk's other main task is the identification of non-attenders and then making sure that they are followed up. 'At risk until seen' should be the motto of every child health clinic.

The overall decline in consulting workload in a practice running such a service is between five and ten per cent as the confidence of mothers increases and they learn to use the services provided intellingently.

The effects of conflicting advice have already been mentioned and nowhere is this more important than between doctor and health visitor. 'The health visitor said' a mother remarks after she has drawn advice from the doctor and the doctor then becomes irritated for it is often different from his own. This need not happen – when it does, patients notice and their confidence in both health visitor and doctor diminishes. Doctor and health visitor must be prepared to invest time to talk regularly to discuss common policies and strategies for the management of commonly occurring conditions, particularly in the first year of life: nappy rash, feeding, sleeplessness, separation anxiety, etc.

What should be the aims of a programme of care for the child under 5?

Morley (1973) identified the corner stones of under 5 child care, as, immunization, weighing (and nutritional guidance), health education (and developmental guidance) and treatment (including the early diagnosis of handicapping conditions). In the UK today, these are still the corner stones. Yet over 100,000 cases of pertussis in the latest epidemic, with a handful of deaths (prevented from being hundreds by the intervention of special care baby units unavailable in the last great epidemic in 1951 when 437 died), is a gruesome reminder of our failure to commit ourselves wholeheartedly to immunization and a reflection of the DHSS's and the profession's lily-livered approach to the scaremongering in the media. The continuing disgrace of inadequate measles immunization is caused by lack of will to immunize and a disbelief on the part of parents and health professionals in its efficacy. We must decide either to immunize twice, at nine months and 4½ years (WHO recommendation) or once at two years. At the moment, except in a few enlightened areas, less than half of the children are immunized at all and older children with declining immunity, caused by immunization at the wrong age, are increasingly at risk.

Weighing in clinics has recently become unfashionable yet with the rise in the number of breast fed babies, the satisfied breast fed baby who fails to gain weight is a new problem that will be missed unless mothers are urged to weigh their babies regularly (Davies and Evans, 1976).

Nutritional guidance is important. No less than 50 of 286 mothers in a recent survey of infant feeding were making up bottle feeds dangerously inaccurately. Nobody had bothered to show them how because they had all left hospital breast feeding and health visitors were not making contact often enough to see what was happening, and do something about it. In addition, 25 per cent were already giving regular solids at two months.

Health education is something to which we all pay lip service, yet 50 per cent of infants are reported to be sleeping 'badly' at one year according to their parents. They sleep less than their parents think they should sleep and it is doctors and their medicines that perhaps help convert 'little' into 'bad' by offering treatment to the infant. Separation anxiety, which sometimes causes an eight-month-old child to scream with terror each and every time he's left, can make mothers' lives a misery, particularly when others advise her that she's made the child behave that way in the first place by spoiling. Such situations as these deserve accurate and informed help. An up to date doctor and health visitor with an adequate grounding in the elements of developmental psychology can transform the picture and parents can be very grateful. Books like *Babyhood*, by Leech (1974) should be required reading, not just for literate upper middle class parents, but for every doctor and health visitor involved in child care.

Developmental checks, birthday checks, screening, developmental assessment are all terms used to describe much the same thing and I prefer the term developmental surveillance examination – a service offered as part of the package of care in the first year of life which consists of three meticulously performed routine examinations of the well child covering all fields of behaviour in the neonatal period, preferably within the first 14 days of life, at 7 months and at 12 months.

The first examination carried out by the general practitioner in the home is the most important of all. At this time, the mother is at her most vulnerable and most willing to accept guidance and help. A carefully and delicately carried out examination, demonstrating to the mother her baby's abilities as a person, to follow the mother's face across a room, to turn through 180° to the parent's voice, the baby's ability to copy the examiner's tongue out and open mouth, will make a lasting impression on any parent seeing these things for the first time. A demonstration of the primitive reflexes never fails to impress and a repeat full physical examination occasionally turns up heart murmers and other congenital abnormalities missed at birth.

When carried out in the home in the way I have described elsewhere the mother sees clearly your interest in her well child – and your expertise (Curtis Jenkins and Newton, 1981). You are also able to reiterate the assurance so anxiously needed by all mothers that her child is normal and at the same time demonstrate to her skills that she never knew the baby had.

In addition, if carried out on a baby less than 14 days old, the visit attracts a post-natal visit fee. About 20 per cent of these babies require a further consultation for a variety of reasons and lastly, a very clear impression can be gained of the sort of baby he is and also of the mother's ability to cope. This examination renders the traditional six week examintion superfluous; by this time anyway many of the effects achieved by an early visit can no longer be achieved – such as switching on an unlikely or unmotherly mother to her baby who often denies that her baby could see, hear or smile in the newborn period.

Visiting all newborn babies in our practice adds just 15 per cent to my visiting work load in the year.

The main aim of the examinations at 7 and 12 months is to confirm for parents' peace of mind that their children are growing normally. Luckily, between 80 and 85 per cent are doing just that. The rest have a multitude of problems ranging from multiple major handicapping disorders to a depressed mother unable to care for her behaviourially disturbed infant. These examinations are described elsewhere (Jenkins and Newton, 1981). How to perform them is a more complicated matter than most people realise. Some still prefer that the examinations should be carried out at six months (too early for reliable Stycar vision and hearing tests) or eight or nine months old (when a combination of stranger and separation anxiety in many infants makes the examination a pointless misery for infant and doctor alike) but many authorities would now agree that seven months is an excellent age for an overview examination. The examination is, of course, only half the object of the consultation. To ask a mother what sort of person her seven month old child is may sound strange, yet her answer to this question will probably reveal more about the mother and her abilities than any other. As Hall (1980) has described, a mother who does not see her child as a person at four months identifies herself at one stroke as someone who is failing to cope and unable to establish a working relationship with her baby, so placing the baby at great risk.

'Is he happy?' may sound a trite question to those doctors whose middle class attitudes rest on the assumption that people enjoy their children. To discover the mother who resents her child, disapproves and reacts violently to her seven month old infant's imagined misdemeanours is vital if you wish to maintain that child's future well being.

The further examination at 12 months is a last ditch chance to detect congenital disorder and it also offers the examiner his first opportunity to raise with the parent suspicions about an infant's developmental deviation or delay.

Figures from our own surveillance programme show that although in terms of yield of disorders found the 12 month examination is the least fruitful, a closer look reveals that in terms of seriousness, they are as important if not more so than those found at any other age (Table 13.2).

Table 13.2 Results of a surveillance programme in general practice

	aged 7 months	*aged 12 months*
Number of children examined	384	410
Percentage with suspected disorder	11%	5%
Numbers of suspected disorders		
strabismus	13	8
myopia	2	3
suspected hearing loss	6	1
cerebral palsy	0	4
motor delay	5	2
overall developmental delay	1	0
battered baby	0	1
maternal deprivation	1	0
others	14	4

Our figures are probably about average for a well-favoured part of southern England. As the Court report stated, in areas of deprivation, the rates for deafness, squint, fits and bed wetting are twice that of areas like ours.

Surveillance is, therefore, many things. To the general practitioner paediatrician it is comprehensive child care carried out in general practice along the lines I have described. However, for any practice that wishes to start improving the quality of its child care as a first step it would be wise for all members of the team to answer these very provocative questions posed recently by the Children's Committee:

1. Do all your patients know your practice arrangements?
2. Do you know when one of your children is seen in an accident and emergency department or by a deputy?
3. Do you find out why?
4. Do you visit your local paediatric department?
5. Do all children get regular surveillance?
6. Are you angry with trivia?
7. Do you explain to parents how to use your service that you provide – and make sure they understand?

If you can answer 'yes' to all except question 6, then you have no need to spend much time on this chapter. I suspect, however, none of us can give all the correct answers all the time.

But the striving towards such standards will make an excellent start in providing a comprehensive preschool child health service. Morley (1973) working in Nigeria was able to achieve the results shown in Table 13.3 when he had built his child health service from those corner stones mentioned earlier.

Table 13.3 Local variations in vital statistics of infancy – Nigeria (Morley, 1973).

	Village A	*Village B*
live births	327	302
infant deaths	26	14
mortality rate/1000 at risk	80	46
child population aged 1–4	987	896
child deaths aged 1–4	48	16
positive malaria films	55%	15.5%

Village A and B were matched for climatic similarity and other variables but village B had a care programme for children under five years, and village A a curative paediatric service only. If the practice of comprehensive child care can achieve such effects in a Nigerian village, is it expecting too much to hope for similar results even in that inner city ward in a certain provincial city in the UK?

REFERENCES

Bryant, G. (1979) *Child care in the suburban environment*. Paper read at Symposium Child Care in the Community, Camberley, Surrey.

Court, D. (1976) *Fit for the future*. The report of the committee on child health services. London: HMSO.

Curtis Jenkins, G. & Newton, R. (1981) *The First Year of Life* Chs 3, 6, 16. Edinburgh: Churchill Livingstone.

Davis, D.P. & Evans, T. (1976) Failure to thrive at the breast. *Lancet*, **2**, 1194–1195.

Hall , F. (1980) Personal communication

Heward, J. & Clayton, D. (1980) The point accuracy of paediatric population registers. *Journal of the Royal College of General Practitioners*, **30**, 412–416.

Ismail, H. (1980) *The school entrant*. In press.

Jackson, B. & Jackson, S. (1979) *Childminder: a study in action research*. London: Routledge and Kegan Paul.

Jackson, (1980) Paediatric primary care in London. *Journal of the Royal College of General Practitioners*, **30**, 520–524.

Morley, D. (1973) *Paediatric priorities in a developing world*. London: Butterworth.

Pringle, M.K. (1974) Social adversity and its effects on the intelligent child's achievement. *Proceedings of Royal Society of Medicine*, **66**, 1203–1204.

Richards, I.D.G. & McIntosh, H.T. (1972) Confidential inquiry into 226 consecutive infant deaths. *Archives of disease in childhood*, **47**, 697–706.

Tudor Hart, J. (1980) *Hypertension*, p. 124. Edinburgh: Churchill Livingstone.

Zinkin, P.M. & Cox, C.A. (1976) Child health clinics and inverse care laws. *British Medical Journal*, **2**, 411–413.

14

Surveillance in the pre-school years

Paul Hooper

Developmental surveillance as a concept seems to have replaced developmental screening in the past few years. The term was coined by the late Ronald McKeith to include not only the routine examination of children for congenital defects or developmental delay, but also the monitoring of their upbringing and the education of parents in achieving this. To what extent can this function be considered as part of the work of the general practitioner? Many will argue that it has no part but it belongs to the purview of the health visitor or the grandmother and that the general practitioner is only of relevance when things go wrong. Anything else is unwarranted interference. But those of us who have attempted to monitor our young patients over the years find it difficult to know where 'screening' finishes and 'surveillance' begins. The one seems to merge into the other and when, at the formal developmental examination, one asks the mother 'Is there any problem you would like to discuss?', as one always should, the questions of present and future management are bound to arise and can hardly be considered unwarranted interference. But nevertheless the only foundation upon which any surveillance programme can be built must be the routine developmental examination divorced from the management of episodic pathological conditions and seen, not only as a diagnostic process for the child, but as an educational process for parent and doctor, particularly for the latter because it is only by the regular observation of the normal that the abnormal can be identified. It must never be forgotten that in examining children we are looking not only at structure but also at function. An ear drum may look normal but does it hear?

FIT FOR THE FUTURE

In *Fit for the Future* (1976) Professor Court and his colleagues made it quite clear that 'health surveillance is in practice essentially a function of primary health care' and he went on to detail what should be the content of this. No one concerned with the primary care of children can afford to ignore his recommendations and not be challenged by them. General practice as a whole has been very slow to recognise the vital place of surveillance in primary care and to take any practical steps to implement it, being willing to abdicate its responsibilities to others. While the Royal College of General Practitioners (1978) has pronounced its support for 'a comprehensive curative and preventive service, including health surveillance through general practice' it has failed to delineate the content of such a service and to give a firm lead in introducing it. It is a great shame that the College, in rejecting with valid reasons the idea of the general practitioner paediatrician, should have given the impression of rejecting the whole of the Court report, for this it certainly did not do. Nevertheless, unless general practice stirs itself and accepts its responsibilities in this field it may well be that the siren voices calling for the removal of child care from general practice will be hearkened to, to the detriment of both children and the medical service.

THE PRIMARY HEALTH CARE TEAM

Both the Court report and the Royal College of General Practitioners have emphasised the importance of the primary health care team in the delivery of primary child care and no general practitioner can function in isolation in this respect. The health visitors and the practice administrative staff are an integral part of the team. The work of the health visitor is considered in Chapter 7. She is usually the one whom parents will approach in the first instance over problems of management and behaviour and her special expertise and training are well suited to deal with them. Yet it occurs from time to time that problems come to light in the developmental examination of which neither the parents nor the health visitor were aware. It is essential that the health visitor and the doctor do not give conflicting advice to parents and that they should work together closely as an integrated and complementary team. As it is a truism that good work cannot be done without good records, the practice staff are essential to see that records are up-to-date and available when needed and that the appropriate appointments for immunisations and developmental sessions are sent out and kept and a note taken of defaulters. In the writer's practice of approximately 12 000 patients and five partners the health visitors keep a birth book in which all expected visits and attendances for immunisation and developmental sessions are recorded and the attendances ticked off at the appropriate time. Two infant clinics are held each week, the health visitors hold an open clinic and anyone can come for weighing and general advice. Those booked to see their own doctor for developmental sessions are weighed prior to the appointment. Those due for immunisation injections go to the practice nurse in a separate room. A lady from the Practice Patients' Association acts as baby minder for the sibs of children otherwise occupied and the whole clinic is kept running by the office staff.

FUNCTIONAL AREAS

It is customary to divide the skills which a child acquires as he grows up into four areas: posture and large movements, vision and fine movements, hearing and speech, social behaviour and play or personal-social (Sheridan, 1960).

Posture and large movements concern the general muscle tone and head control of the small baby, proceeding to sitting, standing, walking, running, balance and co-ordination of gross movements like kicking a ball.

Vision and fine movements concern the development of visual acuity from a baby watching a large ball, to a point source of light and going on to the Stycar tests of vision (Sheridan, 1969) and also eye-hand coordination; the ability to pick up a one inch cube, and manipulate it, to pick up a small pellet, to build a tower of cubes and later, more complex structures such as a pyramid, and later still the ability to draw.

Hearing and speech concern the development of hearing from the small baby's reaction to sounds and progressing to the Stycar tests of hearing (Sheridan, 1958) and the development of speech from a baby's babbling to the production of single words, phrases and then sentences. This double development has been termed input and output communication and clearly is a vital component of the learning ability of a child.

Social behaviour and play is much less precisely defined, for it involves the aptitudes already discussed and the child's ability to apply them in certain situations. It concerns the child's reactions to and comprehension of things and people. A young baby may not recognise his mother's face and voice; is this because he cannot see or hear, or does he see and hear, but fail to comprehend? A child of three may be unable to do up a button; is this due to poor manipulative ability, or just that he does not understand what a button is for? A normal child of eighteen months will obey a simple request, 'Go and fetch your shoes'; if he does not, is this due to inability to hear, or failure to comprehend the meaning of the request? A test of comprehension, his ability to behave and play, must first involve the knowledge that his other abilities, of movement and manipulation, of sight, hearing and speech are intact; we are now in the field of intelligence testing as used by the educational psychologist.

The salient features

Between the ages of twelve months and five years the child undergoes processes of development which largely determine his future achievements. It is said that the period of maximum brain growth is from mid-gestation to the fourth birthday (Lloyd-Still, 1976). We are thus in the age range of development of cognitive functions, intellectual comprehension and communicative ability. Some congenital anomalies may not become apparent till after the first or even second birthday and while these should always be sought, they will be found less frequently. The important fields to consider are vision and eye-hand co-ordination, hearing, comprehension and speech, curiosity, imagination and the ability to concentrate and the child's behavioural functions.

The eye

Distant vision is tested by the rolling ball (Stycar) test. There are those who maintain that this method can be abandoned in favour of the small plastic balls attached to rods with the examiner behind a slit screen (Ch. 41). This, however, involves clumsy apparatus and I think it is unlikely to find favour as a screening test in general practice as opposed to a more definitive test. The cover test is used for squint, but the writer thinks that any child whose mother has reported a transient squint (only when he's tired) should be referred, even though the cover test is normal in the surgery.

Hearing, comprehension and speech

Hearing is tested by the Stycar 4, 5 and 6 toy test. It is fundamental that the examiner should first ensure that the child knows the names of the toys before him (comprehension) and any child who cannot hear the spoken voice across a small table must be very deaf indeed and should have been identified long before. The early detection of deafness is discussed further in Chapter 40. We are concerned here with the lesser degrees of hearing loss at all pitches which delineate the nuances of expression. The range of vocabulary can be gauged by looking at the pictures in a picture book. Pronunciation is noted, as is the degree of interest and power of sustained concentration. Starte, (1976) in an important paper, has shown that of 23 children found to have developmental delay at the age of 4½ years all had delay in speech and/or hearing at the age of two.

At the age of two years the form board (square, triangle and circle) can be used as a test of adaptive behaviour, or a shape box, which can be bought in any toy shop. The Goodenough Draw-a-man test can be used at any age from three onwards and scored appropriately and drawing tests and a variety of others are available. A simple but good test of comprehension and memory at the age of 4½ is to read a short story to the child and ask questions about it afterwards; simply asking his name, age and address is often very revealing. Finally the physical examination must never be omitted, for although abnormal findings are uncommon, they occasionally surprise one and it is for this reason that many of us feel that the time is not yet appropriate for developmental examinations to be done solely by the health visitor.

Increased understanding of behavioural development and its modification

This has been an important advance in recent years in child health care. The identification of children who are shy and diffident, of children who have difficulty in expression although having normal hearing, of children who lack appropriate stimulation at home has led to a search for remedies for these conditions (Pollack, 1972). Many can be helped by attendance at a play group with an understanding and suitable play group leader. The speech therapist is being involved more frequently and at an earlier age. The importance of mothers reading regularly and clearly to children, especially those who have some hearing loss, can be emphasised. Modifications of routine can be suggested and support provided for the parents of children with sleep disturbance. The consequences of isolation and rejection are being better understood and many other instances suggest themselves of ways in which we can help children with these problems.

A STRUCTURED PROGRAMME OF SURVEILLANCE

What is urgently needed is a structured and validated screening programme with specific tests, and there is urgent need for a standard record card to be drawn up to record the result of screening examinations and assessment (Brotherston, 1973).

Such a card could be equally appropriate in general practice, a welfare clinic or a paediatric outpatient department, for there is little doubt that developmental screening must become a routine part of the outpatient interview, if it has not already been done in the primary care situation, and the information forwarded with the referral letter.

Furthermore, such a record card would encourage the adoption of developmental surveillance by general practitioners, but until such time as this discipline becomes an integral part of general practice, a large part of the burden must fall on community physicians working either in welfare clinics or in health centres; there are now plenty of examples of paediatric community physicians working in complete harmony with general practitioners in health centres or welfare clinics (Fisher and Keating, 1973).

There are, of course, certain other screening procedures which, while not strictly 'developmental', should not be overlooked. Testing for phenylketonuria has now become established policy, and screening for metabolic disorders such as hypothyroidism will undoubtedly soon become routine. One condition which is not looked for but which may well repay screening in the future is infant obesity. The plotting of weight gain on the percentile charts of Tanner and Whitehouse (1966) could act as a prophylactic measure for this dangerous condition (Wolff and Lloyd, 1974). Similarly, if height is plotted on similar percentile charts, among other benefits growth hormone deficiency can be detected and corrected at the optimum age (Tanner, 1975).

One other benefit arising from developmental screening in general practice is the high proportion of children who complete their primary immunisation course.

Fisher and Keating (1973) rightly drew attention to the financial aspect involved in developmental screening, and it can be argued that sooner or later the government should finance this on an item of service basis in the same way that antenatal and postnatal care is now financed. Is such expenditure justified? If, as we are assured by our leaders, the future prosperity of this country lies not so much in its natural resources as in the brains and inventiveness of its people, then any policy which will enable future generations to achieve their maximum potential is not only desirable but imperative, and herein lies the importance of screening children. The issue is not so much whether we can afford it, as whether we can afford to neglect it.

REFERENCES

Brotherston Report (1973) *Towards an Integrated Child Health Service*. Scottish Home and Health Department. Edinburgh: HMSO.

Court report (1976) *Fit for the Future*. London: HMSO.

Egan, F., Illingworth, R.S. & McKeith, R.C. (1969) *Developmental Screening, 0–5 years*. London: Heinemann.

Fisher, J.F. & Keating, P.K. (1973) Cooperation in developmental paediatrics. *Community Health*. 5, 153.

Lloyd-Still, J.D. (1976) *Malnutrition and Intellectual Development*. Lancaster: M & P Press.

Royal College of General Practitioners (1978) *The Care of Children*. Journal of the RCGP, **28**, 553.

Sheridan, M. (1958) *Stycar Tests of Hearing*. London: NFER.

Sheridan, M. (1960) *Developmental Progress of Infants and Young Children*. London: HMSO.

Sheridan, M. (1969) *Stycar Tests of Vision*. London: NFER.

Starte, G.D. (1976) *Results from a Developmental Screening Clinic in General Practice. Practitioner*, **216**, 311

Tanner, J.M. (1975) Towards complete success in the treatment of growth hormone deficiency: a plea for earlier ascertainment. *Health Trends*, 7, 61–65.

Tanner, J.M., Whitehouse, R.H. & Takaish, M.C. (1966) Standards from birth to maturity for height, weight, height velocity and weight velocity. British children. *Archives of Disease in Childhood*, **41**, 451.

Wolff, O.H. & Lloyd, J.K. (1974) Obesity. *Medicine*, **27**, 1583.

15

The school health service

John Walker

One of the major problems of the school health service is the fact that its structure and function have survived almost unaltered through seven decades of intense change in the pattern of child health.

Established in 1908, the first organised system of health care for children, the School Medical Service had to deal with the problems of a population, 60 per cent of whom were physically unfit for military service. Through case finding by routine medical inspection, the organisation of treatment by the provision of specialist services and the practice of preventive paediatrics, it played a considerable role in improving child health during the 1920s and 1930s.

By the early 1980s, with the service well over its three score years and ten, few of the problems of schoolchildren are of the type detected seventy years earlier by routine medical inspection. Medical care is provided increasingly by primary care teams, general practitioner, health visitor and home nurse. They are supported by an increasing range of paediatric specialists, and the pathology with which they deal is predominantly functional rather than physical.

Despite these many changes, a small proportion of children still reach school entry suffering from potentially handicapping conditions, some already recognised and treated, others yet to be detected. In addition, many children, apparently normal at school entry, later develop physical, social, emotional or educational problems which require diagnosis and management.

The aim of child care has been defined by the World Health Organisation as 'to give each child the opportunity to achieve his full potential in physical, emotional, intellectual and social terms' – aims remarkably similar to those of the original School Medical Service. Whilst these aims will increasingly be achieved through general improvements in the environment and higher standards of preventive care, a need will continue to exist within a comprehensive child health service for one part to act as a long-stop for those children whose pre-school care has been inadequate, and to deal with those problems of child health specific to education.

Had the proposals of the Court Committee for the development of an integrated child health service been accepted, the staff involved in this work would have been based in general practice and would have provided co-ordinated continuous care throughout childhood. Although many practices are now beginning to organise systems of pre-school health surveillance for children, this will take some time to develop and it is likely that the more specialised care of children in school will remain a separate activity for many years to come.

THE PRESENT SCHOOL HEALTH SERVICE: STRUCTURE AND STAFFING

Until 1974 the school health service was the responsibility of each local education authority, and the medical officer of health held the additional title of principal school medical officer. A senior school medical officer was responsible to him for the day-to-day running of the service and was supported in a hierarchical structure by a number of full and part-time medical staff. In April 1974 the provision of a comprehensive health service for children became the responsibility of each area health authority, and the functions of the principal and senior school medical officers were assumed by the specialists in community medicine (child health).

The role of the clinical medical staff remained largely unaffected by reorganisation. Approximately 4000 doctors work full or part-time in the service (1062 whole-time equivalents) and although no specific training is required, approximately 20 per cent possess the Diploma in Child Health. Many have attended courses in developmental paediatrics, and some, courses required for the 'ascertainment' of the handicapped child.

The absence of a formal postgraduate training requirement nevertheless distinguishes community child health from most other medical work. The Council for Postgraduate Medical Education therefore published in 1978 an outline of objectives and requirements for 'core' medical training for the child health service, the basic elements of which were contained within six months' experience in hospital paediatrics and six months in general practice, community paediatrics and child health. These proposals have been accepted in some regions and elaborated in others, where comprehensive programmes include an appropriate mixture of service experience and academic instruction.

Until 1974 – as a legacy from pre-NHS days – specialist support for school doctors was provided by ophthalmologists, orthopaedic surgeons and other specialists employed by local authorities on a part-time basis. These consultant services are now available in the normal way. Other support is provided by speech therapists, physiotherapists, audiometricians, orthoptists and chiropodists.

In each area the school nursing service is the responsibility of the area nurse (child health). The majority of the 10 000 school nurses possess a health visiting qualification, and many work part-time, with their major role in practice attachment.

Until reorganisation, the child guidance services of the local education authorities employed 111 child psychiatrists directly, and enjoyed the part-time seconded services of a further 293 (114 whole-time equivalents). All these specialists are now employed by the NHS, and are supported by approximately 700 educational psychologists who continue under the aegis of the local authority.

Also integrated within the NHS, the school dental services are under the direction of each Area Dental Officer. They employ almost 2000 dentists and 2700 assistants and technicians. The service, in addition to its major function of routine inspection, is responsible for approximately one fifth of all dental treatment to school children.

Role of the school health service

The tasks of the school health service have been defined in *The Health of the School Child 1969-70* as:

1. To supervise the growth and development of the school child
2. To identify children with specific disorders which may affect their learning and behaviour
3. To identify physical defects
4. To undertake screening procedures
5. To work closely with teachers
6. To supervise at school, children under medical treatment
7. To provide supplementary treatment, e.g. physiotherapy, speech therapy
8. To maintain immunity levels
9. To provide health education
10. To supplement the advisory services for the parents of handicapped children
11. To provide a consultation service for adolescents
12. To work closely with family doctors and paediatricians

The extent to which all of these tasks will be achieved is very dependent upon the attitudes and expertise within each area service. Common to all areas, however, are screening procedures, conducted by the school nurse for the purposes of supervising cleanliness and hygiene; the routine medical examination of children, at or before school entry, and subsequently; the identification of children with specific disorders, their assessment and placement in appropriate schools.

Hygiene inspection

One of the major functions of the school nurse is the inspection of school children for general cleanliness, skin disease and infestation. In 1972 almost 13 000 000 inspections were carried out. Over a quarter of a million children were found to be infested, and appropriate treatment and advice provided. The prevalence of verminous infestation is much higher after school holidays, and without the surveillance of the school nurse would clearly be higher. Other conditions detected and treated at routine hygiene inspections include impetigo, ringworm, scabies and plantar warts.

Routine medical examination

The traditional and most time consuming activity of the school doctor has been the periodic medical inspection of children to detect 'defects capable of correction'. Necessary in the days before the development of the National Health Service, the relevance of examination at school entry when each preschool child should have been under the care of health visitor, general practitioner and child health clinic, is being questioned. The importance of repeated inspections during later years is even more hotly debated.

Although the requirements of a 1945 regulation that each child should be examined on three occasions, at school entry, the last year in primary school, and before leaving secondary school, were modified in 1959, many education authorities were slow to respond. The pattern throughout the country is extremely varied.

All authorities examine all children either just before or just after school entry. Thereafter approximately half continue periodic inspection at specified intervals, despite discouragement by the Department of Education and Science, while the remainder use a more rational system of selective examination, the doctor seeing only those children about whom he, the school nurse, the school teacher or the parent has anxiety. Despite this rationalisation, approximately two million children each year are examined, an expensive activity which must be justified.

In 1968 almost 720 000 children were examined at school entry. The number of defects detected and recorded as requiring treatment proved to be 166 per thousand – those of the eyes 50 per thousand, of the nose and throat 21 per thousand, of the ears 19 per thousand, and of the skeletal system 17 per thousand. By any criterion a screening process with a yield of 16.6 per cent is satisfactory. More recently, the criteria have been widened. In 1976, of the 747 000 schoolchildren examined in England and Wales, 307 000 were found to have visual defects (including squint), 75 000 defects of the ear, nose or throat, 66 000 orthopaedic or postural defects, and 125 000 children were in need of speech therapy. In many cases remedial treatment had been instituted already. These figures, however, are based upon the observations of a large number of school doctors, completing a routine inspection a systematic check list in the school medical record (Form 10M) using a recording protocol:

√ = no defect
O = defect requiring observation
T = defect requiring treatment
RS = defect requiring reference to specialist
RGP = reference to the general practitioner
PD = permanent defect not requiring action

The results of the examination are therefore very dependent upon the interpretation of this protocol by the individual doctor.

In an attempt to evaluate the quality of the problems recorded and their clinical importance, Lowdon and Walker (1975) scrutinised the school medical records of 1255 nine-year-old children. They found after studying the clinical notes of the children that approximately 25 per cent had an abnormality at school entry which could be regarded as clinically significant, and almost five per cent required specialist referral for previously undetected problems. They concluded that routine school entry medical examinations remain an essential screening procedure and recommended that they should continue until completely effective programmes during the preschool years have become established.

However effective earlier care may be, school entry will continue to provide a valuable opportunity for total developmental assessment of each child. Current recommendations of the Department of Education and Science are that the process should begin with a questionnaire seeking information from parents concerning the child's social, medical and family background. A summary of the findings of pre-school medical and developmental examinations and of immunisation should be provided. An assessment of the child's physical growth including measurement of height and weight, and tests of vision, hearing, speech and language should be carried out. An assessment of the child's social and emotional development should be made from observed behaviour, and the recommendations also include tests of fine and gross motor function, tests of hearing by pure tone audiometry, and possibly the culture of midstream urine in girls. The process would be completed by a general physical examination.

During the succeeding years, the school nurse continues to arrange tests of vision, hearing, measurements of height and weight, surveys of hygiene and cleanliness, and the maintenance of immunisation routines. After the completion of the entry medical examination, the school doctor's role is to supervise those children found to be particularly at risk and to collaborate in the care of those being treated. Traditionally the workload of school doctors led to comparatively infrequent visits to individual schools. The Warnock Committee on Special Educational Needs recommended that each school should possess a named school doctor, identified as a member of staff, who would attend for weekly surgery sessions and who would make themselves available to school nurses, teachers, parents, psychologists and others for consultation about the medical educational, or social problems of individual children or of the school population at large. In many areas these proposals are being implemented to considerable effect.

The handicapped child of school age.

As general practice assumes increasing responsibility for the health surveillance of the normal child, the assessment and care of the handicapped will become an increasingly specialised function of the school health service. Whilst the more obviously handicapped children, particularly those suffering from congenital abnormalities, are detected early, many with intellectual retardation are not identified until they have been in school for a term, a year, or even longer, and a high index of suspicion on the part of health visitor, general practitioner, school doctor and school teacher must therefore be maintained. In the Newcastle study, it was found that approximately six per cent of children were referred to the school health service between the ages of five and nine by teachers, parents, social workers or psychologists because of specific problems, the most common of which were educational subnormality, physical handicap, repeated school absence, multiple handicap or emotional maladjustment.

Many handicapped children can be managed within the normal educational system, but some require admission to special classes or special schools, and comprehensive assessment by a panel of family doctor, school doctor, psychologist, social worker, teacher, together with the relevant paediatrician, psychiatrist, ophthalmologist or surgeon is necessary, working together as members of the district handicap team. Formal documentation has been designed to ensure this interdisciplinary collaboration and can be used, if necessary, as the basis for legal action. The importance of close consultation with the parents should ensure that they are in full agreement with any educational placement suggested, but they do have the right of appeal to the

Secretary of State for Education, should this not be the case.

Assessment is followed by educational placement. Originally described as 'ascertainment', assessment under the *1944 Education Act* excluded school children who were unsuitable for education because of a disability of mind. This damagingly negative attitude to mental subnormality began to disappear in the 1950s when 'junior training centres' for the severely subnormal were set up under the *1959 Mental Health Act*. These are now the responsibility of education authorities and have become schools for the severely subnormal.

Whatever the handicap, intellectual, physical or sensory, an appropriate placement can be found within the wide range of day, residential and special care facilities available. As a consequence of Warnock Committee views, the emphasis is moving towards the management of handicapped children in normal rather than special schools.

The school doctor involved in assessment, placement and continuing supervision of handicapped children in any setting, requires a broad knowledge of child development, child psychiatry, the principles of educational psychology, physiotherapy, speech therapy, ophthalmology and social work. To date the only qualification required has been attendance at one of the comparatively short courses on the ascertainment of the handicapped child. It has been suggested that this task might in future be undertaken by a consultant paediatrician with special skills in community aspects of child health, who would play a co-ordinate clinical role and provide support and training for other doctors working with children (Walker, 1968). The identification and supervision of children with handicapping conditions and the management of those in special schools and special classes in normal schools has established a new role for school doctors in continuing care.

In 1979 the number of children in special schools was as follows:

Blind	1100
Partially sighted	2800
Deaf	4100
Partially hearing	7250
Physically handicapped	16 700
Delicate	6900
Maladjusted	22 400
Educationally sub-normal	119 000
Epileptic	1700
Speech defective	2900
	184 850

These children require frequent developmental review, and the staff involved in their care close medical support. Describing the work of the doctor in a school for 200 physically handicapped children, Lowdon and Walker (1975) suggested that the equivalent of four clinical sessions per week were necessary to meet their needs. If those of children in the other categories are to be met, the task is considerable.

The admission of a child to any special school should imply the creation of an active therapeutic partnership between the school, the school doctor, the general practitioner, the hospital specialists involved, the Department of Social Services, and ultimately the Department of Employment. In this context the school doctor should work as a full member of the clinical team, and accept clinical and therapeutic responsibility. At present this is possible only through goodwill and the development of close personal relationships with the other clinicians, for the school doctor is still theoretically inhibited by a restricted and historic job definition from assuming any other than a preventive role.

The major problem faced by the parents of a handicapped child is that of access to authoritative support. The Warnock Committee suggested that a 'named individual' should be responsible for co-ordinating the continuous care of each handicapped child. In many instances the appropriate individual will be the school doctor.

Educational psychology and child guidance

As the physical problems of childhood have diminished, the relative importance of learning problems and behaviour disorders has increased. Educational subnormality is the largest handicapping condition in childhood, and up to 40 per cent of children demonstrate some symptoms of 'maladjustment' at some stage of their development.

The original recommendations (RMPA, 1960) for the structure of a basic child guidance team designed to serve a school population of 35 000 was for one child psychiatrist, two educational psychologists and a psychiatric social worker. By 1972 this target had been achieved in relatively few parts of the country and although the supply of educational psychologists has steadily improved, that of child psychiatrists is likely to be inadequate for many years to come. As child psychiatry units in hospital continue to develop, the pattern of child guidance in the education service will change and much more responsibility for preliminary assessment will fall upon the psychologist. The continuing shortage of child psychiatrists will mean that general practitioners and school doctors will have to play an increasing part in collaboration with psychologists in diagnosing and managing children with learning difficulties and behaviour patterns. This in turn will require developments in the training programmes for these doctors if they are to function effectively. Lowdon and Walker showed that 60 per cent of children classified as educationally subnormal were also suffering from a variety of medical conditions, evidence reinforcing the importance of multidisciplinary assessment and management.

As behaviour problems increase in frequency, the counselling and support of parents, teachers and others involved in child care may prove to be more profitable than the often protracted and detailed care of a small number of children with complex problems by the classical methods of child guidance. It has been shown that attendance at a child guidance clinic produces no greater improvement than management by supportive care in the community. Each child with a behaviour disorder, however, does require diagnosis in social, medical and psychological terms. If the problem arises in school, the teacher will find it most convenient to refer to the psychologist. One of the immediate tasks of the school health service is to ensure that he has appropriate medical support.

THE FUTURE

Most of those working in the community child health services had hoped that the Court report recommendations would end an extended period of uncertainty. The fact that so few of the recommendations have been accepted for implementation has therefore caused considerable concern.

The development of the service must, in the absence of immediate administrative change, therefore rely upon evolution.

The continued development of the primary care team should allow the implementation of the recommendations of the Sheldon Committee that preschool care of children should be concentrated in family practice. When this is achieved the detection of physical and major developmental abnormalities should be complete by school entry, for as Wintle, Clay and Davis (1972) have shown, the equivalent of the school entry medical examination can readily be undertaken in a well organised group practice. This will liberate the school doctor and allow him to concentrate upon the problems of later childhood and those specific to the school situation. In close and effective partnership with school nurses, teachers, educational psychologists, speech therapists and others, the school doctor should become a specialist in the care of the handicapped child, and in the diagnosis and management of all children who demonstrate physical, educational or emotional difficulties during the school years. This role will require a detailed job description and a specific training programme. Some general practitioners with a special interest in children may accept it on a part-time basis. It may be undertaken by the appropriately trained successors of the present community child health doctor, or by specialist 'community paediatricians'. What is clear is that effective care of children demands increasing expertise, of which educational paediatrics is a part.

REFERENCES

Council for Postgraduate Medical Education in England and Wales (1978) *Outline of Objectives and Requirements for 'Core' Medical Training for the Child Health Service.*

HMSO (1972) *The Health of the School Child 1969–1970.* London: HMSO.

HMSO (1974) *The Health of the School Child 1971–1972.* London: HMSO.

HMSO (1978) *Special Educational Needs: Report of the Committee of Enquiry into the Education of Handicapped Children and Young People*, Cmnd. 7212 London: HMSO.

Lowdon, G. & Walker, J.H. (1975) *Bridging in Health.* Nuffield Provincial Hospitals Trust.

RMPA (1960) *Memorandum on the Recruitment and Training of the Child Psychiatrist.* London: Royal Medico-Psychological Association.

Walker, J.H. (1969) *British Journal of Medical Education*, **3**, 316–318

Wintle, C.J., Clay, S. & Davis, R.H. (1972) *Journal of the Royal College of General Practitioners*, **22**, 118, 327.

16

Ill-treated children

Denis Pereira Gray

DEFINITIONS

The ill-treated child syndrome can be defined as 'children who are ill-treated by adults'. It is also known as 'non-accidental injury in children' and 'child abuse', and is best known as 'the battered baby syndrome'. However, as general practitioners make their diagnosis in three dimensions, physical, psychological, and social, it is particularly necessary for them to include emotional ill-treatment which has also been called the 'parental deprivation syndrome' (Pereira Gray, 1970).

HISTORY

Caffey (1946), an American radiologist, first described a syndrome of subdural haematomata and multiple fractures in infants. Silverman (1954), another radiologist, suggested that the cause could be parental violence. Wooley and Evans (1955) suggested that fractures discovered by radiologists might have been inflicted deliberately by parents. Kempe (1962), also from America, in a classic paper first coined the term 'battered baby syndrome'.

PREVALENCE

The exact prevalence of this condition is not known. Kempe (1971) has estimated it at three per thousand live births which would be equivalent to 1500 to 2000 children injured in the United Kingdom each year. The Registrar General (1971) however, reports 9 deaths from deliberate injury, with and additional 49 classified as 'not certain if inflicted'. In addition there are about 250 'sudden deaths cause unknown' under the age of 4 each year. The Tunbridge Wells Committee (1973) estimated that the United Kingdom has 4600 cases a year.

Many authors like Gambrill (1973) have stressed how relatively rarely practitioners will see this condition: 'Each general practitioner will expect to see an average new case once every ten years.' But these figures are based on the serious cases, and milder forms can be seen much more often in general practice. Those general practitioners who are interested in this condition are now reporting a prevalence of one per thousand of their practice population. In other words among ill-treated children the severely battered form only the tip of the iceberg.

The general practitioner's problem is that he has, as always, to define normality. There are many children in rough households where children, wives and others are hit at times. One big problem lies in defining when this constitutes ill-treatment.

Causes

The causes so far known include:

1. A group of parents who feel less caring towards their children than usual. Characteristically they have a lower than average tolerance to stress and less control over their emotions. Factors which reduce the likelihood of parental feeling developing fully are now beginning to be identified and include: ill-treatment of the parents themselves when they were children, poor education, poverty, a handicapping condition in the parent, e.g. epilepsy, and separation of mother and child at birth.
2. Severe blunting of emotional feeling in the parents, particularly the mother, is sometimes associated with puerperal depression.
3. The psychopathic, a group of parents who express their feelings violently, i.e. who 'talk with their fists'. Some of these patients are alcoholics, see Chapter 49.
4. Psychotic parents (in about five per cent of cases of ill-treatment).

Pathology

The main pathological findings are:

1. Bruises or burns which are often multiple.
2. Ruptured frenulum.
3. Fractures, especially of the long bones, ribs, and skull.

4. Subdural haematoma, which is the classic cause of death, and which is often thought to be associated with shaking and injuries to the skull. Shaking in particular is a much underestimated risk for children under the age of two, because of the pressures set up within the skull.

Natural history

Prognosis

Experts are still arguing about the risk of death. The Tunbridge Wells Committee (1973) estimated up to 17 per cent died derived from Hall's (1975) finding of five deaths from 29 definite cases, whereas Castle and Kerr (1972) found that about one per cent were fatal. Personally, I believe the latter figure is more correct. In one of the surveys of the National Society for the Prevention of Cruelty to Children (NSPCC) over 75 per cent of the initial sample followed up were still living at home with their parents, and only 12 per cent of the children at that time were in care. The sociological danger is that the ill-treatment may form part of the 'cycle of deprivation' and may be passed on from one generation to the next.

Characteristics of the families

The child

Physical battering is most common at an age when a child is immobile and unable to talk. Eighty eight per cent are either first or last children in the family. The incidence in children with a birthweight of less than 2500 grammes is about twice as high as in other children. O'Brien (1974) believes that adopted children are most unlikely to be injured.

The adult

The mother is more commonly responsible than the father, and she is usually aged under 30. General practitioners naturally consider both parents, because even if one causes the injuries exclusively, the other usually gives tacit consent. The mother's pregnancy was often unwanted and the mother may have sought abortion in pregnancy; paternity may be disputed. The NSPCC has shown an association with pregnancy, and marital stress is common.

The identi-kit is of unhappy, aggressive, socially isolated young parents, who may themselves have been injured in their own childhood. There are often absent or inadequate contacts with their own parents, ill-treatment being less common in the extended family.

Such parents often co-operate poorly with authorities, including doctors, for example in failing to attend for antenatal care. In general practice they may be frequent attenders and this may represent a form of 'cry for help'. Selwyn Smith (1974) reports that in one third of cases of ill-treated children, the biological father was absent from home, and in half these cases the mothers were living with some other man.

Social class

The bulk of the evidence suggests a higher prevalence in patients in the lower social classes, who are more likely to be subjected to multiple social pressures (Castle and Kerr, 1972). Perhaps the middle classes may be able to afford to employ a nanny or an au pair.

Clinical features in general practice

Most of the children seen regularly in general practice with bruises and injuries will not have been ill-treated. However, the following features are associated with this syndrome, and particular care should be taken if two or more of these occur simultaneously:

1. *The time of presentation.* Characteristically the battered child is presented late, often some time having elapsed since the injury.
2. *The presentation.* The child may be brought to a doctor other than the usual doctor, for example, an accident and emergency department or another practitioner.
3. *Accompanying adult.* The injury may be presented not by the parent, but by some other person, particularly the grandparent.
4. *Significant inconsistencies in the history.* There are inconsistencies in the history of the injury, i.e. discrepancies when the story is repeated at different times to different people. Sometimes the description of the injury is not compatible with the development of the child at the time. Was the child capable of doing what it was alleged to have been doing?
5. *The nature of the lesions.* Most physically ill-treated children show only bruising, especially when over two years old. Burns and scalds also occur (Keen *et al.* 1975). Fractures are unusual in young children, especially under 12 months, and should in themselves arouse the doctor's suspicions. Dappling of the skin and coldness and blueness of the hands and feet in association with low weight occur in emotionally depressed children.
6. *Site of injuries.* Some sites are more likely than others to be associated with ill-treatment. Bruises particularly on the face, i.e. forehead, mouth and jaw-line are important, as are bruises on the buttock and back. One NSPCC survey found that 73 per cent of 292 injured children had head and facial injuries. A ruptured frenulum of the tongue has been described as the classic injury. On the other hand, bruises on the arms and shins commonly occur through children knocking themselves or falling.
7. *Multiple injuries in area or time.* The presence of multiple bruises increases suspicion of ill-treatment in proportion to the number. Similarly, repeated bruising

over a period of time should arouse suspicion where an individual bruise might not attract attention.

8. *The timing of the injury*. Children are more likely to be hit at times when they create problems for adults. Two of the commonest childhood disorders seen in general practice are – 'He won't eat, doctor' and 'He won't sleep, doctor' and these are reminders of the times where ill-treatment may occur from desperate parents. Injuries are much commoner at meal times and after a child has been put to bed, when he cries and will not sleep.

9. *Reluctance to allow medical examination*. General practitioners may find, especially in mild cases, a reluctance to allow full examination. Sometimes on home visits the child is conspicuous by his absence, and great skill and tact may be needed to achieve examination at all.

The role of the general practitioner

There is at present an interesting debate in the medical profession about this syndrome and the role of doctors and general practitioners in particular. Some of the most distinguished paediatricians in the country have argued that as social service departments now have a statutory responsibility for the care of children and sole power with the courts to remove children to a place of safety, practitioners have no responsibility other than detection and referral to social workers and the 'right doctor' (Court *et al*, 1974). 'The doctor cannot abdicate a responsibility he never had.'

This rather narrow view overlooks the fact that general practitioners have a duty to provide all necessary medical care and attention to children, for both physical and emotional conditions. Furthermore, they have also a responsibility to other members of the household who are usually involved. The role of the general practitioner can be classified as follows:

1. Suspecting the condition.
2. Detection.
3. Management in the home
    - accessibility
    - communications
        - with the family
        - within the practice
        - outside the practice
    - continuous care.
4. Management by removal to a place of safety.
5. Prevention.

Suspicion

The general practitioner and the health visitor working together are the ideal health team to suspect ill-treatment in children. They are in contact with more members of the community than any other medically qualified people and most of the situations where ill-treatment is likely to occur are (or should be) known to the practice. The 'at risk' concept is helpful and it is likely in the future that many families will be identified in general practice before serious injury occurs.

Detection

The detection rates reported so far from general practice are not high. The Battered Baby Research Unit of the NSPCC reported 370 children, of whom ten were referred by general practitioners directly (only 2½ per cent). Furthermore, it was noted that at least 60 of these had been children treated for the referred injuries by general practitioners only. 'Without further evidence, it is only possible to speculate as to whether general practitioners are slow to identify or to refer cases of child abuse' (Castle and Kerr, 1972). Practice well-baby clinics and regular surveillance should improve detection in general practice in the future.

Management

Accessibility

Accessibility is an important feature of general practice in the United Kingdom. Open-access surgeries and baby clinics can represent an important 'life-line' for patients in trouble (Waine, 1974). The extent to which families under stress turn to their general practitioner is one index of the doctor/patient relationship. Methods by which accessibility can be improved, including some flexibility in appointment systems and tolerance by doctors and their staff to late calls and aggressive behaviour from parents, could prove fruitful subjects for research similar to Stockwell's (1972) nursing study of the *Unpopular Patient*.

Communication and the co-ordination of medical care

The communication necessary in general practice can be subdivided into communication with patients, communication within the practice, and communication outside the practice.

Communication with patients. This is the essence of the doctor/patient relationship. In the ideal consultation the patient feels free to talk to the doctor about his problems even when these are intense, emotional and severe. Creating a relationship in which patients feel they can talk about the things that matter to them without pressure of time is one of the biggest organisational challenges confronting general practice today. Furthermore, general practitioners and health visitors must be skilled in identifying and understanding non-verbal communication.

The ordinary consultation in British general practice lasts on average only six minutes. On the other hand, general practitioners have an average of five contacts a year with each of their patients, and therefore have an average of 20 contacts with families with two children each year. In five years this is equivalent to over ten hours of doctor time and provides a good base both for communication and professional understanding by the doctor (*Journal of the Royal College of General Practitioners*, 1973).

Communication within the practice. Internal communication is often still difficult in general practice. Although communication with health visitors and nurses is improving, it is sad that even in 1973, as many as 21 per cent of health visitors in the United Kingdom were not yet fully attached to general practitioners (Department of Health, 1974a). If health visitors are not attached, communication within the practice must suffer. Record keeping is attracting increasing attention in general practice and the various medicosocial factors listed need to be recorded. Detailed records are in any case wise when a future appearance in court is possible.

Communication outside the practice. General practice has also been weak in relationships with social workers, partly because of lack of clarification of the practitioner's role. Nevertheless, it is going to be necessary, if adequate surveillance is to be achieved in the community, for general practitioners to be able to communicate outside the practice when they suspect or detect ill-treatment in children.

Continuing to care

One of the most difficult roles in the management of these families is in providing 'support'. Meetings in the surgery with the health visitor and NSPCC worker can be most useful and the family should normally be told about them. Continuity of care for the child means that the general practitioner goes on and on, month after month and year after year. The medical surveillance system must be good enough not to let the child slip through the system. A few parents will go to prison, some children will go into care, but the great majority of parents and children will remain in the home.

One of the most difficult skills in management is for the doctor and health visitor to maintain a detached and professional approach to the many problems which arise in these families. Continuity of care for the patients means being accessible, making contact somehow, and creating a counselling relationship. This takes time and is particularly skilled with rude and aggressive parents. However, the doctor, if he can treat such patients with dignity, may be offering the only model of civilised and caring behaviour available to the family.

Behaviour is infectious; violent, intolerant actions induce similar reactions, even among professionals in the caring professions. Sometimes the behaviour of the professionals is impulsive, impatient, rigid, and authoritarian, and exhibits unreasonable expectations of the family, and so mirrors closely the behaviour for which the family itself is being blamed.

Removal to a place of safety

Most authorities have assumed in the past that if a child who has been ill-treated needs to go to a place of safety, then that place ought to be a hospital bed. However, this need not be so. It depends on the individual child and his needs at the time. If the child has been injured and has, for example, a fracture, then of course, immediate hospital care is required. But if no such injury has occurred and the removal is prophylactic, then other possibilities such as a children's home or a foster home need discussion.

The advantages of hospital admission are:

1. Constant availability of a bed.
2. Specific treatment e.g. for cranial injuries or fractures.
3. Investigations e.g. whole body X-rays and other tests.
4. A consultant opinion may be most helpful.
5. Hospitals can resist parents more easily than a foster parent.

The advantages of admission to a children's home or placing with foster parents are:

1. It is more natural for the child.
2. Investigations, e.g. X-rays, and blood tests can often equally well be done on an outpatient basis.
3. Communication difficulties are minimised. In hospital there is often difficulty
   a. co-ordinating what is said to the family
   b. co-ordinating communication between doctors.
4. A community problem is contained in the community.
5. A hospital bed costs about twice as much per week as a place in a children's home and about ten times as much as a local authority-approved foster parent.

Removal of the child to a place of safety does not 'take the heat out to the situation' as is sometimes said. Often it raises the emotional heat, and it may well place other siblings or members of the household at risk. In all cases temporary removal anywhere represents only a short-term solution, and the general practitioner's role is never to take his eye off the long-term questions: 'Is this child eventually going to go home? If so, how can I promote his future physical and emotional health?'

Prevention

The general practitioner should be chiefly concerned with prevention (McConaghey, 1974). Of the various levels of care, the prevention of illness is the highest and most important. The prevention of physical and emotional harm to children must rank as one of the most rewarding and essential services to society, if the quality of life of future generations is to be improved. The general practitioner operating as he does on the boundary between medicine and society (Marinker, 1973) is ideally placed, particularly when working with home-based social workers, to undertake long-term prospective research within the National Health Service.

Donovan (1974) is leading groups of new mothers in his general practice. This has enabled many of them to share with the group their doubts and anxieties about their maternal feelings, and so learn that such mixed feelings are common. Such methods may lead to hostile feelings towards children being contained, and future injuries prevented.

Legislation protecting ill-treated children

The legislation affecting children in relation to ill-treatment is described in Chapter 3.

Registers of ill-treated children

The advantages and disadvantages of keeping registers of children who have been injured, or who are at risk of ill-treatment, can be summarised as follows:

Advantages

1. Professionals when confronted with an injury can check quickly if the child is on the at-risk register, e.g. accident and emergency departments.
2. Registers help to ensure follow-up when families with children at risk move from one area to another.
3. Data are generated about incidence, prevalence, and the characteristics of families with the condition.
4. Such statistics identify trends and highlight the need for changes in organisation.
5. Such statistics also educate all the caring professions in the area.

Disadvantages

1. Loss of confidentiality. Intimate information about families is made more widely available.
2. A poor example of relationships is given. The creation and use of secret files to which patients/clients have no access, is undesirable, unless absolutely essential. The onus of proof always rests on those who wish to use such registers/files to show that there is no better system available.

On balance, in my view, the advantages clearly outweigh the disadvantages and at-risk registers should at present therefore be supported. These registers are normally maintained by the local social services department, and general practitioners should note that the ethical code of social workers has not yet been agreed or implemented.

Case conferences

Case conferences are fashionable. They are widely put forward as the ideal method for the management of this condition. They have many advantages and many disadvantages. The technique of clinical decision-taking by multidisciplinary teams has not been based on any controlled trial of decision-taking. It has developed through anecdotal evidence of errors. The method therefore depends on, as yet, unconfirmed value judgements.

The objectives of case conferences are:

1. Communication. To inform, more competently than by any other method available, all those involved in the problem.
2. Decision-taking. To take, more effectively than would otherwise be possible, decisions in the interest of the child and family.

The advantages of case conferences are:

1. They bring people together who might not otherwise meet.
2. They educate those involved about the nature and extent of the problem.
3. They support the field workers by sharing the burden of responsibility (the hand-holding role).
4. The police may agree not to act without first consulting the conference.
5. Pressure from the conference may force other professionals or relevant departments to provide more readily resources like housing.
6. Many heads may be better than a few.
7. The problems are more likely to be fully documented.

The disadvantages are:

1. They disrupt the work of many professional people by being held at fixed times in the day.
2. They take time, often one or two hours.
3. They inevitably spread confidential information about people.
4. They offer a bad model of behaviour by being formal, by dealing with personal problems impersonally, and by being held without the knowledge of, and usually without the consent of, the people who are being discussed.
5. They are expensive. Each conference is likely to cost the various government departments (through the staff involved, administration, and transport) about £100 (1980 rates). General practitioners are usually entitled to a fee for attending.
6. Professional responsibilities may become blurred or diminished.

A typical case conference consists of a total authority social worker, an NSPCC representative, a consultant paediatrician, a paediatric registrar, the general practitioner, the health visitor, a police officer and perhaps a representative from the housing department. It is often organised by a district community physician or a member of his staff. General practitioners should establish before attending, who will be present and, if the police will be there, what principles govern police action in that area.

Quite often several members of the case conference do not know all the members of the family personally and many have never visited the home. If this happens then two unfortunate consequences tend to occur. Either these members of the conference stay silent, which is a waste of time and money, or they participate and take the decision, with the effect that the decision-making process moves from those who do know the family as individuals to those who do not.

Evolving a policy of care

Policy-making bodies

No single person, no group of people, no organisation, and no government in any country yet knows how best to organise the medical and social care of children being ill-treated in their homes.

The origins are rooted in the very nature of society itself and many of the causative factors have not yet even been discovered. Factors which are already known like the experiences of the parents themselves as children, education, and poverty will not be soluble in the foreseeable future. The ill-treated child syndrome is therefore a complex medicosocial family problem which will so continue for many years, perhaps for ever.

In medical care normally only well-proven treatments become standard throughout the country, and new methods of management are normally subjected to prospective controlled trials. I believe this is not the time to standardise treatment; on the contrary there is an urgent need for experimentation with different methods in different areas, and for objective evaluation of the different methods.

The *principle* of dealing with the family must be to provide a flexible, tolerant, compassionate and highly-skilled professional medical and social service where it is needed – in the home. The professionals must be able to cope with the parents and simultaneously care for the child. Such a team must always have the power to apply for removal of the child, by a court order, to a place of safety.

Yet all the efforts of central policy-making bodies at present seem to be directed in the opposite direction. The policy of the Tunbridge Wells Study Group (1973) and the Department of Health (1974b) is to admit the child to hospital immediately on the least suspicion, to hold case conferences every time, and to promote case conferences as policy-making and decision-taking bodies.

Thus the authorities are seeking to standardise a remote, formal, impersonal and multidisciplinary solution to a local inter-personal problem in a family. The policy of some NSPCC units of providing local family support in the home on an open access and continuing basis may in the long term prove a more important model.

In 1980, the Department of Health issued new guidelines on the use of risk registers which have moved nearer to the policy advocated in this chapter in the first edition. The Department of Health now recommends that parents should be told when their child is put on the register and the scope is extended to include mental and emotional abuse and failure to thrive. It is suggested that each area should appoint one officer as 'custodian' of the register.

An alternative role for central, regional, and area health service authorities could be to build up and support field workers in the three caring professions (social work, nursing, and medicine). There is a particular need to promote education and also to ensure that executive departments like social security and housing are flexible and respond to local needs. Central policy-making bodies may also be able to support prospective, long-term, home-based research on families where ill-treatment of children may occur.

Life-threatening emotional crises in the home

Ill-treatment of children should not be considered as a problem in isolation. It is a condition of society itself, and police statistics reveal a society where offences against the person are becoming more common. Generalist doctors, working in the field, see such problems in perspective in relation to the whole range of life-threatening emotional crises occurring in the home.

It may be helpful to consider ill-treatment of children as a crisis like abortion and attempted suicide. In all conditions, a life is at stake, usually a young one, and injury to a person occurs. All cause fundamental conflict between the rights of individuals, the duties of the state, and the responsibilities of the medical profession. All create intense emotions among lay people, among the caring professions, and among members of Parliament.

Experience has shown that in the interests of the patient(s) involved, it is often wiser for decision-taking and continuing responsibility to rest with field workers. Only field workers who know the home, and all those in it, can assess the emotional and social pressures (such as personality difficulties, marital problems, housing, and poverty) which drive patients to seek violent solutions to the problems of their lives.

Above all the responsibility for preventing such events lies not in hospital, but in the home. Slowly, shakily, but progressively, general practitioners are awakening and rising to the challenge of the care in the community of such major life-threatening medical and social crises. Attempted suicide is no longer a crime, but is rightly regarded as an acute emotional crisis – usually involving the family. Abortion is also now not usually a crime and is similarly regarded as another acute personal emotional crisis.

I believe that in the future, ill-treatment by a family of its children will similarly be recognised as a serious life-threatening distortion of the family's emotions. If this is so, future management will depend less and less on police prosecution and legal restraint, although these will always be necessary for more severe cases, but will come to depend more and more on highly skilled, and caring social workers, doctors, and health visitors working together in the community.

CONCLUSION

I believe that the care of the ill-treated child will continue in the years ahead to be one of the most difficult and complex clinical problems in family practice. Few conditions are so challenging in the physical, psychological, and social dimensions; few are potentially so serious; few are more difficult to manage. This is a family disease and will always involved the family doctor.

ACKNOWLEDGEMENTS

I would like to thank the large number of general practitioners and several Faculties of the Royal College of General Practitioners who sent me information and comments in reply to my letter in *The Journal of the Royal College of General Practitioners* (1974). I would also like to thank Mrs Mavis Huckle for typing the manuscript.

REFERENCES

British Medical Journal (1969) Editorial, **3**, 667–668.
Caffey, J. (1946) *American Journal of Roentgenology*, **56**, 163–173.
Castle, R. & Kerr. A. (1972) *A Study of Suspected Child Abuse*. London: NSPCC.
Court, D., Lister, J. & Franklyn, A.W. (1974) *British Medical Journal*, **3**, 801.
Department of Health and Social Security (1974a) *Annual Report*. London: HMSO.
Department of Health and Social Security (1974b) *Memorandum on Non-accidental Injury in Children*. London: DHSS.
Department of Health and Social Security (1980) *Guidelines on Risk Registers*. London: DHSS.
Donovan, C. (1974) Personal communication.
Gambrill, E. (1973) *Update*, **7**, 1163.
Gray, D.J. P. (1970) *Transactions of the Hunterian Society*, **28**, 121–175.
Gray, D.J. P. (1974) *Journal of the Royal College of General Practitioners*, **24**, 496.
Holl, M.H. (1975) In *Concerning Child Abuse*, pp. 2–20. Edinburgh: Churchill Livingstone.
Journal of the Royal College of General Practitioners (1973) Editorial, Continuity of care, **23**, 749–50.
Kempe, C.H. (1962) *Journal of the American Medical Association*, **181**, 17–240.
Keen, J.H., Ledrum, J. & Wolman, B. (1975) Inflicted burns and scalds in children. *British Medical Journal*, **4**, 268–9.
McConaghey, R.M.S. (1974) Personal communication.
Marinker, M.L. (1973) *Journal of the Royal College of General Practitioners*, **23**, 83–94.
O'Brien, P. (1975) Personal communication.
Silverman, F. (1954) *American Journal of Roentgenology*, **66**, 413.
Smith, S.M. (1974) *British Medical Journal*, **2**, 443.
Stockwell, Felicity (1972) *The Unpopular Patient*. London: Royal College of Nursing.
Tunbridge Wells Study Group (1973) London: D.H.S.S.
Waine, C. (1974) Personal communication.
Warley, P.V. & Evans, W. (1955) *Journal of the American Medical Association*, **158**, 539.

17

Health education

Cyril Hart

One of the major developments in general practice in recent years has been the extension of our interests from therapeutic to preventive medicine. No vocational training course is now complete that does not provide some grounding in the epidemiology of primary care. We have become the chief agents in the delivery of immunisation programmes. Our involvement in various aspects of screening and surveillance increases year by year. Only when we come to health education, the fourth cornerstone supporting the edifice of preventive medicine, does any slackening of our enthusiasm become apparent.

Cynics will be quick to supply an explanation of the deficiency; there is no money in it for the GP, nor is there ever likely to be. Those more benevolently inclined point to the stresses arising from an increasing workload and an open-ended service commitment. Others argue that in an age of retrenchment and concentration on priorities, it is hard to make a convincing case for putting health education high on the list of our activities.

Yet such a case can be made out, particularly on behalf of our younger patients. How often are we exasperated when a parent brings up a child with a simple cut finger, to dress which requires only the most elementary knowledge of first aid? Or when a late call comes to attend Sally's raging toothache, the end result of too little fluoride, too many sweets, and utter ignorance of our good local facilities for preventive dental care? Or when Timothy, aged five, is rushed to the surgery after swallowing all his mother's nice-tasting iron tablets, or when baby Jane's grandma announces complacently that she has just given her a good dose of brandy to settle her little upset stomach? All these are truthful histories of cases encountered in my practice during the past week. All could have been avoided, had parents been sufficiently exposed to concepts of good child care.

It is not difficult to draw up a list of topics about which we would like our patients and their children to be better informed. My own list runs as follows:

Basic education
- human biology
- hygiene
- sex education
- family planning

Self help
- accident prevention
- first aid
- home nursing
- self care of simple disorders
- baby and child care

Dangers of
- smoking
- alcohol
- drugs
- obesity

Knowledgeable use of facilities
- NHS
- statutory social services
- voluntary services (especially for specific handicaps).

Of course it should be the prime responsibility of parents to teach their children about these things. Of course this should be backed up by more formal instruction in our schools. Of course our health visitors must carry the chief professional burden for health education within the practice. Of course our role as general practitioners should be stimulatory and supportive, rather than central.

Nevertheless, our intervention in this sphere is justified on four counts:

1. Parents and schools often discharge their responsibilities inefficiently, or not at all. Here as elsewhere, the Inverse Care Law applies, those children most in need of help and advice receiving the least, and of the poorest quality.
2. A good GP is looked up to by his patients. He knows their background better than any other health professional, and they are more likely to listen to him than to anyone else.

3. Our special expertise is needed to ensure that health education is of the highest quality, and devoted to desirable objectives.
4. Prevention is better than cure.

Indeed, it can be argued that far from being an excursion into new fields of endeavour, for us to interest ourselves actively in health education would merely involve a reversion to our original role. For too long we have forgotten that the word 'doctor' means 'teacher'. Good general practice calls for more than the passive handing out of advice when consulted; we should be prepared to offer our expertise to our patients in a more positive fashion, even on occasion intervening with information when necessary to combat unhealthy attitudes derived from ignorance and prejudice.

Such advice must be soundly based and attractively presented. By careful planning it can be put over with a minimum of effort on our part. First we should formulate planned objectives for our practice, tailor-made to meet specific local needs. Then we should survey our resources, and exploit them to the full. Receptionists, nurses, midwives, and health visitors should all be involved. Help and advice should be sought from the health education officers now attached to local district health authorities. Their resources and display materials can be backed up by posters, pamphlets, and other visual aids from the Health Education Council and from a wide range of voluntary bodies with specific interests. Consideration should be given to encouraging the formation of a patients' association within the practice.

We must be practical in our approach. Most of us put up posters in our waiting rooms. Go and examine yours. The chances are you will find that they cover a vast range of topics, a hotch-potch of exhortation in which the poor patient is hard pressed to see the wood for the trees. Any good advertising man will tell you that the way to sell is to concentrate on one product at a time, to the exclusion of all else.

Tackle smoking first (one third of regular smokers start before they are nine years old; 80 per cent of child smokers continue with the habit as adults). Sweep away all your posters, and call in your district health education officer. Ask him to mount a 'No smoking' campaign to last a whole month. Restrict your posters to this single topic, backing them up with pamphlets from ASH in front of the reception desk – not just scattered about, but obtainable one at a time from an attractively designed dispensing container. In a spare corner place a small modern projector, loaned perhaps by a drug firm, and running a continuous film – no sound, of course. If there is room, invite patients – particularly schoolchildren – to a concentrated evening course aimed at breaking the habit, and run by the health education officer. After a month of this, pause and recover. Leave the waiting room fallow for a few weeks, then start up another campaign – accident prevention, perhaps (see Ch. 24).

Those of us fortunate enough to practice from health centres or other large group practice premises will have relaxation classes for pregnant mothers, run by our practice midwives and health visitors. Here is the ideal milieu for effective preparation for parenthood, which should be central to our programme of health education in child care. After her confinement, mother is encouraged to bring up baby to the surveillance clinic, and here the education continues. How much do we GPs know about what goes on there? We should visit these classes ourselves from time to time, to encourage our colleagues in the primary care team, and coordinate the advice given by its members.

A recent initiative, worthy of emulation, has been the construction by an experienced GP of a booklet for parents of children under the age of five years, in which subjects such as breast feeding, immunisation, home management of simple disorders, and sensible use of medical services are discussed in simple non-technical language (Pike, 1980). Copies were handed out gratis and evaluation showed that it resulted in a more informed use of the general practitioner services.

For advice on the health problems of later childhood, a wide range of pamphlets is available free from the Health Education Council and from specialised voluntary bodies. These can be backed up effectively by authoritative Family Doctor booklets issued by the BMA, which cost the patient only a few pence. I have listed in an appendix to this chapter the main titles currently available, and a further appendix at the end of this book lists most of the voluntary organisations that issue publications related to their special interests. All these pamphlets, and information concerning the voluntary organisations, should be made available to your patients at your practice reception desk.

My chief criticism of this literature is that (with a few honorable exceptions in the Family Doctor series) it is aimed almost exclusively at adults. We badly need attractive material written and illustrated for children from eight years upwards. By the age of ten or so, attitudes have already crystallised on a wide range of issues such as personal hygiene, smoking and alcohol. If we have not tried to influence our child patients by this age, we have failed in our task.

It is important for us fully to appreciate the problems of learning faced by our less able patients, both children and parents. Simple techniques of everyday living that we may consider too obvious to call for comment are beyond the comprehension of some of the least fortunate; for others they come as major discoveries. The patient teaching of elementary hygiene and self sufficiency pays enormous dividends here, and we should never consider ourselves above such tasks, nor perform them in any way that might be thought patronising. How often do we find instructions for treatment handed out to patients employing a vocabulary of technical jargon way above their heads, provoking antagonism rather than cooperation on their part.

Encourage your young patients to join the scouts and guides, or the youth sections of the ambulance associations. There they will learn the elements of first aid and hygiene, and much else about self-sufficiency and healthy living besides. These organisations are of incalculable benefit to children with deprived backgrounds, or with over-protective parents.

Health education, good or bad, is a component of every surgery consultation and every doctor's visit to the home. From about three years onwards, the child listens to (and often misinterprets) everything the doctor says to his parents about him. Too often we forget this. Attitudes are being moulded all the time. Treat the child as a person in his own right. As soon as he is old enough, address your questions to him, rather than to his parent. Not 'how did Willy sleep last night?' but 'did you sleep well?' Not 'whereabout is his tummy ache?' but 'show me where it hurts.' Explain to him what you are going to do, before you do it. Tell him its your job to help him, and you are on his side. When the news is good, tell him so: 'of course you can go to the party', 'your leg should be OK for the school sports next week'. Give him clear instructions about dosage of medicines; warn him to keep to them strictly, and hand him the prescription.

We all of us can remember the powerful influence exerted by favourite teachers in our childhood. When a child learns to accept his doctor as a friend, lifelong attitudes to details of hygiene and healthy living, and sensible use of medical services, can be fashioned by a few quiet remarks during a consultation. Here, at the core of our practice, a minimum of effort produces maximum returns in the health education of our child patients.

ACKNOWLEDGEMENT

Thanks are due to Dr. George Cust, Chief Medical Officer, The Health Education Council, for reading through this chapter and for helpful advice.

REFERENCE

Pike, L.A. (1980) Teaching parents about child health using a practice booklet. *Journal of the Royal College of General Practitioners*, **30**, 517–519. Copies of Dr. Pike's booklet may be obtained from the Birchfield Medical Centre, 95 Birchfield Road, Birmingham B19.

APPENDIX

Family Doctor Publications obtainable from 47–51 Chalton Street, London NW1 1HT, tel. 01 387 9721.

50	You and your pregnancy
2	Babies and toddlers (management from birth to age 4)
40	Feeding your baby
4	Infant feeding (weaning, with menus and recipes up to age 5)
5	Understanding your child (birth to age 5)
9	Speaking and reading (first steps)
13	Infectious diseases of childhood
17	Common ailments in babies
25	Your child from five to twelve
26	Facts of life for parents
30	Facts of life for children (9 years upwards)
69	How your life began
71	So now you know about sex (12 years upwards)
10	Slim safely (older children)
22	So now you know about smoking
23	Foot care at all ages
27	Drinking and alcoholism
36	Dental care at all ages
49	Pot or not (drug dependence)
48	About your eyes
56	Fit to play (training for sport)

Health Education Council Publications obtainable free from 78 New Oxford Street, London WC1A 1AH, tel. 01 637 1881, or from your local health education officer.

CW20	Pregnancy. What you should know
NT2	The best way to feed your baby
NT4	Bottle feeding? Let's do it right
NT5	Starting your baby on solid foods
NT7	Healthy eating for your children
NT8	The overweight child
HS4	Danger! Deadly sweets! (sugar coated tablets)
M7	Sound advice (communicating with the deaf)
HS1	Safety in the home
ID6	Protect your baby (immunisation)
ID8	Is your daughter between 11 and 14? (rubella immunisation)
ID17	What to do about head lice
FH4	Care of young feet
CW3	Your children need you (simple family care)
DH4	Seven steps towards a healthy mouth (dental care)
DH9	The six-year molars
ID4	What to do about scabies

PART THREE

Clinical care in acute illness

18

Acute disorders of the ear, nose and throat

Walter Anderson

Acute disorders of the ear, nose and throat are among the most common reasons for children being brought to the doctor and children with recurrent infections can prove to be particularly difficult to manage in family practice to the complete satisfaction of the parents and the doctor himself.

DIAGNOSIS

The symptoms of ear, nose and throat disease are sometimes confusing, as pain may be referred to the ear from the teeth, throat, parotid gland or temporomandibular joint. Pain behind the ear is nowadays characteristic of eustachian obstruction, but it is well to remember that mastoiditis, although now rare, still can occur in spite of modern antibiotic therapy for acute ear infections.

Aural discharge may arise from the middle ear, from a boil in the external auditory meatus, or from a moist otitis externa. Deafness may be discovered only during the routine screening of school children, and hearing tests constitute one of the few screening procedures which are generally agreed to be of value in school health service routine examinations. Although a cough is usually considered to be characteristic of chest infections, it is also a common symptom of upper respiratory disease and many children with adenoidal enlargement have a postnasal drip and chronic cough.

A clear nasal discharge is characteristic of upper respiratory infections in their early stages, and perennial or seasonal rhinitis; the discharge may become secondarily infected and purulent. A unilateral purulent nasal discharge is characteristic of a neglected foreign body.

For the satisfactory examination of the ear, nose and throat a good light is essential. ENT surgeons always use a head mirror and a powerful lamp to enable them to have both hands free, but few general practitioners possess a head mirror or the necessary expertise to use one comfortably. A small pocket torch together with a wooden disposable spatula or a reversed household spoon allows a satisfactory examination of the teeth, mouth and throat to be carried out, and the anterior nares of a child can be inspected by pressing the tip of the nose upwards and illuminating the interior with the torch or an auriscope.

An auriscope is required for the proper examination of the tympanic membranes, but care must be exercised in small children as the external auditory meatus is very short and the tympanic membrane lies close to the surface. The auriscope is best held like a pen, with the little finger resting against the patient's cheek, so that if the child moves his head the hand moves with it. It is important to inspect the external ear and to remember to look behind the ear at the mastoid region.

Palpation of the neck completes the examination, but it should be remembered that a careful search will reveal a number of palpable cervical lymph nodes in many healthy children.

During this examination struggling small children are best held on their mother's knee, with one arm round them holding their arms firmly and one hand on their head, turning the child to right, left or facing the examining doctor as required.

Every family doctor in this country should by now have access to X-ray and pathology facilities. X-rays of the maxillary antrum may be helpful in assessing the severity of sinusitis in older children by indicating the presence of fluid or pus, and a lateral X-ray of the neck may indicate the degree of adenoidal enlargement but is not considered entirely reliable by some ENT surgeons.

Swabs of the ear, nose or throat may be sent for bacteriological examination and are of particular value in recurrent, chronic or subacute infections, where they may assist with the choice of antibiotics. The culture success rate can be improved by breaking the swab into Stuart's medium for transport to the laboratory.

Audiometry is now becoming available in an increasing number of health centres and group practice centres, and is useful as a screening test, but simple screening tests using a forced whisper or squeaky toys are used by health visitors for small children. A standard box of toys ('Stycar') is available commercially (Sheridan, 1958).

A significant minority of children with recurrent infections of the ear, nose and throat are found to be anaemic, so a haemoglobin estimation and examination of a blood film are valuable adjuncts to the clinical examination and are necessary to confirm a suspected diagnosis of glandular fever in any case of atypical tonsillitis or sore throat. Keep in mind the variation in the normal levels of haemoglobin in childhood when interpreting the results of blood tests (see p. 237).

In the management of acute infections in children it is important to remember to discuss briefly with the mother those general nursing procedures appropriate for the home. Old ideas die hard, and many parents still think that any child with a fever needs extra blankets, a thick woollen vest, a hot water bottle, and a blazing fire in the room even on a hot summer evening. Small children often improve visibly when they are undressed for examination as they can then lose heat freely. The parents need to be encouraged to keep the child cool and give plenty of fluids, and reassured that he cannot be expected to eat much while he is ill. Parents also require reassurance that such children will not suffer from being brought to the surgery by car; indeed they will probably benefit from receiving more prompt assessment and treatment.

Ear drops have little place in therapy except in otitis externa, and oral antibiotics are now used almost exclusively in general practice, injections being retained only for any child who is seriously ill or vomiting.

Acute viral infections usually affect all parts of the respiratory tract at the same time, the actual diagnostic label depending upon which region is worst affected. Thus a child with 'tonsillitis' commonly has a runny nose, generalised pharyngitis, earache, and cough. The actual diagnostic label attached to the patient also depends upon the doctor and his beliefs and prejudices. What is labelled 'tonsillitis' by one doctor may be labelled 'pharyngitis' or 'upper respiratory tract infection' by another.

OTITIS MEDIA

Acute otitis media is one of the commonest diseases of childhood. Over 90 per cent of all cases occur in children and Fry (1966) found a prevalence of 12 per cent in children under 10, while Illingworth (1974) claimed that cases of otitis comprise 10 per cent of all children seen by the general practitioner. In the study *Growing up in Newcastle upon Tyne* (1960) it was found that nearly 20 per cent of the 1000 children had suffered from otitis media by the age of five.

There are variable general symptoms of fever, malaise, anorexia, fatigue, vomiting or headache, accompanied by earache and deafness. The symptoms commonly follow a head cold or a session of swimming and diving, but may occur spontaneously. The tympanic membrane appears dull, red and infected and in late cases it may appear oedematous and bulging and may subsequently perforate producing a profuse purulent discharge, often blood-stained. Many cases of acute otitis media are viral in origin and will resolve spontaneously without much damage occurring, but in practice viral infections are difficult to distinguish from bacterial infections in the early stages. The severity of the general symptoms does not necessarily reflect the appearance of the tympanic membrane or the apparent severity of the local infection.

The decision to administer or withold antibiotics must be made at the initial consultation and depends upon many factors including previous history, social conditions, the dependability of the mother, the severity of the general symptoms in the child, the appearance of the tympanic membrane and the opportunity for further supervision by the doctor. In most cases rapid resolution can be expected following the administration of adequate doses of an oral antibiotic such as phenoxymethyl penicillin or ampicillin, and it is customary to give at least a five day course (the standard 100 ml bottle). The actual choice of antibiotic appears to make little difference to the outcome which seems to depend more upon the social conditions. A harassed mother is said to be the most important adverse factor in prognosis (Paterson and Maclean, 1970). Ampicillin is probably a better choice of antibiotic under the age of five, as haemophilus influenzae is said to be commoner in this age group, but it should be avoided in older children because of the increased risk of the development of a rash in association with glandular fever.

In babies and small children the diagnosis may not be made until the tympanic membrane is examined during the course of the general examination of an ill child and it is therefore vital to remember to use an auriscope in all children with unexplained fever, general malaise or vomiting.

Follow-up is important and the child should be reassessed not later than the fifth day, and subsequently at intervals until complete resolution occurs; it is customary to continue the antibiotic until then. Most acute perforations appear to heal very rapidly leaving surprisingly little disability, but the small group of children who are left with permanent damage and persistent deafness deserve assessment by an ENT specialist, including audiometry.

Recurrent otitis media should raise the possibility of the presence of secretory otitis media or eustachian obstruction, which may be intermittently present during otherwise simple respiratory infections.

Secretory otitis media ('Glue ear')

In modern practice the use of antibiotics has resulted in

the virtual disappearance of the serious sequelae of acute otitis media which used to be so common and which resulted in the frequent performance of mastoidectomy or myringotomy in acutely ill children. However, enlarged adenoids and a blocked eustachian tube may give rise to the classic picture of a mouth-breathing child who snores at night and has constant or intermittent conductive deafness due to the collection of mucous fluid in the middle ear. Repeated attacks of earache and acute otitis media occur, and speech problems may lead to difficulties at home and at school. The tympanic membranes may appear normal but in advanced cases they lose their usual shiny appearance and become grey and lustreless and may be considerably indrawn. Very rarely a fluid level or bubbles may be seen through the drum. Referral to an ENT surgeon for assessment is indicated.

With the delays which may occur in referral procedures nowadays it is worth prescribing a preparation containing pseudoephedrine and an antihistamine (such as 'Actifed') and to encourage nose breathing while waiting for outpatient appointments. There is no doubt that many cases of secretory otitis media subside spontaneously.

Considerable controversy exists about the causation of 'glue ear' and the condition is commonly blamed on inadequate dosage of antibiotics which may be administered for too short a time. However it seems more likely to result from an anatomical defect of the eustachian tube and pharynx resulting in a tendency for the eustachian tube to block more easily, so that normal drainage and aeration of the middle ear is prevented.

With established 'glue ear', adenoidectomy and drainage of the fluid by myringotomy may affect a marked improvement in hearing. If the eustachian tubes remain blocked after this and conductive deafness persists, the insertion of a small flanged Teflon drainage tube known as a grommet into the anterior lower part of the tympanic membrane under general anaesthesia will usually permit ventilation of the middle ear and restores normal hearing in most cases. The grommets are usually extruded spontaneously after a variable period. In many cases there is no further trouble, but if the deafness recurs the grommet is easily reinserted.

The chief drawback of grommets from the child's point of view is that he must not allow water into his ears, and swimming is banned. However, a number of children with 'glue ears' seem to be worse after swimming and diving so that it seems wise to ban swimming anyway, although it may be permissible if they wear a nose-clip.

The tendency to secretory otitis media appears to resolve spontaneously in most cases in the early teens, and the child may be left with a virtually normal ear and normal hearing. However in an untreated case absorption of the fluid may lead to permanent indrawing of the whole tympanic membrane resulting in what looks like a large perforation and ultimately cholesteatoma formation.

OTITIS EXTERNA

Eczema of the pinna is common in small children and especially affects the skin behind the lobe of the ear but it usually seems to worry parents more than the child himself. The application of hydrocortisone cream one per cent twice daily usually results in rapid resolution. Neomycin or aureomycin may be added if infection is present.

A moist inflammation of the external auditory meatus occasionally occurs, and responds to regular cleaning and drying and the administration of ear drops containing a combination of a cortisone derivative and a topical antibiotic such as neomycin or an antifungal agent such as vioform. Boils of this area are common and while they may subside spontaneously may be extremely painful; it is kinder to prescribe a suitable topical antibiotic such as fucidic acid (Fucidin) in the form of ointment or gel, although an oral antibiotic may be indicated if they are particularly severe.

WAX

The presence of wax is less commonly a problem in children than in adults and usually gentle syringing will remove it; it is kinder to instil olive oil or soap ear drops for two or three days first. This is a task which is frequently delegated to the practice nurse (who should have been specially trained in the technique) but in small children it may be better for the doctor to do it himself. It is important to examine the tympanic membrane and the external auditory meatus afterwards, and the canal may need to be mopped dry with cotton wool on an orange stick. In the presence of acute earache it may be better to wait for a few days until the otitis has subsided because of the considerable pain that may be caused by syringing.

FOREIGN BODIES

Small children sometimes present with small foreign bodies in the ear or nose; small pieces of plastic, sugar coated tablets, or pieces of paper are commonly found. Their chief danger lies in their careless removal and in many cases it is better for the general practitioner to refer the child immediately to an ENT surgeon so that the foreign body can be removed under general anaesthesia. However, it is always worthwhile for the family doctor to look himself to see whether the foreign body is near the external orifice and can be grasped easily with forceps or a Jobson-Horne probe or hook. The family doctor is more likely to have the confidence of the mother and child and to obtain their co-operation than a strange doctor in a casualty department who may find a general anaesthetic necessary simply to calm the child.

Repeated attempts at removal should not be made as repeated failure merely upsets the child and the mother, and care should be taken not to fragment friable objects such as peas or other vegetable material. Small objects in the external ear can sometimes be removed by gentle syringing.

A child with an object such as a fish bone lodged in the throat also requires immediate referral for removal under general anaesthesia, but fish bones lodged in the gums or stuck between the teeth can usually be removed by the general practitioner with a small pair of forceps. It may similarly be possible to grasp a fish-bone stuck in the pillars of the fauces, in a fully conscious co-operative child.

TONSILLITIS

Acute tonsillitis is another of the most common diseases of childhood and some six per cent of children under the age of ten are said to suffer from the disease each year (Fry,1966).

The diagnosis of acute tonsillitis in older children is usually easy. The onset is sudden, with sore throat, fever and general constitutional upset of variable degree. Examination of the throat reveals swollen injected tonsils, sometimes covered in yellowish exudate which may be diffuse or localised to the follicles. At a later stage, a membrane may develop. The appearance of the throat does not necessarily reflect the severity of the general symptoms as an apparently less severely infected throat may be associated with very severe symptoms. The tonsillar lymph nodes are often enlarged and tender. Small children with tonsillitis frequently complain of abdominal pain, and as with any febrile child vomiting may occur so that an acute abdomen may be suspected. Progression to tonsillar abscess or quinsy formation still occurs occasionally, but usually the infection responds to high dosage of penicillin and the need for incision and drainage is now rare.

A more subacute form of tonsillitis is sometimes seen where a child has been less severely ill for a week or two.

There has been much discussion in many papers about the indications for giving or withholding antibiotics in tonsillitis. Many cases of tonsillitis have been shown to be viral in origin (some 50 per cent in Everett's series in 1975) and will resolve spontaneously. No present day antibiotics will affect the course of the illness in these cases. It would therefore be logical to treat with antibiotics only those children who have proven bacterial infection on culture, but in practice the clinical situation usually demands action long before reports on bacteriological swabs can be available. The decision to use antibiotics or not depends upon many factors including the appearance of the tonsils, the social circumstances of the family, the dependability of the mother, the availability of the doctor for regular supervision, a history of previous attacks and the child's general clinical state. Thus the decision must be an individual one made by the doctor at the first examination, as with acute otitis media. It has been shown in a number of studies that this clinical assessment of virus or bacterial sore throat is wrong in a high proportion of cases and Everett has suggested that since beta-haemolytic streptococci group A are present in some 36 per cent of cases, a short course of antibiotic should be given to every child. A full 10 day course can be reserved for those patients who have previously suffered from rheumatic fever, or who live in closed residential communities where the rheumatic fever risk is high.

Most cases of acute tonsillitis respond rapidly to oral antibiotics, phenoxymethyl penicillin usually being the drug of choice in the absence of any specific allergy, and ampicillin or erythromycin being the next most frequently used. In severely ill children the first dose of penicillin may be given by injection (as benzyl penicillin), especially if the child has been vomiting.

Recurrent tonsillitis is a frequent problem and parents may demand consideration of tonsillectomy. The indications for this operation are more indefinite than those for adenoidectomy and must again depend upon a careful assessment of many factors. The actual size of the tonsils is irrelevant and the history is paramount, but any child who is suffering from repeated attacks of sore throat resulting in considerable loss of schooling deserves full assessment including haematological examination and hearing tests, which are often most conveniently performed in an ENT outpatient clinic. A number of these children are suffering from chronic sinusitis and if this can be dealt with recurrent tonsillitis may be prevented.

PHARYNGITIS

Acute pharyngitis and acute sore throats are commonly associated with virus infections of the upper respiratory tract and may be associated with enlargement of the cervical lymph nodes (RCGP Survey, 1975). The constitutional upset is very variable.

As with tonsillitis, the use of antibiotics for sore

throats is controversial but it seems indefensible to give antibiotics indiscriminately to every child with a sore throat.

Any case of sore throat or tonsillitis which appears atypical or which does not respond rapidly to antibiotics should bring to mind the possibility of glandular fever which will be confirmed by a white cell count and Paul Bunnell test.

Diptheria is now almost unknown in this country following the establishment of herd immunity by widespread active immunisation in childhood, but it must still be kept in mind when any suggestion of membrane formation is present in the throat.

Scarlet fever is frequently seen in family practice, often before the rash becomes fully established, but with the ready availability of penicillin the disease nowadays holds no terror for parents and doctor, although it is still notifiable.

CERVICAL ADENITIS

Enlargement of the tonsillar lymph nodes is often associated with tonsillitis or pharyngitis, and enlargement of the occipital nodes is associated with rubella.

Acute infection of a cervical lymph node occasionally occurs with minimal throat infection, and rapid enlargement and abscess formation may ensue. Rapid resolution usually follows the administration of an oral antibiotic, but occasionally abscess formation may necessitate incision and drainage under general anaesthesia. It is important to send the pus for bacteriological examination: occasionally one may be surprised to find that it is tuberculous in origin.

EPISTAXIS

Nose bleeds in small children are not usually very severe and are frequently caused by a nasal vestibulitis and subsequent nose picking. A rapid cure usually ensues following local applications such as Naseptin cream which contains chlorhexidine and neomycin. Cautery of Little's area is only occasionally necessary, but general anaesthesia is required in small children.

Rarely, epistaxis may be a presenting symptom of leukaemia or other blood disorder.

HAY FEVER

Symptoms of hay fever may first occur at virtually any age and the typical clinical picture of red running eyes, profuse clear watery nasal discharge, sneezing and in extreme cases wheezing and breathlessness is characteristic. These symptoms usually occur between May and September with a peak in the month of June in warm dry weather when the pollen count is high. The mainstay of treatment is antihistamines, e.g. chlorpheniramine, but disodium cromoglycate in the form of nasal drops or spray may be useful in individuals who are made drowsy by antihistamines. Sprays containing a steroid are now available ('Beconase'), and these are usually very effective.

PERENNIAL RHINITIS

When the typical symptoms of hay fever persist in greater or lesser degree all the year round the diagnosis of perennial rhinitis may be made and some 'catarrhal' children probably have a substantial allergic element in their make-up. Prolonged treatment with an antihistamine may result in considerable improvement but in severe cases careful history taking, subsequent skin testing and a course of specific desensitising vaccine may be considered. The house dust mite frequently constitutes the chief offending allergen and although specific vaccines may be administered considerable improvement may result from the institution of measures to reduce the house dust mite population of the home (e.g. cotton cellular blankets, foam rubber pillows, daily vacuum cleaning of mattresses).

THE CATARRHAL CHILD

Fry (1961) has shown that the 'catarrhal' affections have a peak incidence between the ages of five and six and they are so common that they may be considered a normal part of growing up. There is considerable disagreement about the indications for tonsillectomy but the indications for adenoidectomy are more generally agreed, although traditionally the two operations have been usually combined. The general practitioner frequently finds himself in the position of helping a child along until the age of eight when a spontaneous cure nearly always results, and this must be remembered when considering surgery for any child.

Parents are often comforted greatly when they are told how frequent the catarrhal infections of childhood are and that spontaneous cure can be confidently predicted after the age of eight. It must also be remembered that the recurrent catarrhal infections presented to the doctor may be a symptom of a family problem, and great patience may be needed on the doctor's part to discover this and offer help and advice.

Adenoidectomy is generally recommended for the treatment of secretory otitis media and for recurrent otitis media when the adenoids are enlarged and blocking the postnasal space. Postoperative breathing exercises are usually advised to encourage the child to breathe through the nose and aerate the post nasal space and enable drainage of the middle ear and eustachian tube to occur.

Tonsillectomy is not now recommended as it used to be for mere enlargement of the tonsils. Some normal children have tonsils which meet in the mid-line when they open their mouths wide, without any apparent interference with normal swallowing. Recurrent tonsillitis, chronic infection, quinsy formation, or gross obstruction of the air passages remain the indications for tonsillectomy (Wood, 1973).

There is, however, considerable disagreement among ENT surgeons over the interpretation of the word 'recurrent'; some surgeons consider three attacks of tonsillitis in one year to be an indication for tonsillectomy and others think a minimum of six. It is important for the general practitioner to become acquainted with the views of his local consultants in this matter and to remember that ENT surgeons are specialists in surgical treatment. Fry (1961) highlighted the inconsistencies in the geographical variation in tonsillectomy rates and came to the conclusion that the only explanation was the variation in the customs and beliefs of the doctors and ENT surgeons in the different areas. It is salutary to note how many children undergo spontaneous cure while on a waiting list for operation. Nevertheless adenotonsillectomy remains the most commonly performed surgical procedure in many parts of the world and the controversy continues unabated (Hickish, 1975; Carne, 1975).

Recent work has suggested that children with low levels of serum IgA immunoglobulin are more likely to continue to have sore throats after tonsillectomy and to derive little benefit from the operation, but the decision remains primarily clinical (Donovan and Soothill, 1973).

It seems logical for the modern family doctor to adopt a strictly conservative approach and to refer to ENT surgeons only those children whose general health and schooling are being severely affected, or who are showing signs of deafness due to secretory otitis media. The delay in obtaining an outpatient appointment or admission for operation may be considerable, and the work of Donovan (1973) and Burke (1956) suggests that prophylactic penicillin or sulphonamides may reduce the incidence of sore throats during this period. It seems sensible for the family doctor to review such patients from time to time and to suggest that the operation be cancelled if the need for it appears to have passed.

There is still considerable misunderstanding among lay people over modern ideas about tonsillectomy and adenoidectomy and great patience may be needed in discussing with parents details about the most appropriate management for their child.

The family doctor should try not to abrogate his responsibility by excessive referral to ENT surgeons, or massive and unrecognised collusion of irresponsibility may easily occur (Carne, 1975).

ACKNOWLEDGEMENTS

This chapter owes much to the late John Grant, ENT Surgeon at Scarborough Hospital, with whom I worked as Clinical Assistant for several years.

I would also like to acknowledge the help and encouragement given to me by my wife who, with great patience, typed the manuscript.

REFERENCES

Burke, J.B. (1956) Prophylactic sulphadimidine in children subject to recurrent infections of upper respiratory tract. *British Medical Journal*, **1**, 538.

Carne, J (1975) The case against unnecessary removal of tonsils and adenoids. *Update*, **July 1975**, 82.

Donovan, R. (1973) Clinical and immunological studies on children undergoing tonsillectomy for repeated sore throats. *Proceedings of the Royal Society of Medicine*, **66**, 413.

Donovan, R. & Soothill, J.F. (1973) Immunological studies in children undergoing tonsillectomy. *Clinical and Experimental Immunology*, **14**, 347.

Everett, M.T. (1975) Antibiotics in the treatment of tonsillitis. *Journal of the Royal College of General Practitioners*, **25**, 317.

Fry, J. (1961) *The Catarrhal Child*. London: Butterworth.

Fry, J.(1966) *Profiles of Disease*. Edinburgh: Churchill Livingstone.

Hickish, G, (1975) The case for the removal of tonsils and adenoids. *Update*, **July 1975**, 73.

Illingworth, R.S. (1974) Frequency of children's diseases. *Medicine*, **1972–74**, 1576.

Newcastle Survey (1960) *Growing up in Newcastle upon Tyne*. London: Oxford University Press.

Paterson, J.E. & Maclean, D.W. (1970) Acute otitis media in children: a medical social study from general practice. *Scottish Medical Journal*, **15**, 289.

RCGP Survey (1975) Acute sore throat-diagnosis and treatment in general practice. RCGP East Scotland Faculty and the Department of Bateriology, Dundee University. *Journal of the Royal College of General Practitioners*, **25**, 126–132.

Sheridan, M.D. (1958) Simple clinical hearing tests for the very young or mentally retarded children. *British Medical Journal*, **2**, 299

Wood, C.B.S. (1973) Children's tonsils. *The Practitioner*, **211**, 713.

19

Acute infections of the respiratory tract

Ian Gregg

INTRODUCTION

Acute infections of the respiratory tract are collectively by far the most common form of illness occurring in childhood. In general, they are not serious and are managed entirely by GPs without referral to paediatricians. Therefore, it is regrettable that few good studies have been undertaken by GPs themselves, since paediatric textbooks often provide a distorted account of the pathogenesis and management of these very common illnesses.

Although respiratory infections in children are so commonplace, there are great differences of opinion among GPs regarding their aetiology and treatment. These derive largely from anecdotal impressions and consequently treatment tends to be determined by personal empiricism rather than having a rational basis.

Two circumstances present difficulties in a discussion of respiratory infection whether in children or adults. First, there is only a limited number of ways in which the respiratory tract can respond to insult, whatever its nature. Hence, there is considerable overlap in the symptoms and signs which are the expression of its response to a wide variety of infective and non-infective agents. It follows that some forms of illness caused by infection are closely resembled by others of non-infective origin and it may be very difficult to distinguish between them on clinical grounds. Second, confirmation of an infective cause, let alone identification of the responsible organism, is often impracticable for the clinician, even if the means of doing so were available to him. In passing, it needs to be emphasised that present day techniques of virological and bacteriological diagnosis are far less precise than is generally assumed.

The high frequency of respiratory infections during childhood is readily explicable on two counts. All parts of the respiratory tract must be in intimate contact with atmospheric air in order that the lungs can perform their essential function of gas exchange. Therefore the whole respiratory tract is exposed to any micro-organisms (or other noxious agents) which are suspended in the inspired air. Second, the immune system and other host defence mechanisms of young children are immature.

In a discussion of respiratory infection it is convenient to sub-divide the respiratory tract into three parts. The *upper* part is comprised by the nasal passages, the paranasal sinuses, the middle ear and the pharynx; the *middle* includes the larynx, trachea and large bronchi; the *lower* comprises small bronchi, bronchioles and alveoli.

In this chapter only passing reference is made to acute tonsillitis, sinusitis and otitis media, since these conditions are dealt with fully in Chapter 18. Furthermore, because of the resemblance between asthma and bronchitis, the latter condition is discussed in Chapter 37.

AETIOLOGICAL FACTORS

Ideally the treatment of respiratory infection should be based on identification of the causative micro-organism. Because this is seldom possible for the GP, his approach is necessarily empirical and has to depend on an assessment of probabilities. Often this empiricism is reflected in the provision of a range of treatment which he hopes will cover all eventualities.

Although precision of *aetiological* diagnosis is seldom possible in general practice, knowledge of the micro-organisms which commonly infect the respiratory tract and an understanding of the host's defences which are called into play will enable the GP to make more valid inferences and accordingly improve the quality of his management.

Micro-organisms which infect the respiratory tract

A large number and variety of organisms are capable of infecting the respiratory tract. Some (for instance, the measles virus) do so as part of a generalised infection, but the great majority have a predilection for the respiratory tract itself and, in some cases, for a particular part of it. This chapter will be concerned mainly with infection by viruses, bacteria and *Mycoplasma pneumoniae*. Other organisms which occasionally infect the respiratory tract include *Chlamydia psittaci* (causing ornithosis), fungi and yeasts.

Techniques of viral diagnosis have developed greatly during the last twenty-five years but most are still highly specialised, expensive and time-consuming. If a virus can be identified only by isolating it in tissue culture, a result may not be available for several days or even weeks. An alternative means of diagnosing viral infection by a rise in titre of complement-fixing antibodies is of limited value, since it is inapplicable to many of the viruses which cause respiratory infection and, in any case, a rise in titre is generally not demonstrable until about ten days have elapsed after the onset of infection.

Although viral diagnosis at present is of limited value and relevance to the GP, it has made possible a clearer understanding of the aetiology and epidemiological aspects of acute respiratory infection, especially in children. Many studies in this country and in the United States have shown that viruses are by far the most common agents causing primary infection at all levels of the respiratory tract.

Primary infection by bacteria is less common, the most familiar examples being acute tonsillitis caused by *Streptococcus pyogenes*, otitis media caused by various bacteria, pneumonia caused by *Str. pneumoniae* and whooping cough caused by *Bordetella pertussis*. Whereas in adults, particularly those with chronic bronchitis, secondary bacterial infection by *Haemophilus influenzae*, *Str. pneumoniae* and *Staphylococcus pyogenes* occurs frequently after viral infection of the lower respiratory tract, in children secondary bacterial infection appears to be much less common. One condition in which secondary bacterial infection not only occurs frequently, but is of paramount importance in management, is cystic fibrosis.

Host factors

Host factors can be conceived as the inherited or acquired characteristics of a subject which determine whether he is susceptible, resistant or hypersensitive to a given environmental agent. The outcome of infection can thus be regarded as the resultant of the pathogenicity of the organism and the efficiency or otherwise of the host's defences.

Defences against infection

The mechanisms of host defence called into play by primary infection include interferon, immunoglobulins and macrophages. Their relative importance is less well understood than in the case of re-infection, in which pre-existent immunity, acquired at the time of primary infection, depends mainly on preformed immunoglobulins which are each specific for a given organism. Acquired immunity may be so efficient that reinfection causes no symptoms and is entirely subclinical.

Age-incidence

The age-incidence of acute respiratory infection in childhood is determined largely by factors of host resistance. Placentally transferred passive immunity lasts for about 4–6 months. Thereafter, immunity has to be acquired as a result of primary infection to each of the large number of organisms which can infect the respiratory tract. Consequently, there is a high incidence during the first years of life when the child's immune and other defence mechanisms are relatively immature and he encounters a succession of organisms to which he has no pre-existing immunity.

The highest incidence occurs when children begin school and are repeatedly exposed to infection transmitted by other children. Thereafter, incidence declines as children acquire immunity to a progressively larger number of organisms.

Other host factors

Other factors, of which little is yet understood, must be responsible for the differences between individual children in their susceptibility to respiratory infection. Although inherited immune deficiency is a rare cause, it is possible that in certain children their immunological and other defences are unusually slow to mature and they cannot produce antibodies rapidly in response to infection, or the quality of these may be defective. Spontaneous correction of these factors, as children grow older, would explain the phenomenon of 'growing out' of the tendency to bronchitis. The same factors might also be responsible for the well-recognised difference between the sexes, boys having a higher incidence of bronchitis than girls.

CLINICAL PATTERNS OF ILLNESS AND THEIR ASSOCIATION WITH CAUSAL ORGANISMS

Because of the limited ways in which the respiratory tract can react to insult, infection by quite different organisms can give rise to similar clinical manifestations. Conversely, due to the modifying effect of the host's defences there is no clear association between a given organism and the pattern of illness to which it gives rise. Nevertheless, it is possible to discern certain propensities of individual organisms and knowledge of these will help in attempting to identify the organism most likely to be responsible for a given episode of illness.

Streptococcus pyogenes
This organism causes acute inflammation of the tonsils, pharynx and middle ear. Infection is usually accompanied by a high fever and constitutional illness and in the case of one serotype by scarlatina. Infection is highly transmissible. The appearance of streptococcal infection of the pharynx may be impossible to distinguish from that of infection by adenoviruses.

Streptococcus pneumoniae
Some serotypes of this organism are commonly present as commensals in the upper respiratory tract. Others are the most common cause of bacterial pneumonia.

Haemophilus influenzae
Capsulated forms cause otitis media (especially in children aged less than five years), and the rare condition of acute epiglottitis. Non-capsulated forms, which are the predominant cause of secondary infection in adult chronic bronchitis, are liable to infect the lower respiratory tract in children if this has sustained structural damage, particularly in cystic fibrosis and bronchiectasis.

Bordetella pertussis
This organism, which is the principal cause of the whooping cough syndrome, is difficult to identify. Similar clinical features have been reported in association with infection by adenoviruses and parainfluenza viruses.

Staphylococcus pyogenes
Secondary infection by this bacterium may complicate influenza. In young children it occasionally causes pneumonia with the formation of a large abscess which, if near the periphery of the lung, may progress to pneumothorax.

Pseudomonas aeruginosa (pyocyanea)
This coliform has a special propensity for causing secondary infection in cystic fibrosis.

Klebsiella pneumoniae
This organism is a rare cause of pneumonia, often leading to abscess formation, and it also occurs as a secondary invader in cystic fibrosis.

Influenza A and B viruses
These cause epidemic influenza. Infection by influenza A virus is generally associated with more severe constitutional symptoms. In younger children, high fever and myalgia, which are so characteristic of the disease in adults, are often absent. Influenza A virus has the property of changing its antigenic structure and therefore the population may have only limited immunity against the current strain of virus (Ch. 20).

Parainfluenza viruses
There are four main types. Cough is a prominent feature associated with their infection which is therefore readily transmitted. Infection occurs sporadically or in small epidemics. In younger children parainfluenza viruses are the most common cause of croup.

Rhinoviruses
There are about 100 antigenically distinct serotypes and it would appear that there is no cross-immunity between them. Formerly, rhinoviruses were believed to infect only the upper respiratory tract in which the common cold is the most familiar manifestation. However, it is now recognised that rhinoviruses are a frequent cause of acute bronchitis with wheeze in children and adults. It has been shown that in such episodes they can be isolated from the sputum of children and adults, confirming that rhinoviruses actually infect the bronchi.

Enteroviruses (coxsackie and echoviruses)
These have characteristics similar to rhinoviruses but there are many fewer serotypes. While infection usually gives rise to gastro-intestinal symptoms and sometimes an influenza-like illness, enteroviruses also infect the respiratory tract.

Respiratory syncytial (RS) virus
Respiratory infection caused by this virus is particularly common in younger children. Although there is only one serotype, reinfection is common. The majority of children show serological evidence of previous infection by the age of five years. Respiratory syncytial virus infection is generally confined to the upper respiratory tract but in young children it may cause bronchitis. During infancy infection may cause bronchiolitis or pneumonia. Since this occurs in only a minority of infants who are infected, it is probable that some abnormality of their host defences is a contributory factor.

Adenoviruses
There are some 30 serotypes of adenoviruses which differ in their pathogenicity and in the form of illness to which they give rise. They are a frequent cause of acute pharyngitis which may closely resemble that due to streptococci. They are seldom associated with bronchitis, but are a common cause of viral pneumonia. One serotype causing pneumonia in children has been reported to give rise to the subsequent development of bronchiectasis.

Mycoplasma pneumoniae
This organism has properties intermediate between viruses and bacteria. It resembles the latter in being able to be grown on artificial culture media and is susceptible to certain antibiotics. It is now recognised that

M. pneumoniae is a common cause of respiratory infection, occurring sporadically and in small but prolonged epidemics which may be recognisable by GPs if they are on the lookout for it. In children infection is usually accompanied by prolonged cough and debility. The organism causes pneumonia, less often in children than in adults.

CLINICAL DIAGNOSIS AND ASSESSMENT

The GP should ask himself several questions whenever he encounters a child apparently suffering from an acute respiratory infection.

First, is the episode, in fact, due to infection? There is often a close resemblance between coryza and allergic rhinitis, between croup and stridor due to obstruction of a large airway, and between acute bronchitis with wheeze and asthma provoked by a non-infective agent. The distinction has to be made on circumstantial grounds, such as a history of recent contact with a person who has also had symptoms suggestive of a respiratory infection.

Second, what part(s) of the respiratory tract are involved? The answer to this question provides some guidance in answering two others.

Third, what is the most likely organism causing the infection and is it viral or bacterial? Clearly, this has implications for the decision whether to treat the infection with antibiotics. The likelihood or otherwise of secondary bacterial infection should also be considered in this context.

Fourth, how seriously ill is the child now, or does it seem likely that he may become more so? The two principal factors determining severity are the degree of constitutional illness ('toxicity') and obstruction to airflow in either the larger airways (as in croup and diphtheria) or in the small airways (as in bronchitis with wheeze and bronchiolitis). Restlessness, loss of appetite and high fever are valuable guides to constitutional severity. Assessment of severity of airflow obstruction must be based upon the respiration rate, the use of accessory muscles, recession of the intercostal spaces and hyperinflation. The presence of respiratory distress with indrawing of the alae nasi and high fever is strongly suggestive of pneumonia.

MANAGEMENT – GENERAL PRINCIPLES

Two aspects of management need to be considered – treatment of the infection itself and relief of the symptoms to which it gives rise.

From what has been stated already concerning the relative frequency of viruses and bacteria as primary causes of respiratory tract infection, it will be appreciated that in the great majority of episodes encountered by the GP no specific treatment (in the form of antiviral chemotherapy) is presently available.

The place of antibiotics

Since viral infection is generally short-lived, the only treatment required for most episodes consists of measures of a palliative nature. While accepting the theoretical validity of this proposition, a GP may justifiably protest that its application in practice is unrealistic for several reasons. How confident can he be that in any given episode the organism responsible is a virus? Does not the likelihood of secondary bacterial infection supervening (if it has not already done so) warrant the prophylactic use of antibiotics? He may support this contention by pointing to the frequency with which bronchitis (widely, though perhaps mistakenly, regarded as an indication for antibiotics) follows commonplace upper respiratory infections. A fuller discussion of this aspect will be found in Chapter 37. In further support of his contention he can cite the present-day rarity, compared with the pre-antibiotic era, of bronchiectasis, empyema and other long-term sequelae of acute respiratory infection in childhood.

The decision whether or not to prescribe an antibiotic in any given episode of respiratory infection is one of the most frequent and difficult problems in general practice. Undoubtedly, there are some GPs who prescribe them indiscriminately and without any more rational basis than the notion, expressed in a much-seen advertisement, that respiratory infections 'do better in practice' when treated with an antibiotic.

The majority of more thoughtful GPs would probably defend their prescribing of antibiotics on the ground of their lack of confidence to make a precise clinical diagnosis under the conditions of general practice, especially in young children: recognition of their limitations compels them to 'play safe'. The sincere conviction that without antibiotics secondary bacterial infection would occur more frequently might seem to be another valid justification for their use. However, evidence that this does commonly occur is lacking. At any rate, there are reasons for supposing that in children secondary infection of the lower respiratory tract is less likely to occur than is the case in acute exacerbations of chronic bronchitis in adults.

The limitations of our present knowledge do not permit any dogmatism over the desirability or otherwise of prescribing antibiotics for respiratory infections in childhood. However, honesty should compel us to acknowledge that factors of a highly subjective nature often influence our decisions. Perhaps the most common of these is the wish to satisfy the expectations of parents and to reassure them that their child will receive the conventionally accepted treatment for 'infection'.

MANAGEMENT OF COMMON RESPIRATORY INFECTIONS

These will be considered on an anatomical and symptomatic basis.

Coryza

Coryza, or the common cold, is a syndrome which can be caused by a large number of viruses. Rhinoviruses, because of their many serotypes, are numerically the most important. The incubation period lasts two to three days and the first symptoms are sneezing and rhinorrhoea. This stage is quickly followed by hypersecretion of mucus and congestion of the nasal passages, which generally lasts for a further four or five days. In infants nasal obstruction interferes with feeding, due to the difficulty of sucking and breathing simultaneously.

The only treatment required for uncomplicated coryza is relief of nasal obstruction by means of decongestant drops. This is particularly important in children with a previous history of otitis media or sinusitis, in whom relief of congestion in the nasal cavity and Eustachian passages is essential to prevent secondary bacterial infection.

In certain children coryza is followed within a day or so by bronchitis, an occurence which mothers describe as 'a cold which has gone onto the chest'. Recent studies have confirmed the correctness of this traditional concept which is discussed more fully in Chapter 37.

In some children persistent hypersecretion of mucus follows every cold and catarrh may last for many weeks, often giving rise to consideration of the need for adenoidectomy.

In general, the only indications for antibiotics are a previous history of otitis media or sinusitis or the presence of a purulent nasal discharge.

Cough

This is the most common symptom of acute infection at all levels of the respiratory tract. Irritation of the cough reflex may be due either to inflammation, especially when this involves the middle respiratory tract, or to the presence of excessive mucus. Hypersecretion of mucus may be confined to the nasal passages but if it overflows into the pharynx ('the postnasal drip') it gives rise to a 'rattling' cough which parents often interpret as indicating that the chest itself has been infected.

Infection of the bronchi is also accompanied by hypersecretion of mucus but this rarely causes expectoration since most children swallow their sputum. Simple techniques of physiotherapy, carried out by mothers after they have received instruction, are valuable for clearing the airways of mucus.

Whatever its cause, cough tends to be more pronounced at night and may cause disturbance of sleep. It may be due either to accumulation of mucus in the pharynx or to irritation of the cough reflex by inflammation in the middle or lower respiratory tract. It should be borne in mind that nocturnal cough is a common symptom of asthma, especially in children who are hypersensitive to housedust mites, high concentrations of which are often present in bedrooms.

Some symptomatic relief can be achieved by cough suppressants, such as simple linctus in infants, or pholcodine and codeine linctuses in older children. Attention to nasal secretions and their reduction will prove rewarding. In older children who are able to cooperate, the inhalation of menthol and eucalyptus is soothing and helps to promote clearance of tenacious mucus in the bronchi. There is little evidence that expectorant mixtures are of value.

Acute laryngo-tracheitis and croup

Parainfluenza viruses have a special propensity for causing acute laryngotracheitis. In young children this takes the form of croup, which is a potentially serious condition because of the danger of asphyxia, the risk being greater the younger the child.

The diagnosis of croup is seldom difficult, the characteristic feature being a sudden onset of a harsh barking cough with hoarseness of the voice, typically occuring at night. It must be differentiated from acute epiglottitis, and stridor due to impaction of a foreign body.

It is all-important to assess the severity of obstruction to airflow. Stridor and retraction of the suprasternal tissues during inspiration suggest that a potentially dangerous degree of obstruction is already present. Increases of respiratory and pulse rates are a poor guide, since these rise as a result of fear and excitement. Restlessness is an important sign of hypoxia, while exhaustion or cyanosis should be regarded as an indication of impending catastrophe.

The age-old remedy of steam inhalation is undoubtedly effective and is the best immediate treatment. The child should be taken into the bathroom and the hot taps turned on so that the atmosphere is saturated with steam. Alternatively, a kettle can be boiled continuously as near to the child as is safe. Usually benefit is obvious within half-an-hour of such treatment but if the signs of obstruction persist the child should be admitted to hospital at once.

Primary or secondary bacterial infection of the middle respiratory tract is uncommon. *H. influenzae* is a cause of the rare condition of acute epiglottitis, in which there is a high fever and the child appears 'toxic'. If this is suspected, no attempt should be made to confirm the diagnosis by visualisation of the epiglottis, since this action itself may precipitate acute and fatal obstruction. The child should be admitted immediately to hospital.

Pertussis (whooping cough)

The introduction of immunisation against *B. pertussis* in the 1950s brought about a striking reduction in the incidence of this distressing and formerly very common disease. Many younger GPs had hardly ever encountered it until a few years ago when its incidence began to rise again. This was probably due to the low level of immunity in the population following the alarm over the vaccine's dangerous side effects. It seems likely that the disease will occur with increasing frequency over the next few years.

The importance of *B. pertussis* is threefold – its possession of a neurotoxin, its unresponsiveness to antibiotics and its ability to cause permanent, structural damage of the bronchi.

The disease is most dangerous in infants. Over three quarters of the deaths caused by pertussis occur under the age of six months. Encephalopathy and convulsions, due to the neurotoxin and hypoxia, are the most serious complications of infection and are also the most dangerous of the side effects which occur in certain children after immunisation.

B. pertussis is sensitive in vitro to many antibiotics but none has any effect upon the course of the disease after neurotoxin fixation has occurred and paroxysmal coughing has begun. There is some evidence that erythromycin, if given before this stage is reached, may abort the development of the disease. This and other antibiotics have been recommended as prophylactic treatment for all contacts, especially infants, once it is known that they have been exposed to infection.

Structural damage of the bronchi, due either to pertussis itself or to secondary bacterial infection, was formerly common in young children. The present day rarity of bronchiectasis may be partly the result of immunisation and the reduced incidence of pertussis.

The distinctive feature of pertussis is paroxysmal coughing followed by a prolonged inspiratory whoop, during which the child often becomes cyanosed. Paroxysms are most frequent and severe at night time. Identification of *B. pertussis* from cough plates is unreliable and the best method of bacteriological diagnosis is by means of pernasal swabs but this is not an easy technique to carry out. Confirmation of the diagnosis is readily made by a rise in complement – fixing antibodies about ten to fifteen days after the onset of infection.

Some relief during paroxysms may be obtained by nursing in a humid atmosphere. Anticholinergic drugs, such as atropine methonitrate, are commonly given with the object of preventing paroxysms and recently salbutamol has been advocated for this purpose. There is no good evidence that either confers much benefit. It used to be a common paediatric practice to prescribe phenobarbitone to suppress the sensitivity of the cough reflex but there is little evidence of its value. Because of the likelihood of secondary infection by other bacteria, causing bronchopneumonia, an antibiotic should be given to prevent this. Nursing care is the most important aspect of management and it is a wise policy to admit to hospital all infants and any older children who are severely affected.

The severity of pertussis and particularly the liability to long term sequelae is related directly to age, being greatest in infants under six months. However, pertussis vaccine is far more liable to cause reactions of all kinds (though not necessarily dangerous) if given to younger infants. The best protection of infants aged less than six months lies either in the giving of erythromycin prophylactically, if they have been in contact with the disease, or in reducing the risk of their becoming infected by siblings by maintaining a high degree of immunity in the child population at large. The latter course has been jeopardised by the fear of dangerous reactions, but the policy of the DHSS has been to advocate continuation of pertussis immunisation, provided that high risk children are identified and not vaccinated. This has been ably reviewed by Preston (1981), and is discussed further in Chapter 11.

Bronchitis and 'wheezy bronchitis'

A full discussion of these conditions will be found in Chapter 37.

Bronchiolitis

This is the commonest form of severe lower respiratory tract infection occurring in infants. It is nearly always caused by RS virus, epidemics occurring in the late autumn and winter in this country and in the corresponding seasons in the Southern Hemisphere. Only a minority of infants infected by RS virus develop bronchiolitis but the host factors responsible are not understood. There is evidence that it may be a hypersensitivity reaction in certain infants who are unable to counteract the initial stages of infection because of their immature capacity to produce IgA antibodies.

Bronchiolitis gives rise to respiratory distress with hyperinflation. It is sometimes accompanied by consolidation. The illness begins as coryza, followed by coughing. There is seldom a high fever. The essential signs on examination are rapid respiration rate, hyperinflation, indrawing of the lower intercostal spaces during inspiration and widespread fine crepitations which may be accompanied by wheeze. Severely affected infants are cyanosed and readily become exhausted. Because of its dangers, infants with bronchiolitis should be admitted to hospital for intensive care with oxygen and intravenous feeding.

A high proportion of infants who have had bronchiolitis become subject to asthma later in childhood. Studies have confirmed that about 50 per cent of infants subsequently develop a liability to episodes of wheezing, while in one study it was found that 25 per cent of such infants were later regarded as having unequivocal asthma. The possible role played by RS virus infection and bronchiolitis in the inception of asthma is more fully discussed in Chapter 37.

Influenza

An influenza-like illness with fever, myalgia, headache and cough can occur as a result of infection by a variety of viruses. Infection by influenza A and B viruses usually occurs in easily recognisable epidemics. In young children influenza is a milder disease than in adults and often constitutional features of high fever and headache are absent. By the time adolescence is reached, influenza usually assumes its typical adult form. The reasons underlying the age differences in presentation are not clear. See also Chapter 20.

Pneumonia

Pneumonia occurs in children of all ages but is most common and most serious in infants. It is a frequent cause of death in undeveloped countries. In Western countries its mortality is mainly in infants or children with other diseases or impaired host defences. Pneumonia, which may be lobar, segmental or subsegmental, is caused by a variety of viruses, of which RS virus, adenoviruses and influenza A virus are the most common primary agents. Infection by these may be followed by secondary bacterial infection. Pneumonia is also caused by *M. pneumoniae* and by bacteria, of which the most common is *Str. pneumoniae*. It is seldom possible to identify the causative organism soon enough in the acute stage of the illness to have any bearing on the initial treatment.

The clinical presentation of pneumonia varies according to the causative agent, the age and general health of the child and the extent of consolidation. There is a gradient in clinical features from an apparently mild illness with insidious onset, in which a chest radiograph unexpectedly discloses consolidation, to a severe illness with sudden onset and accompanied by considerable constitutional disturbance. The complications of pneumonia, of which abscess formation and empyema are the most common, also depend upon the causative agent and the host defences.

The most common symptoms are cough, which is painful if associated with pleurisy, and high fever. Commonly present physical signs are a rapid respiration rate, dilatation of the alae nasi and localised crepitations. However, signs of consolidation are often very difficult to detect, particularly in infants, and the diagnosis of pneumonia can generally be made with certainty only by radiography.

Any child with severe constitutional symptoms should be admitted to hospital but older children with milder illness can be treated at home. Although pneumonia is often caused by viral infection, it is a wise policy to regard every case of pneumonia as being of possibly bacterial origin and to prescribe antibiotics. If it is known that infection by *M. pneumoniae* is prevalent in the neighbourhood and the clinical presentation is suggestive of this, erythromycin is the treatment of choice. Otherwise, penicillin, ampicillin or amoxycillin should be given on the assumption that the causative organism is *Str. pneumoniae*.

FURTHER READING

General

Knight, V. (1973) *Viral and Mycoplasmal Infections of the Respiratory Tract*. Philadelphia: Lea and Febiger.

Williams, H.E. & Phelan, P.D. (1975) *Respiratory Illness in Children*. Oxford: Blackwell Scientific.

Epidemiology

Britain

Horn, M.E.C., Brain, E., Gregg, I., Yealland, S.J. & Inglis, J.M. (1975) Respiratory viral infection in childhood. A survey in general practice, Roehampton 1967–1972. *Journal of Hygiene*, **74**, 157.

Horn, M.E.C., Brain, E., Gregg, I., Inglis, J.M., Yealland, S.J. & Taylor, P. (1979) Respiratory viral infection and wheezy bronchitis in childhood. *Thorax*, **34**, 23.

Miller, D.L. (1968) Epidemiological methods for studying acute respiratory disease. *Journal of Clinical Pathology*, **21**, Supplement 2, 17.

Miller, D.L. (1973) Collaborative studies of acute respiratory disease in patients seen in general practice and in children admitted to hospital. Aims, field methods and morbidity rates. *Postgraduate Medical Journal*, **49**, 749.

Pereira, M.S., Andrews, B.E. & Gardner, S.D. (1967) A study on the virus aetiology of mild respiratory infections in the primary school child. *Journal of Hygiene*, **65**, 475.

Poole, P.M. & Tobin, J.O.H. (1973) Viral and epidemiological findings in MRC/PHLS surveys of respiratory disease in hospital and general practice. *Postgraduate Medical Journal*, **49**, 778.

USA

Chanock, R.M. & Parrott, R.H. (1965) Acute respiratory disease in infancy and childhood: present understanding and prospects for prevention. *Pediatrics*, **36**, 21.

Glezen, W.P., Loda, F.A., Clyde, W.A., Senior, R.J., Sheaffer, C.I., Conley, W.G. & Denny, F.W. (1971) Epidemiologic patterns of acute lower respiratory disease in children in a pediatric group practice. *Journal of Pediatrics*, **78**, 397.

Maletsky, A.J., Cooney, M.K., Luce, R., Kenny, G.E. & Grayson, J.T. (1971) Epidemiology of viral and mycoplasmal agents associated with childhood lower respiratory illness in a civilian population. *Journal of Pediatrics*, **78**, 407.

Antibiotics

Howie, J.G.R. (1976) Clinical judgment and antibiotic use in general practice. *British Medical Journal*, **2**, 1061.

Scott, N.C.H. (1979) Management and outcome of winter upper respiratory tract infections in children aged 0–9 years. *British Medical Journal*, **1**, 19.

Pertussis

Preston, N.W. (1981) Pertussis immunisation: half-truths exposed. *Update*, 15 August 1981, 389.

20

Influenza in childhood

John Briscoe

Influenza is the only known remaining pandemic infectious disease in man. The causative virus every so often undergoes change enabling it to reinfect those who have suffered previous attacks. Influenza is prevalent in the winter and spring and epidemics tend to occur in the earlier part of cold spells of weather. The incubation period is from one to three days. According to the orthodox view the virus is transmitted from person to person by droplets shed from the upper respiratory tract for up to 14 days but variations in the rate of spread of the virus and in the geographical attack patterns in schools support an alternative theory that the virus infects people directly from space.

The virus

The influenza virus is roughly spherical with a diameter of 80 to 120 nanometres. Two surface antigens, Haemagglutinin (H) and Neuraminidase (N), which both induce protective antibody formation in man, project as spikes from the viral membrane within which lies the core containing, among other proteins, ribonucleic acid (RNA) in the form of eight distinct fragments. When two different influenza viruses infect a cell their respective RNA fragments are mixed and then recombine to form a new virus. A new pandemic subtype of influenza may arise either in this way, by recombination of a human and an animal virus, or by direct mutation of an existing human virus; it may even emerge from an animal reservoir but there is no direct proof that any of these hypotheses is correct. The emergence of a new subtype means that the H (and sometimes the N antigen also) has undergone a major change (antigenic shift). Each new subtype is identified by its specific H and N antigens according to the classification recommended by the World Health Organization (WHO), and shifts have occurred about every decade since 1946 thus–H_1N_1 in 1946, H_2N_2 in 1957 (Asian 'flu) and H_3N_2 in 1968 (Hong Kong 'flu). An old subtype which has lain dormant for years may appear and cause fairly extensive infection. In 1978 the H_1N_1 subtype of 1946–1956 reappeared as Red 'flu after an absence of about 22 years. In between these major changes the H and N antigens may undergo minor changes (antigenic drift) causing interpandemic epidemics of influenza every one or two years. There are three types of influenza virus; A discovered in 1933, B in 1940 and C in 1947. Antigenic shift only occurs in A, new subtypes of which are therefore the sole cause of pandemics. Antigenic drift occurs in A and B resulting in different strains which cause epidemics. Virus C is relatively unimportant and only causes sporadic respiratory disease.

Influenza surveillance

Global influenza surveillance is carried out by WHO. Knowledge of the extent and severity of prevalent influenza epidemics and of the antigenic composition of the viruses causing them becomes available from the network of laboratories and international reference centres that have been established. This information is used to recommend the composition of the vaccine for the coming year to the vaccine production laboratories.

In England and Wales various indices are used for influenza surveillance. Among these are deaths from all causes and, more specifically, from influenza, bronchitis and pneumonia, returns for clinical influenza from the Royal College of General Practitioners, new sickness benefit claims and laboratory evidence of infection with influenza viruses reported to the Communicable Disease Surveillance Centre (CDSC). The overall incidence in England and Wales, for the period 1976 to 1980, based on RCGP returns, is shown in Figure 20.1. There is a considerable annual variation, with peaks in the early months of each year. The 1977/78 epidemic of influenza A (H_1N_1) which affected mainly children and young people under the age of 22 years had little influence on these indices. To remedy this gap in surveillance the Medical Officers of Schools Association collaborated with the CDSC to initiate, in 1979, a system of weekly reporting of infectious disease, including influenza, in some boarding schools.

Epidemiology

Children bear the brunt of influenza infection in the population at large and are probably the main vehicle by

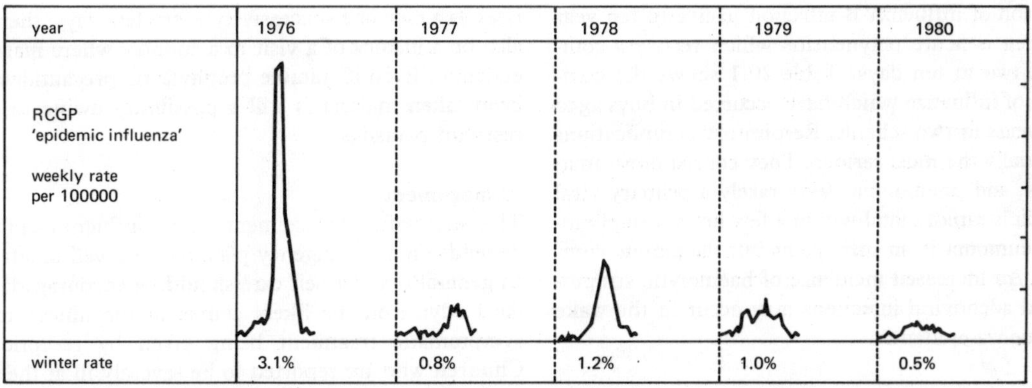

Fig. 20.1 Influenza in England and Wales, 1976–1980. RCGP returns (all ages). Source: *BMJ* 1980, 2, 1649

which it spreads. The younger the child the greater the attack rate. Girls may be prone to develop influenza during the premenstrual week. Influenza A is commonest in children up to four years whereas influenza B mainly attacks school children of five to 14 years. Boarding schools are particularly vulnerable to influenza epidemics, perhaps due to the influence of crowding. Clinical attack rates of up to 40 per cent, rising to 80 per cent when antigenic shift has taken place, have been recorded. Influenza A is twice as common as influenza B as a cause of school epidemics; mixed A and B epidemics also occur.

Clinical features

Influenza starts suddenly with headache, fatigue, sore throat, fever and cough. Inspection of the throat reveals raised pink patches in the oropharynx. The nose is congested and epistaxes may occur. The temperature is high (up to 40°C) on the first day and falls to normal in a few days. The cough is irritating, dry and harsh and may persist for up to two weeks. Nausea and vomiting are common features at onset in younger children. Movement of the eyes may be painful but general muscle aches occur less frequently than in adults. The illness lasts up to eight days and recovery is usually rapid. Mild cases of influenza occur when the child does not become febrile and may only complain of headache, sore throat or cough for a day or so. Subclinical attacks are common. At Christ's Hospital in the 1978 (H_1N_1) epidemic the clinical attack rate was 50 per cent whereas the true attack rate as shown by serological studies was 90 per cent.

Complications

The complication rate is low varying from ten per cent in babies to five per cent in older children, although the rate may approach 30 per cent in some individual outbreaks in schools. Convulsions and respiratory infections affect some children under three years with influenza A. Otitis media is met in older children. A rare

Table 20.1 Complications of influenza. Rugby School data by courtesy of the Journal of the Royal College of Physicians of London

Complication	*Rugby School 1950–1975 (2371 cases)*		*Eton College 1968–1978 (2162 cases)*
Otitis media	57		20
Bronchitis } Pneumonia }	30		33
Asthma	17		16
Tonsillitis	7		6
Stomatitis	7	Sinusitis	15
Peripheral neuropathy	5	Laryngitis	5
Meningism	3	Depression	4
Encephalopathy	2	Urticaria	3
Quinsy	2	Purpura	1
Arthropathy	2	Glycosuria	1
Appendicitis	2		
Pleurisy	1		
Total	135		140
	5.7%		4.8%

complication of influenza B infection in five to ten year old children is acute polyneuritis which recovers completely in two to ten days. Table 20.1 shows the complications of influenza which have occurred in boys aged 13 to 18 years in two schools. Respiratory complications are potentially the most serious. They consist of asthma, bronchitis, and pneumonia. Very rarely a primary viral pneumonia is rapidly fatal within a few hours. Staphylococcal pneumonia is an infrequent but dangerous complication. An increased incidence of haemolytic streptococcal and adenoviral infections may occur in the wake of an influenza epidemic.

Diagnosis

Sporadic cases of influenza cannot be diagnosed clinically with confidence as they are indistinguishable from other viral upper respiratory tract infections. When an increasing number of cases of influenza-like illness occurs in an explosive manner in a community then an influenza epidemic can be diagnosed with certainty. There is no clinical distinction between cases of influenza A and influenza B and many other viruses may cause similar illnesses in the midst of influenza epidemics. In respiratory syncytial virus infections of children under five years bronchiolitis is common and convulsions are rare, whereas the converse is true of influenza.

The only certain method of making an individual diagnosis of influenza is by laboratory investigation. A throat swab and the first sample of ten millilitres of blood are taken in the acute febrile stage of the illness. The swab is placed in a virus-transport medium bottle and conveyed with the blood sample to the virus laboratory as quickly as possible. The virus is most likely to be demonstrated by immunofluorescence or isolated by tissue culture from swabs taken at the beginning of an outbreak, hence the importance of investigation of early victims. A second sample of blood is taken two weeks after the first and sent to the laboratory. Complement fixation (CF) tests carried out on the paired sera can differentiate between influenza A and B and haemagglutination inhibition (HI) antibody tests between the different strains of influenza A or B.

Certain serious diseases, which demand specific treatment for cure, can be confused with influenza. The most important of these are enteric fever, brucellosis and malaria, all of which have been diagnosed in recent school epidemics. An atypical course in a presumed attack of influenza should raise the suspicion of another cause for the illness, particularly if the patient is not recovering after a few days or has been abroad recently. In enteric fever and brucellosis the temperature rises in a step-ladder fashion over several days compared with influenza where the temperature is high on the first day and then falls over the succeeding days. In malaria the temperature having fallen to normal from a high peak rises to a new one successively every few days; there will also be a history of a visit to a country where malaria is endemic. Even if suitable prophylactic precautions have been taken malaria is still a possibility owing to drug-resistant parasites.

Management

The successful management of an influenza epidemic depends on a contingency plan decided well in advance. In general practice self care should be encouraged, standard advice on the likely course of the illness and its symptomatic treatment being given by receptionists. Children who are reported to be severely ill at the onset must be seen then; otherwise parents should be told to contact the doctor again if the child becomes feverish after apparent recovery or develops earache or a worsening cough, suggesting the beginning of complications. Children already suffering from asthma, congenital heart disease, diabetes or any condition requiring steroid therapy must be closely watched so that any complication can be promptly treated.

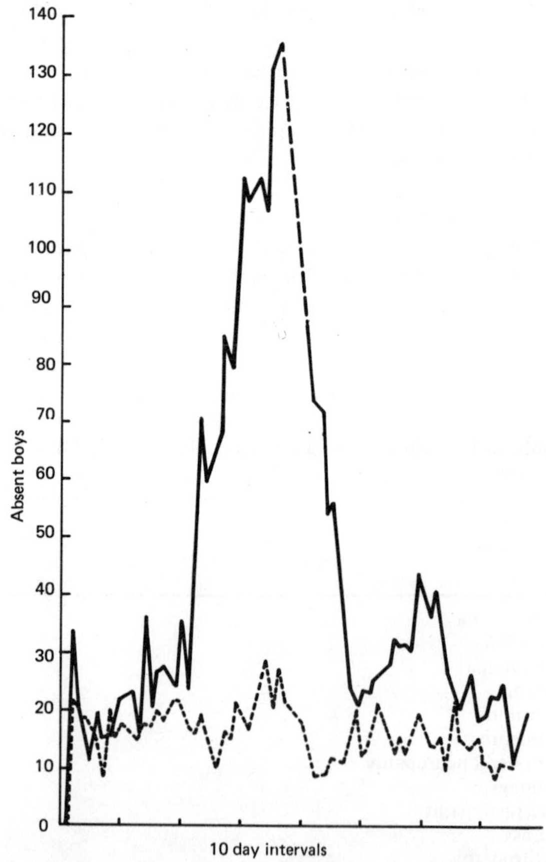

Fig. 20.2 Influenza at Eton: daily total of boys absent for all reasons during the spring term 1973 (dotted lower line) and spring term 1974 (continuous upper line). The interrupted part of the upper line indicates the four-day half-term holiday (by courtesy of *The Practitioner*)

In boarding schools a slight yet sustained rise in the daily total of absent pupils above the usual figure for non epidemic years always heralds an epidemic of influenza. Figure 20.2 shows absenteeism during the 1973 (non epidemic) and 1974 (epidemic) spring terms at Eton College where a daily total of 20 absent boys is considered the top limit of normal. The upper continuous line shows that this number was exceeded continuously for a week before the steep rise in absenteeism started. This warning gives the school doctor time to alert helpers (preferably previously identified) who can take temperatures and perform simple nursing duties. Some dormitories can be converted into sickrooms leaving the sanatorium available for severe and complicated cases. Local parents can be encouraged to fetch their children and nurse them at home.

The child with influenza should be kept in bed until the temperature has been normal for 24 hours as premature mobilization predisposes to relapse. Small children may require tepid sponging to prevent febrile convulsions. Soluble aspirin is useful as an antipyretic and can be given to older children as a gargle to be swallowed for the relief of sore throat. Copious fluids should be given to prevent dehydration. A mixture of glycerin, lemon and honey soothes the cough. Antibiotics should be reserved for bacterial complications such as otitis media, bronchitis and pneumonia. Children with suspected viral or staphylococcal pneumonia must be admitted promptly to hospital for intensive care. Children may return to school only after an adequate convalescence and strenuous games should not be permitted within a week of recovery.

Amantadine, a specific virus inhibitor, can be given prophylactically or therapeutically in a dose of 100 milligrams a day to children over ten years of age who merit special protection but it is only effective against influenza A. Other similar agents are at present too toxic for general use.

Prophylaxis

Influenza vaccination is not recommended for children unless they are over eight years and in hospitals or residential establishments. Vaccination must not be carried out on those who are known to be sensitive to egg products. Protection is variable as vaccines, although updated yearly, may not contain the current virus. Yearly vaccination with inactivated virus vaccine containing the latest strains of two different influenza A subtypes and influenza B is therefore essential.

Whether boarding school children should be vaccinated is controversial. It was shown in 1966 that a regular vaccination programme in schools lessened the likelihood of epidemics of influenza. Experience since then in some schools has confirmed that yearly vaccination has reduced the size of epidemics though not their frequency; serious disruption of school life has been avoided and relapses and complications of influenza have been less common. However, at other schools the protective effect for the individual has been considered insufficient to justify continued vaccination; serological assessment of the value of vaccination in the face of subsequent epidemics has shown that in the susceptible child vaccination protects for a short while but will not affect the chances of an attack of influenza in the long run. Vaccination may therefore be advantageous to the school community as a whole but of no lasting benefit to its individual pupils. Bearing this in mind and taking account of their own experience medical officers will need to decide individually whether they offer vaccination to the schools in their care.

If vaccination is given to a school every effort should be made to obtain an acceptance rate of at least 80 per cent to gain the maximum benefit of herd immunity. Children over 13 years may have the whole virus vaccines (Admune, Influvac) or a vaccine in which the virus is split up and less toxic – disrupted virus vaccine (MFV-Ject). As reactions to these vaccines may occur in younger children those under 13 years should be given purified subunit vaccine (Fluvirin) containing only the H and N antigens. All these vaccines are given by injection or hypojet gun and at present a second dose is recommended four to six weeks later if the child has not previously received a vaccine containing influenza A (H_1N_1). Live influenza virus vaccines, given by nasal spray, may offer a better prospect for the future prevention of influenza but they are rarely available as the safety requirements are strict to ensure that the virus is avirulent, non-transmissible yet immunogenic.

REFERENCES

Belbin, D.J. & Smithson W.H. (1979) 'Red 'flu'; a study of an epidemic in a girls' boarding school in February 1978. *Journal of the Royal College of General Practitioners*, **29**, 151–154.

Birmingham Research Unit of the RCGP (1977) Influenza. *Journal of the Royal College of General Practitioners*, **27**, 544–551.

BMJ Editorial (1980) Influenza 1980–1. *British Medical Journal*, **2**, 527–528.

Briscoe, J.H.D. (1975) Intranasal immunization with inactivated influenza virus vaccine in a boys' boarding school. *The Practitioner*, **214**, 821–826.

Briscoe, J.H.D. (1977) The protective effect of influenza vaccine in a mixed influenza A and B epidemic in a boys' boarding school. *Journal of the Royal College of General Practitioners*, **27**, 28–31.

Briscoe, J.H.D. (1979) Influenza epidemics in two boarding schools for boys. Communicable Disease Report 79/35 insert.

Caul E.O., Waller D.K., Clarke S.K.R. & Corner B.D. (1976) A comparison of influenza and respiratory syncytial virus infections among infants admitted to hospital with acute respiratory infections. *Journal of Hygiene, Cambridge*, **77**, 383–391.

Department of Health and Social Security (1978) *Influenza*. C.M.O. (78) 23. DHSS, Nelson, Lancs.

Fry J. (1979) Influenza. *Update*, **18**, 183.

Hart R.J.C. (1980) Influenza Vaccination. *Update*, **20**, 1071–1082.

Hoskins T.W., Davies J.R., Smith A.J., Allchin A., Miller C.L. & Pollock T.M. (1976) Influenza at Christ's Hospital: March 1974. *Lancet*, **1**, 105–108.

Hoskins T.W., Davies J.R., Smith A.J., Miller C.L. & Allchin A. (1979) Assessment of inactivated influenza A vaccine after three outbreaks of influenza A at Christ's Hospital. *Lancet*, **1**, 33–34.

Hoyle F. & Wickramasinghe C. (1978) Influenza from space? *New Scientist*. 946–948.

Martin A.J., Gardner P.S. & McQuillin J. (1978) Epidemiology of respiratory viral infection among paediatric inpatients over a six-year period in north-east England. *Lancet*, **2**, 1035–1038.

Penny P.T. (1978) Epidemic influenza in schools. *British Medical Journal*, **1**, 298–299.

Pereira M.S. (1979) Global surveillance of influenza. *British Medical Bulletin*, **35**, 9–14

PHLS Standing Advisory Committee on Influenza (1977) Influenza surveillance 1972–75. *Journal of Hygiene, Cambridge*, **78**, 223–233.

Randall C.F. (1975) Temporary paralysis in childhood after influenza B. *Lancet*, **1**, 107–108.

Rose H.J. (1980) The use of amantadine and influenza vaccine in type A influenza epidemic in a boarding school. *Journal of the Royal College of General Practitioners*, **30**, 619–621.

Schild G. (1978) An 'old' flu virus returns. *New Scientist*, 949–950.

Sparks J.P. (1978) Recent experience of influenza. *Journal of the Royal College of Physicians*, **12**, 437–449.

Stevens D., Burman D., Clarke S.K.R., Lamb R.W., Harper M.E. & Sarafian A.H. (1974) Temporary paralysis in childhood after influenza B. *Lancet*, **2**, 1354–1355.

Stuart-Harris C.H. (1959) Influenza and its complications. *British Medical Bulletin*, **15**, 216–220.

Stuart-Harris C.H. (1979) Epidemiology of influenza in man. *British Medical Bulletin*, **35**, 3–8.

Turtle P. de B. (1968) Vaccines in the management of influenza epidemics in schools. *The Practitioner*, **200**, 254–259.

Tyrell D.A.J. & Smith J.W.G. (1979) Vaccination against influenza A. *British Medical Bulletin*, **35**, 77–85.

21

The acute exanthemata

Emanuel Tuckman

Each year nearly 20 per cent of all children under the age of 15 are seen with a rash in the differential diagnosis of which the general practitioner will need to consider the acute exanthemata. Though most of these acute illnesses will be mild, some may be quite severe. Over 99 per cent will be cared for at home by the primary care health team.

Although the acute exanthemata are highly infectious, there is no point in isolating a child in a separate room as it is impossible to prevent infection spreading within the household. The use of disinfectants is sheer waste. The need for admission to hospital arises only when the illness is very severe, usually in a child previously in poor health, or when for special reasons the family is unable to cope with a sick child, even for a few days, in spite of support available from the social services.

School exclusion should follow the advice given in the *Memorandum on the Control of Infectious Diseases in Schools*, prepared jointly by the Department of Education and Science and the Department of Health and Social Security (1971).

When the child is not feeling very ill, there is no objection to his being seen at the surgery provided that there is a room available in which mother and child can be separated from other patients. In 1971, 40 per cent of children with rubella were visited at home by a doctor for the purpose of diagnosis; this is unnecessary.

When the child is first seen and the diagnosis made, the mother should be given full information on the expected course of the infection. When further children in the family develop the illness most mothers are able to recognise it and cope without further medical help. Children with measles or scarlet fever are seen by the doctor on average 1.4 times, whilst the child with rubella is seen only once.

Children who are febrile can be nursed in a downstairs room, provided that it is well ventilated and not filled with cigarette smoke, and may be allowed to watch television. There is no need to darken a room because of the conjunctivitis in children with measles though drawn curtains during the day may well make photopobia less distressing. Special diets are unnecessary but fluids should be given liberally as required.

Generally, the younger the child the higher the fever and the more likely it is that vomiting will occur. Convulsions occur occasionally in measles and in roseola infantum, but are virtually unknown with the other exanthemata. Where there is chilliness, rigors, headache or restlessness, aspirin may be given, particularly in the early afternoon and evening, and when the fever is high tepid sponging is helpful. If a child becomes delirious, he will need to be pacified and gently restrained to prevent him from hurting himself. During the febrile period the child will probably wish to remain in bed but as soon as the temperature falls he will want to get up and should be allowed to do so.

Measles

Its distribution is worldwide. In this country the illness is mild but in countries where malnutrition in children is common it may be severe and have a high mortality. When measles virus is introduced into a community which has had no experience of the disease for many years it usually spreads with great rapidity in both children and adults, causing a severe epidemic. There are no carriers of the virus, infection being transmitted directly from case to case.

The illness is often brought into a household by a child at school and susceptible siblings will almost invariably be infected. School exclusion is for seven days from onset of rash.

The baby of a mother who has not had measles is susceptible from birth, but in urban areas most pregnant women possess measles antibodies which pass through the placenta and confer natural passive immunity in the first six months. The national vaccination scheme started in 1968, and it is not yet known whether the babies born to mothers who were vaccinated in childhood will have similar immunity.

The pattern of incidence in England and Wales in recent years is shown on Figure 21.1. Since vaccination was introduced, measles has affected older age groups. Nearly half the notifications in 1977 were of children aged 5 to 14 years.

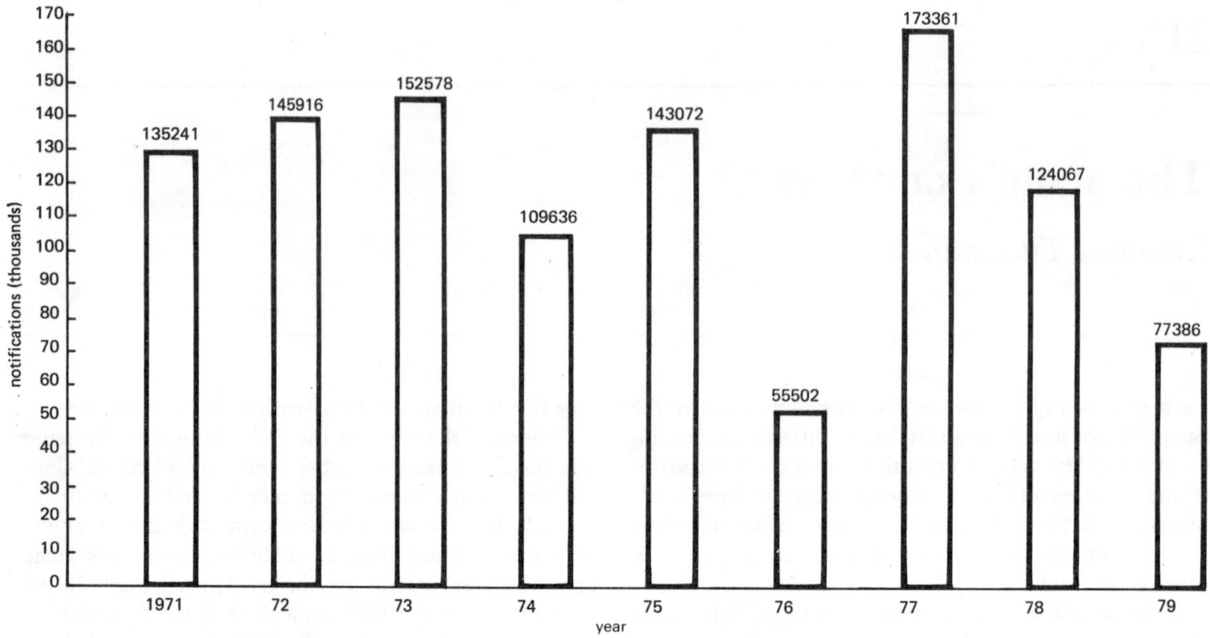

Fig. 21.1 Notification of measles in England & Wales (all ages) 1971–1979 (Galbraith, N.S., Forbes, P. & Mayon-White, R.T. (1980) Changing patterns of communicable disease in England and Wales. BMJ, 2, 489–92)

Clinical features

The incubation period between infection and the onset of symptoms is 8–11 days and the rash begins to appear 2–3 days later. The onset is characterised by fever, coryzal symptoms and a harsh unproductive cough. Koplik spots, which are pathognomonic of measles, may be seen. Pathologically, they are small patches of necrosis in the basal layers of the mucosae with infiltration by mononuclear cells, while clinically, they resemble coarse grains of salt on the background of a reddened mucosal surface. They may be difficult to see in artificial light, but in natural light they are readily seen on the buccal mucosa, particularly opposite the molars, and the diagnosis of measles can be made before the rash appears.

The prodromal stage is accompanies by irritability and conjunctivits and sometimes by vomiting and diarrhoea. Acute appendicitis may be mimicked. The ear drums are oftened inflamed, though earache is not a common symptom. During the two or three days of catarrhal symptoms the child is usually not very ill and is up and about. There is then a rise in temperature, he begins to feel much worse and the cough becomes more pronounced. The rash begins to appear, first behind the ears, and spreads to the face, trunk and limbs. Koplik spots fade as the rash develops.

The rash itself consists of dusky red macules or maculopapules which cover the body and which coalesce to form irregular blotches. Some degree of laryngitis and bronchitis is present in every case. The measles virus itself is responsible for both the respiratory symptoms and the abnormal signs in chest and ear drums, and they are not the result of bacterial infection. Chest X-ray will show enlarged mediastinal lymph nodes and penumonitis.

After two or three days the rash fades, leaving a brownish stain which may last for up to ten days. Occasionally fine desquamation occurs. As the fever subsides the child's condition rapidly improves. The cough may persist for some weeks even though the child is perfectly well, but if the fever lasts for more than a few days and the child remains unwell in himself, secondary invasion by bacteria has probably taken place.

Cerebral complications

Changes in the EEG are commonly found in the acute stage – the transient encephalitis may explain why the child with measles is so often miserable – but EEG changes disappear within a week in uncomplicated cases. Postinfectious encephalitis occurs in one in 1000 patients, usually developing three to four days after the rash. It may be mild with only transient drowsiness and irritability but at the other extreme, coma with a mortality of 10 to 20 per cent and severe neurological disability can occur. Subacute sclerosing panencephalitis (SSPE) may occur several years after an attack of measles and is possibly due to persistence of 'slow' virus in the brain. There may also be an association between measles and the later development of multiple sclerosis.

Diagnosis

During an epidemic there is usually no difficulty in making a diagnosis. The rash in mild sporadic cases, and in those who have been vaccinated, may be confused with rubella or with drug eruptions, particularly those due to ampicillin. However, the rash of rubella is finer and paler than that of measles and does not run into blotches, whilst the ampicillin rash lasts longer and does not evolve from above downwards; an urticarial element in the rash excludes measles. In both rubella and drug eruptions, the total clinical picture is very different, there being no catarrhal phase, fever, irritability, or cough. Occasionally there may be a maculo papular rash suggestive of measles in an older child with infectious mononucleosis.

Laboratory tests are not indicated except when bacterial pulmonary infection is suspected and the diagnosis is not clear. A leucocytosis will then be found, as opposed to a leucopenia in an uncomplicated viral infection. Chest X-ray will be required only if suspected secondary bacterial infection does not rapidly respond to treatment.

Treatment

No drug treatment is required. Linctuses are contraindicated as they are respiratory depressants and any sedative action occurs only with large doses. Antibiotics if given routinely or prophylactically do not decrease the incidence of bacterial otitis media and pneumonia; they may increase it.

When bacterial otitis media does occur as a complication, penicillin V is the antibiotic of choice in children over five years of age and it should be given for ten days. In children under five, *H. influenzae* is frequently the causal organism. Bacterial pneumonia is commonly caused by *Strep. pneumoniae, H. influenzae* or staphylococci; ampicillin is the drug of choice and good clinical recovery should have occurred when the child is seen 48 hours after the start of treatment.

There is no specific treatment for encephalitis, both gammaglobulin and corticosteroids being of little value.

Prevention

Passive immunization is indicated in exposed susceptible children who already have an illness or who are on steroids. For complete prevention, 500–750 mg immunoglobulin is given intramuscularly as soon after contact as possible and for attenuation, the dose is 250 mg. Protection by immunoglobulin lasts about three weeks and a second dose may need to be given if the child is re-exposed. Modified measles is usually mild; it is infectious, and the immunity is for life.

Active immunization is discussed in Chapter 11.

Rubella

This would be an insignificant illness were it not for the harmful effects which may follow infection in pregnancy. Probably one attack confers permanent immunity and the low infectiousness may be due to the high frequency of subclinical attacks. Since the illness is not notifiable in England (except for a few large towns), its epidemiology is not very well known. Recent peak years have been 1968, 1971, 1978 and 1979. In the United Kingdom about 85 per cent of adults have rubella antibodies, indicating previous infection; since the introduction of active immunisation in schoolgirls, this percentage has increased. It is quite common for second attacks of rubella (or rubella-like illness) to occur in children. This may be due to the difficulties of clinical diagnosis, or to their being more than one antigenic type virus.

Incubation is about 16–18 days. The virus, which was first isolated in 1962, is present in the blood and nasopharyngeal secretions during the acute phase of the disease, and infection is spread by droplet spray from these secretions. The minimal period of school exclusion is four days from the onset of the rash.

Clinical picture

Rubella may commence with mild malaise and fever but frequently the child feels quite well and is active and lively. Usually it is the rash that is noticed first; this is variable in distribution and character but usually it emerges on the face and behind the ears, then spreads downwards to trunk and limbs. It may be fleeting and fade rapidly. It is fully developed within 24 hours and seldom persists more than a few days. The predominant lesions are small, pale, pink macules which sometimes coalesce to produce a rash somewhat like measles. Occasionally the rash is similar to that of scarlet fever, but lacks its punctate character.

The rash is preceded by slight enlargement of the lymph glands, particularly those in the posterior triangle of the neck, and suffusion of the conjunctivae is very common. The throat may be inflamed but exudates are not present. The tongue is normal, the buccal mucous membrane pale and clean, and Koplik spots are never found. The coryzal prodromata which occur in measles are completely absent.

Rubella without a rash is impossible to diagnose on clinical grounds, as its features – mild fever, reddened throat and lymph node enlargement – are common to many virus infections in childhood.

The complications sometimes seen in adults – arthralgia, myalgia, peripheral neuritis and purpura – do not occur in childhood, though encephalitis has been described.

Congenital rubella

Active infection during pregnancy gives rise to a viraemia and dissemination of the virus to fetal tissues. The effects are varied and unpredictable, ranging from fetal death in about ten per cent, to birth of an infected but otherwise normal child. The infant mortality rate after maternal rubella occurring in the first trimester is three times the normal, and major defects occur in nearly a fifth of the affected children. When rubella occurs during the first month of pregnancy, over 50 per cent and perhaps as many as 95 per cent of fetuses are affected and defects are usually multiple and severe. As pregnancy progresses the risk of defect diminishes, and the type of defect becomes less severe. By the fourth month the risk is still twice the normal rate. Even after the first trimester there is considerable risk of defects, especially of hearing, but these may be noted only after some years of surveillance. It is important to get these figures into proportion. The number of babies born in England and Wales in 1975 who have been confirmed as rubella damaged is about 50. Details of the defects produced by congenital rubella are given in other chapters.

Diagnosis

Clinical diagnosis is notoriously unreliable, and is frequently made on insufficient grounds. Many virus infections, particularly those due to some of the Echo and Coxsackie groups, mimic rubella. There is need for accurate diagnosis only in patients exposed to or developing a rubella-like illness during pregnancy.

Ideally the level of rubella antibody, as estimated by the haemagglutination inhibition (HI) test, should be known in all woman of childbearing age. At present, the HI test should be done as early as possible in all pregnancies. If an antibody titre of 1/32 or more is present there need be no concern if the woman is in contact with, or is herself developing a rubella-like illness. If antibody is absent repeat the test in two weeks, and again if necessary two weeks later. If reliance has to be placed on only one test to differentiate present from past infection, determination of rubella-specific IgM antibody may prove helpful. If no antibody develops, there has been no infection with rubella virus. If antibody does develop, the risk to the fetus must be explained to both parents and termination of pregnancy offered. Where seroconversion has occurred without any clinical illness, the risk to the fetus is probably less than with overt rubella.

Immunoglobulin given to susceptible contacts does not give protection against infection. However, a serologically negative pregnant woman who has been in close contact with rubella and who will refuse termination of pregnancy, should be given a large dose (3000 mg) of immunoglobulin intramuscularly.

Active immunization

See Chapter 11.

Chickenpox (varicella)

This is caused by a specific virus, identical with that of herpes zoster, and chickenpox may on occasion follow exposure to zoster. It is transmitted by droplet infection. It is usually mild, often no more than a nuisance, but may be dangerous especially in neonates and in children on immunosuppressive therapy. It is highly infective and is most commonly introduced into a family by a school child. Once introduced into a household, all the children are likely to get the disease. Second attacks in childhood do not occur.

Incubation is about two weeks and the infectious stage is confined to the first few days, when there are lesions in the mouth and virus is present in the saliva. Infectivity falls rapidly and ceases once the lesions have crusted, usually after three or four days. The minimal period of school exclusion is six days from onset of rash. Children with scabs are usually sent home from school by head teachers, even though they are not infectious.

Clinical features

The appearance of the rash is usually the first sign of the illness, prodromal symptoms being rare. The characteristic lesion is the vesicle, which is unilocular and lies on the skin like a drop of water. It may be round, oval or elliptical and is surrounded by an erythematous areola which fades as the vesicle dries. Within a day or two the vesicle fluid becomes pustular (not the result of secondary infection) and as it is absorbed a scab forms. The scabs fall off within a few days leaving superficial scars, a few of which may become permanent. Lesions have a centripetal distribution, being heaviest on the trunk and frequent on the proximal parts of the limbs, face and the scalp. In nearly every case there are one or two lesions in the mouth, especially on the hard palate, fauces or uvula. On the skin there may be any number of spots, from only two or three to a profuse rash covering most of the body.

Crops of lesions develop at intervals of up to four or five days so that in any one area of the body, vesicles, pustules and scabs may be present at the same time. A low-grade fever often occurs as the rash is coming out and there may be complaint of a sore throat. Itching is common but it is rare for a child to be acutely ill.

Complications such as haemorrhagic chickenpox and encephalitis are rare in children. Secondary infection of skin lesions with haemolytic streptococci or staphylococci are usually the result of scratching, and occasionally this produces a tangled mass of infected lesions in the scalp which needs the attention of the practice nurse.

Serious complications occur in children undergoing steroid therapy, and passive immunisation is indicated. Immunoglobulin (zoster-immune globulin if available), should be given immediately after contact. If lesions of varicella appear in children on steroids, admission to hospital will be needed with a view to treatment with an antiviral agent.

Congenital chickenpox, the result of infection in the child's mother at or near term, may be severe.

A vaccine for active immunisation against varicella is being developed, but its general use is unlikely unless the virus becomes much more virulent than at present.

Diagnosis

Mild chickenpox, especially when seen on the first day, is sometimes difficult to distinguish from papular urticaria or insect bites in which lesions may be capped by tiny vesicles. However, these are not like drops of water on the skin, they may have been present for many weeks, and there is an irregular distribution without cropping. There are no lesions in the mouth. In cases of doubt, if the child is seen the next day the diagnosis becomes clear. There is little difficulty in distinguishing impetigo, which is usually clustered at one site, commonly the face, does not occur in crops and does not involve mucous membranes. Scabies does not occur above the neck and does not produce vesicles.

As smallpox has been eliminated as a disease, there is no longer any need to consider it in the differential diagnosis of chickenpox. Nevertheless one or two countries still unreasonably require travellers to have International Certificates of Vaccination against smallpox. Eczema vaccinatum may therefore still occur.

Treatment

To allay the irritation, calamine lotion, to which may be added a one per cent solution of coal tar, is used. Sedation may be needed for a few days, promethazine syrup 10 mg given late afternoon and repeated as often as necessary to help the child settle, being most commonly prescribed. Antibiotics are of no value in uncomplicated cases and are required only for secondary infection in children with disturbed immunity.

Scarlet fever

The illness results from invasion by an erythrogenic strain of streptococcus, 90 per cent of which are Lancefield Group A. Entry is usually via the throat, but can follow infection of a wound, skin lesion or the genital tract. Sore throats in children under the age of two are rarely due to streptococci, and scarlet fever is uncommon in preschool children. Spread is by droplet infection but there have been recorded outbreaks in which infected dairy products have been the source of infection.

As haemolytic streptococci may be found in the throats of 10 to 20 per cent of normal children, routine swabbing within a family is pointless. When an outbreak occurs in a boarding school, swabbing of contacts may be advisable. School exclusion is required until appropriate treatment has been given.

Clinical features

The incubation is about three days with limits of one to seven days. Onset is usually abrupt, with headache, sore throat, fever and sometimes vomiting. However, the illness may consist of little more than a mild rash in a child with a mild sore throat.

Classically, the tongue, after a day or two of furring, has a red glazed surface with prominent papillae (the strawberry tongue), and the tonsils are red and swollen with possibly patches of white exudate. There is tender enlargement of the cervical lymph glands and the ear drums are often inflamed. The rash appears on the second day, beginning on the face then spreading to neck and chest, down the trunk and to the limbs. It consists of a background of erythema with intensely red punctate spots which may condense to form discrete macules. It gradually fades after two or three days and as it does this, the fever disappears and the general condition of the child improves. At the end of a week from the onset of the illness the epidermis begins to peel and patches of desquamation appear, firstly on the neck and trunk and then over the rest of the body in the same order as the rash evolved. The hands and feet may be the most involved and coarse strips may be shed from these two areas. However, desquamation is seldom a feature with the mild illness that is usually seen nowadays. The shed skin is sterile and not infectious.

Within a week most children have recovered and complications are rare. Nephritis occasionally follows, particularly if the organism was Type 12 or Type 49. There is no point in the routine testing of the urine once the child is better; even if acute glomerulonephritis does occur, recovery from this usually takes place within a few weeks without treatment. The complications of purulent otitis media, rheumatic fever, arthritis and carditis are now rarely seen. Erythema marginatum may follow scarlet fever.

Diagnosis

Swabs taken in the home or surgery must be inoculated into a transport medium for despatch to the laboratory. A pure growth of *Str. pyogenes* from the throat supports the diagnosis but is not conclusive. The white cell count is usually raised, which is helpful in differentiating mild cases from rubella, but this investigation will rarely be required in general practice. The measurement of antistreptolysin 'O' in the patient's serum is of no value in the diagnosis of scarlet fever.

Many viruses, particularly the Epstein-Barr virus, produce an illness resembling tonsillitis and often it is impossible to distinguish between these and streptococcal infections on the appearance of the throat and the other clinical features. These viral infections may be accompanied by a rash, but this is not often similar to that of classical scarlet fever.

Treatment

Intramuscular penicillin is not necessary and the drug of choice is phenoxymethyl-penicillin (Penicillin V) 250–500 mg orally every six hours for ten days. Erythromycin or a cephalosporin should be used in those children known to be allergic to penicillin. The haemolytic streptococci disappear from the throat within 48 hours from the start of treatment, but may reappear if the penicillin is given for only five days. Mothers should be told this.

Control

Removal to hospital is undesirable, even when there is gross overcrowding in the home or mother has recently been confined. Where a member of the family works in a dairy or a confectioner's, he or she should be swabbed and given prophylactic oral penicillin. It is not necessary to give prophylactic penicillin to other children in the family unless one already has an illness such as chickenpox or is on steroids.

Erythema infectiosum

This is rarely reported, though it is probably not uncommon. It occurs in localised outbreaks, often in school children, and does not affect those under the age of two. Probably it is caused by a specific virus, and it has an incubation period of 4-14 days.

The rash is most prominent on the cheeks, where it first appears as bright macules which finally run into one another. It does not run across the mouth, which gives it its American name 'slapped cheek disease'. Later, the rash appears on the limbs, and sparsely on the trunk, where it is usually less bright. It persists for a week or ten days. Other symptoms are slight and vague – malaise, a few aches, headache – and there are no after-effects.

Roseola infantum

Its origin is unknown, but probably it is due to a specific virus. It may possibly be a slow febrile immunising reaction to many different viral pathogens. It occurs only in children between the ages of six months and three years.

It commences with high fever, which then continues without localising symptoms and signs for three to four days. In spite of the fever the infant is bright and alert. When the fever subsides, a scattered rash consisting of small pink macules, often surrounded by a pale areola, appears on the trunk and may sometimes spread to neck and limbs. The rash does not itch and fades rapidly, usually within 24 hours, to bring the illness to an end.

Administration

Under the *Public Health (Infectious Diseases) Regulations 1968*, measles and scarlet fever must be notified to the local authority (now the community physician) by the first medical practitioner attending. The local authority is responsible for the fee. In some local areas rubella may be notifiable. When scarlet fever is notified, a public health inspector usually visits the home in case a member of the household is involved in food handling.

The Health Services and Public Health Act (1968) makes it an offence for a parent to allow a child suffering from a notifiable disease to expose others to risk of infection by the child's presence in any street or public place. Nor may an article exposed to infectious disease be sent to a laundry or cleaners unless it has been disinfected. There is no record of a prosecution having been brought for such offences.

Supplies of immunoglobulin are obtainable from the public health laboratory service, either directly or via the local district general hospital.

FURTHER READING

Hoeprich, P.D. (ed.) (1977) *Infectious Diseases*, 2nd edn. New York: Harper & Row.

Krugman, S., Ward, R. & Katz, S.L. (1977) *Infectious Diseases of Children*, 6th edn. St Louis: C.V. Mosby Company.

Parry, W.H. (1979) *Communicable Diseases*, 3rd edn. London: Hodder & Stoughton.

Warin, J.F. & Ironside, A.G. (1980) *Lecture Notes on the Infectious Diseases*, 3rd edn. Oxford: Blackwell Scientific.

22

Some common viral infections

Cyril Hart

The viral infections of childhood are responsible for a substantial section of the daily workload of the general practitioner. Those causing acute respiratory infection are dealt with in Chapter 19, influenza in Chapter 20, and the acute exanthemata are discussed in Chapter 21. Some skin disorders of viral origin are described in Chapter 29. It is my purpose in this chapter to discuss some of the remaining common viral infections of childhood, namely those due to herpes simplex virus, myxovirus parotidis, the Epstein-Barr virus, the hepatitis A virus, various neurotropic viruses, and finally the rotaviruses and other diarrhoea viruses. The chapter also deals with gastroenteritis and meningitis of bacterial origin, since these are sometimes difficult to differentiate from viral infections. The episode rates for some of these conditions encountered in general practice in 1970–71 are shown in the accompanying table (Table 22.1), but the figures would be very different today.

HERPES SIMPLEX VIRUS INFECTIONS

The herpes group are large (150-200 nm) viruses which replicate in the nuclei of infected cells and contain a core of double-stranded DNA in a glycoprotein envelope. Herpes simplex viruses form a major component of this group, and are classified into two chief subtypes, HSV1 and HSV2, distinguishable antigenically and biologically. HSV1 affects mainly the oral cavity, eye, skin and brain. Usually the primary infection occurs in childhood, and therefore it is with this virus that we are chiefly concerned here; what follows concerns HSV1 unless otherwise stated. HSV2 affects mainly the genitalia. Usually it is acquired venereally, and is encountered therefore from adolescence onwards; but neonates can be infected during passage through the birth canal.

Epidemiology

HSV1 is one of the commonest of all the infections of mankind, having a worldwide distribution; one third at least of the human race is currently infected. In this country there is a striking correlation of incidence with social class, and grades IV and V tend to contract the disease at a lower age than grades I and II; moreover, the incidence generally has been falling as living standards rise. Serological studies show a high prevalence of neutralising antibody in infants under six months, derived from passive transfer *in utero*. The general prevalence then falls to the region of 20 per cent at 6–12 months, rising shortly thereafter to around 65 per cent at 15–25 years, and 97 per cent at the age of 60.

Almost all mammals can be infected experimentally, but they play no part in transmission, man alone being the natural host. Primary infection occurs chiefly by mouth; the peak incidence of gingivostomatitis occurs in infants of two or three years, and it seems likely that

Table 22.1 Episode rates for some viral and bacterial infections in selected practices in England and Wales in 1970–71*

Infection	Episodes per 1000 patients All ages	Ages 0–4	Ages 5–14
Mumps	1.6	1.7	5.2
Infectious mononucleosis	1.3	0.8	1.8
Infectious hepatitis	0.8	0.6	1.8
All meningococcal infections	0.1	0.3	0.1
Aseptic meningitis due to enteroviruses	0.20	0.5	0.4
Intestinal infections	19.0	63.1	16.8
Acute vomiting and/or diarrhoea	32.7	111.9	30.7

* From *Morbidity Statistics in General Practice* (1974) HMSO

this is usually caused by adults with cold sores of the mouth kissing them; it has been called one of the 'viruses of love'. The eye is also an important portal of entry; HSV1 infection is said to be the commonest identified cause of conjuctivitis in infants in Britain today.

Clinical features

Most individuals get their primary infection of HSV1 in childhood or youth. Incubation takes on average six days. In two out of every three cases, the primary infection is subclinical, and most of the remainder are trivial, especially in the younger age groups. Nevertheless, the general incidence of infection is so high, that clinical manifestations are frequently encountered in general practice.

Gingivostomatitis, the commonest presenting lesion, tends to be more severe in older children, who may exhibit fever and malaise for two to five days, sometimes with marked foetor oris and salivation. The tongue is heavily coated, and the gums are inflamed and friable. Infants become acutely miserable, with continuous drooling. Greyish-yellow vesicles appear on the lips and in the mucous membrane of the mouth, breaking down to form small shallow ulcers with red inflamed bases. Regional lymph nodes become enlarged and tender.

Primary ophthalmic infections are less common, and usually take the form of an acute oedematous conjunctivitis. Herpetic vesicles may be present in the eyelids, and are an important aid to clinical diagnosis. In about half the cases the cornea is involved, and a diffuse epithelialitis occurs. Linear dendritic ulcers are comparatively rare at this stage.

Other sites of primary infection are mostly cutaneous. Infants may develop herpetic vulvovaginitis and napkin rashes. In older children, the cutaneous lesions may be extensive and mimic zoster, but characteristically they are of bilateral distribution, and pain-free. Herpetic whitlows in children result from touching infected lesions on companions, or pricking the finger with infected material. Eczematous children are particularly susceptible to cutaneous herpes; should it happen that topical steroids are being employed for treatment of the eczema at the time, severe infections can occur.

Primary systemic involvement is not unknown. Acute encephalitis carries a high mortality, and residual brain damage is common in survivors. Fortunately, it is exceedingly rare. Hepatitis is another rare complication.

The incidence of HSV2 infection in adults is rising steadily. Unless some form of preventive action is taken, HSV2 infection occurs in 50 per cent of neonates whose mothers have genital herpes at the time of delivery, and half of these babies are killed or severely damaged by it. However most of the reported cases of neonatal infection have been in the American literature; the condition is still rare in the UK. General practitioners should be aware that genital herpes at term can be an indication for Caesarian section, though in recent years the tendency has been to allow normal labour to proceed, under close consultant supervision.

The primary infection of HSV1 virus is self-limiting, and constitutional symptoms when present usually subside within a week. Once acquired, however, the infection persists throughout life, the primary phase being followed by an asymptomatic latent stage, during which the virus integrates with the host cell genomes to form a stable relationship, in which the virus may be protected from circulating antibodies. The old controversy as to the precise habitat of the virus during this period of latency now appears to be resolved. As with zoster, the large size of the herpes simplex virus prevents its spread through connective tissue, and the commonest sites of hibernation appear to be the nerve sheaths and the posterior root ganglia of the sensory nerves supplying the area in which the primary vesicular rash occurs. (The author has a patient in whom surgical ablation of the trigeminal ganglion for neuralgia provoked a severe herpetiform eruption of trigeminal distribution.) CSF antibodies have been recovered from patients with latent HSV1 infections.

The precise mechanism by which latency ceases and the virus is reactivated is unknown. Reactivation of the virus may occur sporadically throughout the lifetime of the infected person, though such recurrences are commoner in adult life than in childhood. Attacks are triggered off by a wide variety of stimuli leading to local metabolic upset; characteristically attacks are provoked by febrile illness, exposure to cold or to sunlight, menstruation, and physical or emotional trauma.

At the onset of a recurrence, the virus is thought to migrate from the root ganglia to the end organs of the sensory nerves at the site of the primary infection, typically the mucocutaneous junction of the lips, though each susceptible individual has his or her characteristic site. Here the virus replicates at a remarkable rate; it has been estimated that about 100 000 copies of viral DNA are manufactured in each host cell. Eventually lysis of the cell membrane occurs, with release of the virus. The characteristic vesicles of the eruption are therefore highly contagious. Recurrences have a high nuisance value, but are less often accompanied by constitutional symptoms than is the primary infection.

Recurrent ocular infection leading to keratitis is not uncommon.

Diagnosis

The illness accompanying primary infection is often undiagnosed or misdiagnosed clinically. In infants, gingivostomatitis may be passed off as being due to thrush or teething; in older children, tonsillitis or Vincents infection may be suspected. In the absence of characteristic vesicles on the eyelids, herpetic conjunctivitis may be thought to be allergic or bacterial in origin, or due to dust or other small foreign bodies. The herpetic vesicles of localised mucocutaneous recurrences are easier to recognise, though occasionally they may be mistaken for zoster or vaccinia.

Laboratory support is rarely necessary in the management of common mild infections, but occasionally the general practitioner needs help when some unusual feature makes precise diagnosis important, for example with eczematous children or those or immunosuppressive therapy.

Skin scrapings from both primary and secondary lesions show multinucleate giant cells, but this does not differentiate herpes simplex from zoster. The virus can be grown in tissue culture, but it is very labile and requires to be kept at low temperatures, so rapid transport of specimens to a laboratory is essential. Where an electron microscope is available, the virus particles themselves may be visualised. Primary infections by HSV1 and HSV2 produce both type-specific antigens and one or more common antigens. These are detectable in scrapings material by fluorescent antibody technique.

Neutralising antibodies are also type-specific, but they are rarely detectable serologically in blood samples taken before the end of the first week of the primary infection. They persist throughout the latent phase, so that often the serological diagnosis of primary HSV1 or 2 infection is made only retrospectively, from a fourfold rise in titre in serial specimens. Complement fixation antibodies also occur, but being non-specific they are of little use in diagnosis.

Management

Simple supportive measures are all that is usually required. Severe stomatitis calls for careful and persistent cleansing of the mouth, and maintenance of an adequate fluid intake. Hyperimmune globulin in sometimes effective, if given soon enough. Vesicles may be treated topically with 5-iodo 2 deoxyuridine (IDU), an inhibitor of DNA synthesis, of which a 5 per cent solution in dimethyl sulphoxide (Herpid) is available. It is painted on to early lesions four times daily. While very effective, this however is too expensive for routine application, and its use is best restricted to ophthalmic complications, and only under consultant supervision. IDU does not eradicate the virus when it is latent, and does not therefore prevent recurrences. IDU can also be used systemically in treating encephalitis, but this is essentially a hospital procedure.

In general practice it is of great importance to avoid using steroids in all HSV infections, particularly when there is ocular involvement, or with eczematous subjects. Children with active eczema should be kept away from known cases of herpes simplex or zoster infection.

The suspect cancer risk associated with HSV infection of the oesophagus, cervix and lips has inhibited experimentation with vaccination. Nevertheless, recent work at Birmingham may lead eventually to the production of a safe vaccine against the HSV2 virus. Killed virus vaccines have been found useless in the treatment of recurrent herpes infections.

MUMPS

Myxovirus parotidis, the causal organism of mumps is a RNA virus approximately 150 nm in diameter, but variable in size. The paramyxovirus group of which it is a member includes the organisms responsible for measles and parainfluenza.

Epidemiology

Man is the only reservoir, the sexes being equally affected. Infectivity is low. Spread is by droplet infection, or occasionally from saliva or close contact with fomites. Entry is gained through the mouth and nose, or rarely by the conjunctivae. The disease is not notifiable in the UK, so its incidence is unknown, and likewise the percentage of the child population affected, but this must be high; before the introduction of mass vaccination in the USA, over 90 per cent of children there were infected before the age of 14.

Mumps is endemic in urban communities, with occasional epidemics, usually in the winter and the spring. Recently there has been a well-marked three year cycle in the UK. In virgin communities, serious and widespread outbreaks may occur.

Clinical features

Mumps is usually a mild disease, and serology shows that up to 40 per cent of infections are clinically inapparent. Commonly the 5–15 age group is affected. Incubation takes 14–21 days, occasionally longer. During this period there is local spread to the salivary glands, and in particular the parotids; the virus is neurotropic and there is also widespread blood-borne infection.

A prodromal malaise, with headache, anorexia, and fever up to 40°C (104°F) is common, but not universal. Swelling of the salivary glands occurs a day or two later. The parotids are nearly always involved, either unilaterally (in 30 per cent of cases) or bilaterally, often sequentially. In 10 per cent of cases the submandibular glands are also affected, and uncommonly the sublingual glands may be seen to be enlarged beneath the upturned tongue. The parotid swelling may be tense and painful, displacing the ear upwards and outwards, and sometimes cellulitis and trismus may be present. The orifice of the parotid duct (opposite the crown of the second upper molar) is seen to be swollen and inflamed.

A dry mouth is common, leading sometimes to difficulty in mastication. Occasionally the early stages of mumps in infants and young children can lead to febrile delirium and convulsions. Fever may persist for up to a week.

Complications

The mumps virus disseminates widely in the host tissues, but outside the salivary glands infection is usually subclinical. The commonest complication in childhood is an aseptic meningitis coincident with or shortly after the parotid enlargement. In epidemics this can occur in up to 2.5 per cent of cases, but usually the reported incidence is considerably lower than this. One authority quotes 0.26 per cent of all cases of mumps. If all cases of mumps were to be subjected to lumbar puncture, evidence of mild meningitis might be found in many more. However, this procedure is rarely indicated in the absence of meningism. Mumps meningitis occurs more commonly in boys than girls. Usually the meningeal irritation and toxic symptoms are mild enough for the experienced practitioner to treat the child at home, but in cases of doubt or parental anxiety a domiciliary visit by a consultant paediatrician is advisable. Admission to hospital may be indicated in a few cases. Lumbar puncture then reveals an opalescent fluid, with a lymphocyte count up to 1000/mm^3, and a normal protein and glucose content.

Encephalitis, fortunately rare, is a much more severe condition. Unlike meningitis, its onset is commonly delayed until 10 to 14 days after the prodromal illness. It may lead to demyelination and residual nerve damage, and should always be treated in hospital.

The only other complication likely to be encountered in a general practitioner's clinical lifetime is orchitis, which is very rare before puberty but occurs in about three per cent of cases of mumps in adolescents, and up to 25 per cent in adults. Commonly the orchitis develops about ten days after the parotid swelling. Usually it is unilateral, but it is now believed that even in bilateral cases, subfertility and sterility are rare sequelae. There is no evidence of a high incidence of congenital defects in the offspring of affected patients. Nerve deafness, diabetes mellitus, pancreatitis and myocarditis (sometimes detected by a friction rub) are extremely rare complications of mumps in childhood. Mumps has the lowest mortality figures of all the childhood virus diseases. In Britain, of 48 deaths due to mumps reported in the decade 1968–1978, 28 were in patients over the age of 64.

Diagnosis

Mumps is easy to diagnose clinically, especially during epidemics. Usually it can be differentiated anatomically from cervical lymph gland enlargement, but oral inspection for tonsillitis should be routine, and a Paul Bunnell test may be necessary to eliminate glandular fever in a few cases. Suppurative parotitis, with or without calculi, is uncommon in childhood, but may occur in an ill, dehydrated and febrile patient with poor oral hygiene. Pus can usually be expressed from the salivary duct in such cases, and a stone may be palpable. When in doubt, mouth washings or a salivary swab should be sent to the laboratory, when the mumps virus may be isolated. It is usually best to consult the virologist first for advice on collection and transport of specimens.

Sometimes mumps is suspected when meningitis occurs in the absence of parotid swelling. Here a complement fixation test on a sample of serum may be helpful, but decision on whether or not to treat the case at home must rest on clinical judgement. Retrospectively, mumps may be diagnosed by a four-fold rise in antibody titre in samples of serum collected two weeks apart in the acute and convalescent stages of the disease.

Management

Treatment is non-specific. Many children are hardly affected by an attack of mumps, but when there is a severe febrile phase, rest and copious fluids are essential, with straw feeding if necessary. For parotid pain local warmth from a flannel round the head and neck is comforting, and simple analgesics such as paracetomol suffice for all but the severest cases. Meningitis may require up to 10 days rest in bed or on a couch, with slow mobilisation. The CSF may not become normal for up to three weeks. Sequelae are rare, but a hearing test is advisable. Orchitis should also be treated by rest. Prednisone in a dose of 15 mg six hourly orally for four days produces dramatic relief from testicular pain. A scrotal support is unnecessary. Reassurance about future sexual performance should always be given.

Prophylaxis

Mumps is infectious for one week before and two weeks after the onset of glandular swelling, but infectivity is low, and cases should be isolated only until the last gland subsides. Quarantine of contacts is unnecessary.

Although the fetus can be infected transplacentally, there is no evidence that this leads to adverse effects, and mumps in a pregnant woman is not therefore an indication for therapeutic abortion.

Transplacental antibodies give most babies passive immunity for the first year of life. One attack of mumps in childhood gives lifelong immunity in nearly all cases. In Britain now, 95 per cent of adults are immune following natural infection in childhood. Live attenuated vaccines have been developed in the USA in the last two decades, and these have now been combined with measles and rubella vaccines, given routinely to children of both sexes at the age of 15 months. As a result of mass vaccination, the number of USA cases notified fell from 120 000 in 1966 to 20 000 in 1977. The overall incidence there is now said to have been cut by 90 per cent. Mumps vaccine gives high protection for a long period. A monovalent vaccine has been available in this country since 1971, but the disease is so mild that vaccination has been severely limited. It is worth considering in the case of a child with cystic fibrosis. It is sometimes given, after primary antibody screening, to post pubertal boys before admission to residential institutions, or to hospital for serious operations. However, in view of the success of vaccination in the USA, we need to look again at this issue in the UK. It is all a question of priorities.

GLANDULAR FEVER (INFECTIOUS MONONUCLEOSIS)

The Epstein-Barr virus (EBV) is now firmly established as the principal cause of glandular fever. It is a herpes virus, rather smaller than the rest of the group, the mature particle having a diameter of c. 110 nm. Another virus of the herpes group, the cytomegalovirus, also causes occasional outbreaks of a disease resembling glandular fever, with a negative Paul Bunnell test.

Epidemiology

EBV infection is common, and worldwide. Man is the only reservoir, the sexes being equally affected. Early descriptions of the disease suggest that at the turn of the present century children were more often affected than young adults, and epidemics were described. More recently, clinical infections have involved increasingly older age groups, and in this country less than ten per cent of cases now occur in children before adolescence. It is rare in infancy. Childhood infection is commonest in low socio-economic groups where there is overcrowding and poor personal hygiene. It is thought that infection is mainly oral-faecal in children, but that kissing is the commonest mode of spread in adolescents and young adults. The virus is thought to be harboured in the salivary glands, and is found in the throat washings of patients for many months after clinical signs and symptoms have disappeared.

Infectivity is low, and epidemics no longer occur in Britain. There is little seasonal variation in incidence. The incubation period is surprisingly uncertain, recent estimates varying between 5–10 days and 6–12 weeks. It seems likely that the lower figures are more common in childhood infection.

Clinical features

Most childhood infections are subclinical, and when symptoms do occur they are usually milder in children than in adults. Glandular fever presents in many different ways, and the severity and the length of the disease are likewise very variable. Insidious onset is common. There may be a prodromal illness lasting up to one week, and characterised by tiredness, malaise, generalised muscle pains, frontal and retro-orbital headache, and pyrexia, particularly at night. Lymph node enlargement then occurs; often this is the presenting symptom. Characteristically the postcervical glands are most affected, and then the upper deep cervical chain beneath the sternomastoid. The glands are large, soft and usually painless unless secondary bacterial infection is present, when they may become tender. Axillary and inguinal glands are also usually palpable, and a minimal soft splenomegaly may be detected. Clumsy palpation of the spleen is said to carry the risk of rupture.

Petechial haemorrhages at the junction of the hard and soft palate are an early diagnostic sign. Sometimes the buccal mucosa is similarly affected. There is usually a sore throat, and many cases present with this, sometimes accompanied by a troublesome dry cough. A grey tonsillar exudate is common. A transient generalised maculopapular rash may occur in children during the first week of the disease. If ampicillin is given, a morbilliform rash nearly always results, and this can be severe.

Complications

Liver involvement, with or without jaundice, is much less common in children than in adults. Meningism is found occasionally in children, and an aseptic meningitis may occur at any stage, but is very uncommon. Encephalitis and polyneuritis are rare. Mesenteric adenitis occasionally causes pain in the right iliac fossa.

Perhaps the commonest complication in childhood is a coexistent streptococcal throat infection, which causes problems both in diagnosis and treatment.

Diagnosis

Glandular fever may mimic many childhood infections, and can be confused with exanthemata, tonsillitis, leukaemia, lymphadenoma, toxoplasmosis, mumps and infective hepatitis. One of the commonest presentations is the apparent acute tonsillitis that does not respond to antibiotics. Examination of the throat is important, and requires a spatula and good light, when the characteristic petechiae at the junction of the hard and soft palate will often be detected. The fundamental investigations are a differential white count and a Paul Bunnell test. The former will usually show a relative and absolute mononuclear leucocytosis, after which the disease is named. Mononuclears may form up to 60 per cent of the total white count. The Paul Bunnell test for heterophile antibodies to sheep red cells is diagnostic when positive but in the early stages of the disease a negative result may be obtained, and a repeat test after one week should always be asked for when the diagnosis remains in doubt. The test is nearly always positive by the third week of the disease and false positives, though well recognised, are uncommon.

In recent years commercial kits such as the Monospot slide agglutination test have become available, which offer a convenient and rapid screening test to back up a clinical diagnosis without reference to a laboratory. It is too soon to be sure, but it looks as if these will eventually supplant the Paul Bunnell test in general practice.

Management

Once the diagnosis is established, nearly all children with glandular fever are best cared for at home. Occasional follow-up by the practice nurse or health visitor is usually all that is required. Parents should be warned that the illness, although mild, is occasionally a long drawn-out affair. Treatment is symptomatic, with bed rest and fluids in the febrile stage. There is little need for drugs. When tonsillar inflamation is present a swab should be taken, especially if the cervical glands are tender. If a streptococcus is isolated, the best antibiotic is usually penicillin V. Drug rashes in glandular fever are commonest with ampicillin, but can also occur with other broad spectrum antibiotics.

Occasionally intermittent fever, sweats, anorexia, and debility can drag on for months, but this is uncommon in children and when it occurs the diagnosis should be reviewed. Concurrent ENT bacterial infection should be sought for, and a chest film is advisable. Serum SGOT and SGPT are commonly raised after the first week of the disease, but hepatic involvement should not be blamed for slow improvement until other possibilities are eliminated. The normal course of EBV infection in children is complete recovery within three weeks.

Occasionally problems arise when children contract glandular fever just before or during examinations. There is no doubt that performance can be seriously affected. Fortunately most examination authorities are well aware of this, and take it into account, but on occasion the GP will be called upon to make representations on the child's behalf.

INFECTIVE HEPATITIS

Acute viral hepatitis is now known to be due to at least four distinct viruses, the two best known and most important being labelled A and B. A is a cubically symmetrical picornavirus 27 nm in size, whereas B is double-shelled and measures 40 nm. Virus A, which was isolated from faeces only as recently as 1973, is the causal organism of most cases of infective hepatitis, and virus B of most cases of serum hepatitis. The two diseases share many features in common, but the A form, which has the shorter incubation period, is the more prevalent in children in this country. Fortunately, it is also the more benign of the two.

In recent years the picture has been complicated by the discovery of at least two different non A-non B viruses by chimpanzee inoculation studies, but as yet no routine laboratory tests are available to identify them. They may be responsible for some cases of both transfusion-associated hepatitis and sporadic hepatitis. In some patients non A-non B hepatitis progresses to chronic liver disease. However the commonest cause of acute viral hepatitis in British children is virus A, and our account will therefore be mainly concerned with infection by this organism.

Epidemiology

Virus A is of world-wide distribution. Transmission is oral, by faecal contamination of hands or formites, or (in the case of epidemics) of water supplies or food. Children are the principal vectors of endemic disease. Parenteral infection from the serum of those having the disease can also occur, but this is unusual.

The epidemiological picture in the UK is changing rapidly, and for the better. Characteristically, infective hepatitis due to the virus A used to be encountered chiefly in children and adolescents, being much less common in those under 5 or over 20 years old, but the decline in incidence for the past decade has been much greater in children than in adults, resulting in an age-shift in incidence towards older people. Moreover, the decline was first noticed in rural areas, particularly in Eastern England, but now this improvement has reached the towns and conurbations. In Britain, the incidence of hepatitis A is still highest in the autumn, and the disease occurs mainly in small clusters, often with only one or two identified cases. Outbreaks are mostly indigenous, but occasionally the infection is brought in from overseas. Travellers and holiday-makers from the UK who swim in sewage-infected waters along the Mediterranean littoral are particularly at risk.

Infective jaundice from A and B viruses became notifiable in England and Wales in 1969, and the steady decline in incidence since then is shown in Figure 22.1. This reflects the real improvement in our standard of living over the past decade, and it is also a triumph for preventive measures in public health. The decline is however, limited to virus A infection, and has not been accompanied by any appreciable reduction in the UK incidence of serum hepatitis due to virus B. Laboratory reporting of hepatitis B antigen and antibody began in 1972, and is now running level at about 1000 cases annually. In November 1980, as this was being written, it was reported that there had been an increase of 37 per cent in the notifications of infectious hepatitis during the first 40 weeks of the year. Most if not all of this

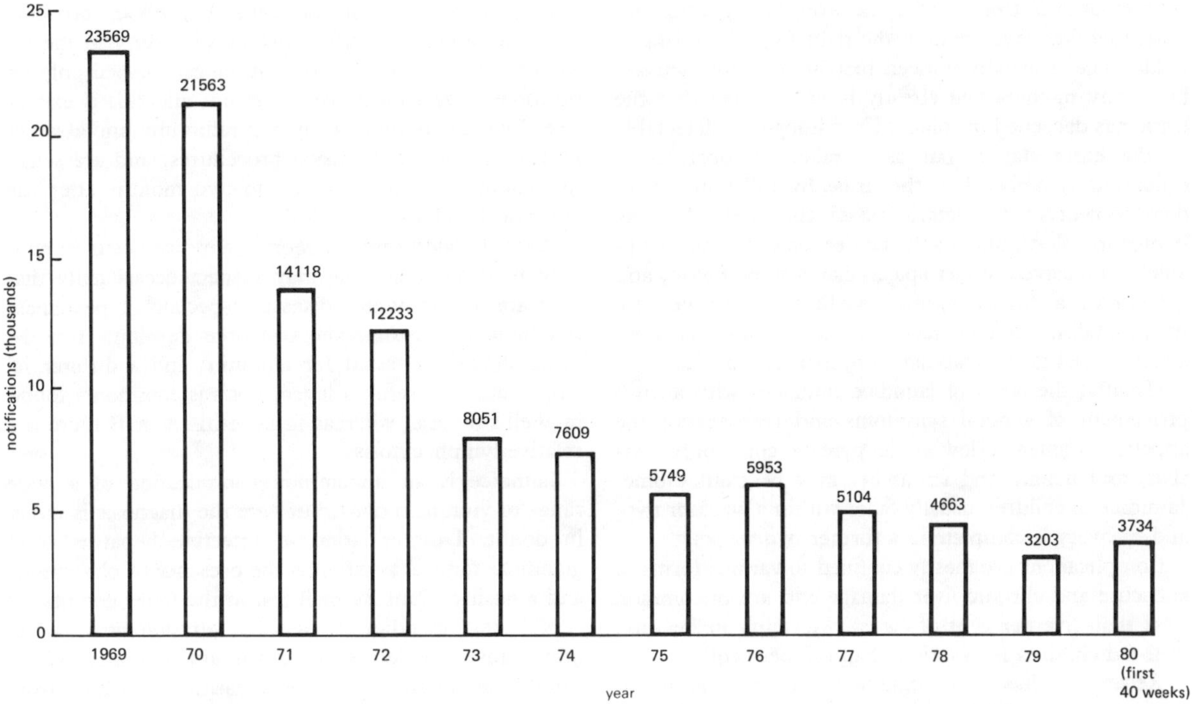

Fig. 22.1 Infective jaundice in England and Wales (all ages) 1969–1979. Source: Communicable disease surveillance centre, reported in *BMJ* 1980, 2, 490

must be due to an increase in virus A infection. This serves to warn us that the reduced incidence over the decade is not an inevitable biological progression, and that the figures will worsen again if standards of hygiene are not maintained.

Virus A has an incubation period of three to four weeks, during which it undergoes blood-borne spread throughout the tissues of the host. Jaundice occurs a few days later in about 10 per cent of cases, the remaining infections being mostly subclinical. The virus appears in faeces as the transaminases begin to rise, and shedding ceases at or soon after the onset of jaundice. The virus has been transmitted experimentally to marmosets and chimpanzees, but it seems unlikely that mammals other than man harbour the virus naturally.

Pathology

Virus A infection is generalised, and changes may demonstrated in such tissues as the lymph nodes, spleen, kidneys, pancreas, gut and brain, but the organ mainly affected is the liver. The centrilobular cells distend, and may become multinucleate. A spotty non-fatty zonal necrosis occurs, leading to hepatocellular jaundice. Specific antibodies must be formed, but have not been identified. Inflammatory invasion by leucocytes, mostly mononuclears, leads to swelling of the parenchyma and compression of the small intrahepatic biliary ducts, sometimes resulting in cholestasis and intrahepatic obstructive jaundice. The intralobular ducts and canaliculi leading to the portal tracts are similarly invaded, and become dilated. Complete regeneration of the liver cells nearly always occurs, and subacute necrotic changes and cirrhosis are rare sequelae.

It is worth noting that this description of the microscopic changes depends largely on specimens obtained from severe cases by liver biopsy or in the post mortem room. Changes may be less marked in the milder forms of the disease encountered in general practice. Nevertheless, cholestasis leading to obstructive jaundice occurs only when there is appreciable swelling of the parenchyma. Macroscopically, these changes lead to a temporary hepatomegaly. Swelling may occur also in the lymph nodes and the spleen, but this is much less marked.

Clinical features

In the normal, well-nourished child, infective hepatitis is a benign illness, being subclinical in up to 80 per cent of cases. In those patients in whom the disease proceeds to an icteric stage, a prodromal feverish illness lasting up to two weeks may occur, with symptoms of shivering, muscle pains, headaches and malaise. Alimentary symptoms are common, with marked nausea and anorexia, and sometimes vomiting and diarrhoea. As the liver enlarges, stretching of the overlying peritoneum leads to a non-colicy pain in the right hypochondrium.

Jaundice is usually noticed first in the conjunctivae, but many mothers will already have observed that the urine has deepened in colour. Urobilinogen is detectable in the early stages, but as intrahepatic obstruction occurs, it is replaced in the urine by bilirubin. With development of the icteric phase the stools become lighter in colour, and a soft, tender liver becomes palpable. An enlarged tender spleen may also be found, and sometimes a corresponding swelling of the cervical lymph nodes. Jaundice may be preceded on occasion by a generalised maculopapular rash, usually transient.

Usually, the onset of jaundice coincides with an improvement of general symptoms and recovery of the appetite, though a low-grade pyrexia commonly persists, and itching and irritability may be troublesome. Jaundice in children usually fades within a week or two, and recovery is complete in a further two weeks.

Complications are mostly confined to various forms of subacute and chronic liver damage and are uncommon (less than five per cent of cases). Mortality in healthy, well-fed children is rare (less than 0.2 per cent).

Recently it has been suggested that there is an increased risk of developing transient or permanent diabetes mellitus following an attack of infective hepatitis, due to pancreatic damage. More studies are needed before one can make a confident pronouncement on this.

Diagnosis

This can be difficult in the prodromal stage, if there is no epidemic or history of contact with jaundiced patients. Gastroenteritis or influenza may be suspected. Unfortunately, as yet no simple and inexpensive specific laboratory test for A virus is generally available. In general practice, the most useful investigations when hepatitis is suspected as the cause of an unexplained febrile illness are the urinary urobilinogen and the serum aminotransferase. Their use in such cases should be early and routine. Ictotest can be employed without having recourse to the laboratory; in some cases it gives positive results five or more days before diagnostic clinical signs and symptoms supervene. These tests do not, however, distinguish between the A and B viruses.

Once jaundice becomes apparent, in most mild cases it is safe to assume that virus A disease is present. When in doubt, differentiation between A and B infection is helped by the longer incubation period, history of risk of parenteral infection (e.g. from transfusions and other procedures), and above all the presence of hepatitis B surface antigen (HBAg), all of which are characteristic of virus B disease.

If these simple considerations do not lead to a definite diagnosis, and if for some particular reason differentiation between A and B infection becomes important, serological tests for the hepatitis A antibody are now available. Since antibody develops very early in the infection, serological diagnosis can be established only by titrations of serial samples of serum, and this is expensive. Enzyme immuno assay and radio immuno assay of IgM antibody are the usual procedures, and are sensitive enough for detection up to two months after the onset of the illness.

When isolated cases of febrile jaundice occur in children in rural areas, one may suspect occasionally that they are due to Weil's disease, especially if petechiae, muscle pains, or toxic manifestations develop. Here the urine should be tested for albumin, and a differential white count is useful; a leucocytosis is commonly found in Weil's disease, whereas in hepatitis A or B there is a relative lymphocytosis.

Jaundice is an uncommon complication of a wide range of viral infections, but here the diagnosis is rarely in doubt. Differentiation of infective hepatitis from glandular fever is assisted by the presence of pharyngitis and a positive Paul Bunnell test in the latter condition.

Neonatal jaundice is usually physiological; when other causes are suspected, consultant paediatric advice should be sought. Infective hepatitis can occur from placental transmission during parturition, but it is rare.

Management

The great majority of children with infective hepatitis are best cared for at home. Bed rest is rarely necessary, and drugs of all kinds are contraindicated, except possibly small doses of analgesics if liver pain occurs, and occasionally an antihistamine as a sedative when itching is intense. During the febrile stage, fluid intake should be encouraged. Fat restriction is unnecessary, and as soon as the nausea and anorexia subsides a high calorie diet rich in protein should be offered.

Once the diagnosis is established, domiciliary follow-up by the health visitor or practice nurse obviate the need for repeat visits by the general practitioner, but persistence of symptoms should be reported back to him. Prolonged jaundice, or the onset of toxic symptoms, are indications for seeking consultant advice.

We tend to be too casual in general practice about containing infection. Isolation of cases from other members of the household is impracticable, but human gamma globulin is valuable in prophylaxis, and should be given to those contacts in whom it is advisable to prevent disease. It is also useful when outbreaks occur in a closed community, and for travellers to areas where the disease is endemic. A single intramuscular dose of 0.04 ml of gamma globulin per kg body weight is usually sufficient for infants and children, and gives protection for about four months. Hypersensitivity reactions are rare provided there is no IgA deficiency.

Visiting an infected household by pregnant women is

best discouraged. A high standard of hygiene should be insisted upon, with particular care in disposal of faeces, and hand-washing after toilet. The health visitor can help here. Parenteral spread is prevented by burning examination gloves and disposable syringes, and by steam or hot sterilisation of instruments. Thermometers also require attention. Finally, it should be remembered that both virus A and virus B hepatitis are notifiable diseases, and that those who are known to have suffered from them within the previous 12 months should not donate blood.

VIRUS MENINGITIS AND ENCEPHALITIS

Virus meningitis is a disease syndrome encountered not very uncommonly among the younger patients of the general practitioner. Usually it is a mild disease, and once the diagnosis is established it can best be managed at home. The difficulty lies in the diagnosis. We have first of all to differentiate between true meningitis and the meningism which commonly accompanies acute febrile illness in childhood. Then we have to ensure that the meningitis is not caused by an acute or chronic bacterial infection. Finally, management is assisted if a reasonable guess can be made as to the identity of the virus concerned.

In general practice, solution to all three problems has to rely on clinical assessment alone, for lumbar puncture outside hospital can no longer be defended as a reasonable procedure in Britain today, except in the most unusual of circumstances. Yet lumbar puncture is the key to accurate diagnosis, and many would argue that because of this, every case in which meningitis of any type is suspected should be admitted immediately to hospital. There is however a case to be made for the domiciliary care of children (but not infants) with virus meningitis. It is a mild, self-limiting disease, and for every case of bacterial meningitis encountered by the general practitioner in Britain he will see perhaps ten or more that are viral in origin. We shall return to this fundamental issue of home treatment later in the chapter.

Aetiology of viral and bacterial meningitis

The viruses commonly implicated in meningitis in this country are *Myxovirus parotidis* (the causal organism of mumps), and enteroviruses of the Echo and Coxsachie groups. There is, in addition, a whole range of viruses which we encounter only very occasionally or rarely as the causal organisms of meningitis; these include the Eptein-Barr virus of glandular fever, measles and rubella, herpes simplex and zoster and varicella, smallpox and vaccinia, and finally poliovirus, now virtually eliminated as a pathogen because of immunisation, but always to be borne in mind, especially in children recently returned from holidays in warmer climates.

Almost all pathogenic bacteria can cause bacterial meningitis, but in normal healthy children in Britain the meningococcus is by far the most common cause, with *Haemophilus influenzae* Type B virtually the only significant runner-up, particularly in infants between the ages of six months and two years. It is as well to remember however that this latter infection is conta-

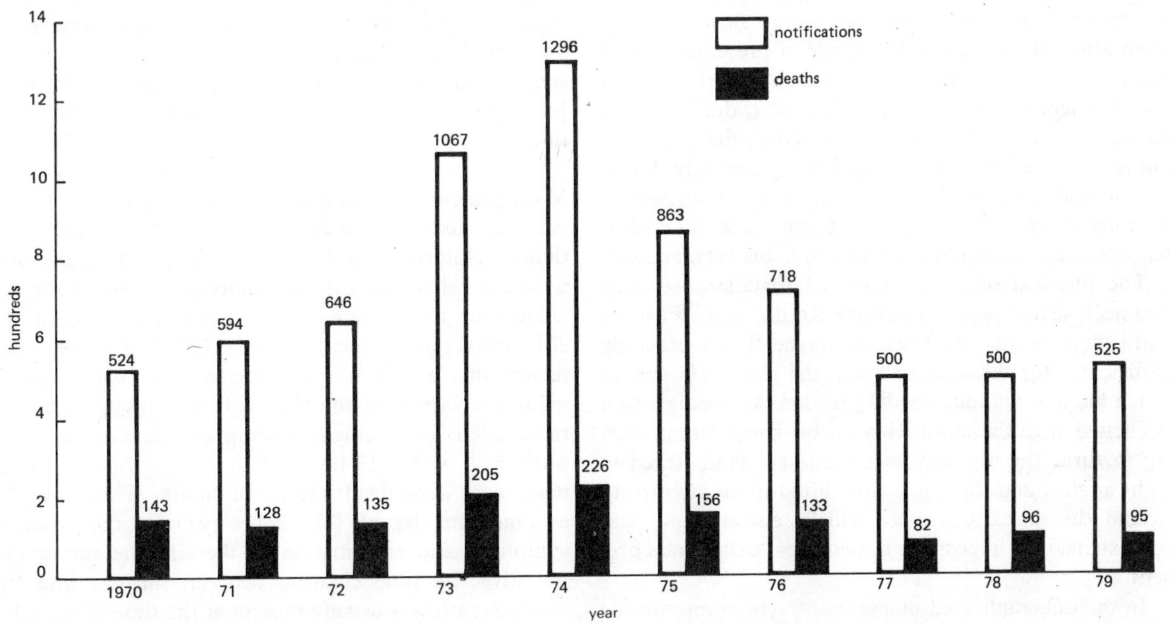

Fig. 22.2 Acute meningococcal meningitis England and Wales (all ages) 1970–1979. Source: Communicable disease surveillance centre, reported in *BMJ* 1980, 2, 490

gious, and siblings should be monitored for a whole month after a primary case has been identified.

In this chapter we are not concerned with bacterial meningitis occurring in the neonatal period in babies with neural tube defects, for their management is essentially a problem for the hospital-based paediatrician. Tuberculous meningitis is now rarely encountered in Britain, and for completeness pertussis vaccination should also be mentioned as a rare cause of meningitis. If it spreads to Britain, rabies will also have to be considered.

Epidemiology of meningococcal meningitis

The known incidence of meningococcal infection in Britain peaked in the mid-1970s, and 52 children under the age of five are known to have died of it in Britain in 1974. The number of notifications has now fallen, and with it the death rate, but the disease is still too prevalent for complacency (Fig. 22.2). Furthermore, it is likely that a significant number of cases of meningococcal infection are undiagnosed and unreported. Some children with undiagnosed petechial rash, with or without pyrexial illness, treated at home with penicillin, undoubtedly fall into this group. Nevertheless it is unlikely that a general practitioner will encounter more than a single case of acute meningococcal meningitis in his clinical lifetime. The problems arising from this are discussed below.

Clinical features of viral meningitis

Virus meningitis can occur at any age, but for the most part it is a disease of youth, being encountered most commonly in the 1–10 years age group. Boys are more often affected than girls. The mode of presentation and degree of severity are both somewhat variable, but usually there is a short prodromal illness, during which mother notices a fall-off in usual activity, the child taking to bed or a couch and lying down voluntarily. Often the temperature is little raised. The characteristic meningitis symptoms of headache, nausea with or without vomiting, irritability and photophobia then appear.

The physical signs of meningeal irritation are back and neck stiffness, and a positive Kernig sign. With the child lying down, the head cannot be flexed passively sufficiently for the chin to touch the chest. He cannot touch his toes without bending his knees. Kernig's sign is elicited with the child lying on his back; taking each leg in turn, the hip and knee joints are both flexed to right angles, and the leg is then lifted in an attempt to extend the knee. Resistance will be encountered, and full extension is impossible if meningeal irritation is present.

In the uncomplicated illness, most symptoms subside within two or three days, but residual lassitude, headache, and anorexia may persist for some weeks.

Differential clinical diagnosis of bacterial and viral meningitis

Meningism without inflammatory reaction occurs quite often in young children with acute specific fevers, otitis media, pneumonia, and other febrile illness. Careful history taking and clinical examination will usually enable its significance to be assessed correctly. Special care is needed with the acute exanthemata when a rash is present. Other causes of neck stiffness, such as acute torticollis and cervical lymphadenitis, are easily eliminated.

If there is a clear history of contact with mumps or if the usual manifestations of this illness are present, then the diagnosis of virus meningitis is seldom in doubt. Knowledge of local outbreaks of Echo and Coxsachie infections will also put the practitioner on his guard; these are particularly prevalent in the summer months, and should be suspected if meningitis develops in a child with diarrhoea, myalgia, rash, or pleurodynia. Quite often, however, there is neither history nor symptomatology to point to a particular virus, especially with enteroviral infections. Here experience comes into its own, important factors requiring clinical assessment being the degree of meningeal irritation, and the degree of toxicity. Usually viral infections of the meninges run a much more benign course than bacterial.

Untreated, a fulminating meningococcal infection leads to death within a few hours, and requires considerable alertness for its early detection. Signs of meningeal involvement in such cases are rarely found before the appearance of a rash. When meningeal signs or symptoms are present in a febrile illness therefore, all types of coexisting rashes require careful examination, particularly petechiae or small crops of purpura, which suggest the presence of meningococcal septicaemia. Joint pains are also suggestive of meningococcal infection.

Management of meningococcal meningitis

A recent survey of ten deaths from meningococcal infection in children under two years old in England and Scotland brings out the very short time-scale of the development of the infection, and the urgent need for effective action on the part of the GP. The survey confirmed that a rash is a much commoner early sign of meningococcal infection than is head retraction, due to meningism. On average, these infants developed a purpuric rash within 13 hours of the first symptoms of illness, and were dead within 21 hours. There was an average time lag of 11½ hours between the onset of symptoms and examination by the GP (the survey did not give the time elapsing between the call and the visit). A rash was usually present at the time of the GP's visit, but sometimes only in its initial petechial stage, before the development of confluent purpura. None of the GPs had seen the rash of meningococcal infection before, so that it is not surprising that its presence did not lead to immediate diagnosis. Nevertheless, with one unfortunate exception, all children were admitted to hospital within seven hours of being seen by the GP, the average time interval being only 2½ hours. Yet this was insufficient to save them. Intramuscular penicillin should be given therefore as soon as suspicion of meningococcal infection is aroused, and before or during transport to hospital, which should be immediately by car, without wasting time waiting for an ambulance. Penicillin should also be given prophylactically to all siblings and other close childhood contacts of confirmed cases of meningococcal infection.

Head retraction, a bulging fontanelle in infants, persistent vomiting, convulsions, and marked drowsiness progressing to coma are all late pointers to severe meningeal involvement, whether viral or bacterial, and these are clear-cut indications for immediate hospitalisation. Similarly, the acutely toxic child, who lies still and looks ill and perhaps dehydrated, should not be nursed at home.

Serological investigations and blood and stool culture play no part in early diagnosis of meningitis in a general practice setting, though retrospective diagnosis from a rise in antibody titre is of course useful epidemiologically.

Home management of viral meningitis

We return now to consideration of the much commoner and much milder viral meningitis. In the first edition of this book a case was argued for home management of selected cases of mild viral meningitis in children, without hospitalisation and lumbar puncture. There is little doubt that many such cases have been correctly diagnosed clinically, and managed competently by experienced general practitioners in the past, with a high degree of safety for the child. However, with the decreasing overall incidence of meningitis, and with the expectation and imposition of ever-higher standards of care, I am reluctantly persuaded that this practice can no longer be defended. During the 1977 Echo 19 epidemic in Birmingham, for example, the large majority of children admitted with meningitis were shown by lumbar puncture to have infections which were clearly viral, but among them were two with meningococcal meningitis, with symptoms in the early stage barely distinguishable from the remainder (Flewett, personal communication).

It must therefore be stated categorically that in the UK today, every child with suspected meningitis of any kind should be admitted to hospital immediately for lumbar puncture. If this establishes the presence of an aseptic lymphocytic meningitis (as in the great majority of cases it will), then consideration should be given to the early return of the child to his home environment, for care by his own general practitioner. There will be less reluctance shown by the GP in referring these children, if he can trust the hospital clinician to return suitable cases speedily to his care. There is just as much need for informed and responsible judgement on the part of the paediatrician in sending these children back home, as there is by the GP in admitting them to hospital in the first case.

When clinical doubts are resolved, and home management is decided upon, parents require reassurance and advice, and nurse can help here. Even the mildest cases however require daily visiting by the doctor until all meningeal signs disappear.

Home treatment is non-specific, and largely a matter of good nursing, and ensuring adequate rest, quietness, and fluid intake. Antibiotics are avoided, for fear of masking bacterial infection. Analgesics may be required for headache. Visits by those outside the family are best discouraged for the first few days, and hygiene needs particular attention when enteroviral infection is suspected. Meningitis is a notifiable disease, but the milder viral forms encountered in general practice are considerably under-reported.

Virus encephalitis

All the causal organisms of viral meningitis may go on to produce a frank encephalitis. Clinically the distinction between the two illnesses is largely a matter of degree. Severe headache and vomiting, cranial or peripheral nerve pareses, ataxia, convulsions, impaired mental function, personality changes, and coma, all raise the question of encephalitic involvement, and such cases require of course immediate hospital care.

It is usual to divide viral encephalitides into two groups: those considered to result from direct invasion of the brain, and those that may result from an immunological response in the nervous tissue of the host. The former arises usually from blood-borne spread of the virus, and is characterised by neuronal destruction of cells in the grey matter; generally it is closely related in time to other manifestations of the systemic illness. The latter affects the white matter and the cord, and the characteristic histological picture is one of demyelinisation; it tends to present clinically at a later stage, as the initiating illness is subsiding. Encephalitis due to direct viral invasion may arise from enteroviral and herpes virus infections, whereas mumps and the acute viral exanthemata, together with immunisation reactions, tend rather to cause the demyelinating or postinfectious type of encephalitis.

Fortunately, both forms of encephalitis are rare. They carry however a high mortality, and a high percentage of residual brain damage in those children who survive. In England and Wales each year about 175 deaths (at all ages) are attributed to encephalitis, of which perhaps 20 are proven virologically. Those due to herpes simplex virus carry the worst prognosis.

ACUTE GASTROENTERITIS

Acute gastroenteritis is one of the commonest of childhood illnesses throughout the world, and is still a leading cause of death in many under-developed countries. In Britain, according to a recent estimate, the average general practitioner sees one in ten of his infant patients with gastroenteritis each year. Of these, nine out of every ten are managed successfully at home.

Many different bacteria and viruses have been implicated as causing both sporadic and epidemic gastroenteritis in children. Until recently, however, no organisms at all have been found in the majority of cases, when searches have been made in patients with the disease. Moreover, the issue is not settled by the discovery of a particular pathogen in an individual case, for very often further investigation has shown the suspect organism to be found as frequently in controls as in patients.

The most prevalent pathogenic bacteria found in diarrhoeal stools are various strains of *Escherichia coli*, *Shigellae*, and *Salmonella*. *Shigella* causes dysentery, which is notifiable. The remarkable decline in incidence over the past two decades is reflected in Figure 22.3. This decline is due to a fall in the number of *S. sonnei* infections, as a result of public health measures. *S. sonnei* is mainly a disease of school-aged and younger children. The fall in this age group has been much greater than that in adults.

Of the viruses, those most commonly encountered until recently have been enteroviruses from the Echo and Coxsachie groups. Late in 1973 however the situation changed dramatically when Bishop and her colleagues in Melbourne reported the detection of reovirus-like particles in the duodenal mucosae of six out of nine babies in the symptomatic phase of acute non-bacterial gastroenteritis. Originally they were classified as orbiviruses, but reports of the discovery of similar particles in diarrhoeal stools soon appeared from centres in many parts of the world, and further study showed that they differed antigenically as well as structurally from the orbiviruses and reoviruses. Flewett and his colleagues at Birmingham have coined the term 'rotaviruses' to describe these organisms. It is apparent already that the detection of these viruses has revolutionised our understanding of the aetiology of acute infantile gastroenteritis, and it is likely that in the near future there will be important repercussions both in prevention and in management of this condition.

The human rotavirus

Rotaviruses may now be included in the list of those

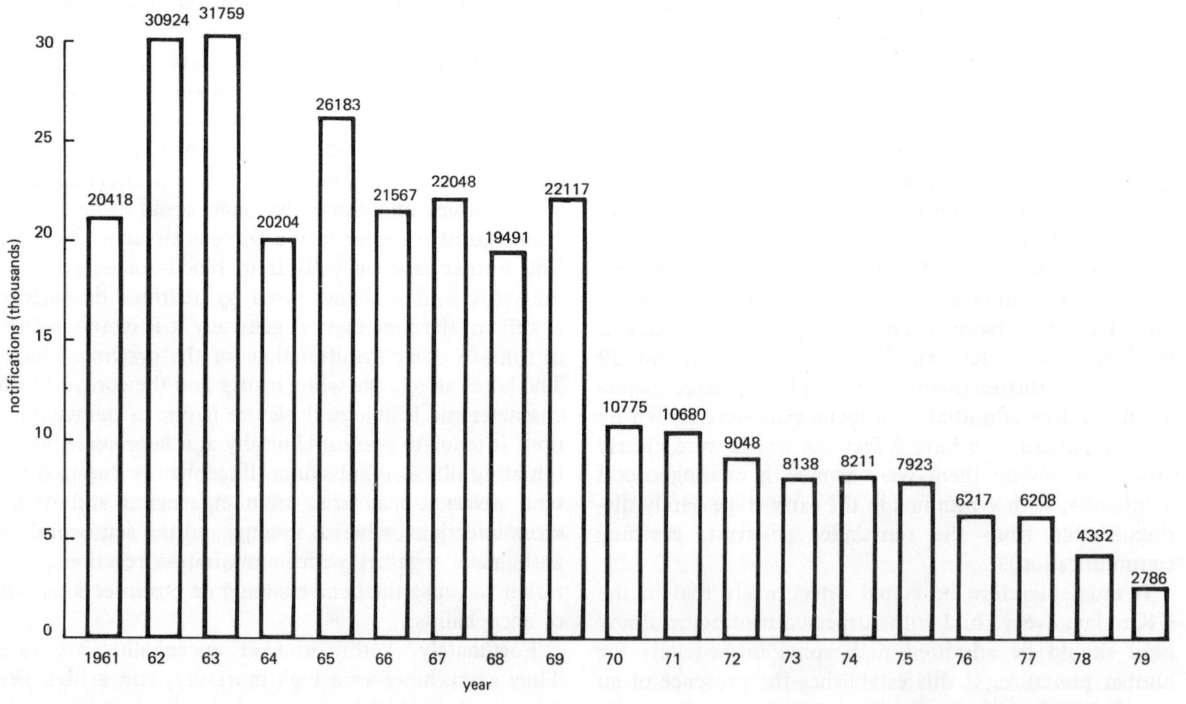

Fig. 22.3 Notifications of dysentery in England and Wales (all ages) 1961–1979. Source: Communicable disease surveillance centre, reported in *BMJ* 1980, 2, 490

viruses such as the herpes group and hepatitis B, which may reliably and rapidly be detected in clinical specimens by electron microscopy. The human rotavirus consists of a core about 38 nm in diameter, surrounded by an inner layer of capsomeres which radiate outwards like the spokes of a wheel. An outer layer of capsomeres appears to be attached to the top of the inner ones, giving rise to the characteristic well-defined rim (diameter 65–68 nm) surrounding the virus particle. It was this wheel-like appearance that suggested the name *rotavirus*, from the Latin.

Viruses indistinguishable morphologically from the human rotavirus have been found in diarrhoeal stools and gut washings of many wild and domesticated mammals, including dogs, rabbits, apes, mice, pigs, sheep, foals, and calves – characteristically in the younger age-groups of each species. Some if not all of these are also related antigenically. The calf virus antibody reacts with the inner but not the outer capsid layer of the human rotavirus particles. Complement fixation and immunofluorescent tests reveal group-specific antibodies common to human, calf, mouse, and monkey viruses, whereas the outer capsid antigens are probably type-specific or species-specific. Much of course remains to be done, before the full epidemiolological implications of all this are worked out.

Recently, a newly described technique has been applied to the diagnosis of rotavirus infections–enzyme linked immunosorbent assay. The test is highly sensitive, and also economical, because the reagents are stable and can be used in high dilution. It may soon be used extensively for diagnostic purposes.

The human rotavirus is thought to be transmitted by the faecal-oral route; there is no firm evidence of droplet infection via by the respiratory tract, although in two-thirds of infections in young children, diarrhoea is preceded by a respiratory illness. The virus is very stable in faeces for prolonged periods at ambient temperatures. Stools may contain up to 10^{11} rotavirus particles per g of faeces. Rotaviruses are rarely detectable in children over the age of six years, by which age most children have developed antibodies. The age-groups most frequently infected are infants between six and 24 months. Subclinical infection has been found in neonates; perhaps maternal antibody may mitigate the disease in the very young.

Rotaviruses are most often found in winter, during which season they may be detected in up to 73 per cent of young children with infective diarrhoea. The disease has an incubation period of one to three days. IgM antibody to the virus has been observed as early as two days after the onset of symptoms. Virus excretion is greatest during the third and fourth days of illness, and is rarely detectable after the eighth day.

Rotaviruses are found only rarely in specimens from children who have had previous attacks of gastroenteritis, so that it is likely that some immunity persists. There is considerable hope that in the foreseeable future a vaccine will be prepared. However, it has recently been shown that there are at least three antigenic subtypes of rotavirus, two with world-wide distribution, although clinical differences have not been established. Children who undergo more than one attack of acute gastroenteritis are sometimes the victims of attack by different subtypes – there is no complete, long-lasting cross-immunity. This has important implications for the manufacture of vaccines.

It seems clear from the foregoing that rotaviruses are the most important single cause of infantile gastroenteritis throughout the world today, and perhaps before long vaccination may give us the means to bring this scourge under control.

The 'Norwalk' viruses and winter vomiting disease

Recent studies have implicated a further type of virus as the causative organism of outbreaks of gastrointestinal upset which follow a characteristic pattern, described below. These are small (33 nm) particles resembling enteroviruses, but separated from them morphologically and antigenically. They have been isolated in the USA and the UK. The USA strains are named Norwalk, Montgomery County and Hawaii after the places where they have been isolated, but strains detected in UK outbreaks are not related to these antigenically.

Epidemics cause by these viruses are much less common than those due to the rotavirus, though both occur more often in the winter months, and both affect children more often than adults. 'Norwalk' epidemics are characterised by family or community outbreaks, schools being particularly affected. There has recently (1980) been a widespread outbreak in Australia. In some UK cases infected cockles have been implicated, presumably from contamination by sewage.

Symptoms include nausea, vertigo, vomiting (sometimes projectile), abdominal pain and diarrhoea, leading to the rather inadequate clinical label of 'winter vomiting disease'. The incubation period is one to two days, and symptoms rarely persist for more than three days. Most cases are quite mild.

When outbreaks are suspected, stools of affected individuals should be sent for electron microscopy, when the characteristic small virus particles may be identified. In contrast to rotavirus infection, immunity develops only slowly, and sero-epidemiological studies in temperate climates have shown that only 50 per cent of adults have acquired resistance. However, in tropical countries, early sub-clinical infection is common.

Because several different strains of the organism have been isolated, it is unlikely that vaccines against viruses of the 'Norwalk' group will be developed in the foréseeable future. Since the illness is usually mild, and outbreaks are relatively uncommon, vaccine research must have low priority.

Clinical features of infective gastroenteritis

In infants and young children most forms of infective gastroenteritis, whatever the causal organism, tend to present with a similar clinical picture, which varies in severity according to the virulence of the strain, and the age and immunological and nutritional state of the patient. At one extreme, the healthy baby may be stricken suddenly with vomiting and diarrhoea, become severely dehydrated with astonishing rapidity, and die within 24 to 48 hours. At the other, the illness is trivial, with only a few loose stools and no constitutional disturbance. This, of course, is by far the commonest experience.

In the early stages of the more severe infection, the clinical picture is often non-specific. Mother may report the recent onset of irritability, crying and insomnia. Normal activity – play in particular – ceases and the infant becomes apathetic and lies down voluntarily. He may or may not be thirsty. The bottle is often refused, and the infant may become pale and distressed.

Vomiting is a common early symptom, especially in rotavirus infections, but may be absent in some cases, particularly with older children. Characteristically, its onset precedes the diarrhoea. In the more severe infections it continues through the diarrhoeal stage, and becomes persistent and distressing.

When diarrhoea commences, the stools become semiformed, then watery, and change in colour from yellow to green. Frequently they contain mucus, and (except in rotavirus infections) they may become bloodstreaked, but frank blood is uncommon. The stools become acid in reaction, and a napkin rash may develop.

Fever is a variable sign of infantile gastroenteritis. Often the temperature is subnormal in the milder cases, but sometimes it rises with the onset of dehydration.

Dehydration with its consequent upset of electrolyte balance is by far the most important complication in infantile gastroenteritis, and requires careful clinical assessment. The very young baby, particularly if thin and under-fed, is extremely vulnerable to fluid loss. With better nourished infants, excess body fat may mask the early signs of dehydration to some extent, but the experienced practitioner will readily distinguish between the flabbyness of fatty subcutaneous tissue and the elastic feel of well-hydrated skin.

The parched mouth and tongue, sunken, dark-rimmed eyes, prominent skull, depressed fontanelle, and thin, dry, inelastic skin of the severely dehydrated infant are well-known signs which the prudent general practitioner will not allow to develop in a case under his care, for he will have admitted the infant to hospital long before things reach this stage. Still later signs are the absent peripheral pulses, mottled cyanosed skin, and icy-cold hands and feet which point to peripheral circulatory failure. Half of these babies die.

Diagnosis of infective gastroenteritis

Some paediatric textbooks claim that the diagnosis of acute infective gastroenteritis in infants and young children presents no considerable difficulty. By the time the infant reaches hospital this may be so, but in primary care one encounters several conditions which may mimic the disease, and delay early diagnosis.

In the early stages, other infections causing vomiting have to be considered. Otitis media is missed too often in the very young, from failure to complete a thorough examination. It is important to visualise the eardrums in every case, and to inspect them carefully. If the drum is obscured by wax, this should be removed gently with cotton wool on an orange stick. Patience, persistence, and skill may be required. In the case of rotavirus infections, diagnosis is further complicated by the frequent presence of upper respiratory symptoms in the early stages. A red throat or eardrum may be due directly to the rotavirus in many of the pyrexial illnesses of infancy in which diarrhoea developes after a day or two.

Severe infective gastroenteritis is rare in breast-fed babies, and if they develop diarrhoea some other cause should be suspected. Hypernatraemia in bottle-fed babies from wrongly made-up artificial feeds is described further in chapter 27. Over-feeding of bottle-fed babies is a common cause of gastric upset, and some misguided mothers put their babies at risk still further by introducing mixed feeds far too early. The gut is a very sensitive organ in the first few months of life, and may react strongly to any freshly-encountered food or drug. Diarrhoea may develop when infants and young children are given oral antibiotics for acute infections outside the gastrointestinal tract. In particular, broad spectrum antibiotics such as ampicillin may upset the normal gut flora and lead to the development of thrush diarrhoea.

Differentiation between infective gastroenteritis and acute abdominal conditions is considered in Chapter 23. Other rare causes of diarrhoea in infants, which may be misdiagnosed as infective gastroenteritis are hookworms (see Ch. 28) and Hirschsprung's disease.

Most cases of infective infantile diarrhoea encountered in general practice are too mild and short-lived to warrant active search for the causal organism. Occasions do arise, however, when precise identification of the pathogen is desirable. This rests in the first place on careful enquiry into possible modes of infection. Epidemic summer diarrhoea is unlikely to be due to the rotavirus or to viruses of the 'Norwalk' group. Adenoviruses have been implicated in some outbreaks.

It is best to consult the local bacteriologist and virologist before sending up faecal specimens for examination. Always request microscopy as well as culture. Often it is advisable to collect stools from all members of the family. The cooperation of the nurse and the community physician should be sought here.

Various cheap immunological techniques may soon be available at local laboratory level for the identification of specific viral organisms causing acute gastroenteritis, but until vaccines are developed immunological diagnosis is best restricted to the necessary gathering of epidemiological information.

Home management of acute infective gastroenteritis
The home care of infants with mild infective diarrhoea of over 24 hours duration should be an exercise in cooperation by the practice team. The general practitioner, nurse and health visitor each have a part to play, and each should know what the others are doing.

Usually the preventive and hygienic aspects are best managed by the health visitor. Her work is especially important when home conditions are sub-standard, when the mother is unable to cope without advice, and where there are other infants in the family.

Nurse should weigh the baby daily and keep a chart so that the degree of fluid loss can be accurately measured. She should also help to implement the doctor's advice on feeding, which is the crucial issue in management. It is most important that doctor and nurse should be of one mind in this matter, and that advice to the mother should be clear-cut and unambiguous.

The clinical care is of course the responsibility of the general practitioner. Kaolin mixtures and antibiotics have no place in domiciliary care of this condition, nor have drugs designed to reduce intestinal motility, e.g. lomotil. These are dangerous in a young child with diarrhoea. As a first measure in the mild case, mixed feeding is stopped, and the sugar content of bottle feeds diminished. Sterilisation of feeds is reviewed, and additional feeds with boiled water advised. If the baby will take a little added salt with these so much the better, but the amount must be carefully regulated to avoid overloading. If this regime does not bring about rapid improvement with cessation of diarrhoea and vomiting, it is best to switch immediately to hourly feeds of small quantities of Dioralyte. This is a balanced formula of sodium and potassium chloride, sodium bicarbonate, and dextrose, conforming to the BPC supplement 1976. The contents of one sachet of Dioralyte are dissolved in 200 ml (7 fluid ounces) of freshly boiled and cooled water. An infants feeding bottle is a convenient way of measuring this volume at home. A total daily intake of at least 180 ml per kg will be required, and more if the weight is dropping. Mother must be warned to keep strictly to the instructions printed on the sachet. Any solution unused within an hour of reconstruction should be discarded.

All practices should stock a small reserve supply of this valuable product, so that treatment can be started when necessary, without delay.

Doctor and nurse should be visiting frequently at this stage, to maintain a close watch on the degree of dehydration. The following table by Professor H.B. Wong may be useful in aiding the clinical assessment; in practice I have found that some fontanelle depression often occurs at an earlier stage than suggested here (Table 22.2).

Ideally, the decision to admit to hospital should be taken whenever the degree of dehydration moves from mild to moderate on this scale. Infants who are anorexic or persistently vomiting belong in a hospital. Other factors to be taken into account include the age and nutrition of the baby, the rapidity of development of symp-

Table 22.2 Symptoms in gastroenteritis according to degree of severity (Wong, 1973)

	Degree of dehydration		
Symptom or sign	*Mild*	*Moderate*	*Severe*
Fever	mild or high	mild or high	high
Oliguria	nil	present	anuria
Fits	nil	nil	may be present
State of consciousness	fully conscious	drowsy	may be in coma
Acidotic breathing	nil	may be present	usually present
Fontanelle	normal	normal	depressed
Eyes	normal	slightly sunken	obviously sunken
Skin turgor	normal	slightly reduced	markedly reduced
Skin colour	normal	normal	mottled, cold and clammy

toms, home conditions, and the ability of the mother to cope. When in doubt, the child is best admitted.

The child whose condition improves under home care should be visited by nurse daily until diarrhoea and vomiting have ceased, and feeding has been restored (by stages, of course) to normality. The infant should be back on a full diet by the end of the fourth day.

ACKNOWLEDGEMENTS

I am greatly indebted to Dr T.H. Flewett for reading through this chapter and giving valuable advice and to Dr J. K. Anand for kindly providing statistics. Responsibility for errors that remain is of course wholly my own.

REFERENCES

Herpes simplex

Cooper, (1979) A new vaccine against HSV2 virus. *World Medicine*, **14**, 26–31.

Higgins. P.G. (1974) Recurrent herpes simplex virus infections. *British Journal of Dermatology*, **91**, 111–113.

Juel-Jensen, B.E. & MacCallum, F.C. (1972) *Herpes Simplex, Varicella and Zoster: Clinical Manifestations and Treatment*. London: Heinemann Medical.

Knox, J.D.E. (1976) *Primary herpetic gingivo-stomatitis. Clinical studies from general practice*. MD thesis, University of Edinburgh.

Lancet Editorial (1973) Herpes simplex encephalitis. *Lancet*, **2**, 1426–1427.

Nahmias, A.J. & Roizman, B. (1973) Infection with herpes simplex viruses 1 and 2. *New England Medical Journal* , **289**, 667–674.

Russell, A.S. & Saertre, A. (1976) Antibodies to herpes simplex virus in 'normal' cerebrospinal fluid. *Lancet*, **1**, 64–65.

Skinner, G.R.B. *et al* (1979) *Herpes Virus Workshop*.Society of General Microbiology, Cambridge.

Mumps

Association for Study of Infectious Diseases (1974) A retrospective survey of the complications of mumps. *Journal of the Royal College of General Practitioners*, **24**, 552–556.

BMJ Editorial (1977) Mumps. *British Medical Journal*, **1**, 1489–1490.

BMJ Editorial (1980) Prevention of mumps. *British Medical Journal*, **4**, 1231–2.

Gamble, D.R. (1980) Relation of antecedent illness to development of diabetes in children. *British Medical Journal*, **2**, 99–101.

Lancet Editorial (1974) Mumps vaccine. *Lancet*, **2**, 326–327.

McLean, D.M. (1971) Mumps. In *Progress in Clinical Medicine*, pp. 24–31, 6th edn. Ed. R. Dayley & M. Miller. Edinburgh and London: Churchill Livingstone.

Practitioner Editorial (1978) Adolescent Mumps Orchitis. *Practitioner*, **221**, 162.

Research Unit (1974) The incidence and complications of mumps. *Journal of the Royal College of General Practitioners*, **24**, 545–551.

Weibel *et al* (1973) The persistence of immunity following monovalent and combined live measles, mumps, and rubella virus vaccines. *Paediatrics*, **51**, 467–475.

Westmore G.A. *et al.* (1979) Mumps and sudden deafness. *British Medical Journal*, **1**, 14–15.

Glandular fever

BMJ Editorial (1980) Tests for infectious mononucleosis. *British Medical Journal*, **1**, 1153–1154.

Cameron, D. & MacBean, L.M. (1973) *Infectious Mononucleosis and Toxoplasmosis*. Bristol: John Wright.

Epstein, M.A., Achong, B.G. & Barr, Y.M. (1964) Virus particles in cultured lymphoblasts from Burkitt's lymphoma. *Lancet*, **1**, 702–703.

Evans, A.S. (1974) The history of infectious mononucleosis. *American Journal of Medical Science*, **267**, 189–195.

Henle, W. *et al.* (1974) Epstein-Barr virus specific diagnostic tests in infectious mononucleosis. *Human Pathology*, **5**, 551–565.

Neiderman, J.C. *et al.* (1976) EB virus in the saliva and oropharynx. *New England Journal of Medicine*, **294**, 1355–1359.

Infective hepatitis

BMJ Editorial (1977) Hepatitis viruses–old and new. *British Medical Journal*, **1**, 985.

Goldberg, D.M. (1971) Diagnosis of infectious hepatitis in general practice. *Lancet*, **1**, 641–643.

Feinstone, J.M. *et al.* (1973) Hepatitis A: detection by electron microscopy of a virus-like antigen associated with acute illness. *Science*, **182**, 1026–1028.

Oli, J.M. & Nwokolo, C. (1979) Diabetes after infectious hepatitis: a follow-up study. *British Medical Journal*, **1**, 926–927.

Rowland, A.J. & Skone, J.F. (1972) Epidemiology of infectious hepatitis. *British Medical Bulletin*, **28**, 149–155.

Stewart, J.S. *et al.* (1978) A three-year survey of viral hepatitis in West London. *Quarterly Journal of Medicine*, **47**, 365–384.

Tygstrup, N. (1974) Viral Hepatitis. In Tygstrup, N. (ed.) *Clinics in Gastroenterology*, Vol. 3, No. 2. Philadelphia: Saunders.

Weinbren, K. & Stirling, G.A. (1972) Pathology of viral hepatitis. *British Medical Bulletin*, **28**, 125–130.

Zuckerman, A.J. (1975) *Human Viral Hepatitis*, 2nd edn. Amsterdam: North Holland.

Zuckerman, A.J. (1978) The three types of human viral hepatitis. *Bulletin of the World Health Organisation*, **56**, 1.

Zuckerman, A.J. (1979) Specific serological diagnosis of viral hepatitis. *British Medical Journal*, **2**, 84–86.

Virus and bacterial meningitis and encephalitis

Glode, Mary *et al.* (1980) Haemophilus influenzae type B meningitis: a contagious disease of children. *British Medical Journal*, **1**, 899–901.

Goldacre, M.J. (1976) Acute bacterial meningitis in childhood. *Lancet*, **1**, 28–31.

Gray, J.A. *et al.* (1969) Viral meningitis: a 10 year study. *Scottish Medical Journal*, **14**, 234.

Hambleton, G. & Davis, Pamela (1975) Bacterial meningitis. *Archives of Disease in childhood*, **50**, 674–684.

Illis, L.S. (1975) *Virus Diseases of the Central Nervous System*. Ed. L.S. Illis. Wessex Neurological Centre. London: Balliere Tindall.

Kennard, C. & Swash, M. (1981) Acute viral encephalitis. *Brain*, **104**, 129–148.
Lambert, H. (1975) Virus infection of the central nervous system. *Medicine*, **2**, 82–85.
Miller, D.L. & Ross; E.M. (1978) National Childhood Encephalopathy Study: an interim report. *British Medical Journal*, **2**, 992–993.
Oakley, J.R. & Stanton, A.N. (1979) Meningococcal infections during infancy: confidential enquiries into 10 deaths. *British Medical Journal*, **1**, 468–469.
Rosenthal, M.S. (1974) Viral infections of the central nervous system. *Medical Clinics of North America*, **58**, 593–603.
Smith, H. (1981) Acute viral encephalitis. *British Medical Journal*, **2**, 936–7.
Taylor, Margaret (1980) Paediatric emergencies: meningitis. *Update*, **21**, 167–175.

Gastroenteritis

Banatvala, J.E. (1979) The viruses causing acute gastroenteritis. *Pulse*, 5 May, pp. 35–37.
Bishop, R.F., Davidson, G.P. Holmes, I.H. & Ruck, B.J. (1974) Detection of a new virus by electron microscopy of faecal extracts from children with acute gastroenteritis. *Lancet*, **1**, 149–151.
BMJ Editorial (1975a) Virus of infantile gastroenteritis. *British Medical Journal*, **4**, 555.
BMJ Editorial (1975b) Feeding sick babies. *British Medical Journal*, **4**, 539.
BMJ Editorial (1980) Rotavirus infections in infancy. *British Medical Journal*, **4**, 1162–3.
Cutting, W. (1979) Oral treatment of diarrhoea in children. *Journal of Maternal and Child Health*, **4**, 276–281.
Davidson, G.P., Bishop, R.F., Townley, R.R.W., Holmes, I.H. & Ruck, B.J. (1975) Importance of a new virus in acute sporadic enteritis in children. *Lancet*, **1**, 242–245.
Drachman, R.H. (1974) Acute infectious gastroenteritis. *Paediatric Clinics of North America*, **21**, 711–737.
Flewett, T.H. *et al.* (1974) The relationship between viruses from acute gastroenteritis in children and new born calves. *Lancet*, **2**, 61–63.
Flewett, T.H. *et al.* (1975) epidemic viral enteritis in a long-stay children's ward. *Lancet*,**1**, 4.
Galbraith, N.S., Forbes, Pat, & Mayon-White, R.T. (1980) Changing patterns of communicable disease in England and Wales. *British Medical Journal*, **2**, 489–492.
Lancet Editorial (1975) Rotaviruses in man and animals. *Lancet*, **1**, 257–259.
Wong, H.B. (1973) Infantile gastroenteritis. In Forfar, J.O. & Arneil, G.G. (eds) *Textbook of Paediatrics*, pp. 1295–1301. Edinburgh and London: Churchill Livingstone.

23

The acute abdomen in childhood

Paul Hooper

The essential aspect of the acute abdomen for the general practitioner is diagnosis; management then follows as a matter of course. This chapter therefore will be concerned mainly with the diagnosis of common conditions. Many conditions which give rise to acute abdominal pain in adults are rare in children. In twenty-five years of practice the author has never seen, in a child under 14 years, a perforated peptic ulcer, acute pancreatitis, impacted ureteric calculus, mesenteric artery occlusion, pericolic abscess, aortic aneurysm, twisted ovarian cyst or ruptured ectopic pregnancy. Acute cholecystitis we have seen twice, both in girls. A general review of the symptoms and signs will be first considered.

SYMPTOMATOLOGY

Pain

Abdominal pain in children is usually poorly localised, but when the site is well defined, it follows the adult pattern; that is to say, pain arising from the embryonic endoderm (the gut, gall bladder and liver) is felt in the midline; pain arising from mesodermal structures (genitourinary tract) is felt on the appropriate side. Thus pain arising in the right kidney is felt in the right side of the abdomen or loin and never crosses the midline, but pain arising in the gall bladder will be felt centrally and may pass to the left side. Furthermore, pain originating in the foregut (supplied by the coeliac axis) is felt above the umbilicus, pain arising in the midgut (superior mesenteric artery) is felt around the umbilicus, and that arising in the hind gut (inferior mesenteric artery) is felt suprapubically. Once the parietal peritoneum has become involved in the inflammatory process, the pain is felt over the inflamed peritoneum. For example, in acute appendicitis the pain is initially midgut and felt at the umbilicus; once the parietal peritoneum is inflamed the pain is felt in the right iliac fossa.

Vomiting

Any sudden onset of severe abdominal pain can cause vomiting, but this then ceases and does not recur except in the presence of obstruction or recurrent severe pain, or gastric inflammation. A child with gastritis will vomit with, or even before the onset of, abdominal pain and continue to vomit anything passed into the stomach, whereas in appendicitis the vomiting, when it occurs, always follows the onset of pain by about an hour, continues for a while and may then cease, only to return with the onset of peritonitis. In acute obstruction the onset of vomiting will depend upon the site of the obstruction; the higher the obstruction the earlier the vomiting. In high obstruction the vomiting is early and not faecal, in obstruction of the lower ileum or colon it appears after several hours and becomes faecal.

Diarrhoea

This is present in gastroenteritis and may precede or follow the onset of vomiting; it is never blood stained except in fulminating cases. In intussusception there may be a blood stained discharge per anum, but not true diarrhoea. Diarrhoea is absent in other acute abdominal conditions.

SIGNS

Fever and tachycardia

These are unreliable signs in children. They can be caused as much by the dehydration of gastroenteritis as by the inflammation of acute appendicitis. But generally they are present to a moderate degree, 38–38.5°C, and pulse 100–120 in inflammatory but not in other conditions. However I would not allow their absence to influence the diagnosis in the presence of other convincing signs.

Fetor

This is present in acute appendicitis, constipation and acute tonsillitis causing adenitis; usually it is associated with a furred tongue. It is also present in the later dehydration stages of other conditions.

Palpation

Tenderness can be a very confusing sign because it is so

subjective. Some children will wince wherever you touch them, others are so stoical that no matter how much it hurts, they will not concede. In general it can be said that the site of maximum tenderness is over the site of the inflammation. If the peritoneum is generally inflamed then the tenderness will be generalised. In acute appendicitis tenderness will be maximum over McBurney's point, as it will in mesenteric adenitis. In gastroenteritis it will be difficult to find a point of maximum tenderness and in fact there will often be none at all, nor will there be in abdominal upset due to threadworms or migraine. In constipation there will be slight tenderness over the pelvic colon; in intussusception it may be anywhere. In cholecystitis maximum tenderness will be under the right costal margin; in pyelitis, in the loin or renal angle posteriorly. In torsion of an ectopic testis the tenderness will be in the inguinal canal where there may be an acutely tender lump – to be distinguished from a strangulated hernia.

Auscultation

This can provide useful confirmatory evidence. In obstructive lesions such as strangulated hernia, or in intussusception, there will be increased sounds and commonly, audible borborygmi in the earlier stages and before the onset of paralytic ileus. Sounds may be increased in constipation and in gastroenteritis. In the early stages of appendicitis and mesenteric adenitis bowel sounds are normal, but they diminish as the condition progresses.

Rectal examination

This is surprisingly well tolerated by children. In the very small child the little finger may be used in place of the forefinger and gives equally accurate information. In some conditions it will reveal only negative information as in migraine, mesenteric adenitis, threadworms, cholecystitis, pyelitis. If the inflamed appendix lies in the pelvis there will be marked tenderness, but if it is retrocaecal the examination will not be painful. In gastroenteritis there will be no pain, but a squirt of liquid faeces may follow the finger as it is withdrawn. In constipation the rectum will be felt to be loaded with hard faeces, though they may be present only in the upper rectum. 'Spurious diarrhoea' in children seems to be a rare occurrence. With an intussusception it is said that the tip of the intussusception may be felt and there is blood (red currant jelly) on the finger; in the author's experience these signs are rare and their absence does not rule out the diagnosis.

ACUTE MESENTERIC ADENITIS

Aetiology and pathology

This is probably not a single disease entity in itself, but a syndrome with several different causes. Any viraemia or bacteraemia may cause an inflammatory reaction in lymphoid tissue; certain organisms are thought to be more likely to do so, such as the adenovirus and the Epstein-Barr virus which causes glandular fever, in which a mild degree of abdominal pain is not uncommon. Acute tonsillitis and pharyngitis with their accompanying cervical adenitis are often associated with abdominal pain, which is due to mesenteric adenitis, presumably. Every general practitioner is familiar with the child who presents with a mild upper respiratory infection, sore throat, a few shotty glands in the neck, anorexia, slight nausea and vague central or generalised abdominal pain which resolve in a few days without treatment. It is to be hoped that with the increasing efficiency of virus isolation in the laboratory it may be possible to elucidate further the causal organisms in mesenteric adenitis, and it would seem that this work would have to be done in general practice in association with a good virus laboratory. In many of these conditions there is diffuse lymphadenopathy with enlarged and tender lymph glands in both triangles of the neck, the axillae and the groins. Presumably the mediastinal and para-aortic glands are involved but cause no symptoms, and the mesenteric glands give rise to abdominal symptoms.

The mechanism by which inflamed mesentric glands cause pain is uncertain, but that they should do so is hardly surprising; inflamed cervical glands may be very painful on neck movement, and so painful as to cause neck rigidity. It is thought that the inflamed mesenteric glands cause irritation of the overlying mesenteric peritoneum or that, lying alongside the small bowel, particularly the terminal ileum, they irritate the bowel and thereby cause increasingly strong peristalsis sufficient to cause the pain, which is nearly always colicky.

When seen at operation, the lymph glands in the mesentery of the terminal ileum are readily visible; they are of variable size, discrete and pale pink in colour. When palpated they feel exactly like the glands palpable in other areas – moderately soft, and moderately mobile. If one is removed for biopsy the pathology report will be 'non-specific or catarrhal inflammatory change'.

Incidence

This is unknown – the condition is not even recorded as an entity in *Morbidity Statistics in General Practice*; perhaps this is wise in the absence of specific diagnostic criteria.

History

This is usually one of two to three days' listlessness associated with slight rhinorrhoea and sore throat, going on to anorexia, slight nausea, perhaps a vomit and vague generalised colicky abdominal pains. During an attack of pain the child may look pale. The bowel habits are unaltered, or there is a slight tendency to constipation. The child is thought by the parents to be suffering from a mild 'tummy upset' but as the symptoms persist for more than 12 hours, and perhaps even get worse, the possibility of appendicitis arises and the doctor is summoned.

Examination

The child is lying comfortably in bed, and does not appear unduly distressed. The respirations are normal, the alae nasae are at rest but the pale yellow crusting around the nose or the sore upper lip betray the upper respiratory infection. There is no significant tachycardia and the temperature is only slightly raised, 37–37.5°C. The tongue may be clear or furred and there is no fetor, except in cases of purulent tonsillitis. The abdomen moves with respiration and can be blown up to touch the hand, it is soft to the touch. Pressure in the right iliac fossa or below the umbilicus causes mild to moderate discomfort which is not accompanied by guarding. Rectal examination is normal. A search will reveal lymph glands in one or more sites. Examination of the pharynx will vary from mild injection and enlarged lymphoid follicles on the posterior pharyngeal wall to gross follicular tonsillitis. There may be adventitious signs in the chest secondary to the upper respiratory infection.

Investigations are not helpful. The white count is normal, the erythrocyte sedimentation rate normal or slightly raised, the urine is normal. Virus studies are never done because by the time the results are back the crisis is passed and a decision must be made on clinical grounds. When the day comes that we can get a rapid result from nasal swabs or faeces, this will be a most valuable investigation.

Management

Except in the presence of a coexisting suppurative condition (e.g. follicular tonsillitis) there is no call for antibiotics. The child is kept at home in bed or resting on a couch and is allowed fluids only by mouth. The parents are reassured, but where there is the slightest doubt in the mind of the doctor a second visit in four to six hours is mandatory, to exclude the possibility of appendicitis. The condition resolves spontaneously in 24–36 hours, by which time the child has entered the stage of convalescence.

ACUTE APPENDICITIS

Aetiology and pathology

Acute inflammation of the appendix is usually caused by the coliform bacteria normally resident in the bowel, usually in association with an obstructing factor which may be a kink in the appendix, or an impacted faecolith. The mucosa above the obstruction becomes generally inflamed and the process spreads quickly to the underlying lymphoid tissue; at this stage the abdominal pain is central and colicky. The inflammation then spreads to the muscle layer and the peritoneal covering of the appendix and a localised peritoneal reaction occurs. At this time the pain moves to the region of McBurney's point which is situated on a line between the umbilicus and the anterior superior iliac spine, two-thirds of the way out from the umbilicus. The omentum moves down in an attempt to seal off the lesion and in the absence of surgical intervention, the inflammation proceeds to pus formation and a local abscess. If the sealing off process is not successful a generalised peritonitis follows after a variable period of time.

The picture may be influenced by the position of the appendix. In 5 per cent of cases (Bailey and Love, 1968) the appendix lies in the region of the caecum and terminal ileum, giving the classical picture. In 74 per cent it lies in the retrocaecal position in which case the site of maximum tenderness lies more laterally, and may extend out to the right loin causing confusion with acute pyelonephritis; the tenderness and guarding in the right iliac fossa is less marked, though still present. In 21 per cent it lies in the pelvis and there is minimal peritoneal reaction in the region of the caecum; hence the signs in the right iliac fossa will be minimal, but rectal examination will reveal acute tenderness on the right side of the pelvis.

Incidence

The national morbidity survey gives an annual incidence of 3.5 per 1000 children at risk. This correlates well with the author's practice, where with 2250 children at risk (total list 11 500) there were 9 cases in one year; an incidence of 4 per 1000. Of these five were males and four females. It can occur at any age, but is rare before 12 months of age.

History

A previously well child complains of central colicky abdominal pain which gradually becomes more severe; within an hour of the onset he starts to vomit and may continue to do so. After about four hours the pain moves to the right iliac fossa, becomes constant and gradually more severe. The vomiting may cease for a while, but as the condition progresses and peritonitis becomes established, it returns. There may be an initial bowel movement after which constipation is absolute. Micturition is unaffected except in the occasional case where a pelvic appendix irritates the ureter or bladder, when there may be frequency and dysuria.

Examination

The child is usually found lying curled up in bed looking flushed and ill. The pulse rate may be raised to 100–120 and the temperature to 38–38.5°C, though not necessarily so. The tongue is furred and the breath smells fetid. Extreme gentleness and tact may now be required to examine the abdomen. There is no movement on respiration or on being requested to 'blow out your tummy'. In the early case gentle palpation may reveal some rigidity in the right iliac fossa and on deeper palpation tenderness and guarding are always present. Rebound tenderness may be present. In a later case there may be signs of generalised peritonitis with generalised tenderness, guarding and rigidity. Rectal examination may be normal or extremely tender. Other signs such as tenderness in Sherren's triangle or the psoas spasm test or Rovsing's sign may be attempted but should not be depended upon in isolation. It cannot be stressed too emphatically that any child who presents with a history of central abdominal pain, followed by vomiting, followed by the pain moving to the right iliac fossa and who has tenderness and guarding in the right iliac fossa has appendicitis until proved otherwise by laparotomy. Never be put off by the absence of fever and tachycardia; the author has removed more than one gangrenous appendix in a child with a normal pulse and temperature. If in doubt, the child is left at home in bed, the parents instructed to give nothing by mouth and a second visit about four hours later is mandatory.

Investigations

Blood count will reveal a leucocytosis of anything up to 30 000. Urine culture is negative. Abdominal X-rays play no part in the diagnosis.

Treatment

This is appendicectomy at any stage of the disease.

MECKEL'S DIVERTICULITIS

Usually this presents as appendicitis and the diagnosis is made at operation. Owing to the thin wall, the condition progresses more quickly than appendicitis and the maximum tenderness may be medial to McBurney's point.

GASTROENTERITIS

Its importance here lies in its distinction from other acute abdominal conditions. The salient features are that the vomiting comes before or with the pain and persists, there is diarrhoea at about the same time, and the abdomen is mobile, soft and not tender. See Chapter 22 for full description.

INTESTINAL OBSTRUCTION

Aetiology

In children this is rare and presents somewhat differently from the adult. It may be caused by a wide variety of congenital abnormalities, adhesions, malrotations and strictures, which in the neonatal period can rapidly be fatal (Ch. 25). In the older child incarcerated inguinal hernia, intussusception and adhesions are the commonest causes.

History

A previously well child suddenly gets central colicky abdominal pain, followed by vomiting at an interval depending on the site of the obstruction; the higher up the intestine the site of the obstruction, the earlier the vomiting. In the intervals between pains the child is at first fairly well, but as the condition deteriorates the pain becomes more persistent until with the leakage of bacteria through the damaged bowel wall and the onset of peritonitis, the pain becomes severe, continuous, and generalised, and the child becomes extremely ill. At first there may be one or two bowel actions, but thereafter constipation becomes absolute.

Intussusception in the older child can be very difficult to diagnose, presenting as it does as an atypical gastroenteritis which fails to settle on a clear fluid regime. Attacks of colicky abdominal pain may continue for two or three days during which the child is in great pain and looks very ill, pale and frightened. Between attacks he appears quite well and runs around playing. Vomiting may be minimal and bowel actions only diminished. Eventually an extremely severe attack which does not subside produces a very ill child with vomiting and possibly signs of peritonitis and blood in the rectum.

Examination

Between attacks of pain the abdomen is frequently normal and this can be very confusing. In intussusception distension, tenderness and guarding may all be absent and the globular swelling usually felt on the right side may not become apparent for 36 hours or more after the onset of the illness. An impacted hernia may be felt at an external ring, but may be quite small. Rectal examination may reveal the empty ballooned rectum of obstruction, but may well be normal.

Management

The combination of colicky abdominal pain and vomiting of sudden onset, with a normal abdomen, is much more commonly due to gastroenteritis than any of the above conditions, but the practitioner may be faced with the difficult choice of admitting a possible gastroenteritis to a surgical ward (where it would not be welcome) or keeping a possible acute obstruction at home until abdominal signs develop – very awkward, and there is very little to help him. The passage of a liquid stool may indicate gastroenteritis; blood in the rectum, intussusception. The length of the history or the general condition of the child may be of some help. The only way may be to keep the child at home, instruct the mother to give nothing by mouth, and revisit two or three hours later in the hope that the situation will have clarified. The very rarity of these conditions makes the diagnosis yet more difficult, but once in hospital, a straight X-ray of the abdomen in the erect or lateral position renders everything easy.

INTUSSUSCEPTION IN A CHILD UNDER ONE YEAR

Aetiology and pathology

The exact aetiology is unknown, though certain facts are known. It occurs most commonly between the ages of four and eight months, in boys twice as commonly as in girls, and there seems to be a seasonal peak in the spring and in December. The commonly held theory is that a swollen lymph follicle or Peyer's patch gets squeezed into the bowel lumen by a vigorous peristaltic wave. This then forms the apex of the intussusception which gets pushed further along the receiving bowel or intussuscipiens. It may be ileo-ileal, ileo-colic or colo-colic.

History

Usually a previously healthy, well-built boy suddenly becomes severely ill with abdominal pain, screaming, drawing up his knees and vomiting. The attack then ceases suddenly and the child appears well again. After a varying interval the pain recurs, and continues to do so, gradually becoming more severe. Vomiting may or may not be present in the early stages, and only later becomes continuous.

Examination

The appearance of the child may be very characteristic. Intussusception is the only condition I know in which a small child really looks frightened; he is pale, sweating and afebrile. In the later stages the skin is flaccid and the eyes are sunken from dehydration. Between attacks the abdomen is soft – perhaps unnaturally so, and examination is not resented. The intussusception is felt as a globular (not sausage shaped) swelling in the right side and this on palpation may be felt to harden as a further attack of pain develops. The abdomen is not distended and the usual signs of intestinal obstruction are absent. Rectal examination reveals an empty rectum and usually a bit of blood. It has recently been pointed out that the classical description of this condition is erroneous (Dennison, 1967) in the following respects:

1. The tumour is globular and not sausage shaped and may not be palpable.
2. The classical triad of obstruction – colic, vomiting and distension, are absent in the early stages, the latter two may be absent altogether.
3. In older children rectal bleeding may be absent.

CONSTIPATION

This occasionally comes into the diagnosis of the acute abdomen; often the parents have no idea that the child has not been defaecating regularly. Sometimes direct questioning will reveal that the child has not had a proper bowel action for several days but merely the passage of a few rabbit pellets, sometimes the answer is untruthful – perhaps for fear of later parental reprisal. The child usually presents with a history of six to twelve hours colicky central abdominal pain, usually without vomiting. The child does not look ill, is afebrile, and the tongue is frequently clean. The abdomen is soft and not distended, there is tenderness in the left iliac fossa, with perhaps some guarding through which it is possible to feel the loaded sigmoid colon. Rectal examination reveals a mass of hard faeces, although the lower part of the rectum may be empty.

Management

A Dulcolax suppository, or if this is not available late on a Saturday night, a slice of toilet soap inserted into the rectum, followed next day by a gentle enema given by the nurse will usually suffice to empty the bowel. A follow-up appointment is arranged so that the parents can be advised how to prevent a recurrence. It may be that the constipation is part of a wider behavioural problem and this will then need to be dealt with (see Ch. 45).

THREADWORMS

These may present as acute colicky abdominal pain (see Ch. 28); they are said to inhabit the appendix and cause this. The child is well, has no vomiting or diarrhoea, no physical signs in the abdomen, but one may be lucky enough to see a threadworm on the perianal skin or in the faeces. The attack subsides spontaneously, and the cause may only be determined by subsequent investigation.

HENOCH-SCHONLEIN'S PURPURA

This presents with colicky abdominal pain due to haemorrhage into the bowel wall. Usually there is a preceding history of sore throat and fever and the symptoms are not so severe as appendicitis or obstruction; indeed it most nearly resembles mesenteric adenitis until the presence of purpura elsewhere, or blood in the rectum or stools clarifies the diagnosis. See also Chapter 36.

HYPERTROPHIC PYLORIC STENOSIS

This affects boys more than girls in the ratio of four to one and most commonly occurs in the first-born male infant. A family history is sometimes elicited (Carter and Evans, 1969). It usually presents between the second and fifth weeks of life with the insidious onset of unexpected vomiting, which progresses over two or three days and becomes projectile after every feed. The type of milk is changed or even replaced by glucose water in an effort to correct matters, but without avail. The infant ceases to gain weight, then loses weight and finally becomes dehydrated. Little is passed per rectum. In the early stages in a well-nourished infant the diagnosis may have to be made on a history alone. Later a test feed will show visible peristalsis in the upper abdomen and the pyloric tumour is felt to harden under the palpating finger below the right costal margin. The vomit is always free from bile.

Management

A trial of Eumydrin (methylnitrite) is sometimes successful in mild cases, but usually surgical intervention is required. Once a case is suspected it is best to transfer the infant to hospital.

CHOLECYSTITIS

Though rare in children, perhaps this is becoming more common in association with the increasing incidence of obesity. It is not usually associated with gallstones (*BMJ* Editorial, 1975). The presentation in children is similar to that in the adult, with the moderately sudden onset of upper abdominal pain, nausea, vomiting, fever and perhaps slight jaundice. The parents may remark that the urine looks dark. On examination there is a moderate fever (37–39°C) and tachycardia, the abdomen shows tenderness and guarding beneath the right costal margin and Murphy's sign is positive. The guarding usually prevents the gall bladder from being felt. Elsewhere the abdomen is normal.

Management

The child is kept at home on a regime of glucose containing fluids, no fats and antibiotics. If there is much vomiting then the antibiotics should be given parenterally. Analgesics such as Paracetamol may be given but are not usually necessary. If there is no improvement within 48 hours then it is reasonable to transfer the child to hospital.

TORSION OF THE SPERMATIC CORD (TESTIS)

Incidence and pathology

The incidence is probably about 0.3 per 1000 patients at risk. Torsion can occur on either side. Incomplete descent or an ectopic position is said to predispose to torsion, and injury or a sudden strain are supposed to precipitate it. The last case in this practice occurred in a normally placed testis in bed at night.

Clinical picture

There is a sudden onset of pain felt in the testis, suprapubically or even referred to the ipsilateral loin. There may be an initial vomit. On examination the patient is afebrile and in obvious pain. The testis, if it is in the scrotum, is swollen, intensely tender to touch and the overlaying skin will be red, if seen an hour or two after the onset. The differential diagnosis is from acute epididymo-orchitis which is exceedingly rare in children. If the testis is in the inguinal region there will be an acutely tender inflamed swelling there and the condition must be differentiated from an impacted inguinal hernia; this will be helped if a hernia is known to pre-exist, but to confuse things, it is possible to have a torsion of the cord adjacent to a hernial sac.

Management

In either case, immediate admission to hospital is mandatory, for operative reduction is the only treatment. Epididymo-orchitis should never be accepted as a preoperative diagnosis in a child and, in the case of impacted hernia, operation is equally essential. In the adolescent it may be possible to reduce the torsion by manipulation and this has been well described by Dr. J.P. Sparks, the Medical Officer of Rugby School (Sparks, 1971).

ABDOMINAL MIGRAINE

This seldom comes into the diagnosis of the acute abdomen, but occasionally a severe attack will bring a request for an urgent visit.

Aetiology and pathology

These are unknown. There is often a family history of typical cerebral migraine, and the child may have had such attacks. Episodes are sometimes triggered off by by the child having to face unwelcome situations such as going to school, or a lesson he dislikes, or excitement such as going on holiday.

History

The story is one of repeated attacks in which there is colicky abdominal pain, perhaps with nausea or even vomiting. The child is listless, may complain of a headache and looks pale. The presenting attack differs only in severity and duration resulting in an increased degree of parental anxiety.

Examination

This will reveal no physical abnormality.

Management

The attack usually resolves spontaneously without treatment in about 24 hours, by keeping the child at rest on a fluid diet and management is directed to the prevention of further attacks. Stress situations are investigated and where possible, alleviated. Domestic tensions may need to be explored and the parents reassured and counselled in the management of future attacks. Drugs play a minimal part in the management, but where attacks are frequent or very disabling, a tranquilliser such as Diazepam may be worth a trial; once embarked upon, it should be continued over a prolonged period of several months, for instance until the child has been symptom free for three months, and then gradually withdrawn. The condition does not necessarily disappear at puberty (Apley, 1974) but it may be replaced by ordinary migraine.

REFERENCES

Apley, J. (1974) *The child with Abdominal Pain*, 2nd edn. Oxford: Blackwell Scientific.

Bailey, H. & Love, M. (1968) In Rains, A.J. & Ritchie, D. (eds) *Short Practice of Surgery*, 16th edn. London: Lewis.

BMJ Editorial (1975) *British Medical Journal*, **2**, 239.

Carter, C.O. & Evans, K.A. (1969) Inheritance of congenital pyloric stenosis. *Journal of Medical Genetics*, **6**, 233.

Dennison, W.M. (1967) *Surgery in Infancy and Childhood*, Ch. 12. Edinburgh: Livingstone.

Sparks, J.P. (1971) Torsion of the testis. *Annals of the Royal College of Surgeons of England*, **49**, 89.

24

Accidents and poisoning in childhood

John Lewis

'Optimism is the greatest analgesic, hope is the most certain tranquillizer'. Sir Heneage Ogilvie.

THE SIZE OF THE PROBLEM

In the last 30 years, accidents have replaced infectious diseases as the main cause of death in childhood, and they now account for one third of all deaths of school children. Nearly half of these deaths occur on the road, but a further third occur in the home. Figures 24.1–24.5 show some of the epidemiology of accidental death in childhood. There is a considerable social class linkage, the incidence of both home and motor vehicle accidents being far higher in children from classes IV and V families than those from classes I and II. There is also a regional increase from south to north of the country, which is not wholly class related (McFarlane and Knox, 1978; McFarlane, 1979). In 1974 for every child killed there were 80 more admitted to hospital. Various local studies in areas such as Liverpool and Glamorgan have shown that one in every hundred children had an accident requiring admission to hospital, and one in ten children received medical treatment for injury each year. Some idea of the extent of GP involvement in this sphere may be obtained from published morbidity statistics (Tables 24.1, 24.2).

Other children who survive injury will be left permanently disabled. As many as 16 per cent of a younger disabled unit may be suffering from the effects of head injury (Mulroy, 1979). The GP who is unfamiliar with such statistics will, however, be acutely aware of the misery of the individual tragedy.

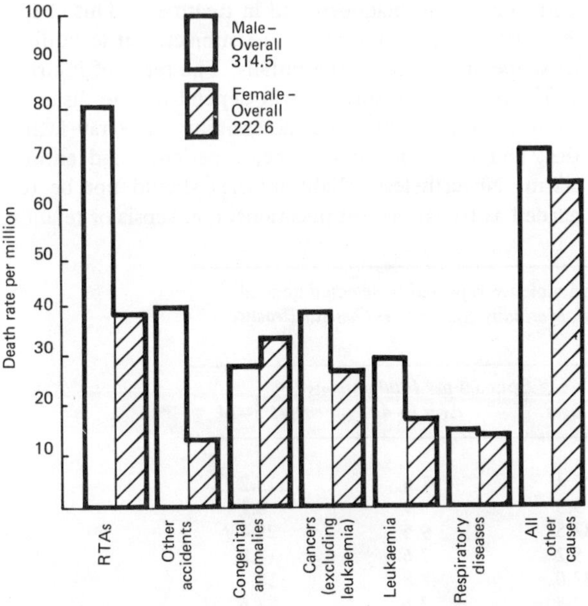

Fig. 24.1 Death rates by main causes per million population in the five to 14 years age group; England and Wales, 1978

THE PART PLAYED BY THE GP IN ACCIDENT CARE

Most major injuries, and many minor ones, will be

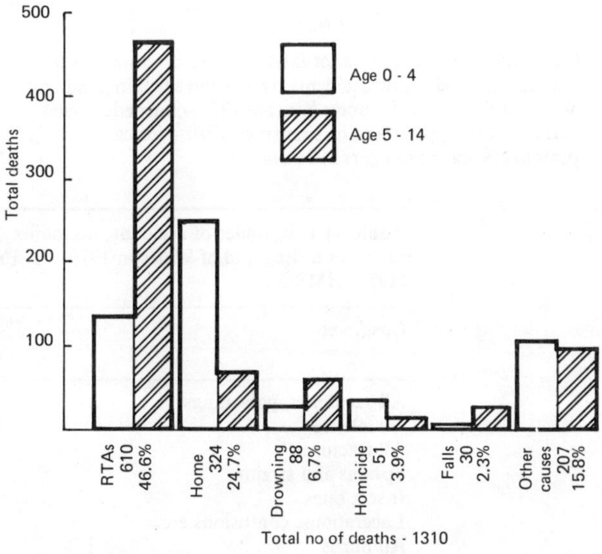

Fig. 24.2 Main causes of accidental death in childhood, England and Wales, 1978

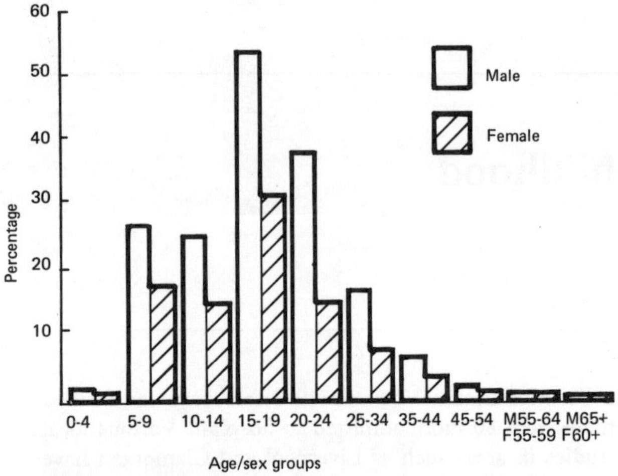

Fig. 24.3 Road traffic deaths as a percentage of all deaths by age/sex groups, Great Britain, 1977. Source: Department of Transport, 1978

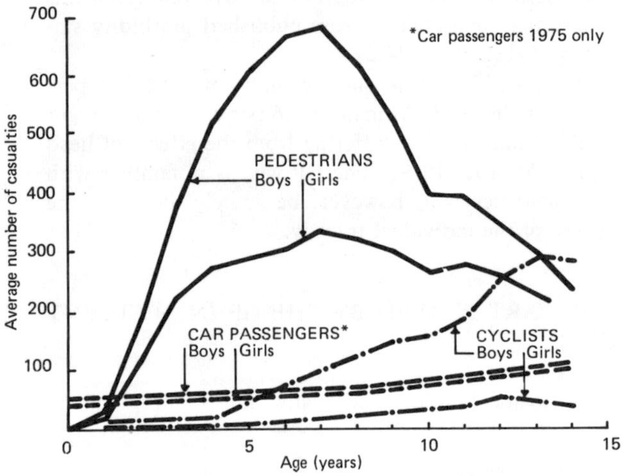

Fig. 24.4 Average number of fatal and serious casualties to children in road traffic accidents by age and sex, England and Wales, 1973–1975. Sources: Russam 1977 – for pedestrians and cyclists. Department of Transport 1976 – for car passengers (car passengers 1975 only)

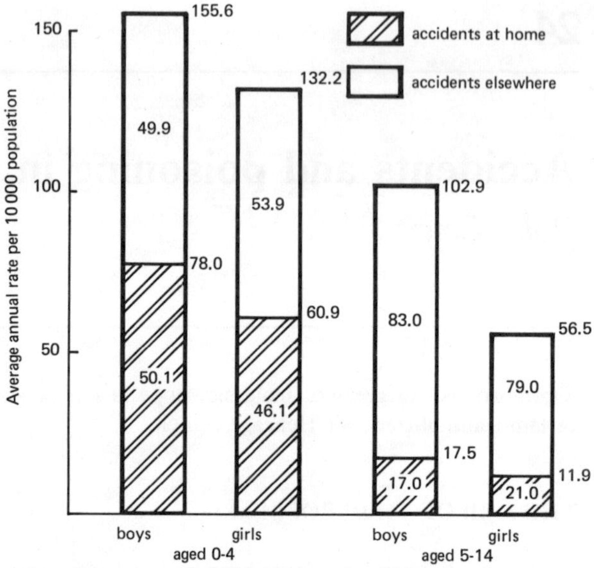

Fig. 24.5 Location of childhood accidents, England and Wales 1968–1974. Estimated total discharges and deaths after hospital inpatient treatment for non-traffic accidents. Source: McFarlane, 1979

treated in hospital, and usually in such cases the family doctor is unable to test his clinical acumen. Rarity is a relative term, and whereas a GP may expect to give life-saving first aid, at least several times in his life, he would need a working life of many hundreds of years before he sees the rarities taught him in medical schools, e.g. mucopolysaccharidosis; one new case every 2400 years (Illingworth, 1979). Unfamiliarity may lead to errors in diagnosis and in treatment. This chapter aims not to summarise a vast subject, but to outline its scope, and some of the pitfalls. The types of injuries a GP treats in his surgery will depend on the distance from an accident unit, the accessibility of X-ray facilities, and his own competence, experience and enthusiasm. Nevertheless, slight injuries should not be regarded as trivial, as complications, e.g. sepsis or tetanus

Table 24.1 Episodes of accident, poisoning, and violence reported to selected general practices in England of Wales in 1970–71. From *Morbidity Statistics in General Practice* (1974) HMSO

Condition	*Episodes per 1000 patients*		
	All ages	*Ages 0–4*	*Ages 5–14*
All accidents, poisonings, violence	107.4	91.6	113.2
All fractures	9.5	3.9	8.1
Sprains and strains	32.5	9.5	28.4
Insect bites	5.2	7.6	7.8
Lacerations, contusions etc.	47.0	48.8	58.4
All burns	3.3	7.6	2.6
Adverse effects of drugs	2.3	3.4	1.0

Table 24.2 Episodes of accident, poisoning, and violence reported to selected general practices in England and Wales in 1971–72. From *Morbidity Statistics in General Practice* (1979) HMSO

Condition	*Episodes per 1000 patients*			*Consultations per 1000 patients*		
	All ages	*Ages 0–4*	*Ages 5–14*	*All ages*	*Ages 0–4*	*Ages 5–14*
Accidents, poisonings, violence	105.2	84.3	103.1	165.3	108.4	126.7
Burns – first degree	1.4	3.7	0.8	2.0	5.2	1.2
second degree	1.2	2.8	0.9	2.2	5.2	1.2
third degree	0.1	0.2	0.0	0.3	0.7	1.1

may follow, and are often a source of much distress to the family.

The care of a serious injury involves many stages beginning with first aid and ending with rehabilitation, recovery, care of the disabled, or even comfort of the bereaved. Skilled surgery is not enough, and the GP knowing the personal and family history plays an important role in this long and often harassing chain of events. He is ideally suited to co-ordinate and liaise with the various people and the departments involved. The diagram illustrates this.

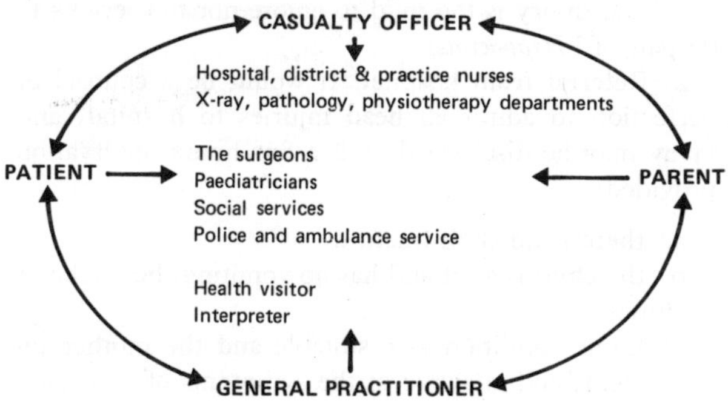

The difference between a child's response to injury and that of an adult

Immaturity and growth influence the response of a child to injury, so that many of the principles and techniques of surgery must be adapted to the young. Conservative treatment often suffices, and the surgeon has a difficult task to decide when to interfere with natural repair. A guillotine amputation of a finger tip in a child heals with the use of a sterile dressing, yet would require surgery in an adult. Excessive manipulation of a supracondylar fracture of the elbow may lead to a Volkmann's ischaemic contracture (Roaf, 1965).

The spectrum of injuries in childhood differs from that of adults. Alcohol and self-poisoning are seldom to blame, and the cause is often found in immaturity and being unprepared to live in a world designed for adults.

Some of the differences between the child's and an adult's response to injury are listed below:

1. The excellent power of tissue healing in the young.
2. The vulnerability of the child to blood and fluid loss e.g. a child who has eight per cent of surface area burnt requires transfusion, yet an adult may tolerate up to 15 per cent before this is necessary.
3. The greenstick fracture and epiphyseal injury is, of course, confined to the young, and usually responds to simple immobilisation. Occasionally damage to an epiphysis may lead to deformity from failure of bone growth afterwards.
4. Injury in infancy may cause a haematoma closely resembling an infection.
5. The ill effects of separation of a child from his parents may modify response to injury, e.g. the abnormal behaviour of a child observed in hospital for head injury. Children under the age of six are more likely to be emotionally disturbed and should be admitted to a children's ward where the mother may stay or at least visit at any time.
6. Underlying disease such as rickets, haemophilia and fragilitas ossium, may make diagnosis and treatment difficult. Often a child's behaviour may be blamed on a coincidental minor injury rather than a febrile illness.
7. The child may be too young to describe his symptoms, or he may conceal his injury for fear of parental reproach.
8. Non accidental injury (NAI) should always be considered as a possible cause of any accident or poisoning (see Ch. 16).

The management of serious injuries

The GP should know the principles of first aid, and their adaptation to the young. His aim is to make a tentative diagnosis, and prevent deterioration on the patient's journey to hospital.

A clear airway

Lay the unconscious child in a semi-prone position with the head slightly extended; a Guedet type airway, size one for children, and size two for adolescents may be needed. It is worth carrying an infant airway in the bag as a routine. Easton (1970) describes a method for blind intubation.

Obstructed airway
A FB in the larynx will cause cough, stridor, cyanosis, choking, hoarseness, and aphonia. Methods in likely order of use to relieve this are:

1. Scoop object from back of mouth with finger
2. Hold child upside down and slap back
3. The Heimlich manoeuvre. Stand behind the child, wrapping arms around waist, and grasping one fist with the other hand, press the fist into the abdomen just below the xiphisternum and give a quick upward thrust
4. Crico-thyroidotomy. A large needle or several smaller ones are inserted obliquely downwards through the avascular crico-thyroid. A last resort for the rare desperate emergency.

When acute epiglottitis is suspected the throat should not be examined as this may cause respiratory obstruction or cardiac arrest.

Blood loss
External blood loss should be controlled by local pressure or bulky dressings. Tourniquets should not be used. Birdwood (1971), in his excellent summary of first aid, emphasises the value of reassurance, raising legs and prevention of heat loss in stopping shock. Ideally an intravenous infusion of a plasma expander should be put into a mid-forearm vein, but this may be technically difficult in a child.

Cardiac massage and artificial respiration
This will not be described here.

Immobilisation of fractures
Support with a sling or the use of a good arm support is usually sufficient for arm fractures. Splintage of leg fractures can be made with an adult arm insufflatable splint.

Burns
Cool immediately with cold water and cover with sterile dressings. Alternatively, a burn may be enclosed in an ordinary plastic bag e.g. cling film, or snappies (Lendrum, 1978). It is important to consider whether or not skin grafting may be required, as morbidity statistics show a surprisingly high proportion of second and third degree burns in children (Table 24.2).

Spinal injuries
These may be suggested by sensations of electric shock, tingling, or numbness. When there is paralysis, the patient is treated in the supine, and not in the recovery position. The neck is held in the neutral position with slight traction. A spinal board may be applied, or the child moved with great care on an orthopaedic stretcher (Hoskins *et al*, 1979).

Relief of pain
Reassurance, gentle handling, and the use of Entenox (50 per cent oxygen and 50 per cent nitrous oxide) are effective. IM injections are ineffective and the risk of miscalculating the small doses of analgesics IV make it unwise to relieve pain in this way outside hospital.

Head injuries
These account for 15 per cent of all children's surgical admissions, and happily most will survive. They present many difficult decisions in selecting the few in danger from the rest.

1. Referral to hospital. Hypoxia, CO_2 retention and hypotension in the unconscious cause further brain damage, and can be prevented by ensuring a clear airway. The following memory aid may be found helpful in assessing the condition of a head injury patient and in giving first aid (Table 24.3).
'No head injury is too mild to ignore nor too serious to despair of.' *Hippocrates*.

2. Referral from hospital. It would be a counsel of perfection to admit all head injuries to hospital, and many may be discharged after a few hours observation provided:

a. there is no skull fracture
b. the child is alert and has no vomiting, headache or amnesia
c. home conditions are suitable and the mother intelligent, and is aware of the symptoms of deterioration
d. there is a telephone in the house or nearby
e. the GP is informed by telephone about the discharge.

Follow-up
Many of these children will be well the next day, though it is wise for them to be seen again. Epilepsy may follow trivial head injuries, and in some a change in temperament is noted. Often this behaviour is influenced by the pre-accident condition of the child, and by parental over-protection afterwards. Behaviour changes may also occur as a result of the head injury itself; the brain takes time to recover, and behaviour may then be restored to normal. The GP knowing the family can often advise and reassure.

Penetrating injuries of the skull may be missed at the time of an accident and not suspected until meningitis follows. The hair around all scalp injuries should be cut before proper suturing, and if in doubt, the skull should

Table 24.3 Assessment and management of head injury

	Coma	*Confusion*	*Coherent*
Condition	Check and record level of coma. Check for other injuries e.g. spinal	Commands not obeyed. Cannot remember accident	Clear about accident. Commands obeyed
Care	Clear airway coma position control bleeding control fits	Check and record condition	Check and record condition
Outcome	Admit to hospital	Admit to hospital	Observe and record condition, usually in Casualty, with early discharge
Complications			
CSF leakage from ear and nose, convulsions, cyanosis, compressed fractures, contusions overlying orbital and mastoid fractures			

be X-rayed. Chronic subdural haematoma can occur weeks after an accident and present as a behavioural change at home and school.

Drowning
About 300 children are drowned in this country each year, mostly in inland waterways. The need for teaching children to swim, and their constant supervision near water is well known. Children with verrucae should be allowed to swim wearing a suitable slipper or soon after starting treatment. Asphyxia, inhalation, and hypothermia are the commonest causes of death. Death may occur from secondary drowning in up to 25 per cent of those who have been apparently resuscitated. Children are prone to hypothermia and when on boats should always wear life jackets and be told not attempt to swim if they fall in, as the effort will lower their temperature considerably. Harries (1979) describes simple first aid.

1. *Airway*. Clear the airway.
2. *Breathing*. Establish breathing using the expired air method.
3. *Circulation*. Maintain circulation using closed cardiac massage. Cardiac massage may however precipitate ventricular arrythmias in patients with hypothermia.
4. *Diagnose hypothermia*. Rewarm with blankets or a warm bath. Avoid massage or movement of the limbs since this will cause cold blood to return to the core of the body.

Eye injuries
Penetrating injuries with arrows, pellets, or fire-works lead to blindness in 50 per cent of cases. Examination of the eye may cause further damage. It should be lightly covered and the child referred at once to hospital. Sometimes a small cut over the eyelid or eyebrow may be the only evidence, and these children need expert attention and X-rays.

Blunt injuries may cause damage to all parts of the eye and orbit. Damage may be caused by swimming goggles, either hitting the eye or being incorrectly removed. Referral to hospital is necessary. Retinopathy and orbital bruising may be found in children with NAI from blows or excessive shaking.

Foreign bodies
These may enter every orifice in the body or penetrate the skin. Illingworth (1977) gives an excellent review of the subject. The GP must decide:

1. If there is an immediate risk to life e.g. FB in larynx (see above).
2. If less urgent referral to hospital is needed e.g. a swallowed coin.
3. If he can remove the object e.g. a bead in the nose or ear. This is possible if the object is visible, the child held still, and a finger placed behind the nostril, and the object removed with blunt forceps. If difficulty is anticipated no attempt should be made since an ENT surgeon welcomes an undisturbed patient. The parents should be warned that anaesthesia may be needed and the child should not be fed (see Ch. 18).

THE MANAGEMENT OF MINOR INJURIES

The doctor with a good bedside manner will have little difficulty in winning the co-operation of his small patient. A gentle friendly voice and unhurried movements will help. Equipment should be prepared out of sight of the patient, and a mask not worn. Parents, too, need reassurance, and to be allowed to sit lest they faint. The frightened child may be securely wrapped in a blanket.

Many cuts can be closed with steristrip, but if suturing is necessary, local anaesthetic should be injected slowly and dexon dissolvable sutures used. Wounds should be dressed as infrequently as possible. Melolin or tulle gras which do not stick are covered with gauze, tube gauze, or netalast. A cling bandage should be used if there is a risk of bleeding, since blood may dry in tube gauze, and cause in effect, a tourniquet round a finger. Prophylactic antibiotics are not usually needed. Adequate notes are made for practical and medico-legal reasons and the future care explained to the parent.

Tetanus. 'Spasm following injury is fatal.' Hippocrates. Macrae describes five children aged nine to 12 years who had had full infant immunization but no booster, and developed tetanus after injury. If enquiry shows that the child is not protected, he should be given HUMOTET one ml (human tetanus immunoglobulin), and a diphtheria tetanus toxoid or tetanus toxoid injection according to age (see Ch. 11).

THE MANAGEMENT OF MAJOR INJURIES PRESENTING WITH THE SYMPTOMS OF APPARENT MINOR INJURIES

Soon after an accident there may be little evidence of serious injury. This is a problem for the GP who may be the first to see the child, and it is hoped the following observations may lessen the risk of misdiagnosis:

1. Listen to a full history from the child, parent or bystander.
2. Observe the child, and be especially suspicious of the pale quiet one who may have internal bleeding. Poor light may make pallor and cynosis difficult to detect.
3. Examine the whole child for evidence of NAI, or multiple injuries, and do not be misled by referred pain.
4. Return and re-examine a child when uncertain or unhappy about his condition.
5. Consider what the most serious diagnosis could be.
6. Make good notes, and give details of the accident, clinical condition, and relevant medical and social history in any letter sent to hospital.

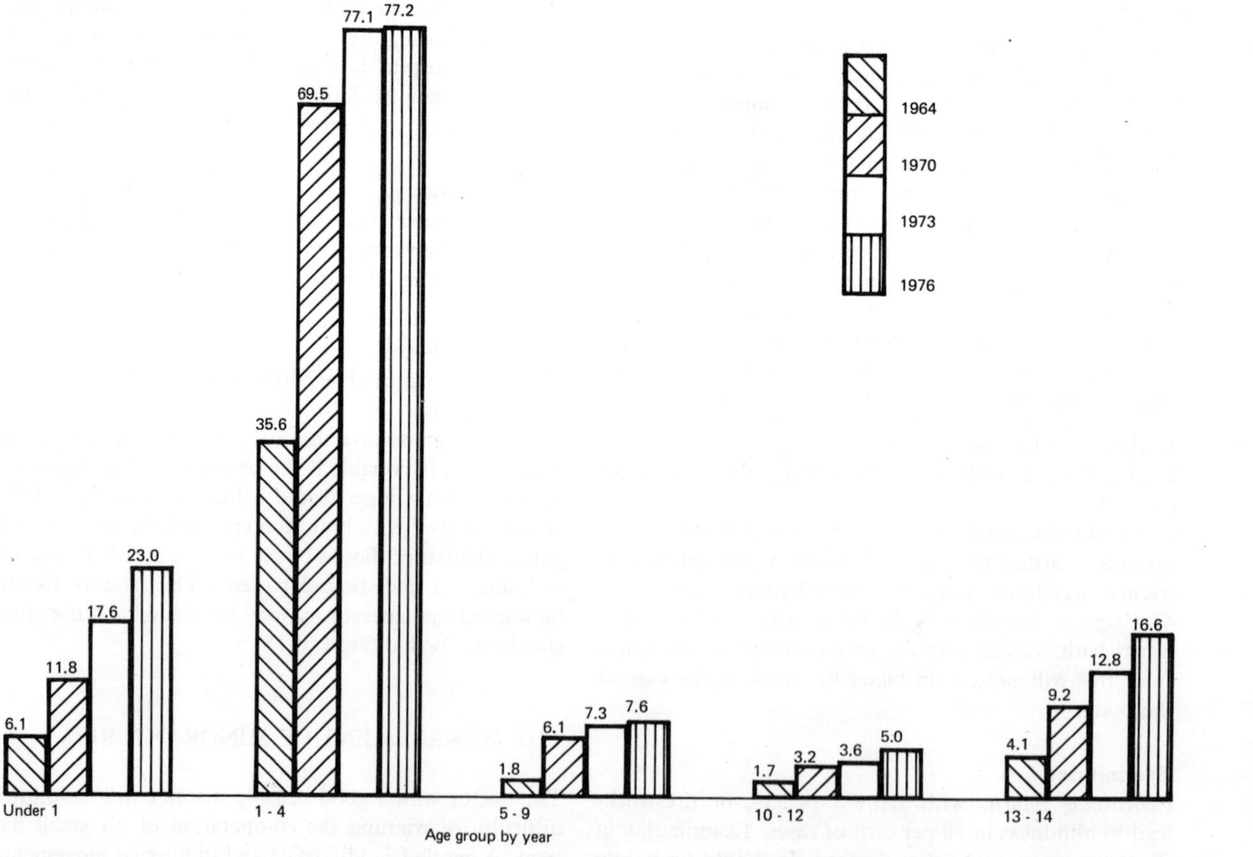

Fig. 24.6 Poisoning in children in England and Wales by age group: admission rates per 10 000 related population, 1964, 1970, 1973, 1976. Source: hospital inpatient enquiry, quoted in McLean, 1980

7. Accompany a seriously injured child to hospital.
8. Seek a second opinion when in doubt.
9. Advice to parents should be simple, clear, and understood.

Printed instructions following head injury and the application of plaster will also warn parents of possible complications.

THE MANAGEMENT OF POISONING

'Let not an apothecary shop thy stomach be.' 16th century advice.

Epidemiology
Each year about 11 000 children in the UK are admitted to hospital with suspected poisoning and about 20 will die. 80 per cent of those admitted are under four years of age (Fig. 24.6). It is estimated that at least another 30 000 children are seen in casualty. A quarter of these will have symptoms of toxicity. Tricyclic antidepressants have now replaced aspirin as the commonest cause of death from medicinal poisoning, followed by opiates (including Lomotil) and barbiturates. Carbon monoxide is particularly lethal to children, being responsible for nearly 80 per cent of the deaths from poisoning by non-medicinal substances in children under four years old in the UK in 1976. The great majority of these were due to fires and explosions (McLean, 1980). Many of the smaller children are poisoned by household products. The number of deaths is of course only a small fraction of those admitted to hospital; it has shown a steady decline in recent years, but there is still room for improvement (Fig. 24.7).

Prevention
This logically follows an understanding of the size and nature of the problem. Detailed studies have already led to changes in the presentation of drugs and household products (see Appendix). Since 1973 there has been a gradual fall in the number of cases reported annually.

The doctor has a paramount responsibility, since his prescribing habits may lead to poisoning (see Ch. 34). Points to be remembered are:

1. Alternative and safer drugs exist to replace barbiturates and tricyclics.
2. Some drugs should not be prescribed to children e.g. lomotil (diphenoxylate) which can be very dangerous. Bain (1973) has questioned the need for tricyclics in the management of enuresis. The phenothiazines may produce symptoms easily confused with tetanus and should be prescribed with care.
3. Tablets should be prescribed in blister packs or child-proof containers. Unfortunately many drugs resemble sweets. There is also a problem, recently identified, that older patients often find child-proof containers difficult to manage, and transfer the drugs to alternative containers (Burns and Jenkinson, 1980).

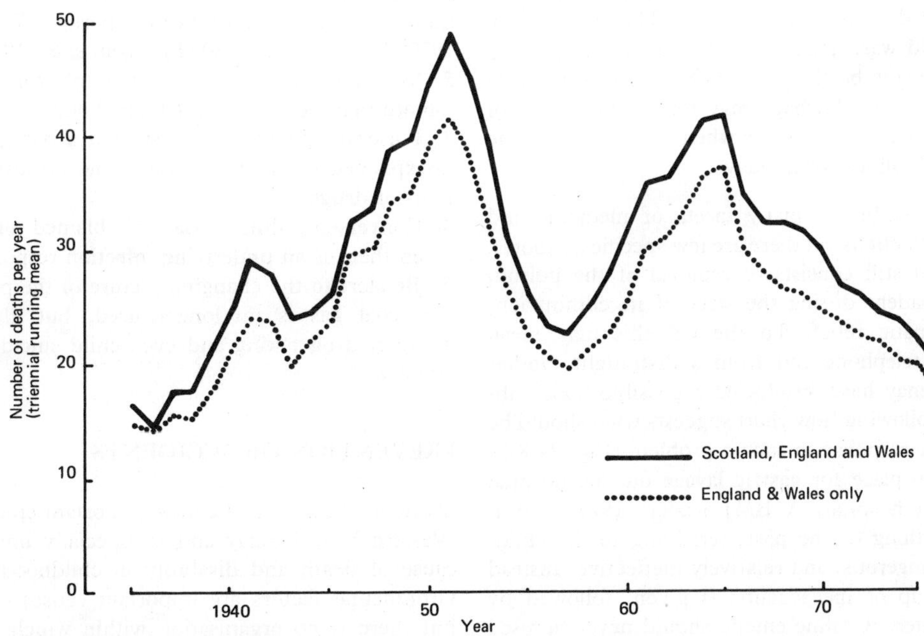

Fig. 24.7 Accidental poisoning in children under ten (Scotland, England and Wales, 1935–77). Number of deaths shown as a triennial running mean (Fraser, 1980).

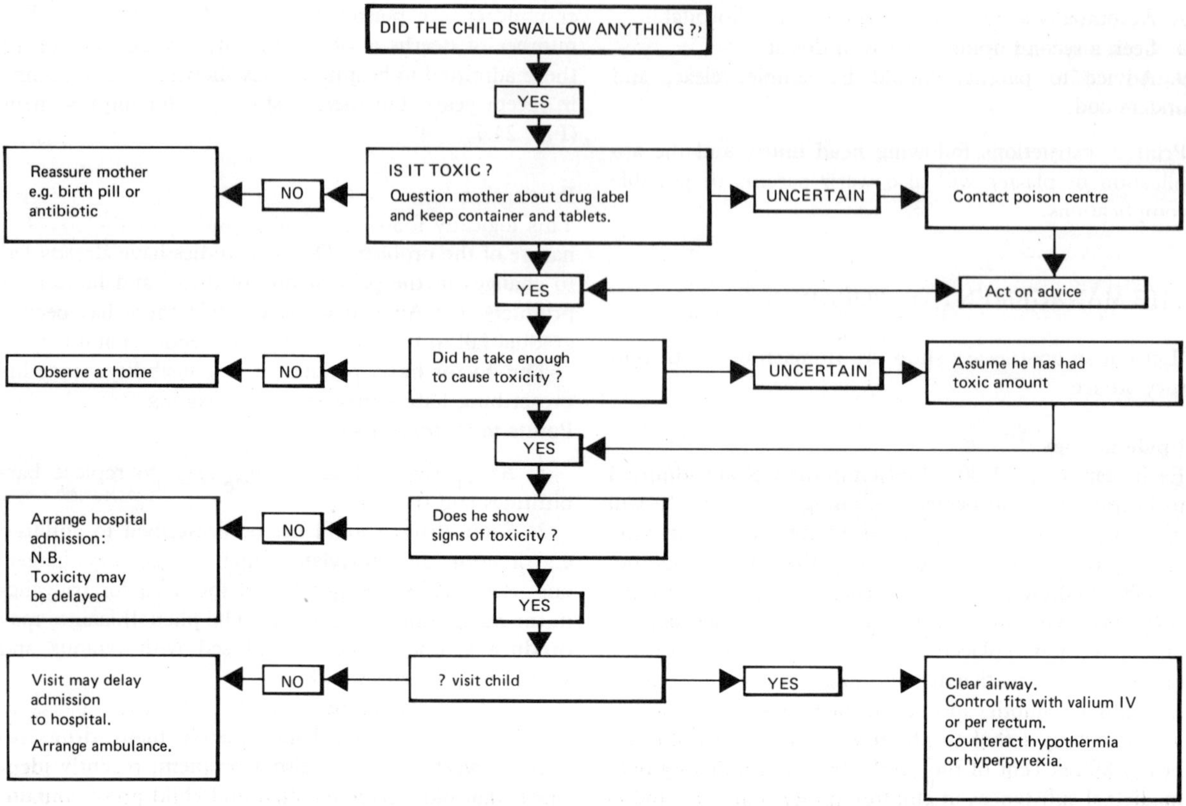

Fig. 24.8 Assessment and management of poisoning

4. Parents should be advised of the potential danger of all drugs and advised on their care. The doctor when visiting should warn parents of the dangers of putting turps in lemonade bottles, or paraffin heaters in poorly ventilated caravans. Mishaps may follow the arrival of an aged parent in the home or when the family routine is disrupted by illness or holiday.

Toxicology embraces many facets of medicine and pharmocology, but as yet there are few specific antidotes, and treatment still consists of removal of the poison, care of the patient during the stage of its elimination, and symptomatic relief. To the GP this may mean answering a telephone call from a distraught mother whose child may have swallowed a possible toxic substance. The following flow chart suggests what should be his immediate response to such a problem (Fig. 24.8).

There is no place for gastric lavage outside hospital and rarely in hospital. A BMJ leader (1975) said it should be a thing of the past, terrifying to the child, potentially dangerous, and relatively ineffective. Instead 15 ml of syrup of ipecacuanha is given, followed by 200 ml of water. A saline emetic should never be used because of the risk of hypernatraemia and even death.

Dr Cynthia Illingworth (1979) stresses that:

1. Poisoning may be a form of child abuse. A growing number of cases have been reported (Watson *et al*, 1979; Lorber *et al*, 1980; Flanagan *et al*, 1981).
2. Symptoms following ingestion of iron, aspirin, or lomotil may be delayed for many hours.
3. Poisoning should be considered a possibility in any unexplained ill child because of the protean manifestations of drugs.
4. Conversely, illness may be blamed on poisoning when there is an underlying infection responsible.
5. Be alert to the changing picture of the poison scene: e.g. coal gas is no longer used, but glue (solvent) sniffing, drug taking and even child suicide are now a problem.

PREVENTION OF ACCIDENTS

'Accidental injury is the most important epidemic in the Western World today and is especially important as a cause of death and disability in childhood. Many environmental factors are important causes of accidents, but there is no organisation within which doctors, official bodies, industry, and voluntary bodies can pool their experience and co-ordinate their efforts to reduce these environmental risks. A joint committee on childhood accident prevention should be formed in this country similar to that which exists in Sweden.' (R.H. Jackson and A.W. Wilkinson, 1976).

Collecting data

Since the above-quoted article was written a joint committee on childhood accident prevention has been established in this country, and hopefully it will help in reducing the numbers of fatal and serious accidents. Two surveys of the Department of Prices and Consumer Protection are of considerable interest to the GP, viz: *Childhood Poisoning from Household Products*, and *The Home Accident Surveillance System* (see Appendix). Other reports have covered such diverse subjects as playground accidents, rugby football, skate board, lawn mower, farm tractor, wringer and spin dryer injuries. The emphasis in the past has been more on accident prevention on the road than in the home, and there is no doubt that continuing attention to the problem of road accident prevention is still needed, particularly for boys in social classes 4 and 5, where the risks are greatest (Jackson, 1978). A recent USA survey revealed the very much greater risk of death to infants than to older children while car passengers (Karwacki and Baker, 1979).

However in 1971 558 children under the age of five years were killed in the home against 245 killed on the road, and of these latter only 46 were passengers. Between 1970 and 1973 a detailed survey of accidents in the home involving children under the age of five years was made in a sector of Bristol by the Medical Research Division of the Health Education Council. Fractures and concussion from falls in the bedroom, lounge and stairway accounted for most of the serious injuries, and it was suggested that more emphasis be placed on accident prevention in the home.

Education

Accidents are usually the result of an interaction of *human factors* e.g. disobedience, poor sight or immaturity, and *external factors* e.g. poorly designed homes or electrical equipment. The infant and toddler should be completely under the protective care of the parents, and at his own pace, and mother's discretion, will assume increasing responsibility for his own safety. The intention is not the complete removal of all hazards but the development of judgement and skills to deal with them. Parents, teachers, police and organisations like the HEC and the Royal Society for Accident Prevention (Rospa) will all help. Since 1968 the HEC has placed increased reliance on promoting health through the mass media. Teaching aids, such as a school safety pack, and Project Fire, are supplied to schools where talks are given by home safety officers. Suitable posters may be put up in doctors' waiting rooms.

Enforcement

The child benefits indirectly from many laws applying to adults, e.g. road traffic acts, and directly from laws laying down the minimum age at which a child may for instance, buy fireworks, firearms, or drive a motor cycle. Regulations made under the *Consumer Protection Act of 1961* and the *Consumer Safety Act 1978* cover standards needed in the design and manufacture of goods such as toys, carrycots, babies' dummies, night dresses and fireworks. We need to consider urgently the introduction of legislation concerning the carriage of children in the front seats of motorcars, and the provision and wearing of safety harness.

Engineering

Responsible manufacturers have set their own high standards of safety design, while legislation and ill effects of bad publicity have encouraged others to seek this goal. Labels such as Kitemark, BEAB, and British Gas Corporation have been helpful to the consumer. The British Standard Institution (BSI) has published many standards for consumer goods relevant to the safety of children, and some of these have been supported by regulations. Improvements in road design have followed investigations done by road safety units and led to a fall in the number of accidents on certain roads.

THE GP'S ROLE IN ACCIDENT PREVENTION

The GP can reinforce the advice given by the mass media, especially when visiting his patients. He may lobby his MP to bring about changes in the law, such as the compulsory use of safety harness, and he can teach first aid in the community. Many doctors combine an interest in a sport or outdoor activity with medical supervision of participants, e.g. boxing, though this has been stopped in some schools, because of the risk of brain damage. The Medical Officers of Schools Association have suggested ways of lessening the risk of rugby football, e.g. by ending matches against adult teams and curbing violent play (Hoskins *et al.*, 1979). School parties should be advised on how to lessen the risk of hypothermia when fell walking. Subaqua diving has become popular but Bickmore (1971) warns against children under 16 using breathing apparatus and going deeper than the use of a schnorkel allows. Children learning to ride ponies should wear proper safety hats and riding boots, remove pierced earrings and keepers, and be taught by competent instructors. The Pony Club teaches accident prevention when riding, and riders should be encouraged to join their local branch (British Horse Society, 1980). Head injuries are a risk in many sports, including horseriding, cycling, and cricket. Now that professional cricketers use protective headwear it is hoped that similar headwear will be used by children for cricket and other sports. The British Cycling Bureau carried out a trial on child cyclists wearing helmets and their reactions were favourable (BMJ, 1979). Boys aged seven upwards are at much more risk of serious or fatal accidents while cycling than from car accidents, either as passengers or pedestrians (Avery, 1980). Helmet propaganda should be directed particularly at this group. Parents should be advised concerning safety harness for children in cars (Avery, 1980).

Haemophiliacs may become crippled by bleeds into joints and muscles unless given an IV injection of freeze dried antihaemophiliac factor (AHF) soon after injury. This may be done at a haemophiliac centre, or the parents taught to give it at home (Levine and Britten, 1973). The expense of AHF is forcing some centres to use cryoprecipitate.

Tetanus may be prevented by immunisation (but see above).

Epileptic children should be encouraged to lead active lives. Medic-alert bracelets may be worn by children with allergy to drugs or who have certain diseases or are taking steroids.

Dog bites are sufficiently common for the doctors to advise mothers on the physical as well as medical risks of keeping pets near children.

POSTSCRIPT

It is encouraging to learn that the rate of accidental deaths in the UK is the lowest of 27 European countries. Nevertheless there can be no complacency, and the GP can expect to be more and more involved in nearly every aspect of accident care.

ACKNOWLEDGEMENT

I wish to acknowledge the help I have had from reading Dr Cynthia Illingworth's book *The Diagnosis and Primary Care of Accidents and Emergencies in Children*, Blackwell Scientific Publications, 1979.

APPENDIX

Poison centres: telephone numbers:
London 01-407600
Leeds 9532-32799
Newcastle 0632-25131

Home safety: publications and teaching aids source list obtainable from The Health Education Council, 78 New Oxford Street, London WC1A 1AH.

The Home Accident Surveillance System and *Child Poisoning from Household Products* is obtainable from The Department of Prices and Consumer Protection, Consumer Safety Unit, Millbank Tower, Millbank, London SW1P 4QU.

REFERENCES

Avery, J.G. (1980) The Safety of Children in Cars. *Practitioner*, **224**, 816-821.

Bain, D.J.G. (1973) A Criticism of the use of anti-depressant drugs the treatment of childhood enuresis. *Journal of the Royal College of General Practitioners*, **23**, 222.

Bickmore, G.H. (1971) Subaqua Diving. *Practitioner*, **206**, 651.

Birdwood, G. (1971) Medical First Aid – A matter of life and death. Folia Traumatologica Geigy 3.

British Medical Journal (1979) Head injuries and head gear for cyclists, **1**, 39.

British Medical Journal Editorial (1975) Head injuries and first aid management, **4**, 483-484.

British Horse Society Booklet (1980) *The Safety Code for Riding*. The National Equestrian Centre, Kenilworth, Warwicks.

Burns, P. & Jenkinson, D. (1980) Hazards from the use of child resistant drug containers. *Journal of the Royal College of General Practitioners* **30**, 555-556.

Easton, K.G. (1970) Road Accidents and the Family Doctor. *British Medical Journal publication.*

Flanagan R.J. *et al* (1981) Value of toxological investigations in the diagnosis of acute during poisoning in children. *Lancet*, **2**, 682-5.

Fraser, N.C. (1980) Accidental poisoning deaths in British children 1958-77. *British Medical Journal*, **1**, 1595-1598.

Harries, M.G. *et al* (1979) Special Report on Drowning. *Practitioner*, **222**, 511-527; 662-667.

Hoskins, T. *et al* (1979) Prevention of rugby football injuries in schoolboys. Medical Officers of Schools Association Report Health Education Council Medical Research Division Reports (1974) Nos 63, 75, 86, 89.

Illingworth, M. (May 1977) Techniques to remove foreign bodies. Mims *Mims Magazine* 49-54.

Illingworth, M. (1979) The Incidence of disease in General Practice. *Practitioner*, **222**, 701-702.

Jackson, R.H. (1978) *Archives of Disease in Childhood*, **53**, 807

Jackson, R.H. & Wilkinson, A.W. (1976) Why don't we prevent childhood accidents? *British Medical Journal*, **2**, 1258-1262.

Karwacki, T.J. & Backer, S.P. (1979) Children in Motor Vehicles. *Journal of the American Medical Association*, **242**, 2848.

Lendrum, J. (1978) Recent advances in plastic surgery. *Practitioner*, **221**, 496.

Levine, P.H. & Britten, A.F.H. (1973) *Annals of Internal Medicine*, **78**, 195.

Lorber, J. *et al* (1980) Non-accidental poisoning: the elusive

diagnosis. *Archives of Disease in Childhood*, **55**, 643–47.
Macrae, J. (1974) Tetanus. A new look at infectious diseases. *British Medical Journal* publication.
McFarlane, Alison (1979) Child death from accidents: place of accident. *Population trends*, **15**, 10–15.
McFarlane, Alison & Knox, J. (1978) Child deaths from accidents and violence. *Population Trends*, **12**, 22–27.
McLean, Wendy (1980) Child Poisoning in England and Wales: some statistics on admissions to hospital, 1964–76. *Health Trends*, **12**, 9–12.
Mulroy, R. (1979) Letter in *British Medical Journal*, **2**, 673
Ogilvie, H. (1960) Symposium on accident management. *Journal of the Royal College of General Practitioners*, **4**, Supplement 1.
Watson, J.B. *et al* (1979) Non-accidental poisoning in childhood. *Archives of Disease in Childhood*, **54**, 143–44.

PART FOUR

Continuity in clinical care

25

Care of the newborn

Colin Waine

INTRODUCTION

There are many excellent texts on the care of the newborn, and it would be both foolish and impossible to try and emulate them in the space of one chapter. However, there are aspects of care of particular importance to the general practitioner, and these I have tried to cover.

The examination of the newborn, and the appreciation of the unique relationship between mother and baby and those symptoms or signs which indicate a departure from the norm, have been given priority over producing detailed descriptions of diseases and treatments. These are covered adequately in other works to which reference can be made if necessary. Infant feeding is dealt with in Chapter 27 and I have, therefore, only given it a brief mention.

I have not referred specifically to any other works, but clearly my approach must have been influenced by books which I have found of particular value. These are listed at the end of the chapter, and I would recommend them to any reader who wishes to pursue the subject in greater depth.

MOTHER AND BABY

The doctor approaching the care of the newborn could well begin by considering the continuum of fetal and neonatal life. To the mother someone has emerged who has lived inside her already for about 40 weeks and who has certainly never been far from her thoughts. Thus the successful management of the neonate demands sensitivity to her feelings as well as knowledge of the physiology and pathology of the newborn.

Most people would agree that a loving, stable mother/child relationship provides a major part of what a child requires to achieve his potential. This relationship can be under threat from many factors, so the doctor should be on his guard not to add to these and should endeavour to achieve a working partnership with the parents.

Factors which prejudice the mother/child relationship before birth and in the neonatal period can, for ease of description, be divided between mother and baby.

Consider the mother first. Is the baby the result of a warm and caring relationship, or does he represent a failure of contraception, or even an indiscretion? What was the mother's childhood experience? Did her parents provide a good model? Is she socially isolated by distance from her family or by being a single parent? Financial difficulties and housing problems bring added stresses.

The baby too can provide difficulties by being a poor feeder, or by having an unpleasant congenital abnormality (e.g. cleft lip and palate). In a poor marital relationship, the child may appear to have inherited the most obnoxious characteristics of the other partner. Babies, though often lovable, can be irritable, restless, cry a lot, be messy and baffling. Mothers and fathers, though usually tolerant and loving, can be tired, irritable, puzzled and at times even angry.

It is important to try and find out what the child means to each parent. Over-concern may be the repair patch on a precarious marital situation. The advent of a child, though often provoking joy, can produce jealousy – a father can even be jealous of the baby at the breast.

The last two decades have seen enormous advances made in the field of neonatal paediatrics. These have often involved the use of highly sophisticated techniques which have necessitated separation of the mother from the baby and, therefore, the vital early contact so necessary for effective bonding has been prejudiced.

The family doctor should, therefore, be particularly observant for a disturbed mother/child relationship when the baby has, of necessity, spent the first part of his life in a Special Care Baby Unit. Extra attention by the health visitor would, perhaps, be the most appropriate way initially of dealing with the problem.

The family doctor who accepts and acknowledges these facts and accepts parents and babies, warts and all, will be in a stronger position to help. It is hoped that he will work in close partnership with midwife and health visitor.

Visiting

Visiting of the mother and baby on their return home from hospital at once indicates an interest in their well-being, but it can also give the mother a chance to ventilate any worries. This she is more likely to do in the security of her own home than in the more awesome environment of the hospital.

Whilst it is perfectly permissible to visit say a six year old with tonsillitis, prescribe penicillin and leave the mother to call you back if worried, such a system is indefensible in the neonate. Each abnormal symptom or sign must not only be evaluated but then observed until it has clearly resolved or a decision has been reached to seek specialist help. This continued surveillance need not always be wholly the responsibility of the doctor, who can share his observations with the health visitor. Such sharing can be beneficial, not only to the health visitor who becomes an acknowledged partner, but also to the parents who can see her commitment to the welfare of the child in sickness or health.

Resuscitation

Nowadays, with virtually 100 per cent hospital confinement, many general practitioners will never attend a birth. However, many others attend confinements of their booked cases at GP units. Moreover, in an emergency any of us could be called to a newborn with respiratory difficulties. Also, there seems to be a growing move by some mothers to opt for home delivery and, therefore, a review of the resuscitation measures which may be needed for a newborn would seem to be justified.

The baby's condition at birth can usefully be assessed by five simple tests, known collectively as the Apgar score, to commemorate Virginia Apgar who invented it in 1952 (Table 25.1).

A score between five and seven calls for close observation, with intervention if the baby's condition worsens. A score of four or less indicates something is seriously wrong, and resuscitation should be attempted.

If the baby fails to cry at once, gentle stimulation such as a light flick on the soles of the feet, is worth trying. More vigorous stimuli are unnecessary and if this fails, the nose and pharynx should be cleared with a mucus extractor.

This manoeuvre will stimulate many babies to breathe spontaneously, but if the baby fails to do so, and if the doctor has the necessary expertise and equipment, endotracheal intubation should be carried out. However, many doctors will have neither the equipment nor the expertise, and for these mouth to mouth assisted respiration is probably safer; but remember to use mouthfuls and not lungfuls of air. The newly born baby is equipped to withstand anoxia better than at any time in its subsequent life. He can metabolise anaerobically for a limited period and care should, therefore, be taken to ensure that he does not suffer more from the enthusiastic efforts of an untrained doctor than from anoxia.

During these procedures the infant should be kept warm, and if a decision is made to transfer the baby to better equipped surroundings, this is better done by bringing help and an incubator to the baby rather than by wrapping the baby in a towel and taking him by car to a hospital unit. Incidentally, if a mother is to be confined at home, an environmental temperature of around 21°C (70°F) is highly desirable.

As soon as all necessary procedures have been carried out the baby should be given to the mother, and if she desires he can be put to the breast. Close bodily contact is highly desirable, as it promotes bonding. Apart from that it would appear to me to be natural and desirable on purely humanitarian grounds. The mother wants to hold her baby, and it is to be hoped that father will not be forgotten!

Initial examination

Most mothers will want to know if their baby is normal, so why not examine the baby in front of her? Whilst the initial examination will in many cases be carried out in hospital, early discharge of mother and baby seems to be growing increasingly popular and, therefore, the

Table 25.1 The Apgar score

Score	A Appearance (colour)	P Pulse (heart rate)	G Grimace (response to stimulation)	A Activity (muscle tone)	R Respiration (respiratory effort)
0	Blue, pale	Absent	No response	Limp	Absent
1	Body pink, extremities blue	Below 100	Grimace	Some flexion of extremities	Slow, irregular
2	Completely pink	Over 100	Cry	Active motion	Good strong cry

initial examination may well fall within the province of the general practitioner.

It helps to work to some sort of routine, and doctors should develop their own. What I will describe is my own approach, which is offered purely for guidance.

Begin with a review of the maternal history. For instance, known exposure to rubella in early pregnancy should put one immediately on the alert. Details of the delivery are relevant – whether labour was prolonged, which could lead to excessive moulding of the skull – and a knowledge of what drugs were used in labour is particularly useful.

Take a general look at the baby, noting colour, and remembering that cyanosis should be looked for centrally, i.e. of the lips and tongue, ignoring slight blueish discolouration of the extremeties if central cyanosis is absent. Look at the facies, which can give the first clue in the diagnosis of Down's syndrome. Observe the respiratory rate, which should lie below 60 per minute and be in the region of about 30–50 breaths per minute.

Look at the head and allow for the effects of moulding. The posterior fontanelle should be nearly closed – if widely open look for patent temporal fontanelles and separated sutures, which can be indicative of hydrocephalus. Look at the ears and observe whether they are low set, i.e. lying below a line drawn backwards from the lateral angle of the orbit. Such low set ears can occasionally be indicative of a renal abnormality. Check the eyes for congenital cataract and coloboma of the iris. Most babies will open their eyes if held up to the light; don't try and force their eyes open.

The baby should breathe easily with a closed mouth. Failure to do so could indicate obstruction of the nostrils. This is important, for infants, unlike adults, do not invariably open the mouth when nasal obstruction is present. Inspect and palpate the mouth for cleft lip and palate, and look to see if the chin is hypoplastic. This abnormality, associated with cleft palate, constitutes the Pierre Robin syndrome. Babies suffering from this are in danger of asphyxia from swallowing their tongue and should be placed in the prone position as a preventive measure, and then admitted to hospital.

Inspect and palpate the neck, chest and abdomen, then turn the baby over and palpate for the integrity of the spine and check the patency of the anus. Next consider the limbs and test for tone and mobility.

In the lower limbs look for talipes deformity. Quite frequently moulding of the feet can occur in utero, especially associated with oligo-hydramnios, and can give rise to confusion. In most instances the foot is acutely dorsiflexed on the leg and at times can look suspiciously like a talipes deformity. However, if gentle stroking on the sole of the foot can stimulate it to come down to an angle of 90° with the leg, no talipes is present, and all that is required is passive stretching of the foot – this can be performed by the mother herself.

Next test for congenital dislocation of the hips. Though rarely diagnosed by the GP (perhaps once in a professional lifetime), this condition is of paramount importance and the examination justifies description. The baby is examined lying on his back. With the hips flexed to a right angle and the knees flexed to about the same degree, abduct the hips, when the femoral head, if dislocated, will be felt to *clunk* into position in the acetabulum as the dislocation is reduced. The hand grip of the examiner is important. Each thumb should lie across the medial aspect of the flexed knees with the fingers lateral to the hip joint, the tip of the middle finger lying in the region of the greater trochanter. Dislocatability can be tested for by using the same grip and rocking the thigh when flexed to 90° and abducted to 45°. This rocking is achieved by alternate medial and lateral pressure from the middle finger and thumb respectively. Beware of bilateral dislocation!

Auscultation of the chest and heart follows. Murmurs heard soon after delivery, and in the absence of other significant findings, should only be noted and the baby re-examined a few days later. Many will by then have disappeared.

Palpate the femoral pulses and check whether the genitalia are normal. Remember that in a new born female the labia minora are relatively prominent compared with the labia majora. In the male it is quite normal for the prepuce to remain non-retractile until the age of three.

Finally, check the cord for haemostasis and determine the number of vessels. Remember that a single umbilical artery can be an indicator of abnormality in the cardiovascular and renal tracts.

Working to a planned routine the examination, carried out more or less as detailed above, can be achieved in a few minutes. In the absence of any significant abnormality the mother can justifiably be reassured as to the normality of the baby. What to do if abnormalities are discovered will depend upon the type and its significance. For instance, congenital dislocation of the hips must be explained at once to the mother, as it justifies immediate treatment, whereas an asymptomatic heart murmur should only be allowed to trouble the doctor and not the mother, as in a day or two it may have disappeared.

Texts on neonatal medicine describe several reflexes which can be tested for in the newborn. I use only three – namely the Moro reflex, the grasp reflex and the rooting reflex.

The *Moro reflex* can be elicited as follows. The baby is supported by the examiner's hands – the right hand of the examiner supports the baby's head and the left hand and forearm of the examiner supports the trunk and lower limbs. The baby is held in a horizontal position and on sharply lowering the head some 2 – 3 inches, the baby is stimulated to produce a symmetrical embracing movement. This reflex should be present in all normal new born babies and its absence usually indicates either brain damage or excessive sedation – the same being true for the other reflexes. Occasionally a unilateral Moro reflex will be elicited and it is worth, here, bearing in mind the possibility of a fracture of the clavicle on the non-moving side.

The *grasp reflex* is tested for as follows. Each forefinger of the examiner is placed across the baby's palm. Normally the infant will then grasp each forefinger with a grip strong enough to permit the weight of the infant's head and trunk to be pulled off the bed.

The *rooting reflex* is easily tested for by the examiner touching the corner of the baby's mouth with the fingertip. Normally the baby's head will be turned towards the examining finger.

The average weight of a new born male is about 7½ lbs (3.4 kg) and the female 7 lbs (3.18 kg). The average length is in the region of about 20 inches (51 cm), and the head circumference 13.8 inches (35 cm).

The optimum environment

During the first hour the infant shows alert and exploratory behaviour, and then usually sleeps for about three or four hours. During the first hour he will follow objects with the eyes and head. Thereafter the baby tends to sleep most of the time, except when fed or handled. The baby will cry when hungry or disturbed, and failure to behave in this way should alert the doctor.

The new born is especially prone to cooling, and generally speaking an environmental temperature persistently below 70°F (21°C) is unsuitable. The baby's cot should be close to the mother's bed, so that she can not only satisfy her desire to look at and touch her baby, but can also observe his general wellbeing. She should be encouraged to pick him up, and the myth of spoiling him should be exploded forever. Babies can see, smell and hear, just as do children and adults, and they are capable of enjoying a cuddle.

Observation of the mother and child interaction at this time can provide much valuable information. Failure to make eye to eye contact, disinclination to handle the baby, complaints about messy feeding or nappies, or about the sex of the baby, can be looked on as possible early warning signs of a disturbed mother/baby relationship and, therefore, of a potential battering situation.

Extra support and supervision by the doctor, midwife and health visitor would then certainly be justified, as would care in the subsequent prescribing of drugs to the mother. (Benzo-diazepines, e.g. Valium, can release inhibitions sufficiently to allow violent behaviour to explode.)

The Toilet

The mother should be encouraged to undertake all necessary tasks for her baby, such as bathing and changing, as soon as she feels capable of so doing. It is tempting, in the interests of speed, for nursing staff to do these jobs themselves, but the result can easily be loss of confidence by the mother who, especially if this is her first baby, will be in need of support and encouragement. The daily bathing period should be an enjoyable time for both mother and baby. It should be unhurried, and the mother encouraged during this time to talk to the baby. It seems traditional that after the drying the baby is thoroughly powdered, but how necessary this is has so far escaped me. However, it certainly makes a baby smell nicer, and anything which improves his attractiveness is probably worthwhile.

The cord should be checked daily for haemostasis, and in most instances will have separated spontaneously by about the seventh day. It is traditional to dab it daily with surgical spirit, but I think normal hygiene alone would suffice. The napkin area merits regular attention, not only at bathtimes, but at each napkin change. A thorough wash with soap and water is highly desirable, and this measure alone should prevent the majority of napkin eruptions. I am not in favour of routinely using creams or ointments when the skin is normal and intact.

Feeding

I firmly believe in the value of breast feeding, but even more firmly in the right of the mother to determine breast or bottle. It is important that the mother who elects to bottle feed should not be made to feel second-rate. Hopefully the advantages of breast feeding will have been explained to her in the antenatal period, and if she still prefers the bottle the only stipulation I would make is that she uses a modified (humanised) low solute formula, e.g. SMA Gold Cap.

The mother wanting to breast feed should be encouraged to put the baby to the breast as soon as she desires. Thereafter, whether she feeds on demand or uses a four-hourly routine, will depend much on her make-up. Some mothers are perfectly happy with the demand regime – others appreciate the security of a tighter schedule. The same remarks really apply to bottle feeding. Correct mixing of the formula is highly important and should be stressed by both midwife and health visitor. It is only human to think that if one is good, two will be better, and the dangers of over-concentrated feeds in producing obesity, and also the danger of hypernatremic dehydration should fluid loss occur, need to be explained to the mother and repeated ad nauseam by the health visitor.

I also believe that over-concentrated feeds can produce restless babies by making them thirsty, but must admit that this is more of a hunch that a scientifically proven fact.

We know that obese babies have the potential to become obese adults, so that there is an opportunity here to practise preventive medicine. By the end of the first weeks the baby can have lost up to ten per cent of his body weight, but thereafter a weight gain of some 6 oz (180 g) per week is perfectly satisfactory. Mothers should be warned that each time the baby cries it is not necessarily a sign of hunger. Also that a drink of boiled water will often suffice to calm him, and that even just being picked up and cuddled can provide sufficient reassurance to stop crying.

Neonatal disorders

Whilst the neonate is subject to his own peculiar pathology, often the presentation is less clear cut than in the adult or older child. Obviously there is a certain lack of cooperation but this is not all. Rather than categorise diseases I will now attempt to deal with the presenting symptoms or signs of disorders that can occur in the neonatal period, as this is more likely to be the way the GP meets them.

1. Cyanosis

Remember that to be significant this must be central, i.e. present in the lips and tongue. If cyanosis is accompanied by rapid respirations and retraction of the thoracic cage, it is likely to have a respiratory cause. It can also, however, be secondary to intra-cranial haemorrhage, and then respirations are often weak, irregular and slow. Cyanosis which persists after several days is very likely to be due to cyanotic heart disease. Episodic cyanosis can be a presenting sign of hypo-glycaemia, when it will usually occur in the first 24 hours.

2. Lethargy

If this occurs soon after delivery it can indicate effects of analgesia or anaesthesia, but can also arise from anoxia or cerebral defect. Lethargy occurring after the second day should alert the doctor to the possibility of infection. The baby going off feeds and lethargic could well be in the early stages of an infection, even meningitis.

3. Fever

High temperatures can well result from overheating, but remember the dehydration fever which can occur at about 48 hours. This is usually not accompanied by other abnormal signs and responds to adequate fluids. Early feeding probably helps to prevent its occurrence.

It is very important to remember that more serious infections in the newborn do not necessarily provoke a febrile response and, in fact, may result in a lowering of the body temperature.

4. Jaundice

If this occurs in the first 24 hours it is due to haemolytic disease unless proved otherwise. No efforts should be made to determine its cause, but the baby should be admitted to an appropriate Unit at once. Rarer causes are toxoplasmosis and cytomegalic inclusion disease, and the congenital rubella syndrome.

5. Vomiting

If this occurs during the first 48 hours it should be

Table 25.2 Disorders in the first week of life

Signs and symptoms	*Days after delivery* 1 – 3	4 – 5	6 – 7
Fits	Hypoglycaemia Birth trauma Hypocalcaemia	Meningitis	Hypocalcaemia* (bottle fed)
Vomiting	Intestinal obstruction (especially if bilious)	Infection e.g. meningitis	
Jaundice	Haemolysis Toxoplasma Cyt. Incl. Dis. Cong. Rubella Syndrome	Physiological	Cretinism
Lethargy	Drugs to mother Birth trauma	Infection	
Bleeding	Inadequate ligation of Cord	Haemorrhagic disease of newborn	

regarded as indicating intestinal obstruction, especially if the vomitus contains bile.

6. Immobility

Failure to move a limb or part of the body, should alert the doctor to the possibility of a fracture or nerve palsy.

7. Fits

In the newborn they do not show the classic grand mal pattern. They can be tonic, clonic or even fragmentary. Although they usually indicate a disorder of the central nervous system, remember that they can also be due to hypo-glycaemia, hypo-calcaemia and even meningitis.

In Table 25.2 these symptoms and signs are related to causes and their presentation on a time scale from birth onwards.

Respiratory and cardiac problems can present shortly after birth, or at any time in the neonatal period. I have taken them together because clinically they often present in the same way with tachypnoea, lower intercostal indrawing and later cyanosis. In addition the baby is often so short of breath as to be unable to suck at the breast or bottle. The general practitioner, recognising the onset of these signs and symptoms, need not be too worried about reaching a definitive diagnosis which often requires a chest radiograph and frequently an ECG. However, he should see that the child is transferred to the Special Care Baby Unit where there are facilities for definitive diagnosis and treatment. If at all possible such a transfer should be in an incubator with a trained person accompanying the infant. Possible causes of the symptoms and signs are respiratory distress syndrome, congenital heart disease, aspiration and diaphragmatic hernia. Each of these conditions requires the facilities of a specially equipped unit for successful management.

A clue to the causation of *fits* can be gained from their timing and the history of the birth. If delivery has been difficult then cerebral oedema or haemorrhage would be likely, especially if the baby is pre-term. In a light for dates baby hypoglycaemia would be a strong possibility. A rarer cause is hypocalcaemia, which can also be associated with difficult delivery.

Again, the niceties of diagnosis need not concern the general practitioner who should, if the fit is still occurring when he arrives, control it with rectal valium and transfer the baby to a special care unit with someone in attendance, armed with suction, to see that the airway is at all times secured. (Rectal valium is given with a Mantoux syringe, or failing that a 1 ml syringe. After drawing up the necessary amount, remove the needle, smear the end of the syringe with KY jelly, insert into the rectum and inject). A response occurs within 10 minutes or less.

Fits occurring at the end of the first week can be due to hypocalcaemia, when they usually arrive de novo in a baby on artificial feeds. Fits occurring after the first 48 hours can be due to meningitis, when they will often be preceded by some of the symptoms and signs already given as indicators of infection. Transfer of the baby to a unit for further investigation is mandatory.

Infection can occur at any time in the neonatal period. The neonate is more susceptible to gram negative and staphylococcal infection than older children. Prevention should be the aim. No elaborate ritual is needed, but merely meticulous hand-washing before handling the baby. Masks are not routinely required but should be worn if the doctor or nurse is suffering from a respiratory infection. In addition, if the membranes have been ruptured for over 24 hours before delivery, prophylactic antibiotics are justified. A combination of Ampicillin 50 mg and Cloxacillin 25 mg (Ampiclox) given to the baby eight-hourly for 48 hours, would be suitable. Oral and intramuscular preparations are available.

Infection is often of insidious onset in the newborn and the doctor should think of it when faced with the baby who is reluctant to feed, vomits, shows temperature instability (often hypothermia), develops abdominal distension or diarrhoea, irritability or jaundice. It is often impossible to localise the infection – therefore, samples of blood, c.s.f. and urine should be taken for culture and sensitivity testing, prior to the giving of chemotherapy. Such procedures are best undertaken by those familiar with them, and this invariably means transfer of the baby to a specialist unit.

Even seemingly trivial infections in the newborn can cause considerable systemic upset. Minor skin infections can put the baby off feeds and it is, therefore, worth taking any infection seriously and treating it vigorously. Staphylococcal skin infections acquired in hospital, should be assumed to be penicillin resistant and Flucloxacillin used in its place. Although the routine of prophylactic drops in the eyes is usually no longer practised, it is worth bearing in mind the gonococcus as the cause of any sticky eye, especially as the incidence of gonococcal infection seems to be rising. Whenever possible, if such a condition occurs, swabs should be taken for culture and sensitivity tests prior to giving treatment, and I usually find that Chloramphenicol eyedrops during the day and ointment at night, are effective in the vast majority of cases.

The general practitioner reading the previous section might understandably be discouraged at having to seek specialist help so frequently. However, I would remind him that by recognising the significance of a particular symptom or sign, he is rendering a great service to his patient. It matters little to have a highly skilled back-up neonatal service if, by lack of early diagnosis, this is never given the chance to deliver skills to a baby before it is in extremis.

Jaundice

It is a pity that the term physiological jaundice of the newborn was ever introduced, as it can produce a false sense of security. Always remember that jaundice occurring in the first 24 hours is never *normal* and should be assumed to be due to haemolysis until proved otherwise. Do not delay by trying to perform any investigations, but get the infant to a centre where an exchange transfusion can be carried out. Jaundice due to rhesus haemolytic disease has certainly fallen with the advent of anti-D prophylaxis. Remember that ABO incompatibility (Group O mother with A or B baby), can produce significant haemolysis.

So-called physiological jaundice usually occurs at about 48 hours after delivery. It should not be taken lightly but watched carefully, as occasionally quite high levels of serum bilirubin can be reached with the dangers of damage to hearing and the basal ganglia. If jaundice is deepening daily it is well worth checking the serum bilirubin, so that if this reaches the level of 12 mg per cent phototherapy can be started. There is a useful tool called an icterometer. This consists merely of a small piece of clear plastic, shaped like a ruler, of some three inches in length. On it is a graduated scale of bilirubin levels matched to a colour chart. The device is pressed against the nose of the baby and the colour compared with the colour chart and scale, and the level of bilirubin read off. Whilst the results are not terribly accurate, they can be used to indicate a rising level of bilirubin so that a laboratory test can perhaps be avoided (as this would invariably mean the baby being taken to hospital). Most cases of so-called physiological jaundice will be mild and fade by the end of the first week. Undue prolongation of the jaundice should make the doctor consider the possibility of thyroid deficiency.

Bleeding

Bleeding can occur from the cord during the first ten days. In the first 24 hours this is most likely to be due to inadequate ligation of the cord at birth. Towards the end of the first week secondary haemorrhage from infection can occur.

Between the second and sixth days bleeding can occur from the bowel, the urinary tract and the cord, when it is likely to be due to haemorrhagic disease of the newborn. The management consists of the administration of vitamin K (Konakion 1 mg) and transfer of the infant to a specialised unit. Usually the condition settles spontaneously without harm to the baby, but close observation is always justified.

The cold syndrome

This merits mention because of two reasons. It is preventable by insuring an environmental temperature of 70°F as a minimum, and secondly because the appearance of a baby suffering from the disorder is deceptive. The baby looks a 'healthy', pinky-red colour, especially about the face and hands. This is due to the lowered body temperature inhibiting the dissociation of oxygen from haemoglobin. Such babies are especially at risk, for if the condition persists pulmonary and gastrointestinal haemorrhages can complicate the picture and prove lethal. Chilling of the baby in the immediate neonatal period can lead to grunting respirations and a picture suggestive of early respiratory distress syndrome. Warming the baby produces spontaneous resolution.

Certain conditions appear to cause worries in the mind of the mother out of all proportion to the significance of the condition.

It is quite normal for the baby to lose weight in the first few days after birth. In fact, up to ten per cent of the bodyweight can be lost. By about the sixth to seventh day, however, this should cease and thereafter the baby should gain at the rate of about 6oz (180g) per week.

Minor problems

Stork marks – a pinkish discolouration of the skin which is situated in the regions of the nape of the neck and in a butterfly shape at the root of the nose – can often create anxiety. The facial lesions invariably disappear in the first year or eighteen months of life, but contrary to the literature those at the nape of the neck do not. However, the growth of hair adequately obscures them.

Milia – small white papular lesions, invariably appear on the nose in particular and on the adjoining facial areas, usually after the end of the first week. They are so common as to be regarded as normal. They do not lead to disfigurement and disappear without trace. No attempt should be made to treat them, but the mother should be firmly reassured that they will disappear without trace.

Breast engorgement can occur during the first week – mastitis neonatorum. This condition is worth watching as occasionally frank abscess formation can occur. This, however, is rare, and the mother can be told that such engorgement is very common, but that the doctor will keep an eye on it until it disappears.

Vaginal discharge. More rarely a blood-stained mucoid discharge can occur from the vagina, presumably due to oestrogen withdrawal. Reassurance as to its normality is all that is required, unless there are other manifestations which suggest haemorrhagic disease of the newborn.

Regurgitation after feeds is very common and often provokes anxiety. It should be distinguished from vomiting – forceful expulsion of the gastric contents. In the vast majority of cases the baby thrives and gains weight, and if this is so no action is necessary. A number of babies continue to regurgitate for several months. As long as weight gain is adequate no action is necessary, and in such cases thickening of the feeds need not be advised.

Talking to parents of a baby born with a disability

Happily most babies are born normal and healthy, but there will be times when the family doctor has to deal with a family who have been less fortunate. Before speaking to the parents try and make sure that you know the name of the child, which at once recognises him as an individual in your own mind and shows this recognition to the parents. Try and find out what has been said at the hospital. This may necessitate a telephone call but it will be well worthwhile.

Try and remember that many parents tend to blame themselves for the child's disability. Encourage them to express their fears, and if possible allay these by factual explanation. It is essential to be truthful at all times. In the end a truthful attitude will ultimately encourage trust. Try to check whether the defect can be recurrent, and if necessary arrange for genetic counselling.

Remember that it will be difficult for parents to take in all the information they require at one interview. Their minds will be in a state of turmoil and it is, therefore, a good idea to offer to see them again after an interval of a week or two.

Some conditions, which in the neonatal period look horrendous, can be cured. For example, cleft lip and palate. Here the attitude of the doctor can be crucial. The mother of a baby with a disfiguring deformity may desperately want to love him and yet be repulsed by his appearance. The doctor who is able to pick up the child and regard him as a whole person, may well act as the trigger which releases pent-up maternal feeling. The situation is rather akin to the nurse who does the first dressing for a colostomy patient. If she shows repulsion seeds can be sown which take years to counteract.

The parents of children born with disabilities require not only explanation but continued support, until they can come to terms with their problems. The job definition of the general practitioner as being one of first contact and continuing presence, is of particular pertinence here. The GP will also, of course, want to bring to the parents the help and expertise of the health visitor and social worker, to help the parents to cope with the many problems that arise.

ACKNOWLEDGEMENTS

Dr J.D. Andrew and Dr A.J.A. Ferguson have kindly read the text and made helpful suggestions. The burden of the typing has fallen on the able shoulders of Mrs N. Clennell and Mrs S. Smurthwaite.
To them all I offer grateful thanks.

FURTHER READING

Clinics in Developmental Medicine (1972) *The Medical Care of Newborn Babies*. London: Heinemann.

Nelson, W.E. *et al* (1979) *Textbook of Paediatrics*, 11th edn. Philadelphia: W.B. Saunders.

BMJ (1972) *Problems of the Newborn*. British Medical Journal Publication.

The Children's Committee (1979) *The reduction of Perinatal Mortality and Morbidity: A discussion document*.

Schaffer, A. & Avery, M.E. (1977) *Disease of the Newborn*, 4th edn.?

26

Problems of maturity

Paul Hooper

If a child is born with a low birth weight, it may because he has been born too early or because, though born at or near term, his intrauterine growth has been inhibited for some reason. The distinction is not difficult when the mother is certain of her 'dates' but quite frequently certainty is lacking and now there is confusion – which is it?

It is important to distinguish between growth in size of the fetus and his developmental maturity. The latter concerns the maturity of function of organs such as the liver, kidneys and haemopoietic system, but particularly of the central nervous system, for this will continue to mature even though growth in size is retarded. So that a small infant can be premature (or better, 'pre-term' or 'short gestation') when his size and maturity are in accord, or dysmature when his size and maturity are not in accord; his size may be less than his maturity as in placental insufficiency ('light for dates', or 'small for gestational age', SGA), or larger than his maturity as in the case of an infant born to a diabetic mother ('heavy for dates' or 'large for gestational age').

Some further definitions are now necessary. The term *premature* which used to indicate an infant of birth weight of less than 2500 g (5½ lb) has now been abandoned and we talk of *preterm* (28–36 weeks gestation), *term* (37–41 weeks) and *post-term* (42 weeks and over) when applied to gestational age and the dates are known. There are now percentile charts of weight for infants in the preterm period similar to those of Tanner and Whitehouse for children (see Ch. 27). Below the 10th percentile the child is *light for dates*, between the 10th and 90th percentile he is *normal for dates*, and over the 90th percentile he is *heavy for dates* (see Table 26.1). Of course, by definition, 10 per cent of normal infants will be below the 10th percentile and so some normal infants will be 'small for dates', but provided it is remembered that 'small for dates' is only a description and not a diagnosis, this is a useful working classification.

MORTALITY IN LOW BIRTH WEIGHT BABIES

A recent discussion document by the Children's Committee identified low birth weight as one of the three principal causes of perinatal mortality. Preterm babies account for over half the perinatal deaths, and a fifth of those who are subsequently handicapped (Children's Committee, 1979). It has been recalculated from the original data of the British Births Survey (1970) that if the deaths of babies under 2500 grams had not occurred, the perinatal mortality would have dropped from the then current rate of 21 to 8 per 1000 total births.

THE AETIOLOGY OF 'LIGHT FOR DATES'

The causes of 'light for dates' infants can be divided into maternal, placental and fetal.

Maternal causes include height, age, nutrition, race and social class; order of pregnancy, pre-eclamptic tox-

Table 26.1 Definitions of maturity (Davies *et al*, 1972)

Birth weight	*Gestational age* Less than 37 weeks	*37–41 weeks*	*42 weeks or more*
Below 10th percentile	pre-term, small for dates	term, small for dates	post-term, small for dates
10th-90th percentile	pre-term, normal for dates	term, normal for dates	post-term, normal for dates
Above 90th percentile	pre-term, heavy for dates	term, heavy for dates	post-term, heavy for dates

aemia and hypertension, cyanotic heart disease and cigarette smoking.

Placental causes include small placenta and multiple microinfarcts. Tests for placental function, such as the serial levels of maternal urinary oestrogens, can indicate placental insufficiency.

Fetal causes include multiparity, congenital abnormalities including chormosomal translocations, and fetal infection by rubella, syphilis and toxoplasmosis.

But how do we know how mature an infant is when we do not know his gestational age accurately?

ESTIMATION OF GESTATIONAL AGE DURING PREGNANCY

This is discussed in more detail in Chapter 9, but a few methods are mentioned here.

1. Bimanual pelvic examination before 16 weeks. Thereafter the fundal height is inaccurate. This is an important reason for early booking.
2. Radiology for ossification centres at the knee. Lower femoral epiphysis appears at 36 weeks, upper tibial at 38 weeks; not consistent and no good before 36 weeks.
3. Ultrasonic measurement of biparietal diameter requires apparatus, a growth chart and serial readings, but probably fairly accurate
4. Amniotic fluid studies. Biochemistry is not reliable and depends on 'biochemical maturity'. Cytology may be helpful in that certain cells appear at 38 weeks and this is independent of placental function and the technique is easy.

Thus there is 'no absolutely accurate method of assessing length of gestation is available to the clinician' (Blastone et al, 1971).

ESTIMATION OF GESTATIONAL AGE AFTER DELIVERY

Remembering that the central nervous system continues to mature, even if growth in size is retarded, certain CNS reflexes have been used as a guide to maturity (Table 26.2).

Table 26.2 CNS reflexes and gestational age (Davies *et al*, 1972)

Pupil reaction to light appears between	29 and 31 weeks gestation
Traction response appears between	33 and 36 weeks gestation
Glabellar tap appears between	32 and 36 weeks gestation
Neck righting response appears between	34 and 37 weeks gestation

Various other tests rely upon the greater degree of muscle relaxation in the mature infant. For instance, if the hand is flexed on the forearm of a full term baby there will be no gap visible between the two; in the preterm infant the degree of flexion will be limited to 60° or 90°, so forming a 'window' (the 'window sign'). Similarly, dorsiflexion of the foot on the shin will be complete in a term infant, but limited to 60° or 90° in a pre-term infant (ankle dorsiflexion test). If the infant's hand is taken across to the opposite shoulder so that the arm is wrapped round the front of the neck like a scarf, it will be found that in the term infant the tip of the elbow does not cross the midline of the body, but in the preterm infant it does cross (the scarf sign). There are several other tests of a similar nature.

Other criteria have also been used, such as the colour and texture of the skin, amount of lanugo hair on the back, size of breast development and firmness and cartilage content of the pinna of the ear. A method of scoring the maturity of these external and neurological signs has been invented and this, combined with the use of a graph plotting the total score against the gestational age in weeks is said to give an accuracy of 95 per cent ± 15 days (Buckler, 1979; Dubowitz et al, 1970; Hancock, 1973).

The postmature infant is defined as an infant born after 41 weeks gestation, and in these days of early induction of labour, is a rarity. He is readily recognised by his dry, peeling skin which tends to crack, and by the lack of subcutaneous fat. The danger lies in his considerably increased mortality during or soon after delivery.

WHY IS ALL THIS IMPORTANT?

Information about size and maturity at birth is important for two reasons:

1. The paediatrician needs to distinguish between preterm and light-for-dates infants because their problems and management can be quite different while they are in hospital. This is a highly specialised field and need not concern us further.
2. It affects the judgement of the doctor who has the continuing care and surveillance of the child. A two week old infant born at 34 weeks will behave differently from a two week old infant born at 40 weeks: for instance his primitive reflexes will be less developed and he may be regarded as a case of brain damage unless his maturity is taken into account. Similarly, a six-month-old infant who shows no sign of weight bearing at six months need cause no anxiety when it is remembered that he was born at 34 weeks and is therefore really only 'four and a half months old'.

An important study by the Newcastle team headed by the late Gerald Neligan called *Born too soon or born too small* was published in 1976. They followed up children who were born too soon (short gestation, born before 36 weeks) or born too small (light for dates) for seven years, using extensive physical and psychological tests. The latter group had to be subdivided into 'very light for dates' (below 5th centile) and 'rather light for dates' (5–10 centile). Their conclusions, very briefly, were that the short gestation and very light for dates developed more slowly physically and intellectually and had more behavioural abnormalities than the control group. Children who grew too slowly in the uterus (light for dates) grew too slowly outside it, whereas those who grew at a normal rate in the uterus but were born preterm grew at normal rate outside.

These findings are indirectly connected with the question of malnutrition and critical periods of growth of certain organs. For instance, it is now known that the critical period of brain growth occurs between 36 weeks of pregnancy and two years of age. Significant malnutrition occurring between these two ages can adversely affect later intellectual performance.

Another interesting conclusion of the Newcastle survey was that 'the most important environmental factor . . . is the quality of the mother's care of her child'.

It is unlikely that the general practitioner will be called upon to make and assessment of maturity, because these very small babies are (or should be) looked after in specialist units until they are big enough to be managed safely at home; but these problems are going to be met with more and more frequently in the future, and it was therefore felt that simple summary might be helpful.

It might be added that a recent study showed that the birth of a baby of low birth weight is emotionally traumatic for the parents, especially when the baby is retained in a special care unit after the mother has been discharged home. Parents of these babies are prone to depression and anxiety, and bonding is slow to develop. Mothers visit their general practitioners much more frequently than the mothers of normal babies, and feel great need for information and sympathetic support (Jeffcoate, 1980).

REFERENCES

Batstone, G.F., Blain, A.W. & Slater, J.M. (1971) *Prenatal Paediatrics*. Aylesbury: Medical and Technical Publications.

Buckler, J.M.H. (1979) *A reference manual of Growth and Development*. London: Blackwell.

Children's Committee (1979) *The Reduction of Perinatal Mortality and Morbidity*: a discussion document.

Davies, P.J., Robinson, R.J., Scopes, J.W., Tizard, J.P.M. & Wigglesworth, J.A. (1972) *Medical Care of Newborn Babies*. Spastics International Medical Publications. London: Heineman.

Dubowitz, L.M.S., Dubowitz, V. & Goldberg, C. (1970) Clinical assessment of gestational age in the newborn infant. *Journal of Paediatrics*, 77, 11.

Hancock, B.W. (1973) Clinical assessment of age in the neonate. *Archives of the Disabled Child*, **48**, 152.

Jeffcoate, J. (1980) Looking at the need for support for families of low birth weight babies. *Health Trends*, **12**, 29–30.

Neligan, G.A. *et al* (1976) *Born too Small or Born too Soon*. London: Heineman.

27

Nutrition in infancy and childhood

Michael Whitfield

PRENATALLY

Nutritionally the prenatal period is one of the safest for the child. In Holland, during 1939–45 war, where the weight gain of most pregnant women was less than four pounds (1.82 kg) over the whole pregnancy the average weight of the newborn babies fell by no more than half a pound (0.23 kg). However, a recent review described the increased risk of complications to mother and child in mothers who were undernourished during pregnancy (*BMJ* Editorial, 1980). It is therefore important to monitor carefully pregnant women who are underweight.

Supplemental iron and a good balanced diet are sensible requirements for any pregnant woman. The rationale for prescribing supplemental vitamins in a present-day relatively affluent society seems questionable with the exception of folic acid in the later months of pregnancy. Recently however the case for vitamin D supplements throughout pregnancy has been reconsidered, and it may be that they should be reintroduced for selected groups of expectant mothers (Cockburn *et al*, 1980).

INFANT FEEDING

Trollope in 1847 wrote: 'How is it that poor men's wives, who have no cooked fowl or port wine on which to be coshered up, nurse their children without difficulty, whereas the wives of rich men, who eat and drink everything that is good, cannot do so?'

In the last few decades this situation has been reversed so that it is now the women in the lower socioeconomic groups who are not breast feeding. The reasons for this change are difficult to pinpoint. The Newson investigation (1965) suggested that the main reason for not breast feeding was 'the vague sense of the inconvenience of breast feeding, frequently connected with considerations of modesty, through feelings of real embarrassment to a deep seated revulsion from the whole process, often quite unexplicable to the mother herself'. This investigation and one by Smith (1969) both denied the commonly held assumption that breast feeding is never started because the mother has to return quickly to work.

Socioeconomic factors are not the only parameters that have been shown to be related to whether a woman breast feeds her baby or not. Prothero (1969) found that if the mother was born outside the United Kingdom she was more likely to breast feed, and two studies, Martin (1978) and Palmer *et al* (1979), have shown that induction of labour and assisted delivery were significantly associated with lower breast feeding rates. Jacob (1968) confirmed that taller women were more likely to attempt breast feeding than shorter women.

Given reasonable motivation, the establishment of breast feeding is the result of reflex interaction between mother and baby. The baby must have the rooting, suckling and swallowing reflexes present and the mother must develop the prolactin reflex and the more important 'let-down' reflex. The prolactin reflex is the main mechanism for milk secretion into the alveoli and is stimulated, as is the 'let-down' reflex, by the amount of suckling that the baby does. The 'let-down' reflex results in the stimulation of myoepithelial cells surrounding the alveoli to 'let-down' the milk into the terminal lacteals. This reflex is inhibited by anxiety, uncertainty and other forms of emotional tension and is therefore of great importance in the establishment of breast feeding.

Practically, the establishment of breast feeding needs encouragement at all stages. In the antenatal period examination of the breasts at the initial examination should be accompanied by an enquiry as to the attitude of the woman to breast feeding. There is little to be gained by persuasion at this stage of a woman's life if she is adamantly opposed to the idea of breast feeding; views can certainly sometimes be modified and misconceptions removed. During the antenatal period the woman should be introduced to the benefits of breast feeding against bottle feeding and the general attitude in classes should be one of breast feeding being the ideal, bottle feeding a good alternative.

The woman should be told of the protective effect against infection of breast feeding as reviewed by Welsh and May (1974) and the decreased possibility of a breast fed baby developing gastrointestinal infections. There is some evidence (Hopper, 1965) that excessive weight gain and increased morbidity are associated in infancy and that obesity is extremely rare in breast fed babies. See further, Chapter 12.

Encouragement to breast feed and continued support during the often troublesome first week or two usually comes from the mother's relatives, the midwife and health visitor. Sometimes this is supplemented by such organisations as the National Child-birth Trust in the United Kingdom, Laleche League International in the USA or the Nursing Mothers Association in Australia. These organisations arrange antenatal and postnatal support, often by mothers who have successfully breast fed their own children, and this can be of great help for the apprehensive new mother. It is of great help if midwife and health visitor, and general practitioner are all of like mind in encouraging breast feeding, and are consistent in the advice they give (Aylett, 1975). Sloper *et al* (1975) were able to demonstrate a marked increase in successful lactation where all the staff of a maternity unit were educated, by seminar, about the benefits of breast feeding. Unfortunately, they were not so successful in ensuring it continued when the mother returned home.

After delivery it is important for the baby to be put to the breast early. Salariya *et al* (1978) showed that the best policy was to put the baby to the breast as soon as possible after delivery, to follow this by two hourly feeding until lactation is established and thereafter to feed on demand. The initial length of time the baby is suckled on each breast should be limited so that the nipples do not get sore. Care should be taken to ensure that the baby takes the areola into the mouth to reduce the likelihood of sore nipples. There is no definite evidence that the manual expression of colostrum or the wearing of Waller's Shells to facilitate later breast feeding really makes any significant difference.

Common problems associated with breast feeding

Cracked nipples

This is often the result of either sensitive maternal skin or not limiting the time suckling takes place in the early stages of breast feeding. The remedy is to apply some soothing cream (e.g. Masse cream), Friars Balsam or Rotersept spray and to discontinue putting the baby to the breast until the soreness disappears. It is important to express the milk regularly from the breast until the nipple has healed. The use of a nipple shield is often a good alternative method.

Breast infection/abscess

The early use of a broad spectrum antibiotic (e.g. Ampicillin) is important. Cessation of breast feeding is not always necessary and should only be used for as long as the breast is too painful to suckle. Analgesics are often required.

Breast engorgement

This usually occurs during the first week of breast feeding and may result in considerable discomfort for the mother. It is important to continue feeding and to use warm compresses and analgesics. The use of alternately warm and cold compresses is also sometimes beneficial. If the discomfort is very great a small dose of Stilboestrol (5 mg b.d.) for one or two days, can prove very beneficial. There is no evidence that this level of dosage is harmful to mother or baby.

Pains in the breast after suckling

This is quite common and is not easily explained. It is best dealt with by analgesics and reassurance. It is not a sign of imminent infection.

Weaning

There is no ideal length of time for breast feeding to continue. When well established four to six months appears a common length of time but the variation is very great. Missing one feed every day for three or four days and then two feeds for three or four days and so on results in little or no breast discomfort. A written out or duplicated sheet indicating in detail how this can be done can be very helpful. There is much to be said for progressing from the breast directly to drinking reconstituted milk from a cup. This can be done from about three months of age if necessary.

Alternative forms of infant feeding

Many formulae are available for artificial feeding. They result in perfectly adequate nutrition for the baby when used correctly and all mothers (and ideally fathers too) should receive adequate prenatal instruction in the preparation of such foods. Fresh cows' milk can be used as an infant feed but it is not ideal in view of its tough protein, coarse fat and high mineral salt content. It can be modified by drying or evaporation and it is in these forms that it is usually used for feeding nowadays. These processes result in a slightly reduced carbohydrate level, so it is advisable to add a level 5 ml spoonful of sugar to each feed to approximate to the carbohydrate level of human milk unless the manufacturer has already added it. The use of dried or evaporated milk depends on the preference of the mother. Dried milk is probably easier to use since it is less likely to become bacteriologically contaminated after the packet has been opened.

Some authorities suggest the use of half cream dried milk for the first week or so of life, gradually increasing the concentration to full cream by four weeks.

Preparation of feed

Simple hygienic principles are important and parents should be reminded of the need for hand washing before preparing feeds. Equipment (bottle and teat, etc.) must be efficiently sterilised. Two methods are commonly used: boiling and chemical sterilisation. The latter is certainly the most reliable and for this reason alone has much to commend it. The greater incidence of gastroenteritis in bottle fed babies compared with that in breast fed babies in sufficient reason to emphasise continually the importance of efficient sterilisation.

The concentration of the feed is important. The powder must not be compressed in the scoop and must be scraped flat, although one well known brand advises that the scoop be packed firmly. The correct scoop must be used as different formulae have different sized scoops. Milk that is made up in too concentrated a form is at risk of being high in mineral content. Two complications may result:

1. *Neonatal hypocalcaemia*, which occurs typically on the sixth day of life and is accompanied by a marked increase in plasma inorganic phosphorus concentration and clinically increased neuromuscular excitability; there may be generalised convulsions.

2. *Hypernatraemia*. Oates (1973) showed that incorrect preparation can increase the value of sodium to six times the average content of breast milk. This can result in a hypertonic or hypernatraemic type of dehydration which is compounded if high concentration reconstituted milk is fed to infants who have become slightly dehydrated with gastroenteritis

The quantity of milk fed to individual babies will vary as different babies have differing requirements. The average infant between two and three months of age will require about 2½ ounces of milk per pound body weight per day (155 g milk per kg body weight per day), assuming the milk contains twenty calories per ounce (700 calories per kg).

Supplements

1. *Iron*. Both human and cows' milk are poor in iron. For the full term baby sufficient iron will have passed into its body transplacentally to maintain stores until the baby is able to take mixed food. Certainly by four to five months of age the baby should be gaining iron from egg yolk, minced meat, sieved vegetables, stewed apple, etc. and some proprietary forms of baby cereal. Premature and low birth weight babies are at special risk of developing iron deficiency anaemia and should receive medicinal iron supplements from the age of four weeks up to one year.

2. *Vitamin C*. Only if the mother has a very high intake of vitamin C will the breast fed baby get sufficient vitamin from breast milk. It is important therefore to ensure the addition of this vitamin to the diets of all infants. Rosehip syrup or concentrated orange juice should be diluted with water to ensure a daily intake of 15–20 mg of vitamin C.

3. *Vitamin D*. An infant should have a daily intake of 400 i.u. vitamin D. All dried milks and evaporated milks in the United Kingdom are fortified with vitamin D and will ensure its adequate level. Supplemental vitamin D is needed if fresh cows' milk is used and also in breast fed infants. The vitamin is contained in cod liver oil and in proprietary multivitamin preparations.

4. *Fluoride*. Tooth enamel which incorporates the fluoride ion into its crystalline structure is more resistant to acid dissolution than is enamel which is fluoride free. Although fluoridation of public water supplies is widely supported, in areas where this is not available the daily ingestion of a fluoride tablet supplies the necessary fluoride. The recommended dosage is: from birth to two years of age 0.5 mg of fluoride per day, i.e. half a tablet daily. This can be dissolved in water and swallowed, or sucked. From two years to 12 years the recommended dosage is one tablet daily. The tablets are prescribable under the National Health Service by general practitioners (Brandt, 1975).

Feeding problems

The co-operation and help of the practice health visitor is of great importance in the problems of the newborn. On occasions she may not be immediately available so it is important for the doctor to learn about some of the problems.

Any experienced mother will know that a crying baby does not necessarily indicate a hungry baby. The dilemma facing parents with their first child is distinguishing when it is appropriate to satisfy the child with food and when it is appropriate to leave the child to settle without feeding. For most mothers it appears that there is no problem and *feeding on demand* works ideally. This form of feeding is undoubtedly the best, especially for the breast fed infant. Unfortunately for some inexperienced mothers this form of feeding can result in tiredness, frustration over the seeming inability to satisfy the infant, and increasing irritability. It is in these circumstances that the rigid *four hourly feeding* schedule comes into its own. The mother then has the security of knowing that the baby is taking adequate food (in breast fed babies this can be checked by test weighing before and after each feed.) Advising the mother to embark upon a rigid schedule enables the doctor to learn how much the baby is being fed and frequently tends to lessen the tension that develops between mother and baby. The middle of the night feed should be omitted if possible, or if started should be discontinued as soon as possible.

Overfeeding used to be thought of as impossible in babies. It was often stated that babies will not absorb excess food. This is certainly so for some babies, especially those who are breast fed. Hooper (1965, 1971) considers that it is the bottle fed baby who is especially at risk for overfeeding, and found that in his practice these babies are consistently heavier than those that are breast fed. It seems that this may be due to the higher protein concentration in cows' milk and to the fact that infants fed on cows' milk retain greater quantities of nitrogen and minerals such as potassium and sodium, but Hooper (1965) considers it primarily due to the fact that bottle fed babies are simply fed more milk 'to keep them quiet'. Helping the mother and father to find alternative ways of ensuring a quiet, contented baby other than by feeding can be difficult, particularly in the midst of the family stresses that are inevitable with the arrival of the first child. The use of a pacifier (dummy) should be considered, but not one that contains fruit juice because of the likelihood of developing subsequent dental caries.

It is important to gain the co-operation and confidence of the young mother in the early months as once poor feeding habits are established, particularly those leading to obesity, they are very likely to become a life long problem (Asher, 1966).

OBESITY

Asher (1966) found that 44 per cent of overweight children had been overweight since infancy and stated that in these children dietetic treatment was particularly unsuccessful. Eid (1970) found that weight gain in infancy was a better guide to the risk of obesity in later childhood than was the weight of the parents. Hirsch *et al* (1966) found in studies of biopsy material that there was a threefold increase in the number of adipose cells in subcutaneous tissues in fat as compared with lean individuals. Once established the cell number remains constant, and only the size of the cell varies with fluctuations in weight. They state that this constancy, despite weight loss, may account for the liability to relapse. The increased cell number appears to occur early in life, but it is not known whether the pattern is inherited or whether it is caused by overeating.

Defining clinical obesity in childhood is difficult and most authors state that if a child looks obese, he is. Measurement of height and weight can certainly be of some use when compared with the weight graphs produced by Tanner *et al* (1966). Unfortunately many obviously obese children will come within normal limits of weight and height. Skinfold calipers can be of use in monitoring obesity and in assessing the efficacy of treatment.

Obese children tend to be taller than normal for their age. This tallness is, however, offset by the advance in bone age and the earlier epiphyseal union results in the height of the obese child being certainly no greater and often is less than that of their thinner companions. There is often earlier sexual maturation with its concomittant emotional problems. Obese children are also susceptible to increased respiratory infections (Tracy *et al*, 1971).

Brook (1973) lists a further series of disadvantages of obesity in childhood:

1. Striking hyperinsulinaemia and increased insulin response to oral glucose load.
2. Few obese children have an entirely normal glucose tolerance curve; it is rare for the blood sugar level at 2½ hours to have returned to base-line value.
3. They have subnormal responses of growth hormone to the usual stimulatory tests.
4. Raised levels of plasma non-esterified fatty acids.
5. Increased production of 17-hydroxycorticosteroids.

He states that these do not appear to be of immediate importance to the child but may contribute to long term morbidity. Hueneman (1968) states that the incidence of diabetes mellitus and cardiovascular disorders is highest in those adults who were obese as children.

In contradistinction to adult obesity, there is little evidence that psychological factors are of importance in the pathogenesis of childhood obesity, but the psychological consequences of obesity can be great (Silverstone, 1973). The obese are the least popular as playmates and companions and such relative unpopularity can lead to severe emotional consequences. In keeping with this is the finding that obese adolescent girls show many traits similar to those found among discriminated-against minority groups.

Prevention of obesity

There is no doubt that prevention is better than cure and certainly it is considered a lot easier. Eid (1970) suggests not introducing cereal until after the first month, advising parents not to start the sweet eating habits and not to encourge constant eating between meals (e.g. potato crisps). Besides encouraging the mother in this way the general practitioner and health visitor together should carefully monitor the weight gain of the young babies in the practice. The use of charts such as the one designed by Dr H.J. Wright which can be obtained from the Royal College of General Practitioners, Central Information Unit, 14 Princes Gate, London SW7 IPV, make such monitoring easier. The knowledge that bottle fed babies are particularly at risk for obesity should alert health visitor and doctor to any excessive weight gain. Many doctors doubt the wisdom of regular weighing of babies, but there is no alternative to this if the prevention of obesity is to be taken seriously.

Dubois *et al* (1979), however, question the above conclusions after comparing a group of obese infants and a group of normal infants. They state that the current stereotype of the obese infant as one who is overfed, is given solids very young, is not breast fed, and whose mother is not responsive to his satiety signals, ought to be challenged. The model developed by Vuille *et al* (1979) to explain the aetiology of childhood obesity may help to explain these varying conclusions.

Treatment of obesity

It has been stated (Everley Jones,1972) that even with enthusiastic treatment only about 15 percent of patients have a five year success rate in the treatment of obesity. Treatment involves instruction in dietetics and restriction or carbohydrate. Most authorities accept that anorectic drugs have no place in the treatment of childhood obesity.

MALNUTRITION

Although mostly a problem for the 'third world', malnutrition may become apparent in a number of situations in the United Kingdom. There it is very rarely the result of insufficient food being available; rather it is poor education as to the ideal diet for the child. A degree of malnutrition can occur in breast fed babies where the mother is striving to achieve the ideal but the baby does not gain weight and cries almost continually. A few test weighings will quickly point to the cause of the problem and increasing the frequency of feeding or the addition of artificial feeding will rectify this problem. The relationship of malnutrition in childhood to poverty is discussed in Chapter 43.

The discovery of rickets in Indian and Pakistani communities in the United Kingdom is another indication of malnutrition. Nordin (1974) describes this as being surprisingly common and alarmingly widespread, and Ford *et al* (1972) found that 24 per cent of the Pakistani adults and children they examined in Glasgow showed evidence of vitamin D deficiency.

Various suggestions as to why this occurs have been made. Some have suggested that the dark skin makes the Asian more dependent upon dietary vitamin D and others that it is because they are more housebound that they receive less solar radiation. The relationships between vitamin D and dietary phytate has also been considered as a cause of rickets – the high phytate content of the Asian binding the calcium and preventing absorption. Ford *et al* (1972) suggest that high phytate intake may produce rickets only when both dietary and non-dietary sources of vitamin D are suboptimal.

In later childhood Lynch (1969) found that 25 per cent of his sample of 10 and 11 year olds went for 18 hours each day without a meal, eating nothing between the evening meal and lunch on the following day. Another study (Richardson and Lawson, 1972) showed that, among children not eating a school meal, only four per cent had a meal of comparable quality; four per cent had no lunch at all and the remainder brought food from home or bought snacks which were low in protein, iron and calcium and high in sugar.

Nutrition of this order is obviously indicative of poor education of parents. Thomas (1975) comments that national statistics on obesity, coronary heart disease, dental health and other nutrition-related health disorders indicate that a considerable amount of health education is required. General practitioners should take every opportunity to prevent poor nutrition in their patients.

REFERENCES

Asher, P. (1966) Fat babies and fat children. The prognosis of obesity in the very young. *Archives of Disease in Childhood*, **41**, 672.

Aylett, M.J. (1975) Who wants to breast feed and who succeeds? *Update*, **10**, 1133.

BMJ Editorial (1980) Nutrition in pregnancy. *British Medical Journal*, **1**, 1154.

Brandt, R.S. (1975) Fluoride and dental caries. *The Practitioner*, **214**, 388.

Brook, C.D.S. (1973) Fat Children. *British Journal of Hospital Medicine*, **10**, 30.

Cockburn, F. *et al* (1980) Maternal Vitamin D intake and mineral metabolism in mothers and their newborn infants. *British Medical Journal*, **2**. 11–14.

Dubois, S., Hill, D.E. & Beaton, G.H. (1979) An examination of factors believed to be associated with infantile obesity. *American Journal of Clinical Nutrition*, **32**, 1979.

Eid, E.E. (1970) Follow-up study of physical growth of children who had excessive weight gain in first six months of life. *British Medical Journal*, **2**, 74.

Everley Jones, H. (1972) The fat child. *The Practitioner*, **208**, 212.

Ford, J.A., Colhoun, E.M., McIntosh, W.B. & Dunnigan, M.G. (1972) Rickets and osteomalacia in the Glasgow Pakistani community. *British Medical Journal*, **2**, 677.

Hirsch, J., Knittle, J.L. & Salans, L.D. (1966) Cell lipid content and cell number in obese and non obese adipose tissue. *Journal of Clinical Investigation*, **45**, 1023.

Hooper, P.D. (1965) Infant feeding and its relationship to weight gain and illness. *The Practitioner*, **194**, 391.

Hooper, P.D. (1971) Infant morbidity and obesity. *The Practitioner*, **207**, 221.

Hueneman, R.L. (1968) *Public Health Reports*, **83**, 491.
Jacob, A. (1968) Infant feeding in East Scotland. *Journal of the Royal College of General Practitioners*, **16**, 327.
Lynch, G.W. (1969) Food intake and the education of children. *Medical Officer*, **121**, 41.
Martin, J. (1978) Infant Feeding 1975: attitudes and practice in England and Wales, H.M.S.O. London.
Newson, J. & Newson, E. (1965) *Patterns of Infant Care in an Urban Community*. London: Pelican Books.
Nordin, B.E.C. (1974) Calcium, phosphorus and vitamin D. In Symposium on nutrition. *The Practitioner*, **212**, 474.
Oates, R.K. (1973) Infant feeding practices. *British Medical Journal*, **2**, 762.
Palmer, S.R., Avery, A., & Taylor, R. (1979) The influence of obstetric procedures and social and cultural factors on breast feeding rates at discharge from hospital. *J. Epidemiology and Community Health*, **33**, 248.
Prothero, R. (1969) Women who still breast feed their babies. *Medical Officer*, **121**, 141.
Richardson, D.P. & Lawson, M. (1972) Nutritional value of mid-day meals of senior school children. *British Medical Journal*, **4**, 697.
Salariya, E.M., Easton, P.M. & Cater, J.I. (1978) Duration of Breast feeding after early initiation and frequent feeding. *Lancet*, **2**, 1141.
Silverstone, J.I. (1973) Psychological and social aspects of obesity. *British Journal of Hospital Medicine*, **10**, 39.
Sloper, K., McKean, L. & Baum, J.D. (1975) Factors in fluencing breast feeding. *Archives of Disease in Childhood*, **50**, 165.
Smith, D.V. (1969) Attitudes to breast feeding. *British Medical Journal*, **2**, 695.
Tanner, J.M., Whitehouse, R.H. & Takaishi, M. (1966) Standards from birth to maturity for height, weight, height velocity and weight velocity of British children, 1965. *Archives of Disease in Childhood*, **41**, 454.
Thomas, J.E. (1975) The nutritional component of health education. *The Health Education Journal*, **34**, 14.
Tracey, V.V., De, N.C. & Harper, J.R. (1971) Obesity and respiratory infection in infants and young children. *British Medical Journal*, **1**, 16.
Vuille, J.C. & Mellbin, T. (1979) Obesity in 10 year olds – an epidemiological study. *Pediatrics*, **64**, 564.
Welsh, J.K. & May, J.T. (1979) Anti-infective properties of breast milk. *J. Pediatrics*, **94**, 1.

28

Infestation with worms and insects

Neville Silverston

'Modern' doctors tend to be preoccupied with sophisticated diseases and it is easy for them to lose perspective that, in many of the tropical and sub-tropical lands of the world in which live the majority of mankind, parasitic infestations are still a cause of untold misery, suffering and even death.

The British general practitioner is frequently presented with parasitised children – indeed, there is little evidence that medicine has changed the situation greatly. Parasites always cause a degree of alarm and revulsion in the mind of the layman and reassurance, although time consuming, is always worth the effort.

WORMS

Parasitic worms have become modified to live within the gastrointestinal tract of the host, resistant to being digested and able to survive in an environment of low oxygen tension. Many worms have fascinating life cycles with stages passing through secondary hosts and one must marvel how such cycles, dependent as they are on a series of chance factors, first began. An intimate knowledge of the life cycle of each species is a prerequisite to its control.

In Britain, family doctors will find their experience of worm infestations to be limited mainly to threadworms but it is always important to bear in mind that immigrant children may be infested with parasites indigenous to their countries of origin (Thompson *et al*, 1972), and British travellers abroad, especially following safaris and overland treks to the East, may return home bringing a 'visitor' or two with them.

Occasionally, eosinophilia will be found when blood investigations of children are undertaken for purposes other than suspected worm infestations. A search for ova in the stools is then well worth while.

Threadworms (Enterobius vermicularis)

'The exceeding ytche in the fundament' Thomas Phaer, 1544.

Incidence

A multi-centre survey (Gatherer, 1978) of the incidence of infestation with threadworms showed the highest degree of infestation in seven to eight year olds – 30 per cent. Figure 28.1 shows the infestation rates for all groups. Interestingly, the prevalence appears to be commoner in girls, a fact noted previously (MacKeith and Watson, 1948; Gatherer, 1973); this suggests that the school lavatory seat may be a source of infestation.

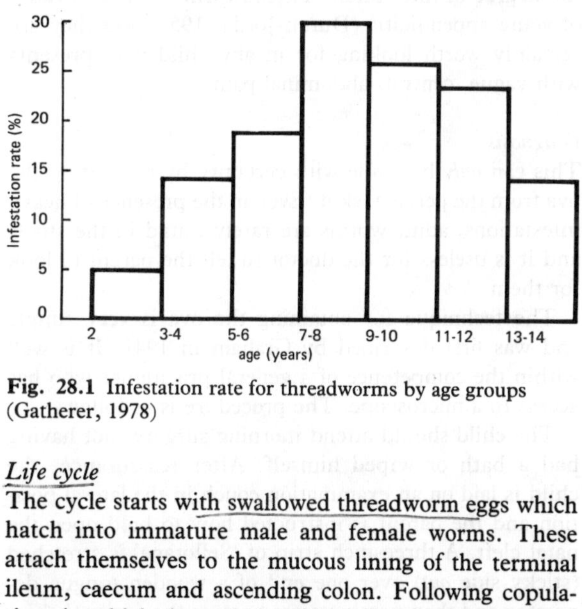

Fig. 28.1 Infestation rate for threadworms by age groups (Gatherer, 1978)

Life cycle

The cycle starts with swallowed threadworm eggs which hatch into immature male and female worms. These attach themselves to the mucous lining of the terminal ileum, caecum and ascending colon. Following copulation, in which the male is said to die, the female worm 8–13 mm long, laden with eggs, migrates down the large bowel and emerges from the anus, usually at night. Here it undergoes violent contractions, finally rupturing and depositing 10 000 to 15 000 ova around the perianal skin. The irritation causes the child to scratch himself and ova adhere to his fingers and also become embedded under the nails.

The ova are not immediately infective and require a minimum period of six hours at body temperature in the presence of humidity and oxygen. At lower temperatures this maturation may take up to 30 hours and in north Europe the ova can survive up to three weeks in dust. In hot dry air it is unlikely that they can survive for more than 48 hours (Gatherer, 1978).

Once transferred to the mouth and swallowed, the cycle starts again. Quite large numbers of eggs become distributed within the bed clothes and are dispersed during bed making into the atmosphere, finally settling with the dust. Counts of 7000 ova per square foot have been made on the floor under dormitory beds.

Symptoms

In the majority of cases there are no symptoms but it is not uncommon for an anxious mother to bring her child to the surgery after she has noticed a few worms in the child's stools or on the perianal skin. Many symptoms such as head banging, nightmares, teeth grinding and fits have been ascribed to threadworms but controlled trials have shown these to have no greater incidence in infested than in non-infested children. The only *real* symptom is pruritis ani and even this is most probably dependent more on the personality of the child than on the degree of infestation. Threadworms may be a cause of acute appendicitis (Duran-Jorda, 1957) and they are certainly worth looking for in any child who presents with vague, central, abdominal pain.

Diagnosis

This can *only* be made with certainty by recovering the ova from the perianal skin. Even in the presence of heavy infestations, adult worms are rarely found in the stools and it is useless for the doctor to tell the parent to look for them

The technique for obtaining the ova is very simple and was first described by Graham in 1941. It is well within the competence of a general pracitioner who has access to a microscope. The procedure is as follows:

The child should attend morning surgery, not having had a bath or wiped himself. After reassurance, the child is laid on an examination couch in the lateral position and the parent is instructed how to hold open the natal cleft. A three inch strip of 'Sellotape' is stretched (sticky side *out*) over one end of a wooden tongue depressor and then firmly pressed across the perianal skin. The 'Sellotape' is then pressed (sticky side *down*) on to a microscope slide. The characteristic oval eggs, looking so regular in the amorphous debris, easily stand out under the low power.

Treatment

The piperazine compounds have been the standard treatment for the past quarter of a century and act by narcotising the worm. In practice, a combination of piperazine phosphate, 4 g, with standardised senna 0.18 g made up in the form of a powder (Pripsen) and dissolved in milk or water to make a palatable drink, is effective in 90 per cent of cases (White and Scopes, 1960). The dose is a complete sachet for children over six years old, two-thirds of a sachet for children between one and six years old and one third of a sachet for infants between three and twelve months. All members living in a household should be treated at the same time, and, in theory at least, the treatment should be repeated a fortnight later in order to eliminate any worms which have developed from ova after the first treatment. Some children do have mild abdominal pain next day and most have three or four loose motions.

The very effective vermicide, viprinium embonate (Vanquin) was withdrawn from the U.K. market in 1979 due to limited demand, price regulations and manufacturing licence legislation factors (personal communication).

The anthelmentic drugs merbendazole (Vermox) and thiabendazole (Mintezol) are very effective against threadworms (Foy, 1977). Merbendazole is well tolerated but should not be given to children of two years or under. Otherwise, it is given in a standard dose of 100 mg bd for three days and should be repeated a week later. Thiabendazole is less well tolerated but does have the advantage that it is ovicidal, dispensing with the need for second treatment. The dose is calculated on the basis of 25 mg per kg and is given for three days.

More recently, a single dose of levamisole (Ketrax) has been found to give a cure rate equal to that of the piperazine compounds but it not without mild side effects (Omer, 1978). The dose is 40 mg for children under three years, 60 mg for children between three and nine years and 80 mg for older children and adults.

Roundworms (Ascaris lumbricoides)

This is the commonest worm found in man for it thrives in areas of poor sanitation and in countries where raw human faeces are used as an agricultural fertiliser. For these reasons, it has become a rarety in Britain. It resembles a pale yellow or pink earthworm, 20–35 cm long, and the passing of one of these is the signal for great alarm. The child, usually wrapped in a blanket, and the worm, wrapped in toilet tissue, are conveyed post haste to the doctor's surgery!

Life cycle

The adult worm lives free in the small bowel and the females are reputed to lay about 250 000 eggs a day which pass out with the faeces. The worms cannot multiply within the host. On the ground, the ova can survive for many years and are not destroyed by the usual methods of sewage disposal. Under favourable conditions they embryonate into the infective forms which are equally resistant to destruction. When swallowed, the larvae penetrate the intestinal wall and are carried in the blood stream to the lungs where they penetrate the alveoli, undergo a moulting stage and finally ascend the trachea as far as the pharynx where they are once again swallowed. In the small bowel they develop into the adult form.

Symptoms

These are in direct proportion to the worm burden which, when heavy, can give rise to intestinal colic or even small bowel obstruction. During the invasion stage, respiratory symptoms in the form of scattered areas of haemorrhagic pneumonitis with haemoptyses, rigors and bronchospasm may occur.

Diagnosis

This is dependent upon finding the ova in a stool specimen. The Public Health Laboratory Service will carry out this examination but, if in doubt about any form of worm infestations, stool specimens should be sent to the laboratories of the hospitals specialising in tropical diseases which are situated in London, Birmingham, Liverpool and Edinburgh.

Treatment

The salts of piperazine are the drugs of choice and Pripsen, given as a single dose without prior fasting, gives excellent results.

Whipworms (Trichuris trichiuria)

These are of world wide distribution and with roundworms and hookworms form the so-called 'trinity of worms'. Their dissemination is related both to the use of raw sewage as a fertiliser and the absence of latrine facilities. It must now be a rare disease among the indigenous population of Britain, but a survey of a village in East Anglia (Silverston, 1962) revealed that 40 per cent of the families who emptied their nightsoil on their vegetable gardens were infested with these worms. The whipworm resembles the threadworm in size but is distinguished by possessing a long anterior whiplike process by which it attaches itself to the mucosal lining of the caecum and the adjacent large bowel.

Life cycle

The females pass great quantities of eggs and counts in excess of 75 000 ova per gram of faeces are not uncommon. On the ground, the ova embryonate until an infective stage is reached after about three weeks. When swallowed, these develop into the adult worms in the small intestine.

Symptoms

There are usually no symptoms unless the child is heavily infested when diarrhoea ('whipworm dysentery') may result.

Diagnosis

This is dependent upon visualising the characteristic ova in the stools. The Public Health Laboratory Service will carry out this examination on request.

Treatment

The anthelmentic merbendazole (Vermox) is the drug of choice and is given to all patients over two years old in a standard dose of 100 mg bd for three days. An alternative drug is thiabendazole (Mintezol) given at a dose of 25 mg/kg bd for three days. The worms are difficult to eliminate completely.

Hookworms

There are two types of hookworms. *Ankylostoma duodenale* which is found around the Mediterranean, the Middle East, the Indian sub-continent and South-East Asia and *Necator americanus* which is found in South America, the West Indies, Central Africa and also in South-East Asia. They are a common finding in immigrant people from these areas and will undoubtedly be an increasing problem in British holidaymakers returning from countries where the disease is endemic.

Life cycle

The hookworm produces ova at a prodigious rate which pass out with the faeces. On the ground, the eggs 'hatch' to produce larvae and these develop rapidly into the infective filariform stage which can penetrate the intact skin, enter the venous blood system and are carried to the lungs where they enter the alveoli, ascend the respiratory tree as far as the pharynx where they are swallowed. In the small bowel they attach themselves to the mucosal wall by their large mouth.

Symptoms

At the point of entry of the larvae into the skin a local dermatitis ('ground itch') may be set up. Once in the large bowel, the symptoms depend very much on the number of worms present. They can cause diarrhoea associated with epigastric pain and tenderness. However, the most important symptom is a debilitating, iron deficiency anaemia, for *each* worm consumes blood at the rate of 0.05 ml per day. A moderate degree of infestation is 100 to 500 worms, i.e. a daily loss of 5 to 25 ml of blood. This causes quite a severe degree of hypoalbumenaemia in children with a development of oedema, puffy facies and a pot belly.

Diagnosis
This is dependent upon visualising the characteristic ova in the stools. This examination will be carried out by the Public Health Laboratory Service.

Treatment
The compound bephenium hydroxynaphthoate (Alcopar) is the drug of choice and is a safe and effective treatment both against hookworms and roundworms. The dose is 5 gm daily given on an empty stomach for three days. Children should be given half this dose. Alternatively, a single dose treatment with 150 mg levamizole (Ketrax) has given cure rates of 100 per cent and 93 per cent for ascarus and A. duodenale respectively (Farid et al, 1977). For N. americanus infestations, thiabendazole is said to be more effective than bephenium to which it has relative resistance (Omer, 1978).

Visceral larva migrans
This disease is due to the ingestion by man of the eggs of the dog and cat roundworm, *Toxocara canis* and *Toxocara catis*. Infestation with this roundworm is common in both animals especially in puppies and kittens which can become infected *in utero* . The combination of a crawling child with an untrained, worm infested puppy must be very common both in and around the house and in public parks. Once in the human gut, the *Toxocara* ova develop into the larval forms which penetrate the intestinal wall and are carried in the blood stream to various organs where they become encysted. Severe *visceral larva migrans* can present with hepatomegaly, eosinophilia and an irregular fever. Should the larva become arrested in the eye, it sets up a granulomatous reaction indistinguishable clinically from a retinoblastoma and the eye may be enucleated. There is evidence that the disease may be a cause of epilepsy (Woodruff, 1970). The diagnosis can be difficult. The indirect fluorescent antibody test or specific skin test can be helpful in making the diagnosis, although these may give a positive reaction in about two per cent of the British population (Denham *et al*, 1971).

INSECTS

Parasitic skin infestations are quite commonly seen in general practice in Britain and, indeed, the incidence would seem to be increasing. The two main types found are the louse of which there are three species (the head louse, the body louse and the pubic louse) and scabies.

Head louse
Infestation with the head louse (Pediculus humanis capitis) is still common. But, because it is not a notifiable disease, the degree of infestation in the community is not accurately known. A survey commissioned by the Health Education Council in 1975 calculated by extrapolation that almost 200 000 school children in England were infested with head lice. The infestation rates by geographical location and type of school are shown in Figure 28.2 and by age and sex in Figure 28.3 (Donaldson, 1976).

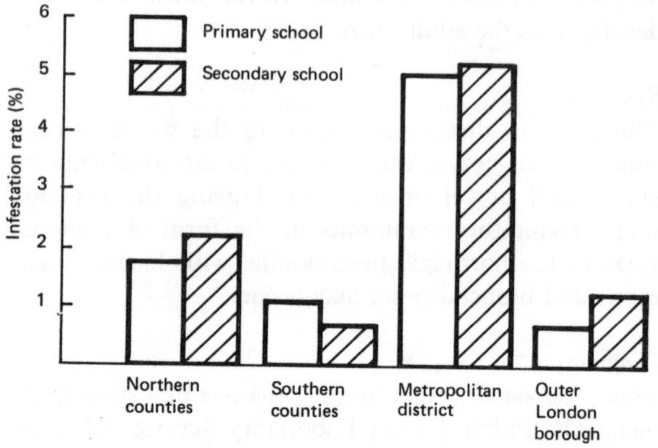

Fig. 28.2 Topographical variations in the infestation rate of head lice (Donaldson, 1976)

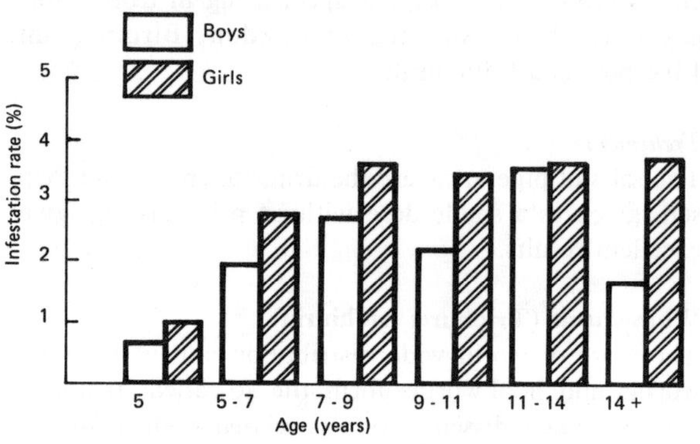

Fig. 28.3 Age and sex variations in the infestation rate of head lice (Donaldson, 1976)

The human louse is specific to man but anatomical differences exist between forms infesting various races (Buxton, 1947). For example those found in negroes' hair are themselves black and their claws are specialised to grip negroes' hair which, unlike that in Caucasian races, is oval in cross section. Even the Chinese and North American Indians have their own specific head lice – a fact of demographic interest.

The louse lives on the scalp from which it sucks blood, injecting saliva in the process. It is probably the allergic reaction to this that causes the irritation which is the principal symptom. The average infestation is remarkably light – about ten adults and a few younger ones. They live for about a month and during this time the female, which outnumbers the male by two to one, lays about 300 eggs (nits). These are about the size of a pin head and are very firmly glued to the shaft of a hair close to the scalp. A minimum temperature of 22°C is needed for hatching which, under optimum conditions, takes seven to ten days.

By carefully measuring the position of the most distant nit on a hair pulled out by its root, the length of time of the infestation can roughly be gauged, based on the assumption that hair grows at the rate of 1.25 cm per month. Hence a nit found 10 cm along the hair was probably laid eight months previously. The spread from one person to another is not fully understood. It is often alleged that hats, shared combs and the backs of chairs can be inanimate vectors but the evidence suggests that such lice are probably dying and constitute little danger (Maunder, 1977).

Secondary infection may supervene with the development of impetigenous lesions and it is important to look for head lice in any child presenting with painful occipital lymph nodes.

Diagnosis

With high degrees of infestation the lice and nits can be seen without difficulty, but in carrying out a survey of children, many of whom may be without symptoms, it is important to use a Sacker comb which is a carefully designed fine metal comb with spaces between its teeth corresponding in size to that of a human hair. At the base of each tooth the metal is ground to form a sharp blade and the nits are caught between the teeth and the hair is cut off painlessly below the egg.

Treatment

For many years DDT and gamma benzene hexachloride (Quellada, Lorexane) were the drugs of choice but there is evidence that many lice in this country have become resistant to these organochlorine insecticides (Maunder, 1971). Furthermore, DDT is now banned as it does not undergo biological degradation and gamma BHC does not kill the louse egg.

The treatment of choice is Malathion (Erskine, 1978). It is an organo phosphate/chlorine preparation widely used in horticulture and is available both in the form of a lotion (Derbac liquid, Prioderm) and also as a shampoo (Prioderm). Whilst a shampoo seems an elegant treatment, higher cure rates result from the lotion being carefully applied and left overnight to be followed by a mild shampoo in the morning. It is not necessary to remove the dead lice and nits with a Sacker comb after treatment. Used in this way, Malathion has a residual effect lasting about six weeks (Maunder, 1971).

An alternative organo phosphate preparation is carbaryl which is also available as a 0.5 per cent lotion (Carylderm) and a one per cent shampoo (Suleo, Derbac shampoo).

In waging war on the louse, the whole family should be treated and the doctor's role, in addition to being a therapeutic one, should also be educational. It should never be forgotten that a reservoir of infestation frequently exists in the pre-school child and the health visitor should visit each home – and not forget to examine granny. Once a case has been discovered in the practice, the general practitioner should inform the Specialist in Community Medicine who should, through the school medical officers, set in motion the examination of the other children in the school.

The manufacturers of Prioderm (Napp Laboratories Ltd, Watford, Herts WD2 7RA) make available very useful pamphlets which can be given to patients and which explain the nature of the disease and its treatment. The manufacturers of Derbac (Bengue & Co Ltd, St Ives House, Maindenhead, Berks SL6 1RD) make a cheap version of the Sacker comb which patients can purchase over the counter (Priddy, 1976).

Body louse

The body louse (*Pediculus humanis corporis*) is larger than its near relative the head louse and lays its eggs in the seams of clothes. Its presence is only found in the families of vagabonds and nomadic caravan dwellers and others who rarely wash or change their clothes. It is susceptible to gamma BHC and Malathion but, obviously, the management should be directed to the underlying social conditions.

Pubic louse

The pubic or crab louse (Phthirus pubis) is the commonest of all the human lice but, being mainly sexually transmitted, it is rare in children. Maunder (1977) maintains that one per cent of head lice infestation in children is caused by the crab louse but the author has yet to see a case. There have been rare cases of the louse being found on the eyelashes and eyebrows of breast fed infants (Ronchese, 1953).

SCABIES

The discovery in 1687 of the itch mite (*Sarcoptes scabiei*) marked scabies as being the first disease of man with a known cause (Friedman, 1947). As an infestation, it has lowered the morale of armies and sapped the initiative of their commanders.

The adult female is 0.3 mm long and slightly resembles a minute tortoise. The male is about one third this size. The female burrows into the skin by raising its posterior end on the bristles of its hind legs until it is almost standing on its head. It burrows vertically through the skin and then continues parallel to the skin depositing eggs behind it. The rate of burrowing is from one to five mm per day and, classically, these are seen as dark grey or black ridges 5–15 mm long, usually curved or S shaped.

After a few days the eggs hatch and the larvae emerge to the surface where they form their own burrows and undergo a number of moults before reaching adulthood. The burrows of these immature forms are frequently associated with the development of discrete vesicles. Thus it can be seen that the infestation can only be spread from one person to another when a gravid female becomes transferred and, therefore, close person to person contact is necessary (Carslaw, 1976).

Incidence

There is a curious cyclical fluctuation in the incidence of scabies throughout the world with epidemics occurring about every 15 years (Orkin, 1971). In this country, towards the end of the Second World War, scabies accounted for 15 per cent of cases attending dermatology outpatients but by 1953 it had fallen to one per cent (Shrank and Alexander, 1967). In the past 10 years, the incidence has increased markedly, suggesting that the immunity in the community has waned. There is also a seasonal incidence with peaks in January, April and November.

Symptoms

Intractable, generalised itching is the most obvious manifestation and starts four to six weeks after contracting the disease. It is probably a hypersensitivity phenomenon (Mellanby, 1943) and is considerably worse at night. The distribution of the mite on the skin is not influenced by the site of the initial infestation. The burrows should be looked for between the fingers, on the volar aspects of the wrists and around the axillary folds. Looked at under a hand lens, a few minute scales at one end of the 'run' indicates the point of entry and a reddish papule at the other indicates the presence of the acarus.

The lesions can be found over a wide area of the body but, *except in the case of infants*, they are rarely found on the palms, soles, face, scalp or on the back. A large variety of different lesions are seen in scabies and the disease can mimic many other conditions. Most commonly, there are papules, vesicles, pustules and the secondary infection resulting from excoriation. Sometimes, the reaction about the burrow leads to the formation of an elongated red papule. Occasionally, eczematization occurs in infants and young children and even bullous lesions resembling pemphigus can be found (Bean, 1974).

Diagnosis

Unfortunately, the diagnosis of scabies in infants and children is often long delayed, the most common reason being the low index of suspicion (Alexander, 1969; Herwitz, 1973). The diagnosis should always be suspected in a child who is itching and, if there is a characteristic distribution of the lesions with some suggestion of symmetry, the index of suspicion is strengthened. A careful history and examination of the parents and siblings should provide the essential clues. The ultimate proof rests on finding the burrows and the discrete vesicles in characteristic sites and extracting the mite from its burrow on the end of a needle. This is not always possible and a useful technique is to 'shave' along the length of a burrow or the roof of a vesicle with a scalpel blade drawing it along and keeping the blade parallel to the skin. The scraping is placed on a slide with a drop of 40 per cent caustic potash and covered with a glass cover slip. The preparation is warmed gently over a flame for a few seconds and then examined under the low power of the microscope when the mite or the eggs are often clearly seen. The whole procedure takes only a minute and the reward can be gratifying and well worth the trouble.

Treatment

This is relatively simple. The following preparations are equally effective:

1. Benzyl benzoate, 25 per cent emulsion.
2. Gamma benzene hexachloride 0.1 per cent lotion (Quellada, Lorexane).
3. Monosulfiram 25 per cent in alcoholic base (Tetmosol) which should be diluted one part to three parts of water immediately before use.
4. Malathion 0.5 per cent (Prioderm, Derbac).

It is important to emphasise to the parent that the whole body surface below the collar and including the external genitalia should be meticulously treated. In the case of infants with lesions on the face and scalp, these areas should be similarly treated with the same strength medication but great care taken to avoid the eyes.

The treatment should be given on two consecutive nights immediately after a warm bath. The application should be allowed to dry on the skin. Following this, clothing and night attire can be laundered in the usual manner. It is important to treat the underlying scabies before paying attention to complications, although, of course, if widespread secondary infection is present, an appropriate antibiotic should be administered.

REFERENCES

Alexander, J.O.D. (1969) Scabies in children. *Clinical Paediatrics*, **8**, 73–85.

Bean, S.F. (1974) Bullous scabies. *Journal of the American Medical Association*, **230**, 878.

Buxton, P.A. (1947) *The Louse*, 2nd edn. London: Arnold.

Carslaw, R.W. (1976) Skin infestation. *The Practitioner*, **216**, 154–158.

Coates, K.G. (1971) Control of head infestation in children. *Community Medicine*, **126**, 148–149.

Denham, D.A., Ridley, D.S. & Voller, A. (1971) Immunodiagnosis of parasitic diseases. *The Practitioner*, **207**, 191–196.

Donaldson, R.J. (1976) The head louse in England. *Royal Society of Health Journal*, **96**(2), 55–57.

Duran-Jorda, F. (1957) Appendicitis and enterobiasis in children. *Archives of Disease in Childhood*, June, 208–215.

Erskine, D. (1978) Dealing with lice. *Prescribers' Journal*, **18**(2), 42–48.

Farid, Z., Bassily, S., Milner, W.F., Hassan, A. & Laughlin, L.W. (1977) Comparitive single/dose treatment of hookworm and roundworm infections with levamisole, pyrantel and bephenium. *Journal of Tropical Medicine & Hygiene*. **80**(5), 107–108.

Foy, J.M. (1977) The Chemotherapy of enterobiasis (threadworms). *Pharmacology Journal*, **218**, 320–322.

Friedman, R. (1947) The Story of Scabies. New York: Froben Press.

Gatherer, A. (1973) Threadworms. *Health and Social Service Journal*. Nov. 10th.

Gatherer, A. (1978) A common problem. *Nursing Times*, **74**(41), 303–304.

Graham, C.F. (1941) *American Journal of Tropical Medicine*, **20**, 377.

Hurwitz, S. (1973) Scabies in babies. *American Journal of Diseases of Childhood*, **126**, 226–228.

MacKeith, R. & Watson, J.M. (1948) The diagnosis and treatment of threadworm infestation. *The Practitioner*, **160**, 264–270.

Maunder, J.W. (1971) Resistance to organochlorine insecticides in head lice and trials using alternative compounds. *Medical Officer*, **125**, 27–29.

Maunder, J.W. (1977) Parasites and Man. Human lice—biology and control. *Royal Society of Health Journal*, **97**(1), 29–32.

Mellanby, K. (1941) Incidence of head lice in England. Medical Officer, **65**, 39–43.

Omer, S.H.A. (1978) Intestinal worms. *Medicine*, **3**(6), 281–288.

Orkin, M. (1971) Resurgence of scabies. *Journal of the American Medical Association*, **230**, 593–597.

Phaer, T. (1544) *Boke of Children*. p. xiii.

Priddy, R.F. (1976) Head lice infestation. A practical approach. *Journal of Maternal and Child Health*, **1**, 38–41.

Ronchese, F. (1953) Treatment of pediculosis in children. *New England Journal of Medicine*, **249**, 897–898.

Silverston, N.A. (1962) Whipworms in a Cambridgeshire village. *British Medical Journal*, **2**, 1726–1728.

Shrank, A.B. & Alexander, S.L. (1967) Scabies: another epidemic? *British Medical Journal*, **1**, 669–671.

Thompson, R.G., Hutchinson, J.G.P. & Johnston, N.M. (1972) Survey of intestinal pathogens from immigrant children. *British Medical Journal*, **1**, 591–594.

White, R.H. & Scopes, J.W. (1960) A single dose treatment of threadworms in children. *Lancet*, **1**, 256–258.

29

Some common skin disorders

Denis Dean

INCIDENCE

Many childhood skin disorders are treated at home without medical supervision. Accurate incidence rates are therefore impossible to determine but some indication of the general practitioner's involvement may be gained from the following table of episode rates in 1970–71 (Table 29.1).

NOTES ON DIAGNOSIS AND TREATMENT

It cannot be stressed too strongly that one should not be pushed into a diagnosis. Because the skin is there for all to see, one is expected to make an instant diagnosis. Although this is often possible, and it becomes more so with experience, if a diagnosis is not obvious it is not an indication for despair. The exercise of history, examination and investigation should be gone through. Treatment should not be undertaken until at least a tentative diagnosis has been made.

In general practice, even more than instant diagnosis, the patient expects instant treatment. The temptation to give this must be avoided. A large element in the successful management of paediatric skin conditions is the gaining and maintaining of the confidence of the parent. If the doctor transmits to the mother the impression that he is uncertain of the diagnosis, and backs this up by the presentation of the latest drug firm sample and a 'try this', the battle is lost.

Table 29.1 Episode rates for some common skin disorders of childhood in selected general practices in England and Wales, 1970–1971. From *Morbidity Statistics from General Practice* (1974) HMSO

Disorder	*Episodes per 1000 patients* All ages	Ages 0–4	Ages 5–14
All skin and subcutaneous disorders	136.5	214.3	149.9
Viral warts	12.0	4.6	42.2
Fungal infections	5.1	4.8	6.8
Boils and carbuncles	12.1	8.8	15.2
Cellulitis of fingers and toes	7.2	8.8	9.2
Other cellulitis and abscesses	7.6	6.4	7.1
Impetigo	8.0	25.8	23.7
Other skin infections	8.2	11.8	10.1
Seborrhoeic dermatitis	4.4	8.4	3.4
Eczema and dermatitis – specific allergens	9.0	21.2	5.6
Other eczema (including infantile)	28.4	79.0	24.7
Psoriasis	3.5	0.7	2.2
Pruritis	7.2	4.1	2.7
Diseases of nails	2.1	1.7	2.2
Diseases of hair	1.9	1.8	1.7
Diseases of sweat and sebaceous glands	3.6	1.5	2.4
Acne vulgaris	1.5	0.1	7.6
Urticaria	8.7	15.1	14.0
Apyrexial rash	7.0	27.0	9.3
Pyrexia with rash	1.0	5.7	1.7

INFANTILE (ATOPIC) ECZEMA

This is an inborn condition and is often associated with asthma in the so-called asthma/eczema syndrome. It is the example *par excellance* where the parents as well as the child have to be treated. It is very important to grasp the nettle firmly when one is first consulted about this problem, which may or may not have been treated before. Two or three consultations will be required to get the situation under control. The child will be fractious, irritable, and tend to sleep badly. If the condition has been going for some time, the mother may well be distraught. If the child is old enough he will realise that he can play up the eczema to gain his own ends. The condition is rarely, if ever, seen before 12 weeks of age, and tends to get better as the child gets older.

Treatment

The mother

The explanation to the mother should indicate that:

1. The doctor knows well the condition with which he is dealing.
2. There is no immediate magic cure.
3. It will improve as time goes on.
4. The symptoms can be kept to a minimum if instructions are followed.
5. It may well, in later life, go completely.

One should make sure that the mother understands the treatment and *how, where and when* the applications should be applied. Advice should be given about bathing, clothing and when to come again and see the doctor (continued care is most important).

The child

Bathing. When the outer layer of the skin has been abraded water may be drawn into the cells by osmosis, disrupting them and producing vesicles and an exacerbation of the eczema. Because of this it used to be common to advise bathing the skin with oil instead of water, but this was of no great help as it reduced the exudation of the normal skin secretions and increased the tendency to superficial infection. The addition of emulsifying ointment BP, to the bath water, gives the water an emollient property. About one ounce of emulsifying ointment should be 'creamed' with a little water and tipped into the bath. This will form a scum on the top of the bath water, which may safely be rubbed into the dry area. Soap should be used very sparingly and any medicated or scented soaps, completely avoided. Dirty areas of the skin may be cleaned by rubbing emulsifying ointment in and 'creaming' by the slow addition of water.

Medication. Generally speaking weeping areas should be treated with a lotion and dry areas with paste. Lotio Plumbi Co BP mixed with an equal amount of boiled milk is a suitable astringent lotion.

The two most suitable pastes to use are one per cent crude coal tar in zinc oxide paste, or half per cent ichthyol in zinc oxide paste. The crude coal tar or the ichthyol may be added to Lassars paste, but it should be remembered that Lassars paste contains a small amount of salycilic acid and is therefore mildly keratolytic. Coltapaste (or in cases of intolerance, Ichthopaste) bandages are most useful for the limbs and may be applied to be worn continuously or just at night to prevent excoriation by scratching. The bandage is originally moist, but even after drying may be used again and again. It is sometimes preferable to put on the bandage in its dry state and one would advise that lengths of bandage are stretched out onto newspaper and allowed to dry before application. If there is *any* sign of weeping, vesiculation or infection, occlusive dressings must *not* be used.

Steroids The overuse and abuse of topical steroids, particularly of the fluorinated variety, has caused dermatological opinion to swing against their use, and in some circles their use at all is openly condemned. They do have a place in the treatment of infantile eczema, but should not be used extensively or over long periods. Use should be confined to the bad areas, or to any bad patches on the face. The principles of treatment with steroids should be:

1. To use the preparation in an acceptable vehicle.
2. When resolution is obtained to tail off the use of the steroid, either by less frequent application or reduction in strength.
3. Not to chop and change the application in the hope that another preparation will do better.
4. Not to persist too long with the therapy.

'Seborrhoeic' eczema of children

This is characterised by weeping, crusting, red patches in folds and behind the ears. There may be a history of cradle cap and intolerance to wool. It arises at any time, and is not constitutional.

Management

Practical points: avoid chafeing and woollen garments.

Therapy:

3% Aureomycin ointment	15 g	mixed
Lassars paste	100 g	together

or

3% Aureomycin ointment	equal parts
1% Hydrocortisone ointment	of each mixed
Zinc Oxide ointment BP	together

Napkin rash

Three broad divisions:

1. Simple irritant dermatitis.

2. Secondary infection, either (a) pyogenic, or (b) fungal.
3. Seborrhoeic.

General care
It is worth pointing out to the mother that this is not caused by 'strong urine', and that fresh urine does *not* smell of ammonia. Bacteria must have had an opportunity to break it down to ammonia, and therefore there must have been bacteria present on the napkin or the skin for some time for this to have occurred.

Advice about washing napkins. There is no substitute for boiling napkins to sterilise them. They should be washed in good quality soap flakes and rinsed thoroughly. Nappy liners or 'Harrington' squares will make things much more comfortable for the child. Rubber or plastic pants should never be used. Care with washing the napkin area should be stressed, paying particular attention to the folds of the skin, drying carefully and using a little good quality dusting powder. Silicone barrier cream may also be used, if the skin is not broken.

If the napkin rash becomes secondarily infected either with pyogenic organisms or with candida it may become successively more red, scaly, vesicular and ultimately ulcerated. A badly excoriated inflamed napkin area may well cause a little secondary eczema to appear elsewhere on the body. This should not be confused with an atopic eczema. The secondary eczema will disappear when the napkin rash has been treated.

Treatment of an infected napkin rash. General care as above (silicone barrier cream not to be used if the skin is broken).

Medication In a mild case half per cent ichthyol in zinc oxide paste may be all that is needed. It should be explained to the mother that the paste is the consistency of putty and should be taken between the finger and thumb, softened and spread directly on to the baby's skin. Removal may be aided by the application of emulsifying ointment during a bath. More severe cases may warrant the use of a topical antibiotic, either three per cent. Aureomycin in Lassars paste as above, or if the infected organism is thought to be candida, Nystatin cream may be used, or a mixture of

Nystatin ointment 3% Aureomycin ointment Zinc oxide ointment	} equal parts mixed together

When the condition begins to settle down, half per cent ichthyol in zinc oxide paste is advised.

Seborrhoeic or 'psoriatic' type of napkin rash. This looks not unlike an adult psoriasis confined to the napkin area; some authorities believe that it is related, and that in later life the child may develop psoriasis.

Treatment for this is as for secondarily infected napkin rash, since there is often a candida element present.

The use of steroids in the treatment of napkin rash. There is no doubt that topical steroids will help to settle an inflammatory condition more quickly, but they should be used over a short time only and with adequate control, i.e. seeing the child again in a few days and turning to more bland applications as the condition improves. Nystaform HC both in ointment and in lotion form is a useful preparation, remembering once more that lotions are particularly useful on weeping areas. Lotio Plumbi Co. mixed with an equal quantity of boiled milk is a very useful bland astringent lotion.

Papular urticaria
The lesions of this very common condition are very easy to recognise, with groups of wheals accompanied by small papules. They persist for a few days and occur in crops. It is generally accepted that they are due to sensitivity to the bite of fleas from dogs, cats or birds. It usually occurs in children between the ages of two and seven. This is thought to be due to the fact that under the age of two sensitivity has not developed, and over the age of seven some desensitisation has occurred due to repeated bites. Local application of calamine lotion with one per cent phenol added as an anti-pruritic is suitable. An antihistamine by mouth will also help. Both are merely symptomatic remedies. If there is a pet in the household its bedding and fur should be dusted with a proprietary flea powder. Birds are more difficult to deal with and some persistent cases have been traced to the mites co-existing on birds nesting in the eaves of the patient's house.

Note: There is no place for local application of antihistamine creams in these cases – or indeed at all. The high degree of sensitivity these preparations produce precludes their use.

Warts
Almost all children have warts at some time. They fall into three categories, the common wart, the plane wart, and plantar warts or verrucas.

Common wart
This is due to inoculation with a virus. The incubation period is long.

Treatment Most warts will disappear on their own if left long enough. Leaving alone is probably the best, but possibly the most difficult, path to pursue. If one is pressed to treat them there are four ways in which this may be done.

1. Paint the wart daily with six per cent Podophyllin in Tinct Benz Co., and after the first two or three applications use pumice or fine sand paper to rub down the surface of the wart and repaint.
2. More persistent warts may be treated with carbon

dioxide snow or carbon dioxide slush. In the surgery carbon dioxide snow may be conveniently made from a small apparatus which takes sparklet bulbs. In the apparatus a stick of solid CO_2 is produced, the end is accurately applied over the wart and held in place until a ring of frozen skin about one millimetre in thickness is seen around the stick. If the wart is small it is worth sharpening the CO_2 'pencil' so that it is accurately applied to the wart and not to the surrounding tissue. After a few days a small blister is formed, which pushes the wart off. If there is too long an exposure to the CO_2 blistering may be excessive, but no lasting damage is caused.

3. If one possesses a cautery machine and feels competent to use it, cauterisation of troublesome warts is a simple matter. A little local anaesthetic is inserted under the wart and the warty tissue burnt away with the cautery. It is worth remembering that the element of the cautery need not be red hot. A heat just less than this is sufficient and the patient will be far less apprehensive if he does not see a red hot cautery element approaching his skin.

4. Occlusion by elastoplast. A waterproof plaster is applied until maceration occurs and the wart is then carefully curetted away, with a small spoon curette.

Plane warts
These are numerous flat warts and because of their number cannot usually be treated as vigorously as individual warts. They are, however, said to be the most susceptible to treatment by charming.

Treatment. A small spot of Pig. Podoph. Co. is applied very accurately with an orange stick to each wart; there should be the strong suggestion that the warts will fall off, often accompanied by a little itching. Other coloured paints, such as Gentian Violet or Castellani's paint may be used in place of the Pig. Podoph. Co., with equally successful results, if it is applied accurately (giving the parent a positive job to do), and accompanied by very strong suggestions that the warts will fall off. It has been reported that itching does, in fact, occur before the warts undergo spontaneous remission and if it is mentioned, the suggestion may help a lot.

Plantar warts (verrucae)
Plantar warts seem to have become much more popular over the past ten years, due almost certainly to the fact that more children now go to swimming baths and indulge in free expression dancing and 'music and movement' in school halls in bare feet. There are two methods of dealing with these warts: (a) to dry them, (b) to allow them to become macerated.

The drying method. The affected area of the foot is soaked in a three per cent solution of formalin each night for 20 minutes. When the surface of the wart becomes dry, it should be rubbed with pumice or fine sand paper or pared down as far as possible, before subsequent soaking occurs. The patient can return to the doctor at fortnightly intervals when a little more energetic paring and reassurance can be carried out. If considerable drying out of the surrounding tissues occurs, a little vasoline is put on the foot, excluding just the area around the wart. If this treatment is to be successful it must be carried out properly and it is worth while having a small handout to give to the parent, pointing out the following:

1. The solution must be applied undiluted.
2. The foot is soaked in the solution in a dish (not dabbed on).
3. Fresh solution is used for each application.
4. The soak must be at least 20 minutes each night.

The advantage of this method of treatment is that the wart surface becomes sterile after the first few applications. It is best to suggest that this is a week and then the child can go swimming again.

The maceration method. A strong ointment of Podophyllin (Posalfillin) may be applied under plaster until maceration occurs and then the wart curretted out. This may well cause a little bit of sterile pus to form, but it does not mean that the condition is getting infected.

Cautery. Treatment with cautery is certainly possible, but it is not the treatment of choice for a child because of the discomfort of putting local anaesthetic into the sole of the foot.

Naevi
There are three common types: cavernous naevus, spider naevus, the port wine stain.

Cavernous naevus
This is usually present at birth and may appear to get larger during the first six months of life. It is best left alone, even if quite large and in a prominent site. Spontaneous disappearance is the rule, though it is often difficult to persuade the parents that this is so. Serial pictures of a naevus which has regressed may help to illustrate the point.

Spider naevus
The odd spider naevus is not uncommon in a child aged between six and twelve and can be treated with trichloracetic acid. The technique of treatment, which requires considerable care, is to sharpen an orange stick and dip it into a very concentrated solution (the acid is obtained in crystal form; it is deliquescent, and only a few drops of water are required to make the solution). The tip of the orange stick is then applied very accurately to the centre of the spider naevus. If the

point of application is correct, slight pressure will occlude the central vessel and the naevus will disappear from sight. The stick is gently rotated for a few moments and then removed. A small white speck is visible where the acid has been applied. Considerable care is required for this application, and trichloracetic acid should not be left around the surgery for anyone, other than the doctor, to use.

Port wine stain
Little can be done to improve the appearance of these, except covering them with a suitable cover cream.

Herpes simplex
Primary attack of herpes simplex is quite common in children and it may affect almost any site on the body. The characteristic herpetic lesions do not need to be described but these should be remembered as a diagnosis when a small crop of inflamed vesicles are seen in a young child. It is usually self limiting and the treatment is just to prevent secondary infection and help the drying process with local calamine lotion. See further, Chapter 22.

Pseudamina
The appearance in a new baby of very small vesicles scattered over the face, which appear to be more prominent at feeding time, is a very common condition. This is often mistaken for the early signs of an atopic eczema and not uncommonly has been treated with local steroids. The vesicles are, in fact, immature sweat glands and treatment is nothing other than regular washing and careful drying accompanied by strong reassurance that this is a normal conditions, and will disappear spontaneously.

Molluscum contagiosum
This is a virus infection, usually acquired at the swimming baths. It can be troublesome and often comes along in crops. It is frequently missed, but it is a once-seen-never-to-be-forgotten condition. The vesicles are characteristically umbilicated, but by no means invariably so. They tend to appear in small crops in a localised area. They should be left alone to regress, or the vesicle may be taken between the points of a Spencer Wells forceps and avulsed.

The ringed lesion
A child may well be brought to the surgery with a diagnosis of 'ringworm', made either by the parent or the school teacher and certainly in an urban practice the lesion is more commonly *not* that of ringworm. The common ring lesions are: granuloma annulare, impetigo, the herald patch of *Pityriasis rosea*, nummular eczema, ringworm.

Granuloma annulare
This is a slightly raised ringed lesion, usually on the hand or the foot, solitary, non-itchy, not scaly. It used to be said that biopsy of this caused regression, but in fact spontaneous remission is the rule and it is best left entirely alone. Some dermatologists inject the edge with a little hydrocortisone. This also is said cause regression.

Impetigo
This is a superficial infection which may be caused by the *Staphylococcus* or the *Streptococcus*. It starts with erythema, which quickly passes to the pustular stage. The pustules may become large blisters. This is usual in the staphylococcal type, (the more commonly seen). The most usual site for impetigo is the face. It is usually a primary infecton but may be associated with scabies, papular urticaria or pediculosis. If impetigo is seen in areas other than the face, the possibility of a concomittant infestation with scabies should be borne in mind.

Treatment. It should be possible to get impetigo under control in two or three days and achieve a very substantial improvement in the first 24 hours. It is wrong to give the latest antibiotic-steroid mixture and dismiss the case. The lesions should be carefully descabbed before the application of a topical antibiotic. I favour three per cent Aureomycin ointment because of its very low skin sensitivity rate. The scab may be removed either by soaking with a strong solution of bicarbonate or by rubbing in an emulsifying cream. Bicarbonate has been found to be the easiest and simplest to apply. The mother is told to make the solution by mixing a tablespoonful of bicarbonate of soda in one third of a cup of warm water. This makes a thin paste with which the lesions should be soaked for about five minutes, and then the scab gently peeled off. An attempt should be made to remove all of the scabs before any ointment is applied. However, in persistent cases the first application may have to be applied after partial removal of the scabs. The ointment should be applied four times a day and any dried ointment, serum, blood, or residual scabbing should again be removed with the bicarbonate solution before applying the ointment. The bicarbonate solution should be sponged off with warm water and the area blotted dry before the ointment is applied. The parents should be instructed that there will be a considerable improvement in 24 hours and except for a mild erythema the lesions should have disappeared within three days. Any source of infection, such as discharging ear, discharging nose, a paronychia or an abscess should of course be dealt with at the same time.

The herald patch of Pityriasis rosea
This will only occur in the older child. It is slightly oval

in shape – non-itchy, slightly scaly with characteristic collarette scales, i.e. gentle scraping towards the centre of the lesion will make the scales stand out like the layers of an Elizabethan ruff. Diagnosis is soon confirmed when other lesions begin to appear. Although this condition may appear to be rather alarming to the patient it is always self limiting. The patient can be told firmly that this is not infectious, will last for somewhere between three and eight weeks, does not recur, never gives any trouble, and will disappear whatever is put on it. Nevertheless, there will quite often be a wish to have something prescribed and half per cent ichthyol in zinc oxide paste is a suitable application.

Nummular eczema

This is a round, universally scaly lesion without any clear centre; it may be single or multiple. Treatment is again half to one per cent ichthyol in zinc oxide paste, and firm reassurance that it is *not* ringworm.

Ringworm

Ringworm of the scalp is easily diagnosed with the use of Wood's light, which causes the hairs which contain the fungus to fluoresce. On any other part of the body diagnosis is made on the appearance and the symptoms. It is a scaly, inflammed, itchy area, usually with a clear centre, and there is usually a history of contact with animals. In most cases Whitfield's ointment is enough to deal with the condition.

Guttate psoriasis

It is not always appreciated that psoriasis occurring in children usually has a different form from the adult. The lesions are small, multiple, round, oval, scaly and red. It may follow an upper respiratory infection by 10 or 20 days, and there may be a family history of psoriasis.

Treatment. One per cent ichthyol or crude coal tar in emulsifying ointment. The parents should be told that the condition is likely to last three to six weeks, when it will regress but there is a substantial possibility that psoriasis in adult form may appear in later life.

FURTHER READING

Godber, G.E. (1974) Diseases of the skin. In *The Health of the School Child 1971–72*, pp.44–47. London: HMSO.
Hart, C.R. (1974) Plantar warts. *Chiropody Review*, **35**, 9–15.
Jacobs, A.H. (1971) Symposium on pediatric dermatology. *Pediatric Clinics of North America*, **18**.
MacDonald, R.H. (1975) Skin diseases in children. *Update*, **11**, 851–863.
Morley, W.N. (1973) Diseases of the skin. In Forfar, J.O. & Arneil, G.C. (eds) *Textbook of Paediatrics*, pp. 1550–1585. Edinburgh: Churchill Livingstone.
Rook, A.J. (1973) *Recent Advances in Dermatology No. 3* Edinburgh Churchill Livingstone.

30

Some common orthopaedic disorders

Thomas Moore

In this chapter it is not proposed to deal with the management of major problems, since these will almost certainly be under the care of orthopaedic and other specialist doctors. Even major problems, however, must usually present to the general practitioner in the first instance. It is here that an early diagnosis or at least a high index of suspicion leading to an early second opinion from an expert can often improve the prognosis and save a lifetime's discomfort and the premature onset of complications in adult life. Thus it is proposed to point out briefly the more common problems in this specialty, to give advice on the diagnosis, and to indicate the management of these conditions.

Since the subject of orthopaedics is concerned with disorders of the musculo-skeletal system the presenting symptoms are usually deformity, pain and an abnormality of joint function. Deformities, especially in infants, present when parents are worried that something doesn't 'look right'. As a general rule easily correctable deformities are less serious than those which are fixed or unilateral, but a sound knowledge of anatomy and the range of normality and the confidence this brings allied to a careful and sympathetic hearing and examination of the problem goes a very long way if only reassurance is required.

Pain is very variable as a presenting symptom. Some adults tolerate it very much better than others and the same applies to children. Some have known nothing else and thus do not complain. Quite young children however can locate very accurately a new pain, and most children will refrain from moving something that hurts, so a child who has an immobile limb almost certainly has something wrong with it. Beware the adolescent who may not be moving a limb for her own, rather than orthopaedic reasons!

Abnormalities of joint function may be associated with pathology involving the joint itself, the supporting structures of muscle and ligament and the neurology, both central and peripheral, of these. This may involve an examination of the whole body and go far beyond peering at what the patient feels is necessary.

Since bones are radio-opaque, plain X-ray of the affected part of the body will demonstrate most problems associated with them and the congruity of joints. The X-ray does, however, have to be of the affected part and it is well to remember some pains can be referred elsewhere, one example being that of hip disease which can present as pain in the knee. Simple blood chemistry and haematology complete the diagnostic armamentarium and should enable the general practitioner to make a diagnosis as competently as an orthopaedic surgeon.

The treatment of orthopaedic conditions must depend on the cause, and is directed at preserving normal development and function. Some problems require only advice and reassurance, others require the services and skills of a hospital and specialist colleagues. It is only by reaching a correct diagnosis that each doctor is able to decide what he can manage himself and what needs to be referred to hospital.

DISORDERS OF THE SPINE

Deformity is the most common presenting symptom in children, only the more serious problems giving rise to pain and stiffness.

Abnormal curvatures

Curves in an antroposterior direction (kyphosis) and a lateral direction (scoliosis) need to be differentiated into postural and structural types, since management depends on this differentiation.

Postural curves, which are the most common, tend to occur among adolescents. The curves are smooth and painless and the deformity will always correct by voluntary movement. The spine always remains mobile; rotation of the vertebrae and other deformities do not occur. The prognosis is good and treatment is directed at reassurance and encouragement to improve the posture by exercise and voluntary effort. It is worth examining the length of the legs to exclude a compensatory scoliosis, which also remains mobile, but which is caused by unequal leg lengths for which a specialist opinion should be sought.

Structural curves in the spine are characterised by a permanent curve which cannot be eliminated. Flexion of the spine will demonstrate the smallest structural scoliosis and remove postural curves.

Reduction of mobility and sometimes pain occur. Rotational changes occur among the vertebral bodies leading to deformities of the back and chest, while compensatory curves develop to keep the pelvis and head upright. Structural kyphoscoliosis may be caused by defects in bone development and collapse due to disease in the vertebral bodies or to pathology in muscles or nerves involved in supporting the spine. The commonest type is idiopathic and can occur at any age. Usually the younger it develops the worse the prognosis, although it has been suggested that those occuring in infants under one year resolve. The remainder may progress to severe deformity. Deformity ceases to increase at about the age of 16 years when growth in the spine is complete.

Cases of structural kyphoscoliosis need careful follow up and the management should be in the hands of a specialist in this subject from as early an age as possible.

One of the commonest forms of localised scoliosis in children is a torticollis or 'wry neck', due to spasm in the neck musculature. This can be treated by manipulation, local heat and analgesics. Other common causes of holding the head to one side are associated with local painful conditions such as earache, tender cervical glands or mumps, which require appropriate measures.

A congenital torticollis presents shortly after birth when a sternomastoid tumour may be palpable, or if this is missed, at a later date with a shortened sternomastoid muscle. Failure to deal with this, which may need anything from passive stretching to surgery, can lead to facial asymmetry.

DISORDERS OF THE BONES AND SOFT TISSUE

Slipping of one vertebral body on another, commonly the fifth lumber vertebra on the sacrum, is thought to be due to a stress fracture of part of the neural arch. This may give rise to local backache or pains due to compression of nerve roots. Often a defect is palpable in the back and an X-ray will confirm the diagnosis. Although most are stable, management should be left to an expert.

A bone defect of the spine which may be associated with skin stigmata such as tufts of hair, angiomata or even just a dimple is Spina bifida occulta. This is a failure of the neural arch to fuse properly and may be totally unsuspected, or there may be neurological deficit of any degree, involving sphincter muscles and lower limb musculature, with or without associated mental defect.

Acute prolapsed intervertebral discs can occur in children. They are managed in the same way as for adults with analgesics and bed rest, after investigations to exclude other pathology have been carried out.

DISORDERS OF THE LOWER LIMB

It is worth remembering that the nerves from the back will influence the musculature of the lower limb, and abnormalities in the upper bones and joints will alter the position of the foot. Thus an examination of, say, pidgeon toes, must exclude problems in the hips and long bones.

The hip

Discussion on hip disorders can be sub-divided into two groups; the unable-to-complain neonates on one hand and older children who can complain of pain or have a disorder of function such as a limp or unwillingness to use a limb on the other.

In neonates it is important to exclude congenital dislocation of the hip, since the degree of improvement secured is directly proportional to the age treatment is commenced. Thus it is important to diagnose the condition as early as possible and all children should be screened at birth.

Ortolani's test for CDH is simple and takes a few seconds to perform. It is described in Chapter 25.

Figures for the incidence of CDH vary between four and eleven per thousand live births while between eight and twenty live births per thousand have unstable hips. The condition is about four times as common in girls and ten times more likely in a breech presentation. The left hip is the more commonly affected joint. Since the incidence would appear to reduce with age some cases must cure themselves spontaneously. These points lend credence to the idea that the majority of cases are due to intra uterine pressures and ligamentous laxity; thus, if the hip is reduced and held so until the ligaments tighten up and allow the acetabulum to develop, it is felt normal development will take place. It is worth remembering that there is a familial incidence. In spite of all this children still get missed and some authorities suggest babies should be screened again at six months.

Older children in whom the diagnosis was missed may present with a limp, classically walking with a bent knee in an attempt to stabilise the opposite hip joint. Lack of abduction, asymmetry of the lower limbs which shows as unequal leg lengths, or a difference in the number of transverse skin creases in the thigh, should lead to a thorough examination of the stability of the hips and an X-ray.

In older children the early signs of hip disorder are pain and limp. These, with spasm and limitation of movement, are all indications for investigation by an X-ray. Since the early signs of disease in the hip are similar, the child must be treated as though the problem were serious. The majority will be suffering from a transient synovitis of the hip probably due to trauma, but that particular diagnosis can only be made if, after 10–14 days bed-rest the hip has recovered, and nothing else has materialised clinically or radiologically.

Other causes of hip disorder in children include Perthe's disease, thought to be due to ischaemic changes in the femoral head, which usually presents in boys of the four to nine age group. Fragmentation of the ossification centre can be seen on X-ray, and this is how the diagnosis is made. The disease runs a two to three year course and treatment is aimed at preserving the femoral head until reossification can occur. Follow-up is thus a long drawn out process and management should be in the hands of orthopaedic surgeons.

Adolescent Coxa Vara describes the untreated deformity which occurs with a slipped upper femoral epiphysis. This condition is more common among rather fat under developed boys in the twelve to fifteen age group. There may be a traumatic history and pain may be referred to the medial aspect of the knee. X-rays of the hip must include a lateral view which will demonstrate even a minor slip.

Treatment is operative and is aimed at fixing the epiphysis, after reduction if that is necessary.

The knee

Disorders of the knee present as deformity, pain or locking of the joint.

The commonest deformity associated with this joint is 'knock knee' or Genu Valgum. Most, if not all children are knock kneed at some stage in their development. Almost all will correct with growth by the age of seven years.

Indications for expert guidance are a failure to correct by this age and if a gap of three inches or more is present at the lower end of the tibiae at the age of three years. This measurement is made between the medial malleoli with the knees together and the patellae facing forward.

Unilateral knock knee is abnormal and must give rise to a suspicion of local epiphyseal damage. The joint should also be X-rayed to exclude bone abnormality if there is an intermalleolar separation of more than four inches at any time.

The opposite deformity is that of 'bow leg' or Genu Varum. Normal tibiae have a slight bow which must be differentiated from the pathological deformities of rickets with the deformity present in the lower third of the bone, or a growth disturbance which usually presents as a varus deformity of the upper third. The normal tibial bow associated with torsion of the bone may contribute to the bow leg deformity. The torsion should have corrected by the age of seven years and should not normally exceed 30 degrees at the age of three years.

The most common form of bow legs is a postural fault caused by a rotation of the legs and may be accompanied by a hyperextension of the knee. The latter is normal in infants and is due to ligamentous laxity and weakness of the muscle support of the knee. Persistance after the age of seven years or any instability are to be regarded as pathological.

Trauma is the most common cause of pain around the knee and in young children is characterised by reluctance to use the limb. Careful palpation can often pin point the site of the lesion. It is worth remembering that fractures especially of the fibula and metatarsal bones can occur without an obvious traumatic history–the stress fracture of excess activity.

A very common cause of pain around the knee in children during the adolescent period of bone growth, and associated with over-activity, is osteochondritis of the tibial tubercle and much more rarely at the lower pole of the patella. This is thought to be associated with stress of the patellar ligament imparted to its bony origin and insertion. Local tenderness, enlargement of the tibial tubercle and radiological changes give the diagnosis. Recovery takes place when the condition has settled which may take two or three years and may leave the tibial tubercle larger than normal. The pain usually settles with the avoidance of physical activity for a time. If this is unsuccessful, injections of hydrocortisone or surgery aimed at improving the vascularity of the area may be indicated.

Chondromalacia of the patella is another cause of pain in adolescent children. This symptom presents as an ache which is worse on movement, especially on climbing stairs. The pain may be reproduced by rubbing the patella on the lower end of the femur. In the early stages rest is all that may be required; more severe pain, however, may require analgesics and splintage.

Locking or clicking, provided it is not the vacuum click, are signs of internal derangement of the joint and are among the indications for exploring the joint surgically. Surgery may also be required for the unstable patellae of girls with a recurrent dislocation of that bone.

The foot and ankle

The functions of the foot and ankle are to provide contact with the ground and support the body and provided this can be done adequately and without pain, the indications for interference are minimal.

Deformities of the feet are usually what cause parents the most anxiety. The most common is probably that of the 'flat foot'. All normal infants have flat feet, partly due to the mobility of the foot and to the presence of a pad of fat under the medial arch.

If the mobility of the foot is retained, as in races which are habitually unshod, the foot can always appear flat. Thus, provided the child can run around with its peers, it is most unlikely anything further need be done.

It is as well, however, to examine the whole limb to exclude a compensatory flat foot due to femoral or tibial torsion which may require advice on improving the posture of the child.

Restoration of the longitudinal arch and straightening of the heel while standing on tip toes will exclude muscular weakness, and if the foot is supple it is unlikely that there will be any abnormality in the tarsal bones, which can produce a stiff flat foot which may require surgery.

Pes cavus or claw foot is associated with flexion deformities of the toes and the primary pathology is neuro muscular.

The common serious congenital abnormality of the ankle and foot, which occurs in between one and four babies per thousand live births, is the club foot deformity of talipes equino-varus. This has elements of plantar flexion and inversion of the hind foot combined with adduction of the fore foot, giving rise to the appearance of a foot with a small elevated heel and a broad twisted forefoot with a curved lateral border.

Club foot deformities fall into two types. The majority which are thought to be associated with intra uterine pressures and positions have, at first, a normal skeleton and will correct fairly easily and permanently if treatment is started early. The others are more severe cases which only correct with difficulty, have skeletal changes at birth and may be associated with other congenital abnormalities.

The earlier specialist treatment is started the better, since this allows less time for bones to become deformed and soft tissues to contract. Thus if there is any doubt about limitation of eversion or dorsiflexion of the foot in a neonate an early specialist opinion should be sought. Normal babies may hold their feet inverted at birth, but there is a full range of passive movement which allows the dorsum of the foot to touch the shin. Treatment of mild cases consists of manipulation to reduce the adduction deformity of the fore foot, then to correct the equinus element. This is maintained by strapping. More resistant cases may require extensive surgery to produce a reasonable foot.

The other deformity of the fore foot which may cause some anxiety is hook foot, or metatarsus primus varus. This may be distinguished from TEV because the hind foot is straight or turned outwards. If the deformity can be passively corrected easily and comfortably it will probably get better. About ninety per cent of these feet will straighten by the age of three years. Wearing shoes on the wrong feet will do no harm and may help to keep parents happy. If the deformity is unilateral or will not easily correct or if it persists beyond the age of three, an orthopaedic opinion should be sought.

The other defect of a congenital nature is that of the congenitally short tendo achilles. A normal baby will allow dorsiflexion of the foot so that the top of the foot can touch the shin. The ability to do this reduces with age or if the tendo achilles is tight. An older child with this condition will be unable to walk on its heels without hyperextending its knees. The condition may require surgery.

It should be remembered that the normal child starts to walk on tip toes but this habit is usually abandoned by the time the child is four or five years old.

Congenital deformities of the feet and toes are often familial and are usually bilateral and symmetrical. Provided these are painless no treatment is required. If adequate shoes and simple symptomatic measures fail, surgery may be indicated.

Pain in the foot is an uncommon complaint in children unless it is due to a locally painful skin condition such as a blister or wart. Deep pain can occur with an osteochondritis of the bones especially of the navicular, and with a stress fracture. X-rays will give the diagnosis, but in the latter case it may need 10–14 days to allow a callus to form before being conclusive.

Hallux valgus is not uncommon in children but only increasing deformity or the development of a hallux rigidus are indications for surgery.

Ingrowing toenails are caused by pressure from tight shoes or encroaching toes. Treatment is aimed at eliminating these causes, treating the infection and trying to prevent a spike of nail growing into the toe. Failure to control the discomfort by simple means is an indication for a radical excision of the nail bed.

Occasionally advice about shoes is sought. Common sense should be the guideline, bearing in mind the foot needs protection, room to spread under load and room to grow without deformity.

DISORDERS OF THE UPPER LIMB

Rounded shoulders are the commonest deformity and usually it is found one or both parents have a similar shape. Occasionally the onset in adolescent girls coincides with the onset of breast development. The elevated shoulders of, the rarity, Sprengl's shoulder are associated with elevated scapulae. This problem is cosmetic and may need surgery.

Trauma can lead to dislocation of the relatively unstable shoulder joint making it more unstable. Recurrent dislocation can be helped by operative measures.

Pulled elbow in toddlers is thought to be due to the head of the radius being pulled through the orbicular ligament when the child is jerked by the hand. Most cases settle after a few days in a sling or by gentle pronation and supination of the forearm while supporting the elbow.

It should not be forgotten that circulatory changes associated with fracture or vascular damage at the elbow require prompt treatment to prevent ischaemic contractures.

Trigger thumbs and fingers in children, due to thickening in the flexor tendeon catching in the tendon sheath may, as in adults, require surgical release. Congenital curly fingers like the similar condition affecting toes very often have a family history and only reassurance is required. Finger sucking can cause a digit to bend and the fingers will straighten out when the habit is lost.

DISORDERS OF THE SKELETAL SYSTEM

Infection

Acute osteomyelitis in children is not a rarity and must be promptly and adequately treated to prevent the miseries of the chronic condition. The infection is usually blood borne from another source and it has been estimated eighty per cent are probably caused by the Staphlycoccus. The organism classically lodges in the cancellous bone under the epiphyseal plate of a long bone, usually the upper tibia or lower femur, but can occur in any bone. The earliest symptoms are local pain and tenderness in a feverish child who may occasionally give a history of trauma. Later redness, swelling and a reactionary joint effusion develop. X-ray changes take 10–14 days before showing signs of the condition.

The blood picture shows a high leucocytosis and blood culture will prove positive in fifty per cent of cases. Because of the high morbidity, hospital admission should be promptly arranged so that bed rest and adequate doses of an appropriate antibiotic, can be given. Further treatment may require surgical drainage.

Acute suppurative arthritis of joints is much less common, the hips of neonates perhaps being the most common. Evidence of infection with pain and spasm round the joint requires hospital treatment if the joint is not to be irreparably damaged.

Tuberculosis most commonly involving the spine is now a rarity in the United Kingdom and is always secondary to infection elsewhere. General malaise and muscle spasm and occasionally pain are the clinical signs. The diagnosis is confirmed by x-ray, and culture.

Tumours

Benign skeletal tumours are rare and malignant tumours even more so. They are associated with local tenderness and swelling; some will cause mechanical problems and some pain. Radiology will demonstrate their presence. The management of them should be in the hands of an orthopaedic surgeon.

Metabolic

Rickets is an uncommon disorder in this country among the indigenous population, but it is now becoming recognised among the Asian immigrant community. Lack of vitamin D in the diet and lack of sunlight associated with a pigmented skin, coupled with a high phytate intake reducing calcium absorption have been suggested as causes.

Lack of vitamin D interferes with calcification leading to soft bones which can then distort under load. In children the epiphyseal plate becomes thicker and enlarges to an extent where this can be palpated. Classic sites are at the wrists, knees and costo chondral junction of the ribs. X-ray changes and the blood biochemistry confirm the diagnosis.

DISORDERS OF SOFT TISSUES

Infection

Infection presents with symptoms of pain, swelling, redness and warmth. If the infection is localised pus is formed and may be visible as the abscess points under the skin. A diffuse infection gives rise to a spreading cellulitis. The treatment of both forms is the prompt administration of antibiotics which usually resolves the infection. When pus begins to form the swelling and pain may increase and treatment at this stage is aimed at draining the abscess as well as giving antibiotics.

Pulp and tendon sheath infections need urgent drainage if they do not appear to be resolving, to prevent osteomyelitis and tendon damage.

Tumours

Any of the soft tissue tumours can occur, the histology being confirmed by excision and biopsy. A common cystic swelling associated with a joint or tendon sheath is the ganglion. A thirty per cent cure can be expected if nothing is done or if the lesion is aspirated or punctured. Surgical excision under general anaesthetic with a bloodless field gives better results, since complete excision often involves opening joint capsules.

FURTHER READING

Fixsen, J.A. (1980) Within normal limits? Borderline orthopaedic abnormalities in children. *Update*, **20**, 13–21.

Hoekelman, R.A. (1975) Paediatric problems; common foot problems. *Update*, **10**, 449–457.

Murley, A.H.G. (1975) The painful elbow. *The Practitioner*, **215**, 36–41.

Pollen, A.G. (1973) *Fractures and Dislocations in Children*. Edinburgh: Churchill Livingstone.

Sharrard, W.J.W. (1979) *Paediatric Orthopaedics and Fractures*. Oxford: Blackwell Scientific.

Tachdjian, M.O. (1972) *Paediatric Orthopaedics*, 2 vols. Philadelphia: Saunders.

Walker, G. (1972) Minor orthopaedic problems in childhood. *The Practitioner*, **208**, 227–238.

Wiles, P. & Sweetnam, R. (1965) *Essentials of Orthopaedics*. London: Churchill.

31

Urinary infection in childhood

David Barton

INTRODUCTION

The diagnosis of urinary tract infection was inexact until Kass (1956) established the necessity for quantitative bacteriological methods. It is accepted that significant bacteriuria is present if fresh urine contains more than 10^8 organisms per litre (MRC 1979), and urinary infection is present if in addition there are excess pus cells. A colony count of less than 10^7 organisms per litre indicates contamination, while intermediate colony counts are inconclusive. More recently Maskell and Pead (1976) and others have suggested that levels of 10^7 per litre should be regarded as significant. Urinary infection and bacteriuria are described as overt if symptoms are present which have necessitated medical attention, and covert in the absence of symptoms or when symptoms have not necessitated medical attention.

NEONATAL URINARY INFECTION

Urinary infection occurs in about two per cent of infants in the first month of life, with a marked male preponderance. This has been established by a number of screening surveys (O'Doherty, 1968; Littlewood, Kite and Kite, 1969; Abbott, 1972). The pathogenesis is thought to be haematogenous and the proportion of urinary infections associated with abnormalities of the urinary tract is lower at this age than later in childhood. Consequently the relapse rate after treatment is lower in the neonatal period.

The majority of cases are asymptomatic and occur in apparently well babies. Symptoms when they occur are non-specific and include: irritability, sluggishness, feeding difficulties, vomiting, diarrhoea, weight loss, failure to thrive, distended abdomen, jaundice, cyanosis, convulsions and fever. These symptoms give no clue as to the diagnosis of urinary infection, and examination of the urine is essential in all unexplained illnesses in the neonatal period. Sometimes urinary infection is one manifestation of coliform septicaemia. Some neonatal urinary infections will clear without treatment, but the majority will cause persisting vague ill health unless treated.

There is no doubt that neonatal urinary infection is underdiagnosed in general practice, owing to unfamiliarity with the symptomatology, and practical difficulties in collecting adequate urine samples.

URINARY INFECTION IN LATER INFANCY AND CHILDHOOD

After the first year of life the sex ratio reverses so that, by the age of six, covert infection is 40 times more common in girls. Overt infection is three times more common in girls throughout childhood, which suggests that bacteriuric boys are more likely to have severe symptoms.

It is difficult to estimate the incidence of urinary tract infection because most hospital series are selected to some extent, and most series from general practice are small and use varying diagnostic criteria. Kunin (1968) and Arneil (1972) suggest that approximately five per cent of children will suffer from urinary infections at some time during childhood. Up to the age of nine years the annual incidence is 2.7 per cent. It falls to 0.4 per cent in the 10-14 age group and subsequently rises during adolescence. This gives an average annual incidence in children of 1.5 per cent (Kunin, 1968). A similar incidence was found by Hodgkin (1973) in his general practice population in the north of England.

No very striking racial, geographical or social class differences have been recorded, and there appears to be no seasonal variation in the incidence of this disease. The pathogenesis is ascending infection, with underlying urinary tract abnormalities present in a large proportion of cases.

Up to the toddler stage symptoms are non-specific: failure to thrive, weight loss, pallor, rigors, pyrexia, convulsions, diarrhoea, vomiting, abdominal distension and abdominal pain. Later in childhood symptoms tend to be referred to the upper or lower urinary tract. A clinical diagnosis of acute pyelonephritis is made when there is loin pain and tenderness associated with pyrexia and rigors. A clinical diagnosis of cystitis is made when there is dysuria, frequency, urgency and strangury. The assignment of urinary infections to one or other category on clinical grounds is unreliable. Even later in childhood symptoms may be absent or non-specific. It should be remembered that haematuria and vague abdominal pain in this age group are commonly due to infection. Urinary infection must be excluded when bed wetting or day time wetting persist after two years, or reappear after a period of being dry. Haskell and Pead (1976) have shown that enuresis is more commonly associated with infection in girls (12 per cent) than in boys (two per cent). A large proportion of children with classical urinary symptoms do not have a urinary infection.

Bacteriological examination of the urine is essential to confirm the diagnosis in every case.

Chronic pyelonephritis

Chronic pyelonephritis is caused by recurrent acute pyelonephritis, and virtually all cases are associated with vesicoureteric reflux.

The radiological features of chronic pyelonephritis were described by Hodson (1968). The minor calyces are dilated and distorted with thinning of the overlying renal cortex, resulting in shrinkage and distortion of the kidney. This scarring may affect the kidney evenly or may be limited to one pole. In unilateral cases with a normal contralateral kidney, nephrectomy may be indicated for persistent infection, loin pain or hypertension. In severe bilateral cases the signs and symptoms of chronic renal failure will appear: polyuria, polydipsia, dwarfism, renal osteodystrophy. Eventually dialysis and renal transplantation have to be considered.

Vesicoureteric reflux

In vesicoureteric reflux the valvular mechanism at the lower end of the ureter is deficient, allowing urine to flow freely from the bladder back into the ureter during micturition. It is present intermittently in some cases, so that ureteric reflux cannot be excluded by a single normal micturating cystogram. The stagnant urine in the bladder predisposes to infection which is then transmitted to the kidney, so it is customary to advise double micturition to reduce the amount of residual urine. If recurrent infection or fresh chronic pyelonephritic scarring occurs despite adequate chemotherapy, reimplantation of the ureter is indicated to cure the reflux; but this operation is less fashionable now than it was a few years ago.

A number of reports have shown that vesico-ureteric reflux tends to be familial. There appear to be several distinct modes of genetic transmission including sex-linked, autosomal dominant, and multifactorial. It follows that relatives of patients with vesico-ureteric reflux are 'at risk'.

Covert bacteriuria

It has been confirmed in a number of surveys in the British Isles and USA, including Kunin, Zacha and Paquin (1962), Savage *et al* (1973), Asscher *et al* (1973) and Edwards *et al* (1975) that bacteriuria is present in about two per cent of schoolgirls and in less than one in 1000 schoolboys.

On direct questioning, over half the bacteriuric children are found to have urinary symptoms, including: dysuria, frequency, urgency, daytime wetting, primary nocturnal enuresis, secondary nocturnal enuresis, nocturia, loin pain and unexplained fevers. Because of the frequency of symptoms in bacteriuric children discovered by routine screening, there is a tendency to use the term 'covert bacteriuria' in preference to 'asymptomatic bacteriuria'(Savage *et al*, 1973). It is surprising that the parents of bacteriuric children do not seek medical advice for these symptoms. There seems to be a need for health education along these lines.

About a third of bacteriuric children have a previous history of overt urinary infection, which confirms the need for prolonged follow-up of all children who have had an episode of urinary tract infection.

About a third of bacteriuric children are suffering from vesicoureteric reflux, and over half of these show radiological evidence of chronic pyelonephritis. Some of the chronic pyelonephritic children are symptom free and have no previous history of overt infection, so that routine screening is the only method of detection.

A case can be made for the periodic screening of all children. Ideally it should start in infancy, when the incidence of bacteriuria is highest. It is necessary to repeat screening at intervals as the age of onset varies. It might be argued that screening is not worth while in boys in view of the very low incidence.

Routine screening could be carried out by the child welfare clinics and school medical services. Alternatively, it could be organised on a practice basis by the GP and attached health visitor. Mond, Gruneberg and Smellie (1970) have established the feasibility of screening for bacteriuria in children within the setting of general practice.

Tuberculosis of the urinary tract

Tuberculosis of the urinary tract is rare in children in this country. It may be associated with tuberculosis affecting other parts of the body, or may be found in isolation.

There may be constitutional symptoms, including fever, malaise, weight loss and raised sedimentation rate. If the infection involves the kidney there may be loin pain or episodes of renal colic as debris passes down the ureter. If the bladder is involved symptoms may include frequency, dysuria and nocturia which become severe in late cases due to contraction and scarring of the bladder. Heavy sterile leucocyturia is usually present and will provide a clue to the diagnosis.

The diagnosis may be confirmed by examining three early morning urine specimens for acid fast bacilli and submitting the urine to Lowenstein-Jenner culture, which takes an average of eight weeks to produce a result. Full radiological investigation and cystoscopy is necessary. Specific antituberculous chemotherapy is continued for two years, and prolonged follow-up is needed.

COLLECTION OF URINE SPECIMENS

To minimise contamination, a mid-stream clean catch urine specimen (MSU) is required. There is disagreement regarding the need for prior cleansing of the genitalia but this is probably not necessary in the absence of discharge or dirt. The specimen is obtained by inserting a sterile container into the stream of urine during micturition. With patience this is possible in the vast majority of children, including neonates. Bacteriological examination of urine decanted from a chamber pot into an unsterile bottle is valueless.

An alternative method of urine collection in male and female infants is to apply an adhesive uribag. As soon as micturition occurs the bag must be removed and inoculation onto the culture medium must be carried out without delay, as contamination is inevitable with this method.

In infants suprapubic aspiration (SPA) may be used to obtain an uncontaminated urine specimen. Urinary infection is confirmed by a colony count of more than 10^6 per litre. After skin cleansing an intravenous needle is inserted without local analgesia 2.5 cm above the symphysis pubis downwards and backwards at an angle of 45° until urine is drawn into the syringe. This technique is useful if the diagnosis remains in doubt after several MSUs have been examined, but will rarely be feasible in general practice.

In older children catheterisation of the bladder will occasionally be required to establish the diagnosis. Full aseptic precautions are necessary because of the risk of introducing infection, and this will normally require hospital facilities.

STORAGE OF URINE SPECIMENS

Urine is a suitable culture medium for most bacteria, and contaminants multiply at room temperature to produce 'significant' levels of bacteria in the urine within two hours. This can be prevented by refrigeration immediately after voiding, or by immediate inoculation onto the culture medium or dip slide.

The main problem in diagnosing urinary infections in general practice is the inevitable delay between voiding and inoculation onto the culture medium. The specimen may be several hours old when brought to the surgery. This problem can be overcome by having facilities at the surgery premises for the practice nurse to supervise the collection of urine specimens, which can then be refrigerated without delay.

Transporting the urine specimen to the laboratory by post, public transport, private car or hospital transport involves further delays. In some practices it is possible for the urine to reach the laboratory within two hours. When distance or organisational problems make this impossible, a large number of false positive results will occur due to multiplication of contaminants.

CHEMICAL TESTS

There is little correlation between proteinuria and urinary infection. Testing the urine for protein has no place in the management of urinary infection.

Indirect biochemical tests depending upon detection of the metabolic effects of bacteria on urine have been extensively reviewed by Constable (1975). None of these tests has proved sufficiently reliable or convenient for routine clinical use in general practice.

URINE MICROSCOPY

The number of pus cells in fresh, well-mixed, uncentrifuged urine can be counted using a microscope and Fuchs-Rosenthal counting chamber.

It is generally accepted that less than 10 pus cells per mm^3 are within normal limits. Over 100 pus cells per mm^3 indicate a probable infection, while between 10 and 100 per mm^3 indicate a possible infection. However, numerous studies, including Houston (1963) and Robins *et al* (1975), have demonstrated the relatively poor correlation between leucocyturia and bacteriuria. About one third of cases of urinary tract infection and bacteriuria have no evidence of leucocyturia. On the other hand, in the absence of urinary infection, leucocyturia is frequently found due to contamination from the external genitalia or to non-bacterial inflammation of the urinary tract.

Robins *et al* (1975) have attempted to increase the reliabilty of urine microscopy as a screening test for urinary infection by combining pus cell counting with examination for motile bacteria in the urine which misses less than 10 per cent of infected urines.

Microscopy for pus cells has frequently been recommended as an aid to the diagnosis of urinary tract infection in children in general practice (Hodgkin, 1973). In view of the large number of false positives and false negatives, the diagnosis must be confirmed bacteriologically.

DIP SLIDES

Owing to the delay between voiding and inoculation of the urine onto the culture medium at the laboratory, quantitative bacteriological methods were impractical in the general practice setting until the development of the dip slide by Naylor and Guttman (1967), based on a previous idea by Mackey and Sandys (1965). The dip slide consists of a microscope slide coated with nutrient medium. This can be inoculated by dipping it into fresh urine or by the dip stream method when it is wetted by placing it in the stream of urine. Numerous studies, including Guttman (1973) have confirmed the reliability of dip slides and their feasibility in general practice. After incubation for 18 hours at 37°C examination of the slides establishes the colony count and the purity of the bacterial growth. Subcultures may be taken for identification and antibiotic sensitivity testing by conventional bacteriological methods. Arneil *et al* (1970) have established that dip slides give a reliable result after 18 hours at room temperature, and that reliable results are obtained after posting the specimen.

The dip slide provides the most reliable method of detecting significant bacteriuria in the general practice setting, as the delay between voiding and inoculation is minimal. In the majority of cases where the clinical situation is not urgent and in screening programmes, the dip slide can be retained in the general practitioner's surgery for reading the next day, so that only the positive dip slides need to be sent to the laboratory for sensitivity testing.

Further investigation of urinary infection

Opinion is divided as to whether full investigation is indicated after a single episode of urinary infection, or after recurrent urinary infections. About half the children in hospital series of infection have radiological abnormalities (Smellie and Normand,1968) but the true incidence in general practice is probably lower. However, even in routine screening programmes, one third of bacteriuric children have radiological abnormalities. Therefore it is easy to justify full investigation after a single episode of urinary infection.

A physical examination should be carried out on all children with proven urinary infection. Abdominal examination may reveal an enlarged kidney or distended bladder. Abnormalities of the external genitalia include phimosis or pinhole meatus in males or ectopic ureteric orifice in females. The central nervous system should be examined to exclude neurological problems. Constipation must be excluded by rectal examination. However, in the majority of cases no abnormality will be detected.

An intravenous pyelogram (IVP) is essential in every case as almost any congenital or acquired abnormality of the urinary tract can be associated with infection (Fletcher and Stephenson, 1975). About 10 per cent of cases will be found to have chronic pyelonephritis.

A micturating cystogram is necessary in every case as approximately one fifth will have vesicoureteric reflux. Contrast medium is injected into the bladder by means of a catheter. X-rays are taken before, during and after micturition to detect any reflux of dye into the ureters.

Cystoscopy is indicated for lower tract symptoms persisting after the infection has been eradicated. Bladder neck obstruction and urethral valves are diagnosed less frequently than in the past. Some urologists carry out urethral dilatation if the urethra appears narrow. Rarely retrograde pyelography is indicated to clarify a ureteric or renal lesion.

Full investigation identifies those cases in which recurrence is more likely or potentially more serious. Without this information it is impossible to plan a rational scheme of treatment and follow-up. A few cases will require surgery for stone, diverticula, ureterocoele and other abnormalities. Without full investigation cases of vesicoureteric reflux or chronic pyelonephritis will be missed, and with inadequate treatment and follow-up, further infection may lead to renal failure.

The majority of general practitioners have direct access to IVP and micturating cystogram examinations. It is possible for the general practitioner to manage all uncomplicated cases of urinary infection, referring to a specialist only one third of cases who prove to have a radiological abnormality.

TREATMENT OF URINARY TRACT INFECTION

In children the bacteriology of urinary tract infection shows a striking sex difference. In girls the vast majority of infections are due to E. Coli, whereas in boys E. Coli and Proteus account for about half each. Less commonly Klebsiella aerogenes, Streptococcus faecalis, Staphylococcus aureus, Staphylococcus albus and Pseudomonas pyocyanea are the causative organisms. The majority of E. Coli infections are sensitive to sulphonomide which is the drug of choice if treatment must be started before antibiotic sensitivities are known. If there are clinical signs of acute pyelonephritis, amoxycillin or co-trimoxazole are more effective because they produce adequate tissue and blood levels.

Nitrofurantoin and nalidixic acid are used when indicated by the results of sensitivity tests. The more toxic antibiotics should probably be reserved for hospital practice.

The choice of antibiotics should be based on the known antibiotic sensitivities in the practice area as there is some regional variation. Furthermore, the bacterial population will alter in the course of time due to changing antibiotic prescribing patterns.

Recurrence is frequent following a urinary tract infection, occurring in at least 50 per cent of uncomplicated cases (Kunin, 1970). When radiological abnormalities are present the recurrence rate is higher. In cases of reflux, repeated infection may lead to chronic pyelonephritis. Phage typing studies have proved that most recurrences are reinfections with a different strain of *E. coli*. Thus there is no basis for very prolonged courses of treatment in full dosage, as the infection is eradicated after a short course of treatment. There is a strong case for continuing prophylactic antibiotics in reduced dosage for prolonged periods to prevent reinfection (Smellie and Normand 1968; Stansfeld, 1975; Katz and Smellie, 1976). The optimum duration of treatment has not been settled conclusively, and policy varies from centre to centre. Initial treatment with antibiotics in full dosage varies from one to six weeks in uncomplicated cases. In ureteric reflux with or without chronic pyelonephritis, the duration of prophylaxis ranges from six months to several years until the reflux has ceased. When other radiological abnormalities are present, prophylactic treatment is continued for between three and twelve months. If infection recurs after stopping treatment, then a further, more prolonged course is indicated.

The follow-up of children with urinary tract infection will normally be the joint responsibility of the hospital and the general practitioner. In the absence of symptoms, the urine should be examined at least four times a year during the period of follow-up to exclude asymptomatic recurrence of infection. It is necessary for a suspected recurrence to be confirmed bacteriologically, to establish the need for reinvestigation and the length of chemotherapy required. Follow-up should be continued for several years in uncomplicated cases, and for several years after reflux ceases in cases of vesicoureteric reflux (Katz and Smellie, 1976).

Childhood urinary infection is liable to recur in adult life. This is more common in females, particularly at the onset of sexual activity or during pregnancy (Kunin, 1970). Antenatal care should include repeated urine culture when there is a past history of urinary infection.

Psychological and social aspects

Parents' attitudes towards urinary infection vary widely. At one extreme they regard it as trivial and are unwilling to bring their child for follow up. At the other extreme they become over-protective and are afraid of renal failure, dialysis, and transplantation. It is important to explore these attitudes and establish a realistic approach to the illness.

Prolonged follow up may lead the child to think of himself as an invalid. The general practitioner must bear this in mind, particularly with older children.

Social problems may arise in relation to incontinence, frequency and enuresis. It may be necessary for the general practitioner to communicate with the child's school if difficulties occur.

CONCLUSION

Urinary infection in childhood is a relatively common disease. In view of its protean manifestations in early childhood it is not sufficient to rely on the classical symptoms of cystitis and pyelonephritis. Urinary infection must be suspected in all unexplained illnesses, particularly if there is a previous history.

The surgery nurse can be trained to use the microscope to examine the urine for pus cells and bacteria, enabling a provisional diagnosis of urinary infection to be made in the majority of cases. However, there will be a proportion of false positives and, before starting treatment, it is essential to obtain a urine specimen to confirm the diagnosis bacteriologically. The most satisfactory method in the general practice setting is the dip slide, which enables specimens to be taken at any time of the day or at the week-end. A reliable diagnosis can be made after 18 hours even without an incubator. In an ill child treatment can be started as soon as the dip slide has been prepared. It cannot be emphasised too strongly that testing for proteinuria has no place in diagnosis of urinary infection.

The scope of the general practitioner's clinical work can be extended by the use of microscopy and dip slides, but additional demands will be placed upon his time, his staff and his resources. It may be possible in some practices to take on this additional diagnostic work load and even to set up routine screening programmes for bacteriuria.

It is suggested that full radiological investigation of every proven case of urinary tract infection is necessary, as it is impossible to plan a rational course of treatment and follow-up without an exact diagnosis. This would put an additional load on the hospital services, but it should be offset in the long term by a reduction in the need for renal dialysis and renal transplantation. This is one area in which early diagnosis and careful management by the general practitioner can help to reduce the incidence of serious disease and mortality in children and young adults.

REFERENCES

Abbott, G.D. (1972) Neonatal bacteriuria: a prospective study in 1460 infants. *British Medical Journal*, **1**, 267–269.

Arneil, G.C., McAllister, T.A. & Kay, P. (1970) Detection of bacteriuria at room temperature. *Lancet*, **1**, 119–121.

Arneil, G.C. (1972) Urinary tract infection in children. *Update*, **November**, 1115–1122.

Asscher, A.W., McLachlan, M.S.F., Verrier Jones, R., Meller, S., Sussman, M. & Harrison, S. (1973) Screening for asymptomatic urinary-tract infection in schoolgirls. *Lancet*, **2**, 1–4.

Constable, P.J. (1975) Urinary Infection. In Hart, C.R. (ed.) *Screening in General Practice*, ch. 16, pp. 163–175. Edinburgh: Churchill Livingstone.

Edwards, Bridget, White, R.H.R., Maxted, Heather, Deverill, I. & White, Patricia A. (1975) Screening methods for covert bacteriuria in school girls. *British Medical Journal*, **2**, 463–467.

Fletcher, E.W.L. & Stephenson, R.H. (1975) The findings reported in patients under-going excretory urography for recurrent urinary tract infection. *Journal of the Royal College of General Practitioners*, **25**, 146–150.

Guttman, D. (1973) Follow-up of urinary tract infection in domiciliary patients. In Brumfitt, W. & Asscher, A.W. (eds) *Urinary Tract Infection: Proceedings of the Second National Symposium held in London March 1972*, ch. 8, pp. 62–73. Oxford University Press.

Hodgkin, K. (1973) *Towards Earlier Diagnosis, A Guide to General Practice*, 3rd edn, ch. 8, p. 497. Edinburgh: Churchill Livingstone.

Hodson, C.J. (1968) Radiological diagnosis of renal involvement. In O'Grady, F. & Brumfitt, W. (eds) *Urinary Tract Infection: Proceedings of The First National Symposium held in London April 1968*, ch. 13, pp. 109–112. Oxford University Press.

Houston, I.B. (1963) Pus cell and bacterial counts in the diagnosis of urinary tract infections childhood. *Archives of Disease in Childhood*, **38**, 600–605.

Kass, E.H. (1956) Asymptomatic infections of the urinary tract. *Transactions of the Association of American Physicians*, **69**, 56.

Katz, G. & Smellie, Jean M. (1976) Urinary tract infections in children. *Journal of Maternal and Child Health*, **1**, no. 5, 24–27.

Kelly, D.G., Duff, F., Diskin, Sheila F. & Cahalane, S.F. (1969) Prevalence of urinary tract infection in Dublin school children. *Journal of the Irish Medical Association*, **62**, 420–422.

Kunin, C.M., Zacha, E. & Paquin, A. (1962) Urinary tract infection in schoolchildren. *New England Journal of Medicine*, **266**, 1287–1296.

Kunin, C.M. (1968) Emergence of bacteriuria, proteinuria, and symptomatic urinary tract infections among a population of school girls followed for 7 years. *Pediatrics*, **41**, 968–976.

Kunin, C.M. (1970) The natural history of recurrent bacteriuria in school girls. *New England Journal of Medicine*, **282**, 1443–8.

Littlewood, J.M., Kite, P. & Kite, B.A. (1969) Incidence of neonatal urinary tract infection. *Archives of Disease in Childhood*, **44**, 617–620.

Mackey, J.P. & Sandys, G.H. (1965) Laboratory diagnosis of infections of the urinary tract in general practice by means of a dip-inoculum transport medium. *British Medium Journal*, **2**, 1286–1288.

Maskell, R.M. & Pead, L.J. (1976) Urinary infection in children in general practice: a laboratory view. *Journal of Hygiene*, **77**, 291–298.

Meadow, S.R., White, R.H.R. & Johnston, Natalie M. (1969) Prevalence of symptomless urinary tract disease in Birmingham schoolchildren. I – Pyuria and Bacteriuria. *British Medical Journal*, **3**, 81–84.

Mond, N.C., Gruneberg, R.N. & Smellie, Jean M. (1970) Study of childhood urinary tract infection in general practice. *British Medical Journal*, **1**, 602–605.

MRC (1979) Medical Research Council Bacteriuria Committee Report. *British Medical Journal*, **2**, 717.

Naylor, G.R.E. & Guttmann, D. (1967) The dip-slide: A modified dip inoculum transport medium for the laboratory diagnosis of infections of the urinary tract. *Journal of Hygiene*, (Cambridge), **65**, 367–371.

O'Doherty, N. (1968) Urinary tract infection in the neonatal period and later infancy. In O'Grady F. & Brumfitt, W. (eds) *Urinary Tract Infection: Proceedings of The First National Symposium held in London April 1968*, ch. 14, pp. 113–122. Oxford University Press.

Robins, D.G., White, R.H.R., Rogers, K.G. & Osman, M.S. (1975) Urine microscopy as an aid to detection of bacteriuria. *Lancet*, **1**, 476–478.

Savage, D.C.L., Wilson, M.I., McHardy, M., Dewar, D.A.E. & Fee, W.M. (1973) Covert bacteriuria of childhood: a clinical and epidemiological study. *Archives of Disease in Childhood*, **48**, 8–20.

Smellie, Jean M. & Normand, I.C.S. (1968) Experience of Follow-up of Children with Urinary Tract Infection. In O'Grady, F. & Brumfitt, W. (eds) *Urinary Tract Infection: Proceedings of the First National Symposium held in London April 1968*, ch. 15 pp. 123–135. Oxford University Press.

Stansfeld, J.M. (1975) Duration of treatment for urinary tract infections in children, *British Medical Journal*, **3**, 65–66.

32

Blood disorders in childhood

Cyril Josephs

Blood differs from other human organs in that its site of origin (the haemopoietic system) is throughout life distant from its working site. To counterbalance the somewhat increased vulnerability which arises from this circumstance, the blood system has remarkable powers of regeneration and recovery.

The haemopoietic system of early life differs from that of the adult in several important aspects. It is relatively larger and more widely distributed in childhood; it needs relatively more blood-building substances because blood volume is increasing with body growth; its responses to toxic agents (including pathogenic organisms) and malnutrition may be exaggerated; its ultimate aim of producing normal adult white and red cells is subject to many genetic factors. The ladder of progress from primitive to mature cell has so many rungs that it is surprising, not that the process of blood formation goes astray sometimes, but rather that this does not happen more often.

The one day old baby has about 20 g of haemoglobin per 100 ml blood; this falls rapidly to about 15 g at one month, then more slowly to about 11.5 g at one year. These falls are normal and not influenced by giving iron. A slow rise follows to about 13 g at between 10 and 12 years, finally reaching the adult level of between 14 and 16 g at puberty (see Table 32.1). Fetal haemoglobin differs in biochemical structure from that produced after parturition. At birth about 80 per cent of the haemoglobin is of the fetal type and 20 per cent adult; at about four months the fetal component has dropped to 10 per cent. It is rarely demonstrable after 30 months.

The number of leucocytes is high in early childhood compared with that of adult life, being about 12 000 per cubic millimetre at two months. Of these, 35 per cent are granulocytes and 60 per cent lymphocytes. These values persist until the fourth and fifth years when the total count drops to 8000 and the differential percentage is reversed to 60 per cent granulocytes and 35 per cent lymphocytes. From the sixth to the fourteenth year there is a gradual numerical shift to adult values of 7000 white cells, with 65 per cent neutrophilic granulocytes and 30 per cent lymphocytes.

ANAEMIA

A child is anaemic if the concentration of haemoglobin or the number of red cells (or both) are reduced below the normal range for age; it is therefore of prime importance to have a working knowledge of the normal. Many children are treated for non-existent anaemia.

Anaemia is a sign of underlying disorder and its treatment is that of the cause. It is the most common haematological disorder in infancy and childhood; approximately one child in seven will be anaemic at some time before he is two years old. Certain points in the history and examination suggest an anaemic child irrespective of the cause. Anaemia of rapid onset is more obvious than that of gradual onset.

History

Enquiries should cover the following items:

1. *General.* Tiredness, breathlessness, poor appetite, failure to thrive.
2. *Infection*, including occasionally chronic bowel infection.
3. *Bleeding* into skin, joints, renal tract (urine), bowel (faeces).
4. *Diet*, particularly malnutrition. A retarded child not uncommonly has a diet deficient in vitamins and iron; occasionally he exhibits pica (dirt-eating); rarely he presents as anaemia due to lead poisoning from pica.
5. *Faeces.* Frequency and appearance of faeces may suggest malabsorption, bleeding or infection.
6. *Drugs.* Microcytic anaemia may be caused by intestinal bleeding due to aspirin; macrocytic anaemia may arise from anticonvulsants such as phenytoin or primidone which interfere with folic acid metabolism; aplastic anaemia (often serious) from cytotoxic drugs (sometimes a necessary hazard when treating neoplasm) or from chloramphenicol. In aplastic anaemia the bone marrow activity may be suppressed beyond recovery.

Examination

Look particularly for:

1. Pallor. Many children look pale and are not

Table 32.1 Mean normal blood values at different ages (modified from Green & Haggerty, 1968)

	Birth (cord values)	*1 wk*	*2 wk*	*2 m*	*6 m*	*1 yr*	*2 yr*	*4 yr*	*10–12 yr*	*Adult males*	*Adult females*
RBC (million per mm^3)	5.7	5.3	5.1	4.5	4.5	4.6	4.7	4.7	4.9	5.4	4.8
Haematocrit (PRCV/100 ml)	56.6	52.7	49.6	38.9	36.2	35.2	35.5	37.1	41.3	47.4	42.7
Haemoglobin (g/100 ml)	13.6 –19.6	19.6	18	13.3	12.3	11.6	11.7	12.6	13.1	16	14
MCV (μ^3)	106	101	96	85	78	77	78	80	81	87	87
MCH ($\mu\mu$g)	38	37	35	30	27	25	25	27	28	29	29
MCHC (g/100 ml packed RBC expressed as %)	38.0	37.0	36.3	34.2	34.0	33.0	33.0	34.0	33.8	34	34
Reticulocytes (% RBC)	4.5	0–1	0.67	1.2	1.4	0.9	1.0	1.0	1.0	1.6	1.7
Nucleated (% nucleated cells)	1.5	–	–	–	–	–	–	–	–	–	–

anaemic. Look at the palms of the hands and the colour of the knuckles as well as the mucosae, conjunctivae and tongue. A pale child may be nervous, or have a pale parent.

2. Bruising, including petechiae and the result of the Hess tourniquet test.
3. Jaundice.
4. Enlargement of liver, spleen and lymph nodes.
5. Koilonychia. Not common in children but when it occurs is likely to be either congenital or due to iron deficiency.
6. Heart murmur. An apical systolic murmur (and less commonly one over the pulmonary area) may be loud enough to be considered of organic cardiac origin, yet vanish when an underlying severe anaemia is treated.
7. Mental retardation, including cretinism.
8. Infection.
9. Urine: infection; haematuria; bile and urobilinogen.
10. Stools: presence of blood; evidence of malabsorption.
11. Blood examination.
12. Racial origin. Certain haemolytic disorders are relatively more common in certain races. Thus thalassaemia occurs more frequently in those from the Mediterranean region, the Middle East and Far East; sickle cell disease in African Negroes and Mediterranean populations.

Classification of the anaemias

There are several ways of classifying the anaemias, each with its protagonists. It is suggested that the most useful is that which depends on the practical and clinical approach, leaving the morphological approach for the haematologist. Thus we can divide anaemias into three broad groups, with appropriate subdivisions as follows:

1. Anaemia due to deficient production of red cells or haemoglobin (dyshaemopoietic anaemia). Underlying causes:
   a. Deficiency in haemopoietic factors, e.g. iron, folic acid, thyroxin, vitamin C, vitamin B_{12}.
   b. Deficiency of haemopoietic tissue (hypoplastic anaemia), arising from marrow hypoplasia, chronic or acute infection, leukaemia, or toxic effects of drugs (e.g. chloramphenicol, sulphonamides and their derivatives, phenylbutazone, phenytoin).
2. Anaemia due to excessive destruction of red cells (haemolytic anaemia). Underlying causes:
   a. Primary abnormality of red cells or haemoglobin, e.g. sickle cell disease, spherocytosis, thalassaemia.
   b. Destruction of red cells by extraneous factors, e.g. Rh or ABO incompatibilities, toxic substances including infection, vitamin B_{12} or folate deficiency.
3. Anaemia due to excessive loss of red cells, arising from:
   a. Simple acute haemorrhage.
   b. Chronic overt haemorrhage, e.g. Meckel's diverticulum, polyps, oesophageal varices, hookworm disease, genitourinary bleeding.
   c. Bleeding diseases, e.g. purpura, haemophilia, leukaemia, scurvy.

The deficiency anaemias

Iron deficiency anaemia

Anaemia due to iron deficiency is the most common nutritional defect seen in paediatric practice; it is particularly prevalent in infancy. Minor degrees of nutritional anaemia are common and severe anaemia is not rare (Moore, 1975). In the infant, it must be remembered that if milk alone forms the diet, there is likely to be a low iron intake because breast milk is low in iron whilst cow's milk is even lower. Diluting the cow's milk makes the iron loading lower still. Most dried milks however, have added iron. The child is growing rapidly, thus his iron requirements increase relatively rapidly. Anaemia seems to predispose to infection, which in turn, by causing loss of appetite and sometimes poor food absorption, may increase the anaemia; thus a vicious circle is set up.

Clinical features. Even with moderate anaemia, some infants seem of good colour and are not overtly ill. A history of repeated upper respiratory infections and gastrointestinal upsets should call for a blood count.

In advanced iron deficiency anaemia the sheet-like or waxy pallor is very striking. The mucosae are pale, the spleen may be enlarged and a soft blowing systolic murmur is frequently heard. Usually the heart is not enlarged, but slight dyspnoea and oedema may occur. The changes in the epithelial structures which form such a good diagnostic aid in adults (such as atrophic glossitis, dysphagia and koilonychia) do not occur in infants and only rarely occur in older children. The child goes off his food and may be irritable.

The blood picture. Characteristically there is a hypochromic and microcytic anaemia (in contrast to the normochromic, normocytic type of physiological anaemia seen in the neonate). Since iron deficiency primarily affects haemoglobin synthesis and to a lesser degree the formation of red cells, the red cell count may be normal or only slightly reduced. Haematocrit levels are reduced. The haemoglobin is reduced out of proportion to the number of red cells. The red cell count usually ranges between three and five million; the haemoglobin may range between three and nine grammes per 100 ml.

Other blood findings:

1. A mean corpuscular haemoglobin (MCH) less than

27 $\mu\mu g$. (The MCH represents the average quantity (by weight) of haemoglobin per single red cell). The normal range is from 27 to 32 $\mu\mu g$.

2. A mean corpuscular haemoglobin concentration (MCHC) less than 30 per cent. (The MCHC represents the average concentration of haemoglobin per red cell, as calculated from the amount of haemoglobin per 100 ml of cells rather than of whole blood. The result is expressed as a percentage). The normal range is from 32 to 38 per cent.

3. A mean corpuscular volume (MCV) less than 78 cubic microns (78 μ^3). (The MCV is the mean or average volume of a single red cell in cubic microns. The normal range is from 80 to 94 μ^3. A MCV of more than 94 μ^3 indicates macrocytosis; 80-94 μ^3 normocytosis; less than 80 μ^3 microcytosis).

4. Characteristically the film shows a predominance of hypochromic microcytes with pronounced central pallor. Irregular shaped red cells (poikilocytes) are common. The platelet count is usually normal but may be raised and in severe anaemia may be reduced.

Treatment: prevention. One should note that premature infants and rapidly growing children require more than the average amount of iron and are thus particularly vulnerable to anaemia. Thus low birth weight infants and twins should receive iron from four weeks of age until mixed feeding occurs. All babies should be encouraged to start mixed feeding from about four months. Strained fruits, vegetables, beef, beef or lamb liver, fortified cereals and eggs are useful sources of iron.

Treatment of the established case. Nearly every case responds well to oral iron. There are many iron preparations on the market, but despite the claims of the manufacturers regarding the advantages of their various iron compounds, ferrous sulphate is nearly always effective, well tolerated and cheap. The simplest oral preparation is Ferrous Sulphate Mixture Paediatric, BPC for infants or in tablet form for older children (remember the tablets are poisonous in large doses). An elemental iron dose of 5 mg/kg/day in three divided doses is adequate for therapy. Ferrous sulphate contains 20 per cent elemental iron.

It is now no longer considered necessary, or advisable, to give iron on an empty stomach. It is adequately absorbed when taken during or after a meal (which includes milk), when it is less likely to irritate the bowel. Mothers should be warned that iron will blacken the stools and the liquid iron preparations may stain the teeth. Both discolourations are harmless and transient and the purist may suggest that liquid iron be taken through a straw (this antic may be the persuading factor in ensuring that the child takes his medicine). The black stools offer the practitioner useful evidence that his instructions are being followed.

It is most important that treatment be continued for at least six to eight weeks after the haemoglobin has returned to normal levels. Before overt iron deficiency anaemia occurs, the total iron stores in the body have been depleted and failure to replenish these will eventually result in recurrence of anaemia.

Response to treatment. After a lag period of seven to ten days the haemoglobin should rise by one gramme per 100 ml every ten days. The child should improve dramatically in temperament, activity and appetite within one week of initiating therapy. Failure to respond to treatment usually means:

1. The patient has not taken the iron.
2. The diagnosis is wrong.
3. There is active infection somewhere.
4. There is undiagnosed bleeding somewhere.
5. Rarely, failure to respond to treatment implies malabsorption of the iron. This would indicate the need for intramuscular iron injections. Such cases are reported in the literature, but I cannot recall an uncomplicated case of childhood iron deficiency anaemia in general practice requiring such injection.

Treatment of iron deficiency anaemia is simple and rewarding. The apathetic child bounces back into robust health. Relapses should not occur: when they do, one should suspect an underlying cause, such as chronic, occult bleeding or chronic infection to which treatment must be directed.

Anaemia due to folic (pteroylglutamic) acid deficiency

Folic acid is of fundamental importance in protein biosynthesis, and in the synthesis of DNA and RNA. Deficiency leads to diminished cell growth and megaloblastic anaemia, but this is uncommon in childhood.

The main causes of folic acid deficiency:

1. Inadequate dietary intake. Folic acid, a member of the vitamin B complex, is found in plant and animal tissues. Potent sources of the vitamin inclтde liver, beef and fresh green vegetables.

2. Defective absorption. Folic acid is readily absorbed from the gastrointestinal tract. Malabsorption may occur in such conditions as coeliac disease, gastrointestinal resections, fibrocystic disease and prolonged diarrhoea from other causes.

3. Increased requirements such as rapid growth, haemolytic disease (e.g. sickle cell disease), infection, leukaemia.

4. Presence of folic acid antagonists such as drugs used to combat neoplastic disease (e.g. methotrexate) or anticonvulsant drugs (particularly phenytoin).

Ascorbic acid seems to be related to folic acid synthesis, and the incidence of megaloblastic anaemia in infancy has dropped precipitously since infant foods have been fortified with large amounts of vitamin C. However, some authorities believe that the occurrence of folic acid deficiency anaemia in infants suffering from scurvy is really due to the fortuitous deficiency of both vitamins, and that the addition of vitamin C to the feeding formula acts as a preservative for the folate content.

Clinical features. The onset is insidious, usually between the ages of 2 and 18 months. The premature baby is particularly liable. The infant presents with the signs and symptoms described earlier in common with other forms of anaemia.

Diagnosis. This is confirmed by the laboratory. The blood film shows moderate macrocytosis and the red cell folate and serum folate are low. Bone marrow examination can usually be avoided, but it may be needed for precise diagnosis.

Treatment. The anaemia responds readily and completely to oral administration of folic acid given in a daily dosage of 5 mg until the blood picture returns to normal (5–15 μg folic acid per cent in serum). A reticulocyte response to treatment confirms the diagnosis and usually obviates the need for further bone marrow examinations.

Vitamin B^{12} deficiency

This is very rare as a primary disorder in children. It is treated by intramuscular cyanocobalamine (or related compounds), a suitable dose being 100 microgrammes three times per week until the haemoglobin is normal, followed by the same dose once per month thereafter.

Leukaemia

'Leukaemia is a major killer of children and is second only to accidents as a cause of death in children between one and fourteen years of age' (Lascari, 1973).

Aetiology. Little is known for certain about the cause of leukaemia. Exposure to ionizing radiations may play a part; after such exposure there is an interesting delay period of from about 18 months to 5 years. Prenatal exposure to diagnostic X-rays appears to increase the incidence. The condition is relatively more common in cases of Down's Syndrome and Turner's syndrome. There is some evidence that a virus may be one of the aetiological factors (Allen and Cole, 1972). Viruses are certainly the main cause of leukaemia in several animal groups, but their causal role in the human disease is not yet proven despite a considerable degree of research directed to this question. The family doctor may well be asked if it be likely that a sibling of a patient with leukaemia will develop the disease. The extreme rarity of this occurrence other than in identical twins permits unequivocal reassurance on this point.

Types. The most useful, somewhat simplified, classification recognises four types, i.e. acute and chronic lymphoblastic leukaemia and acute and chronic myeloblastic leukaemia. There is no clinical difference between acute lymphoblastic and acute myeloblastic leukaemia.

Incidence. Leukaemia is much the commonest malignant disease of early life. There is roughly one case per 2000 children up to the age of 14 years; the condition is slightly commoner in boys. The peak incidence occurs between the ages of 2 and 4 years. About 75 per cent of the cases are of the acute lymphoblastic type; about 15 per cent are acute myeloblastic leukaemias. The chronic forms are uncommon in childhood.

Clinical features. The disease may present at any age but is commonest in children between two and four years old. The onset may be insidious. A previously well child becomes tired, pale and unwell over a considerable period. More usually the onset is rapid with perhaps severe anaemia, bruising, petechiae and haemorrhages.

a. Growth of leukaemic deposits. Enlargement of superficial lymph glands or the discovery of an abdominal mass may be the reason for the child being brought to the doctor. The cervical glands are those most often involved, but they can occur anywhere. Typically they feel rubbery and are discrete and painless. The spleen is enlarged in about 80 per cent of cases; it is smooth, firm and painless unless very big. The liver is often enlarged but usually not as markedly as is the spleen.

Meningeal involvement is commoner in those cases in which systemic remission of months or years has occurred. It is becoming more common nowadays, since treatment is rather more effective than formerly. Papilloedema, nerve palsies and fits may occur, as may other signs and symptoms of increased intracranial pressure, notably headache, papilloedema and vomiting.

Bone and joint involvement. Sometimes the first complaint is of bone or joint pains. Radiological examination shows highly characteristic translucent bands transversely placed just proximal to the metaphyses of the long bones. Less characteristically, periosteal lesions and areas of erosion and pathological fractures may occur.

b. Bone marrow disturbance. This is common, and causes a variety of symptoms. Of importance is the frequent presence of anaemia, often the presenting symptom in leukaemia. Haemorrhages are usually due to severe thrombocytopenia; bleeding may be *overt* and show as purpura and bruises, and bleeding from the nose, gums or gastrointestinal tract, or *covert* such as microscopic haematuria.

c. Enlargement of various organs. Enlargement of the spleen and liver are common (see above). Any organ can be involved: the kidneys, gonads, mediastinum and periorbital tissues are examples. The skin can be involved in a variety of ways. There may be petechiae and bruises as mentioned earlier. More specific are small, yellow, discrete and elevated flat-topped plaques. Skin lesions may become haemorrhagic, necrotic and infected.

d. Infection. Oropharyngeal sepsis with gingivitis and bleeding from the gums is frequently a presenting feature. Thrush of the mouth, intestine or vagina may occur. Systemic infections and septicaemia are also encountered.

Diagnosis. Leukaemia may be suspected on clinical grounds: the multiplicity of symptoms with relatively insidious onset make it a great imitator. A high index of suspicion on the part of the family doctor is essential, especially when the child presents with anaemia, bruising and enlarged lymph glands. The diagnosis is confirmed and the type ascertained by blood and bone marrow examination. Most cases show a low platelet count and low haemoglobin. Immature white cell (blast cells) may be obvious or require repeated searches.

It is important that all cases of thrombocytopenia, unexplained anaemia, and neutropenia undergo marrow examination if leukaemia is not to be missed, as the peripheral blood not uncommonly fails to reflect the grossly abnormal marrow from time to time during the course of the disease.

Treatment. Treatment is a complicated affair and firmly in the hands of the specialists. Results are steadily improving and long remissions of several years have been recorded. It is possible to achieve remission in 4-6 weeks in over 90 per cent of children with acute lymphatic leukaemia using one of the recommended drug regimes. More and more cures are being reported: if children are not cured, they have remained well for over eight years. Keeping these children alive longer than hitherto has yielded the relatively new hazard of more frequent extramedullary presentation of the disease. Presumably the leukaemic child used to die before he could develop these complications. Thus central nervous system involvement is commoner nowadays, and without the appropriate prophylaxis it can be expected in about half the cases of acute lymphatic leukaemia. Meningeal leukaemia will often occur whilst the peripheral blood and bone marrow show good remission.

There is a multiplicity of treatment schedules. New cytotoxic drugs appear at frequent intervals and research in this field is continuous and rewarding. The drugs most frequently used at present are the corticosteroids (such as prednisolone or prednisone in a dose of about 2.5 mg per kg body weight per day, in divided doses), and the antileukaemic drugs, such as methotrexate (which is a DNA antimetabolite), vincristine and aspariginase. The two types of drugs are more effective in producing a remission if used together, but this increased effectiveness is at the cost of increased marrow vulnerability. It can be a delicately balanced decision what to use.

Early central nervous system prophylaxis is now advocated and it has been conclusively shown that either craniospinal radiotherapy or cranial radiotherapy combined with drug therapy administered early in remission will reduce meningeal relapse from 50 per cent to as low as 5 per cent (Simone *et al*, 1972; Aur *et al*, 1973). In boys, the testicles are frequently involved and bilateral biopsy is advocated to detect occult disease. Some centres routinely irradiate the testicles.

Bone marrow transplants have proved a useful adjunct to treatment using marrow extracted from the pelvic bones of a normal individual. The aim is to repopulate the haematopoietic marrow which has been destroyed by the drug therapy. Recently, autotransplantation, that is intravenous transplant to the patient of his own leukaemic marrow (after it has been 'cleaned' of leukaemic cells) seems a promising line of treatment.

Of current interest, too, is the culture of specific cytotoxic cells in vitro – so-called "T" cells (thymus-derived lymphocytes) – which will destroy the leukaemic cells specifically.

Non-specific treatment includes blood transfusions which may be needed to tide the patient over whilst awaiting a remission and to counteract severe anaemia. It would take several weeks for normal red cell regeneration and it is wrong to deny the very definite improvement in symptoms which can be expected after transfusion.

The potential cure of perhaps one quarter of children with acute lymphatic leukaemia with modern therapy makes it very important that none die as a result of the treatment, which is necessarily very hazardous. Whilst awaiting the remission, the child is at risk from infection, haemorrhage and metabolic disturbance. Infection presents the greatest risk and must be energetically treated with antibiotics, often on an empirical basis. The anti-leukaemic treatment causes immunosuppression and death can occur from such usually trivial conditions as chickenpox or measles. Children should have varicella and measles antibodies measured at the start of chemotherapy and parents of non-immune children should be warned of the potential hazards of infection. Contact with these infections should be avoided as far as possible and in the event of contact, zoster immune globulin (for chickenpox) or broad-spectrum immune globulin (for measles) should be given within 1-2 days of contact.

When a child does not improve rapidly with the more commonly used antibiotics, he should be admitted to hospital where fuller investigation is possible. Combinations of antibiotics are frequently needed some of which must be given intravenously.

Children with leukaemia should not receive any live vaccines such as influenza, smallpox, poliomyelitis or measles but diptheria and tetanus toxoids may be given.

It is of the utmost importance that the family doctor is kept informed of the treatment his patient is receiving from the specialist. It is commonplace nowadays for the patient to lose contact with his family doctor whilst attending outpatients at frequent intervals. Just as surely as specialised treatment is firmly in the hands of the specialist so is the day-to-day surveillance firmly in the hands of the family doctor. It is he who will be called upon to treat the potentially dangerous infection – infection which would normally be mild and 'routine'. It is he who is likely to be the first to note signs and symptoms of impending relapse, and to be called upon to counsel and guide the parents through the everyday problems of management.

Management of acute myeloblastic leukaemia is on similar lines. Intensive combination chemotherapy is followed by transfusion and other supportive measures where indicated. Routine cranial irradiation is not indicated but intrathecal anti-leukaemic drugs should be given as C.N.S. prophylaxis. Bone marrow transplants are giving much more promising results but the likelihood of remission is at present much less than with acute lymphatic leukaemia.

Prognosis. It is essential that the family doctor has some knowledge of the risks and hopes which attach to this serious group of disorders. Adverse prognostic features include early central nervous system involvement, a high leucocyte count and the presence of a mediastinal mass or large liver or spleen. The outlook is worse below the age of one and above 10 years, in negro children and in males.

With treatment in special centres and with the closest cooperation between the family doctor, the paediatrician and the treatment centre, more than half the children with acute lymphatic leukaemia should be alive and well after five years and a proportion of these may be cured.

The prognosis with acute myeloid leukaemia is still poor and only about 10 per cent of patients will be alive three years after diagnosis.

The special role of the family doctor. It seems appropriate to discuss here the particular role the family doctor has to play in the management of leukaemia when the tragic situation arises in which a child, hitherto well, may die within a relatively short time. The doctor must be constantly aware of the fact that he is treating not only the blood but the child and his family. In spite of the fact that there may be little hope of cure, there is much to be done.

The child. Previous knowledge of the child is an advantage. He should be told about the various procedures about to be done, such as the drawing of blood or lumbar puncture, but there is little merit in telling him too much at one time or too soon. The child's belief and trust in his doctor is very important. Admissions to hospital can be timed to interfere as little as possible with holidays and school matters. His schooling can be supervised to some extent, as can the desirability of his sitting for examinations. Whilst he should be restricted as little as possible, he should not be overtaxed. Failure to take part in activities of which he is quite capable, will inevitably induce depression, gloom and fear.

The child is far more able to cope with his illness when his doctor presents a degree of hope and an assurance that he not only understands the illness but is competent to deal with the symptoms as and when they develop. It is useless to ask the child to cheer up when he is feeling ill or in pain: it is constructive to alleviate the symptoms whilst offering confident hope for the next few days. The time will come when the child's hopes become more circumscribed and on a day-to-day basis. Should he be depressed and apathetic, he will require constant sympathy and understanding. He must be allowed to do whatever he wishes at this stage, notwithstanding the oft-repeated fears of his parents that he may worsen his condition. If he wishes to do nothing his wish should be respected.

Should the child with leukaemia be told the diagnosis? A child's idea of death is different from an adult's, and below about the age of ten there is probably no virtue in telling the diagnosis. Above ten years, it is very likely that the child will want to know about his condition, and failure to satisfy his wish will induce fear and the conclusion that he is so gravely ill that it must not be discussed. There is a real danger that he will hear odd scraps of discussion whilst in hospital or at home, and be very concerned when these do not fit in with what he is told to his face. I am of the opinion that when the child asks he should be answered as truthfully as possible. The answer must be tempered with hope and the discussion turned towards the great possibility of remission and the constant seeking for new treatments. If the lines of communication are always open between the doctor and his young patient, and the child knows that he can depend on the doctor to attend him when needed, a difficult situation will be the better managed.

The parent. Each parent of a child suffering a fatal illness must adapt to the inevitable loss and final death of his child. The doctor must be aware of the terrible shock to a parent such a diagnosis affords, and of the inevitable sequence of initial numbing followed by the anguish and depression as the truth sinks in. The parent may react by refusing to admit of such a diagnosis, by wishing to seek innumerable 'second' opinions or by deep feelings of guilt regarding his failings as a parent. The fear that leukaemia is hereditary or attributable to some episode in the child's past may put one spouse against the other. They may well seek to lay the blame at someone's door. Often the doctor will be accused of incompetence. 'Should you not have thought of the diagnosis earlier, doctor' may be implied or said.

The doctor must steer his family through all these vicissitudes and discuss problems as they arise, which they surely will, with calmness, sympathy and empathy (MacCarthy, 1975). He must tell them what he can offer and what he cannot. He must be prepared to discuss the questions of schooling, holidays and many other matters which would normally seem outside his remit. He should encourage parents to join the Leukaemia Society (see p. 396). He would be well advised to work in close cooperation with the specialist and seek his advice on details of management so that he has extra help when needed, and in particular so that the parents can see that all that can be done for their child is being done. Above all, he must be ready and willing to help whenever needed and must convince that he is so. Throughout this intimate liaison with the family he must be dispassionate to a degree and avoid being too entangled in the grief situation, lest his judgment becomes impaired.

Despite the relative helplessness of the doctor when treating a disease with inevitable fatal outcome, there can be few more rewarding tasks for the family doctor than helping a family through a fatal illness. Their gratitude will be a measure of his success.

The haemolytic anaemias

In the haemolytic anaemias the red cells are broken down prematurely; that is before their normal life span of about 120 days. The excessive haemolysis is due to (a) abnormal extracorpuscular factors acting on normal red cells, or (b) intracorpuscular defects (usually congenital). The increased haemolysis causes recognisable features common to this group of anaemias.

Clinical features

1. Anaemia – not always present, if the marrow can regenerate the red cells adequately.
2. Jaundice, minimal or marked (always acholuric).
3. Bone hyperplasia (seen on X-rays as radial striations produced by newly formed spicules of bone. Bossing of the skull can occur, due to long-standing marrow hyperplasia).
4. Splenic enlargement.
5. Haemosiderosis, with enlargement of liver and spleen due to storage of excessive iron.
6. Gallstones.
7. Black stools (due to stercobilin).
8. Urine becoming darker on standing (due to uribilinogen changing to urobilin).

Laboratory findings

1. Raised serum bilirubin (giving indirect Van den Bergh reaction).
2. Increased number of reticulocytes.
3. Increased serum iron.
4. Morphologically abnormal red cells (in many cases).
5. Increased urobilinogen in urine and faeces.
6. Methaemoglobinaemia.

Haemolytic anaemia due to extracorpuscular causes

These include haemolytic disease of the newborn (dealt with in Ch. 25), and reactions to blood transfusions. Other precipitating factors include.

1. Infection, e.g. streptococcal, malaria, *Clostridium welchii, Haemophilus influenzae*.
2. Chemical agents: sulphonamides, chlorpromazine, phenacetin, penicillin, to name but a few. NB: individuals whose erythrocytes are deficient in glucose-6-phosphate dehydrogenase have an inborn proclivity to haemolyse upon exposure to drugs or on ingestion of fava beans. This congenital abnormality is not uncommon and can occur in over 10 per cent of certain races, notably Negroes, Jews and Mediterranean races. It is rare in other Caucasian races. It is much commoner in males, as the condition is inherited as an X-linked recessive disorder.
3. Severe burns. Acute haemolytic anaemia may occur within 48 hours of being severely burnt, probably due to a direct effect of heat on the erythrocyte.

Haemolytic anaemias due to intracorpuscular defects

In the main these are hereditary conditions. Hereditary spherocytosis (familial acholuric jaundice) was the first form of familial jaundice defined at the end of the last century. Other forms of inherited haemolytic anaemia have since been described, including thalassaemia and other haemoglobinopathies. All these conditions have two common factors: (a) they are inherited and (b) the abnormality is in the red cell, so that transfused normal red cells survive normally.

Hereditary spherocytosis

Aetiology. Males and females are equally affected. It is a dominant hereditary disorder, much commoner in white Europeans but occurring also elsewhere. The mature red cells are small, thick and spheroidal and the basic defect seems to be an increased permeability of the red cell membrane to the sodium ion. This can be compensated for only by excessive cation diffusion working in the opposite direction. When the cation load into the cell becomes too great, haemolysis occurs.

Clinical features. Most commonly it is diagnosed in children of school age, but it can occur in the neonatal period (so mimicking haemolytic disease of the newborn). Jaundice may be slight, anaemia may be marked, the spleen is palpable and the blood shows a high reticulocytosis. Gallstones can occur in later life. The picture is complicated by periods of crisis when haemolysis is increased and the child becomes acutely ill with abdominal pain, fever, vomiting and jaundice. Occasionally an aplastic phase occurs when the blood picture changes and is characterised by complete absence of reticulocytes (showing that erythrogenesis is not occurring).

The red cells show consistently increased fragility and are spheroidal.

Treatment. This condition is intimately linked with splenic activity, and splenectomy is indicated in all but the mildest of cases where there is an entirely compensated haemolytic anaemia and where no aplastic crises have developed. Operation should be deferred, if possible, until the age of four years because of the danger of severe infections in the earlier years. All cases respond excellently to splenectomy, which cures the anaemia and allows the red cell survival to return to near normal. Transfusion is needed as supportive therapy at times of severe anaemia or aplasia. Transfused cells survive normally. The administration of folic acid during aplasia seems to be useful.

The haemoglobinopathies

Sickle cell disease

Aetiology. Sickle cell disease is a comprehensive term used to include those hereditary conditions in which the underlying pathology is the presence of sickle haemoglobin (haemoglobin S) in the red cells. It is a disease found primarily in Negroes and in white people of Mediterranean origin, particularly people from Italy and Greece.

When haemoglobin S coexists with normal adult haemoglobin (haemoglobin A) the result is *sickle cell trait* – a mild or asymptomatic form of the disease. When all the haemoglobin is haemoglobin S, or when it co-exists with the fetal type of haemoglobin (haemoglobin F), *sickle cell anaemia* results. Thus, both the parents of children with sickle cell anaemia will have the sickling gene, but only one of the parents of children with sickle cell trait carries the gene.

Clinical features. Sickle cell anaemia usually manifests itself between six months and two years. Usually anaemia occurs early in the disease and some children die within weeks of first developing symptoms. Painful crises occur due to intravascular thromboses; a crisis may last up to a week during which time the child complains of pain in any organ, but particularly in the bones and joints, and in the abdomen. In infants and young children, marked pain and swelling of the short bones of the hand and feet, due to infarction, constitute the relatively common 'hand-foot syndrome'. Occasionally complications common to haemolytic anaemia, such as gallstones occur. Throughout childhood there is chronic anaemia with periodic exacerbations and as the child gets older he develops the curious typical sickle-cell appearance: long, thin arms and legs, upper dorsal kyphosis and bossing of the skull. A curious benefit of the disease is that it protects from malaria.

Sickle cell trait causes no symptoms under normal conditions. However, should the child with the trait become hypoxic (such as whilst under an anaesthetic or in a non-pressurised aircraft), he becomes liable to minor crises.

Diagnosis. This is confirmed in the laboratory by the co-existence of haemolytic anaemia and haemoglobin S. Sickled red cells may be seen on the direct blood film in sickle cell disease, but not in the trait, where sickling can be induced by rendering the blood anoxic *in vitro*.

Treatment. There is no specific treatment for sickle cell disease (or for any other haemoglobinopathy) other than blood transfusion during a crisis to counteract severe anaemia. Bed rest, oxygen and analgesics will be required for a painful crisis, and antibiotics if infection supervenes. Regular folic acid supplements are required. Iron has no effect and should be avoided. As treatment is frequently unsatisfactory, genetic counselling should be offered to all parents when both are heterozygous for haemoglobin S. On average, three quarters of the children of such parents have sickle cell trait and one quarter have sickle cell disease.

Prognosis. The outcome is still very unfavourable in many cases of sickle cell anaemia, with a fatal outcome in childhood or early adult life in many instances. However, improved nutrition and better supervision have improved the outlook in recent years. When haemoglobin F coexists with haemoglobin S (found more commonly in children from Saudi Arabia and India) the disease is more benign as the haemoglobin F seems to prevent or restrict the sickling process.

Thalassaemia (Cooley's anaemia, Mediterranean anaemia)

Thalassaemia is a hereditary haemolytic disorder occurring predominantly in persons of Mediterranean origin (Thalas = inland sea), the peoples of Africa and the middle and far East. It comprises a heterogeneous group of syndromes characterised by a deficiency in the synthesis of normal adult haemoglobin. *Thalassaemia major* is the homozygous form and shows the fully developed serious form of the disease. In the major form fetal type haemoglobin (HbF) persists, while adult haemoglobin (HbA) is absent or deficient. *Thalassaemia minor* is the heterozygous form, in which there is a lower proportion of HbF.

There are thus many grades of the disease, ranging from the asymptomatic trait (which is probably of significance only in the risk of a more severe form occurring in offspring) to the fully fledged, serious major form. Except for the marked elevation of fetal haemoglobin, no specific abnormal haemoglobin has been described in patients with this disease.

Thalassaemia may occur in co-existence with another haemoglobinopathy, and sickle cell trait or other haemoglobinopathy should be searched for when only one parent of a child with the severe disease shows the thalassaemia trait. It is likely that an abnormal haemoglobin will be found in the other parent.

Clinical features. Thalassaemia presents a wide and continuous spectrum of severity ranging from the minor to the major forms. The age at which the disease becomes overt depends on the grade. Thus a severe case may require transfusion in the first year of life; in the intermediate group the disorder becomes clinically manifest in later childhood.

In the major form the clinical picture is one of severe anaemia, splenomegaly and a characteristic facies due to prominence of the malar eminences, frontal bossing and a Mongoloid slant to the eyes. Aplastic crises and folic acid deficiency can arise, as with sickle cell disease. The prognosis is poor in the severe form and death in childhood is common.

Treatment. Apart from symptomatic treatment during a crisis, transfusions form the main line of attack. Chronic anaemia is the main hazard and it seems reasonable to transfuse with red cells when the haemoglobin level falls below 6 g/100 ml because of the danger of heart failure. It is unnecessary to maintain the haemoglobin level above 10 g/100 ml as there is then a possibility of depressing erythropoiesis. There is no shortage of iron and repeated transfusion, whilst prolonging life in the short term, carries the real danger of producing haemosiderosis which may itself prove lethal.

When transfusion requirements become excessive, that is at less than monthly intervals to maintain a haemoglobin level above 6 g/100 ml, splenectomy should be considered; this has been found to reduce transfusion requirements. Removing the spleen creates the new hazard of increased liability to severe infection and should be delayed to at least late childhood.

It can be seen that the management of these cases of haemoglobinopathy requires a well balanced judgement and the family doctor has at least as important a role to play as the specialist in dealing with the patient and the family. Close cooperation and communication between the family doctor and the specialist is of great importance. With a more cosmopolitan population present in Britain than in former years, these severe diseases are no longer rare, and it is both necessary and rewarding for the family doctor to understand how to deal with them.

BLEEDING DISEASES

Clinically, the most important of the hereditary bleeding diseases are *haemophilia, Christmas disease* (named after the boy in whom this disease was first diagnosed) and to a lesser extent *Von Willebrand's disease.* Whilst these conditions are still uncommon, it is likely they will become less so as most sufferers now reach adult life and have children.

These three conditions have in common an absence or deficiency of an essential clotting factor: factor VIII in haemophilia and Von Willebrand's disease and factor IX in Christmas disease.

Genetics. The abnormal genes responsible for haemophilia or Christmas disease are recessive, sex linked and carried on the X chromosome. Since the male (XY) has no normal X chromosome to counterbalance the abnormal gene, these conditions usually occur in males. For a female (XX) to have haemophilia or Christmas disease she must have the abnormal gene on both X chromosomes. It will be seen that this could happen in the female offspring of a male with the disease and a female carrier, but this is rare.

For the purpose of genetic counselling it can be stated that an affected male cannot transmit the disease to any of his sons or their descendants, but that any daughter of his will be a carrier. In about one third of cases there is no family history of disease, either because spontaneous mutation has occurred, or because inheritance has been through a long line of female carriers. In Von Willebrand's disease the offending, abnormal gene is not sex linked, but attached to one of the autosomes.

Haemophilia and Christmas disease

Clinical features: the bleeding tendency in haemophilia and Christmas disease affects mainly the deeper tissues and organs (in contradistinction to bleeding in disorders of platelets and capillaries which affects mainly the skin and mucous membranes). Bleeding occurs into subcutaneous tissues, joints, and muscles, or from the kidney. After injury or surgery bleeding may be delayed for several hours, but then it may continue for days and is not controlled by pressure. Bleeding from superficial cuts is not usually excessive because primary haemostasis, dependent as it is on capillary contraction and formation of platelet plugs, is normal (again, this is in contradistinction to thrombocytopaenia and toxic purpura). In the severe forms these diseases show early in life, often in the first year. Such patients are likely later to develop bleeding into joints with resulting haemarthroses which are crippling unless treated promptly. Haemophiliacs do not bleed spontaneously but always as a result of trauma. However, the trauma can be so trivial as to be unnoticed.

Von Willebrand's disease

Clinical features: the bleeding manifestations of this condition illustrate the mixed nature of the disorder, i.e. the deficiency of factor VIII combined with a capillary defect. The clinical picture is dominated by cutaneous and mucosal bleeding (frequently manifesting as epistaxis) but deep intramuscular haematomata may occur. Serious bleeding following surgical procedures is a risk. However, Von Willebrand's disease is usually relatively mild compared with haemophilia.

Diagnosis of bleeding diseases

An abnormal bleeding tendency after such procedures as tonsillectomy or tooth extraction, or 'spontaneous' haemarthroses limited to males, suggests haemophilia. The whole blood clotting time is usually (but not always) prolonged, whilst the bleeding time is normal. In Von Willebrand's disease the bleeding time is prolonged, clotting time is normal and the disease occurs in both sexes.

The final diagnostic proof may result from the assay of the various clotting factors, in particular of factor VIII and factor IX. These tests are becoming more widely used; even so, the diagnosis in the milder case is not always easy.

Management of bleeding diseases

Treatment of bleeding

Minor episodes are treated by compression of lacerations (rather than stitching), cooling, and various local applications. Gelatin sponge saturated in a solution of topical thrombin and adrenalin and applied with firm pressure is valuable. A major bleeding episode must be controlled by giving the deficient clotting factor (usually factor VIII). There must be enough to raise the level in the blood to that required for haemostasis and healing. Fresh whole blood, rapidly frozen fresh plasma, dried human or animal factor VIII or cryoprecipitate can be used. All are given intravenously. Cryoprecipitate is the cold, insoluble fraction of plasma protein obtained by thawing frozen plasma slowly. The resulting precipitate is a potent source of factor VIII and fibrinogen and can be kept refrozen for months.

Large quantities of fresh whole blood may be needed, but cryoprecipitate can be given by syringe and in small volume and is therefore both convenient and less likely to overload the vascular system. It seems a pity to give whole blood when it is a relatively small quantity of missing factor that is required. In the future, one could envisage giving small, daily prophylactic dosages of factor VIII, rather akin to the administration of insulin to a diabetic.

Joint swelling and pain often herald haemarthrosis, which is the single most incapacitating event in the life of a severe haemophiliac. Factor VIII should be given as soon as possible. Should the joint continue to swell, hospital admission is desirable, when the joint should be aspirated and firm bandaging applied until bleeding appears to have stopped. Gentle exercise should then be given.

Pain

Aspirin and other salicylates should not be given because of the real danger of bleeding. Alternative drugs include dihydrocodein (D.F. 118), pentazocine (Fortral), paracetamol and dextropropoxyphene (Doloxene). Avoid the use of addictive drugs.

For necessary surgical procedures one must keep the blood level of factor VIII above 30 per cent for over 24 hours. Cryoprecipitate is probably the preparation of choice.

Specific replacement therapy in Christmas disease

Cryoprecipitate is without benefit in Christmas disease as it does not contain the missing factor IX required. Fresh frozen plasma should be used, and a factor IX concentrate is becoming more readily available.

Home treatment

There has been a marked improvement in the care of the haemophiliac in recent years and it is now possible to teach him to treat himself with intravenous injections of Factor VIII concentrate as soon as bleeding is suspected. This often obviates the need for hospital admission and greatly increases the sense of independence and the confidence of the patient who believes with justification that he will become a self-supporting member of his community. Crippling haemarthroses, so common in the past, have virtually disappeared.

Prophylactic management

The boy with haemophilia has to learn to live with his disease and to find a useful place in society. The family doctor must counsel the boy and his parents, and strike a midway position between that of letting the boy do nothing at all for fear of trauma and doing too much. He must avoid obvious hazards (an extreme would surely be rock climbing) but should attend an ordinary school, avoiding strenuous games. Swimming is good exercise and safer than most for him. He should be steered into a sedentary occupation rather than that of physical labour. On the whole, the doctor should constructively encourage rather than obstructively restrict. Much valuable advice on the practical details of daily life can be obtained from the Haemophilia Society (see p. 396).

PURPURA

The word 'purpura' is derived from the Greek and Latin for purple. The purpuras embrace a group of diseases which have in common spontaneous haemorrhage into the skin, with or without bleeding into mucous membranes and internal organs. Small spots of extravasated blood are called *petechiae*, the larger ones are *ecchymoses*. Petechiae tend to occur where skin tension is low, for example in the supraclavicular fossae and infraorbital areas, are not raised above the skin surface, and do not blanch with pressure on the surrounding skin. This last point is important in differentiating petechiae from erythematous spots such as occur in the exanthemata. Ecchymoses tend to occur over pressure points such as the elbows or sacrum.

Purpuric spots occur as a result of capillary or platelet abnormality or both. The platelet abnormality is either qualitative (with normal numbers) or quantitative (with reduction, i.e. thrombocytopaenia). It is convenient therefore to classify purpuras into two broad groups, those with normal platelet count and those with thrombocytopaenia, for they are quite different groups of diseases.

Thrombocytopaenic purpura

The normal platelet count lies between the range of 150 000 and 400 000 per mm^3. This type of purpura does not occur until the platelet count is below 40 0000 per mm^3. The haemostatic defect is due to the platelets being insufficient in number to form an effective plug for torn capillaries, arterioles and venules. Platelets may also be partly responsible for maintaining normal intact capillaries. The bleeding time is increased and the clotting time is normal in thrombocytopaenia. (This contrasts with haemophilia, where the bleeding time is normal and the clotting time is increased). The commoner causes of thrombocytopaenic purpura are:

1. Idiopathic.
2. Due to infection, e.g. bacterial endocarditis and the acute specific fevers.
3. Drugs and chemicals.
4. Blood disorders which grossly affect marrow function, e.g. leukaemia, aplastic anaemia.

In paediatric practice idiopathic thrombocytopaenic purpura and leukaemia are the two commonest causes of significant thrombocytopaenia, with about equal incidence. Leukaemia we have considered already (above).

Idiopathic thrombocytopaenic purpura

In about two thirds of cases there is a history of recent infection, often of the throat or upper respiratory tract, and it may be that immunological factors are disturbed. However, the cause is far from clear. Bleeding into skin, mucosae and renal tract and less commonly into brain, occurs. Splenomegaly may be a feature. The peripheral blood shows thrombocytopaenia and is otherwise normal. Bleeding time is increased, clotting time normal, and a tourniquet applied to the arm usually increases the petechiae distal to the tourniquet (Hess test).

Course and prognosis

Most children with this condition recover spontaneously within two to three months and it rarely recurs. More rarely the disease assumes the adult form, being more chronic and liable to exacerbations. With these chronic cases, recovery is the rule, however, and haemorrhage into the central nervous system constitutes the only real hazard.

Treatment. Little need be done, as a rule, for the first six weeks of the disease, after which, if the platelet count is still very low, a course of steroids will usually produce rapid recovery. A suitable course would start with 15 mg prednisolone four times daily for ten days, after which gradual reduction over about six weeks is advisable. In children under two years of age, the daily dose should not exceed 40 mg.

In the chronic cases, where bleeding has persisted with exacerbations over a period of a year or longer, splenectomy is advisable, producing cure in about 80 per cent of cases. Splenectomy is reserved for children over four years of age, by which time the risk of overwhelming infection is virtually non-existent.

Purpura with normal platelet count (non thrombocytopaenic)

In these conditions the defect is primarily in the small blood vessels; the vascular endothelium is disturbed, resulting in increased fragility and permeability. The platelets are normal in number.

The causes of non thrombocytopaenic purpura include:

1. Allergic purpura (anaphylactic purpura; Henoch-Schonlein purpura).
2. Drugs, chemical agents, toxins and avitaminoses (scurvy).
3. Infections, e.g. acute fevers, subacute bacterial endocarditis (this can cause purpura with or without thrombocytopaenia), and meningococcal septicaemia. This septicaemia must always be considered in cases of acute purpura.
4. Von Willebrand's disease (discussed earlier).

Allergic purpura (anaphylactic purpura, Henoch-Schonlein purpura)

The term Henoch-Schonlein purpura includes Henoch's purpura (purpura with visceral manifestations) and Schonlein's purpura (purpura with arthralgia).

Aetiology

The aetiology is unknown. About one third of cases follow closely on a streptococcal infection of the throat and upper respiratory tract but a definite association has not been proven and antistreptolysin titre is rarely raised. It is probably a sensitivity reaction to something – but to what is uncertain. Ingestion of a drug may be a causal factor and recurrent attacks have occurred when the drug has been re-administered.

Incidence

It is an uncommon disease but not rare – the exact incidence is unknown. Boys are affected twice as often as girls and it is commonest between the ages of three and seven years with the highest incidence at five years.

Pathology

Acute inflammation of the capillaries and arterioles is widespread and results in increased vascular permeability and haemorrhage into tissues.

Laboratory tests are not diagnostic – indeed any abnormality discovered throws doubt on the diagnosis. It is particularly important to remember that the platelet count, bleeding and clotting times and capillary fragility tests are all normal. The sedimentation rate is usually raised.

Clinical features

Skin manifestations are variable. Classically the lesion begins as a typical urticarial wheal progressing through a small pink punctum in the centre of the wheal to frank purpuric areas which do not blanch on pressure. The petechiae and purpuric areas typically predominate on the extensor surfaces of the limbs, the buttocks and the lower part of the back. The trunk is usually spared as is the face except in infants. The tourniquet test may be positive and sometimes petechiae develop at the site of the tourniquet some hours after its removal.

Effusion into the big joints causes pain and swelling. If the bowel is affected there are abdominal pain and bleeding. Rarely intussusception occurs. About half the children develop nephritis with albuminuria and haematuria and half of these are likely to develop azotemia or hypertension or both.

Diagnosis

This is usually made from the typical distribution of the skin lesions and the absence of haematological abnormalities. Possible confusion may occur with septicaemia (particularly meningococcal) but the septicaemic child would usually be far more acutely ill and toxic with high fever.

Course and prognosis

Most commonly the disease is mild and lasts but a few days being manifest only as a few purpuric spots and transient joint pains. Occasionally symptoms persist for several weeks and may relapse after apparent remissions.

Occasionally death occurs from intestinal involvement and later from renal involvement. Exact figures appear not to be known but it seems clear that about 95% of cases recover completely with no residua.

Treatment

There is no specific treatment and careful observation with simple symptomatic treatment is usually all that is required. Bed-rest in the early stages, correction of anaemia with oral iron, salicylates for painful joints and antibiotics where there seems an infective focus would be reasonable. Surgery will be needed for intussusception. Corticosteroids may occasionally help but there is insufficient evidence that there is real benefit: in any event, they should be reserved for the severe case and there is doubt of their effectiveness in patients with severe renal damage. If one is confident of the diagnosis, the child should be treated at home. It is wise to admit to hospital the child with severe bleeding from the bowel or with worsening kidney involvement manifested by frank haematuria and increasing hypertension.

HODGKIN'S DISEASE

Although not strictly a disease of the blood in that it is a malignancy of lymphoreticular tissue it is convenient to consider this condition here.

Incidence

The disease occurs mainly in adults but can occur in children: it is very rare under three years of age. It is three times more common in males.

Aetiology

The cause is unknown and although a viral aetiology is suspected this has not been proven. One current hypothesis is that the disease starts as a protracted immunological response to a virus infection, later undergoing neoplastic change.

Pathology

The basic lesion is malignant proliferation of reticulum cells in the lymph glands, spleen and bone-marrow the normal structure of which is gradually destroyed. The disease advances to involve other organs such as the liver, lungs, skin and meninges.

Giant cells, called Reed-Sternberg cells, are an important diagnostic feature of Hodgkin's disease and can be found in the affected tissues: without their presence the diagnosis remains in doubt. The cells are large and vary in appearance, usually having large double or multiple nuclei and large inclusion-like nucleoli.

Clinical features

Hodgkin's disease is protean in its manifestations and during its course can resemble both tumour and infection. The most common presentation is that of a painless enlargement of one or more cervical lymph nodes without systemic symptoms. The glands tend to remain firm, discrete and have a rubbery, elastic feel.

Sometimes it presents as a mediastinal mass found on X-ray examination. After a few weeks general symptoms occur, including loss of weight and appetite, dyspnoea, cough and intermittent fever (Pel-Ebstein). Pressure from enlarged glands can cause a wide variety of symptoms. Over half the cases have splenomegaly.

Diagnosis

This is usually made from lymph gland biopsy when a distinctive histological alteration in involved tissue is found. Reed-Sternberg cells and an abundant mixture of lymphocytes and eosinophils form the characteristic picture. Any enlarged gland, present at least six weeks, the cause for which has not been found, should be biopsied.

Treatment

Specific treatment is largely in the hands of the specialist since it entails radiation and chemotherapy. Surgical laparotomy may be indicated to evaluate the extent of the disease in the abdomen.

Once Hodgkin's disease has been confirmed it is of the utmost importance to determine the extent of the disease. An attempt must be made to 'stage' the patient according to the Ann Arbor modification of the Rye staging system (1971). In essence this system recognises *four* stages ranging from the relatively mild Stage I in which involvement of a single lymph node region or of a single extralymphatic organ occurs to Stage 4 which implies widespread disease.

Patients with Stage 1 or Stage 2 disease are best treated by wide irradiation techniques. Those with Stage 3 or Stage 4 disease are treated with various chemotherapeutic agents used in varying combinations. Effective agents include mustine hydrocholoride, vincristine (Oncovin), procarbazine and prednisone. (This constitutes the so-called 'MOPP' combination of drugs.) Several courses of 'MOPP' treatment are given with short periods of rest between courses. New cytotoxic drugs are constantly being produced.

Prognosis

The aim of treatment in Hodgkin's disease is now cure rather than palliation. With the most meticulous planning excellent results can be expected in many cases. Remission can be forecast in about 80 per cent of all cases.

Expected survival rate after appropriate treatment

Pathological staging	*5 year disease – free survival (percentage)*
Stage1	80–90
Stage 2	70–75
Stage 3	45–60
Stage 4	20–40

New protocols of treatment are appearing with regularity and even those cases of widespread disease can look forward to prolongation and improved quality of life with an ever-increasing chance of cure.

This represents a remarkable achievement considering that prior to 1960 a solitary Hodgkin's gland signified certain death.

The role of the family doctor

He certainly need not know all the details of the treatment schedules, but an understanding of the principles involved and the expected outcome will obviously be of considerable assistance in his management of the condition, in the treatment of symptoms and in the support he must give to his patient and the parents. He must liaise closely with the specialists involved, ensuring that he is kept fully informed of progress and set-backs.

ACKNOWLEDGEMENT

I acknowledge my indebtedness to Dr John Apley's *Paediatrics*, from which I have quoted extensively, with his permission. His concise textbook is well suited to the needs of the general practitioner, and I could not myself better his account of blood disorders in childhood.

REFERENCES

Allen, D.W. & Cole, P. (1972) Viruses and human cancer. *New England Journal of Medicine*, **286**, 70.

Apley, J. (1973) *Paediatrics*. Blood disorders, Ch. 20; pp. 305–323. London: Ballière Tindall.

Aur, R.J.A., Simone, J.V., Hustu, O. & Verzosa, M.S. (1973) A comparative study of central nervous system irradiation and intensive chemotherapy early in remission of childhood acute lymphocytic leukaemia. *Cancer*, **29**, 381.

Green, M. & Haggerty, R.J. (1968) *Ambulatory Paediatrics*, p. 246. Philadelphia: Saunders.

Lascari, A.D. (1973) *Leukaemia in Childhood*, Springfield, Illinois: Thomas.

MacCarthy, M. (1975) The care of childhood leukaemia in general practice. *Journal of the Royal College of General Practitioners*, **25**, 286–292.

Moore, R.M.A. (1975) Anaemia. In Hart, C.R. (ed.) *Screening in General Practice*. Edinburgh: Churchill Livingstone.

Oski, E.A. & Naiman, J.L. (1972) Hematologic problems in the newborn. In *Major Problems in Clinical Pediatrics*, vol. 4. Philadelphia: Saunders.

Simone, J., Aur, R.J.A., Hustu, O. & Pinkel, D. (1972) Total therapy studies of acute lymphocytic leukaemia in Childhood. *Cancer*, **30**, 1488.

Willoughby, M.L.N. (1973) Disorders of the blood and reticuloendothelial system. In Forfar, J.O. & Arneil, G.C. (eds) *Texbook of Paediatrics*, pp. 903–963. Edinburgh: Churchill Livingstone.

Willougby, M.L.N. (1977) *Paediatric Haematology*. Edinburgh: Churchill Livingstone.

The teeth in childhood

Gerald Winter and Ruth Holt

In the developed countries of the world, dental disease is probably the most prevalent chronic disease to affect children. On average, in England and Wales by the age of five years, every child has suffered more than three decayed primary (deciduous) teeth and by the age of 15 years, eight permanent teeth have decayed (Todd, 1975). In 1976 dental inspection of 4 893 000 school children in England and Wales showed that 2 495 000 or 51 per cent were in need of treatment (CSO, 1979). Perhaps because it is so widespread, dental disease has often been considered inevitable, but at best, dental decay requires operative intervention and at worst, it may result in severe pain, infection and other more serious sequelae. Against much popular belief, most dental disease found in children is preventable, but these preventive measures have lagged behind others in the field of child health. With the increasing value put on overall positive health, this should be a cause for concern to all those providing health care for children.

Normally, young children are seen by a doctor on a number of occasions before they are seen by a dentist. Mothers may also seek the advice of a doctor as to how they should care for their children's teeth. General practitioners concerned about child care, therefore, have an excellent opportunity to instill good attitudes and habits for dental health.

DENTAL DEVELOPMENT

Early tooth formation

The earliest cellular changes indicating dental development are seen at about 28 days in utero as localised thickenings in the epithelium lining the primitive oral cavity. With continued growth and fusion of the underlying frontonasal, maxillary and mandibular processes these thickenings extend and coalesce until by the 35th day they form continuous bands, termed dental laminae, overlying the future upper and lower jaws. With continued development epithelial proliferations arise at specific sites along each lamina, corresponding to the future positions of the primary (and succedaneous permanent) teeth. These localised proliferations are termed tooth buds. Tooth buds for the 20 teeth of the primary dentition are first seen about the 39th day in utero. Each tooth bud extends downwards into the underlying mesenchyme of the upper and lower arches, which condenses around it. As a result of further proliferative growth involving histodifferentiation and morphodifferentiation of the tooth bud, a bell shape is established and continuity is lost with the overlying parent lamina. At this stage the inner layer of cells of the tooth bud assume a columnar appearance and are responsible for the subsequent formation of the enamel covering of the tooth crown. These cells are also thought to be necessary for the induction of cellular changes in the surrounding mesenchyme of the dental follicle which give rise to the formation of dentine and pulp. Mineralisation (calcification) of the enamel and dentine occurs shortly after the organic matrix is deposited.

Mineralisation

Mineralisation of primary teeth begins at about 14 weeks in utero and follows a definite pattern or sequence starting at the tooth cusps or incisal edges. Mineralisation of the permanent dentition starts later, just prior to birth, and also follows a distint sequence. A summary of average timings for these processes is given in Table 33.1. Mineralisation of teeth, unlike that of bone, is irreversible. Interruptions to the process are marked indelibly on the tooth structure and in this respect are comparable to the growth rings of a tree.

The formation and mineralisation of the crown is largely complete before the tooth erupts, but root formation continues for some time afterwards. Dentine formation on the walls of the pulp cavity within the tooth continues throughout life.

Disorders of dental development

Disorders of tooth formation may be confined to one tooth or group of teeth or they may affect the whole dentition. Defects in tooth structure may take the form of a discolouration, hypoplasia (deficiency of matrix

Table 33.1 Age of initiation of tooth mineralisation (Data for primary teeth from Lunt and Law, 1974a). Copyright by the American Dental Association. Reprinted by permission

		Maxilla	*Mandible*
Primary tooth	A	14 weeks in utero (13–16)	14 weeks in utero (13–16)
	B	16 weeks in utero (14⅔–16½)	16 weeks in utero (14⅔–16½)
	C	17 weeks in utero (15–18)	17 weeks in utero (16–18)
	D	15½ weeks in utero (14½–17)	15½ weeks in utero (14½–17)
	E	19 weeks in utero (16–23½)	18 weeks in utero (17–19½)
Permanent tooth	1	3– 4 months	3– 4 months
	2	10–12 months	3– 4
	3	4– 5 months	4– 5 months
	4	18–21 months	21–24 months
	5	24–27 months	27–30 months
	6	8 months in utero	8 months in utero
	7	30–36 months	30–36 months
	8	7– 9 years	8–10 years

formation), or hypomineralisation. More than 90 causes of developmental dental defects have been described, including both inherited and environmental factors (Small and Murray, 1978). Inherited defects may affect either the enamel (hereditary amelogenesis imperfecta), or the dentine, e.g. hereditary opalescent dentine. These defects may be limited to the dentition and arise from a single gene anomaly. At least 11 types of hereditary amelogenesis imperfecta have been identified (Winter and Brook, 1975). Alternatively, the enamel or dentine anomaly may form part of a complex inherited clinical syndrome, e.g. epidermolysis bullosa dystrophica or osteogenesis imperfecta. However, all these forms of inherited anomaly are rare, the most common enamel defect affecting approximately one in 2000 of the general population (Witkop and Sauk, 1976).

During the pre-natal period, tooth formation appears to be well protected from all but the most severe environmental insults, e.g. maternal rubella, but development occurring after birth is more easily disturbed. Systemic changes associated with nutritional, infective and metabolic upsets may result in areas of hypoplasia and/or hypomineralisation in either primary or permanent teeth. These areas are not haphazard, but have a linear distribution around the dentition, corresponding to the stage of tooth formation or mineralisation at the time of the disturbance. The terms systemic or chronological hypoplasia (or hypocalcification) are commonly applied to such maldevelopments. Discolouration of the dental tissues with a chronological distribution, in either the primary or permanent dentitions, is a frequent sequela to the administration of tetracycline antibiotics either late in pregnancy or during the first seven years of childhood. The colour change may vary from lemon yellow, to yellow brown, to dark grey, and may be associated with clinically evident hypomineralisation or hypoplasia. The resultant defect may be very disfiguring, not easily masked, and produce a considerable cosmetic and psychological problem for the child. Tetracycline drugs are, therefore, contra-indicated during late pregnancy and for children up to the age of seven years, unless there is an overwhelming case for their prescription. Localised hypoplasia or hypomineralisation of individual permanent teeth may result from trauma or infection to a primary predecessor.

Eruption

Eruption of primary teeth usually begins at about six months of age. As with the process of mineralisation of the dental tissues, a chronological sequence is followed with the lower central incisors usually erupting first, followed by lower lateral and upper central incisors. In the primary dentition, however, it is not unusual for this sequence to be varied. Average timings for the eruption of primary teeth are given in Table 33.2. Each tooth

Table 33.2 Eruption dates for primary teeth (from Lunt and Law, 1974)

Tooth	*Maxilla*	*Mandible*
A	10 months (8–12)	8 months (6–10)
B	11 months (9–13)	13 months (10–16)
C	19 months (16–22)	20 months (17–23)
D	16 months (13–19) boys (14–18) girls	16 months (14–18)
E	29 months (25–33)	27 months (23–31) boys (24–30) girls

continues to erupt until it reaches a functional position in the mouth, guided by the activity of lips, tongue and cheeks. The complete primary dentition is usually fully erupted between the ages of 24 and 28 months.

During eruption, the tooth roots continue to develop.

Each primary incisor and canine has a single root, each mandibular primary molar two roots and each maxillary primary molar three roots. The roots of primary incisors and canines are conical and normally straight. Those of the primary molars are finer and widely splayed, enclosing the follicles of the premolar teeth.

Soon after the primary teeth are fully formed, and have begun to function, their roots begin to resorb. Resorption continues until little or no root remains; the tooth then becomes mobile and is exfoliated. Exfoliation is normally associated with the eruption of the permanent dentition, but primary teeth may resorb and be exfoliated even in the absence of a permanent successor, albeit at a slower and extremely variable rate.

Permanent teeth begin to erupt around the age of six years. The first to erupt is either the lower central incisor or the first molar, and in distinction to the primary dentition, eruption follows a more definite sequence. Average eruption times of permanent teeth are given in Table 33.3. Apart from the third molars, formation of the permanent dentition is usually complete by the age of 15 to 16 years.

Table 33.3 Eruption dates for permanent teeth

Tooth	*Maxilla*	*Mandible*
1	7–8 years	6–7 years
2	8–9 years	7–8 years
3	11–12 years	9–10 years
4	10–11 years	10–11 years
5	10–12 years	11–12 years
6	6–7 years	6–7 years
7	12–13 years	11–13 years
8	17–21 years	17–21 years

Disorders of eruption

Tooth eruption (teething) is a normal physiological process. However, in infancy teething may be associated with irritability, disturbed sleep, reduced food intake, increased fluid intake, reddening of the gingival tissues (gum) overlying the erupting tooth, cheek flushing, excessive salivation (drooling), and circum-oral rash. Teething is never the cause of more severe disturbances such as pyrexia, diarrhoea or bronchitis, which may occur coincidentally in children of this age. Biting on a hard object such as a teething ring or non-sweetened rusk appears to relieve the discomfort associated with teething and this may be supplemented by the use of a suitable analgesic for a few days, e.g. elixir of paracetamol. A variety of solutions and gels are also available for local application to the gum. Many of these medicaments contain honey or sucrose, and their prolonged use is potentially cariogenic. Some also contain local anaesthetic agents which carry the additional risk of inducing hyper-sensitivity reactions.

The eruption of primary teeth is frequently preceded by a bluish swelling of the overlying gum, which is most often due to the formation of a localised haematoma, the underlying tooth emerging in to the mouth within the next two weeks without the need for treatment. Less commonly the bluish swelling signifies the presence of a true eruption cyst; these too may rupture spontaneously without treatment with the subsequent emergence of the underlying tooth. Interference with normal feeding may occasionally require surgical excision of a portion of the cyst wall to facilitate tooth eruption.

In common with other developmental milestones, there is a wide range in the timing of tooth eruption in children. Up to 12 months' delay in eruption in a child who is otherwise normal may be of little or no significance. More marked generalised delay in eruption may occur in association with a variety of systemic disturbances, including osteodystrophies, hypothyroidism, hypopituitarism and Down's syndrome, and with oral abnormalities such as hereditary gingival hyperplasia (Winter and Simpkiss, 1974).

Variations in the sequence of eruption may indicate a localised problem such as the presence of dental infection, an additional tooth lying in the path of eruption, or cyst formation. A tooth may fail to erupt if there is insufficient space for it within the dental arch or if it is ectopically placed within the jaws. Trauma to a primary tooth may result in the dilaceration (or malformation) of the succedaneous permanent tooth, which may also fail to erupt in the normal way. All these localised causes of delayed eruption require early diagnosis and treatment if satisfactory results are to be achieved.

Malalignments and malocclusions

Malalignments and malocclusions may affect either primary or permanent dentitions or both. In the primary dentition, one common cause of orthodontic disturbance is dummy or digit sucking. Especially when this type of sucking habit is prolonged, it may be associated with an open bite between anterior teeth and with cross bites of posterior teeth. It is generally believed that anterior open bites of this type will resolve once the sucking habit is discontinued and that the posterior cross bite will resolve with the eruption of the permanent teeth (Winter, 1980).

A more serious cause of disturbance is the premature extraction of carious primary teeth, especially primary molars. This may lead to drifting of adjacent teeth with loss of space for the permanent successors which may complicate a pre-existing malocclusion. In general, crowding is a result of an imbalance between jaw size and tooth size. It may affect any part of the dental arches.

Another common type of malocclusion is seen when the relationship between upper and lower teeth in the sagittal plane occurs anterior or posterior to the usual position. These types of malocclusion may be relatively mild and confined to the dental arches, or they may indicate an underlying malrelationship between the jaws.

Correction of many malocclusions and malalignments may be achieved by the suitable extraction of teeth and/or use of removable or fixed orthodontic appliances. This type of treatment is usually carried out in the permanent dentition. In cases of severe malocclusion, particularly those involving a skeletal malrelationship, more radical oral surgery may provide the most effective means of improving the situation.

COMMONLY ACQUIRED DENTAL DISEASES

The two most commonly acquired dental diseases occurring in children are dental caries and gingivitis.

Dental caries

Dental caries, or tooth decay, is the localised destruction of hard tooth tissues. In the simplest terms, caries initiation is thought to result from the acid dissolution of enamel, produced by bacterial decomposition of dietary carbohydrate within dental plaque on the tooth surface. Whilst the aetiology of dental caries is not fully understood, it would appear to be a multifactorial disease in which there is an interplay of factors between the host and the environment. Factors in the host which govern the disease are both inherited and acquired and include items such as tooth tissue resistance to acid demineralisation, the rate of production and quality of saliva, and the immune status of the individual to plaque micro-organisms. Environmental factors include the nature of the microflora in plaque (Streptococcus mutans is particularly important in this respect), the frequency of dietary intake of refined carbohydrates, especially sugar, and the level of fluoride in the drinking water.

Caries is seen in all age groups, but the first two decades of life represent a period of particularly high caries activity.

In both primary and permanent teeth, caries may occur in pits and fissures (the most common site), on approximal surfaces or on other smooth tooth surfaces. The earliest sign of caries is the development of an opaque white area which represents a zone of demineralised sub-surface enamel. At this stage, the surface is intact, but with time demineralisation increases to the point where the enamel surface breaks down and becomes roughened and stained. Destruction of enamel continues until the less highly calcified dentine is reached. The carious process then becomes more rapid, with bacterial invasion of the dentinal tubules, undermining adjacent enamel and extending towards the pulp. Pulp and dentine are capable of a limited reparative response, but with continuation of the carious process, the pulp eventually becomes inflamed, infected and necrotic. This in turn may lead to acute or chronic abscess formation in the tissues surrounding the tooth.

The carious process is the same in both primary and permanent teeth, but because of the relatively large pulp chamber in primary teeth, caries appears to progress faster, with earlier involvement of the pulp. In very young children, caries initiation and progression may occur so rapidly and extensively that parents believe the primary teeth have erupted decayed. This type of caries, termed rampant caries, has been shown to be particularly associated with the use of sweetened comforters, such as dinky feeders or feeding bottles containing neat syrups, sweetened milk or diluted fruit juices (Winter *et al*, 1971). Rampant caries in the primary dentition is commonly associated with high levels of caries in permanent teeth at a later age. Despite its very high prevalence in the child community, 97 per cent having met the disease by 15 years of age in England and Wales, dental caries is preventable.

Prevention of dental caries

Dental caries is currently prevented by either community based measures, such as water fluoridation, or by measures more suited to the individual.

Community based measures

Water fluoridation. The most effective public health measure available to prevent dental caries is the fluoridation of drinking water supplies, to a level of 0.9 – 1.0 part per million in temperate climates. Numerous independent studies have shown that this single measure will significantly reduce the level of dental caries in children. In Birmingham, with fluoridated water since 1964, the prevalance of caries has been more than halved, and in older children fewer than half as many permanent teeth are being extracted (Whittle and Downer, 1979). Many of these benefits are maintained into adult life (Murray, 1976).

The safety of water fluoridation has been very closely scrutinised by a number of independent authorities in different countries. In Britain, in 1976, both the safety and the effectiveness of this measure were endorsed in a report from the Royal College of Physicians.

Measures for the individual

Measures that are at present available for the individual to prevent caries include (a) the use of fluoride supplements, (b) the professional and self-administration of topical fluoride agents, (c) the professional application of fissure sealants, and perhaps most important (d) the establishment of good dietary habits.

Fluoride supplements. In areas where the fluoride level in the drinking water supply is below optimum, caries prevention can be achieved through the use of fluoride supplements in the form of tablets or drops. In order to gain the best effect, these supplements need to be given daily throughout the period of tooth development (i.e. from birth to the age of 13 years). Scientific evidence of benefit to the fetus is insufficient to warrant their use by expectant mothers.

Recommended daily dosages vary with the age of the child and the level of fluoride present in the water supply. For bottle fed babies dosages for areas with less then 0.3 ppm fluoride in the water are given in Table 33.4. Where fluoride levels are between 0.3 and 0.7 ppm these daily dosages should be reduced by 0.25 mg fluoride. For wholly breast fed babies 0.25 mg fluoride ion/day is required, irrespective of fluoride levels in the drinking water. Fluoride taken in this way requires sustained parental motivation and enthusiasm if it is to succeed. Few studies involving the use of fluoride tablets and drops have been able to demonstrate benefits equal to those achieved through water fluoridation.

Table 33.4 Dosage of fluoride ion recommended for use in areas where drinking water contains less than 0.3 ppm F.

Age of child (years)	*Recommended daily dose (mg of fluoride ion)*
0–1	0.25
1–2	0.50
2–3	0.75
3–14	1.00

Topical fluoride agents. A variety of solutions, gels and varnishes containing fluorides are now available for professional application by dentists. These agents are normally applied to cleaned, dried tooth surfaces either twice or three times a year.

Fluoride is also included in the majority of toothpastes presently sold, forming a further means of topical fluoride application. The regular use of these toothpastes has a definite, if small, caries preventive effect. Fluoride containing mouth rinses for daily or weekly use are available as a further means of topical application. These are not suitable for children under the age of five years who may swallow the solution, but they may be useful for older children, especially those with a high level of caries.

Most topical fluoride preparations achieve their maximum benefit by preventing caries on smooth tooth surfaces. However, the greatest proportion of decay starts in the pits and fissures and it is to prevent this type of caries that fissure sealants were developed.

Fissure sealants. Modern sealant materials are resins or cements that adhere to dental enamel and are used to block the ingress of plaque bacteria to the pits and fissures present on tooth surfaces. To achieve their best effect, sealants need to be applied as soon as possible after tooth eruption. Their application also requires an extremely exacting and meticulous technique. For these reasons, fissure sealants may not be practicable for all children, but this does not reduce their value to the individual, especially for the permanent teeth of children with a high caries experience in the primary dentition, or for those at particular risk from dental infection, e.g. with cardiac disease.

Both fissure sealants and fluorides act principally by diminishing the hazard of bacterial attack on the enamel surface. Hypothetically, this risk can also be reduced by complete plaque removal or by the control of substrates utilised by plaque bacteria, i.e. dietary sugars. Although the efficient removal of plaque by highly trained professional staff has been shown to reduce dramatically the incidence of dental caries, there is little evidence to suggest that plaque removal by children or their parents will have the same effect. By contrast, studies of patients with hereditary fructose intolerance and of institutionalised individuals on strict dietary regimes have shown that the initiation and progression of dental caries can be reduced by the careful restriction of dietary sugars, especially sucrose.

Dietary measures to prevent caries. The most important single dietary measure to prevent caries is to restrict the intake of sugars. In the aetiology of caries, sugar does not affect the teeth directly, but is utilized by plaque bacteria with the formation of organic acids, e.g. lactic acid. Acid production begins within two to three minutes of sugar being taken in to the mouth and absorbed by plaque. Plaque pH is rapidly reduced and remains lower than the critical pH to effect enamel demineralisation for periods of 20 minutes or more. Thus, repeated intake of sugar, or that produced with a retentive form, such as toffees, can result in prolonged periods of low plaque pH throughout the day with the attendant danger to the tooth surface. The frequency and nature of sugar intake, therefore, are dentally of greater importance than the total amount consumed. To discourage a craving for sugar, mothers of bottle fed infants need to be advised against adding sugar to already sweetened milk feeds and from giving repeated sweetened drinks. The association between rampant caries and sweetened comforters has already been described and all mothers should be warned of the dangers of using this form of pacification for their young children.

A considerable proportion of older children consume sweetened snacks and drinks between meals, a habit that is encouraged socially and by advertising. Numerous alternatives are available, such as cheese, crisps, fruit, unsweetened fruit juice and milk. These items should be recommended to parents and children who find they cannot eliminate snacks, and they should be advised to limit sweet foods and drinks to meal times only.

A further source of dietary sugar for a few children is the sucrose contained in medicinal syrups. In the short term, these may do little damage, but a group of children who had been medicated in this way for periods of six months or more were shown to possess a higher prevalence of caries than a control group (Roberts and Roberts, 1979).

The search for an effective and safe substitute for sugar in the diet to reduce the problem of dental caries has been actively pursued during the past decade. Xylitol, produced from the birch tree, has been shown to be entirely non-fermentable by plaque bacteria and therefore non-cariogenic (Scheinin and Makinen, 1974). However, gastro-intestinal side effects are occasionally observed and the cost is high compared to that of sucrose. Total substitution of sucrose in the diet is therefore unlikely at the present time, but such substances may be of value in formulating medicines for children.

Gingivitis

Chronic inflammatory changes in the marginal gingiva surrounding children's teeth are common. Like caries, this chronic marginal gingivitis is related to the activity of the plaque bacteria. Whether both these dental diseases are related to the same species of plaque bacteria is at present unknown.

In adequately nourished and healthy young children the host resistance to gingivitis may be better developed than that to dental caries. Certainly the clinical signs of gingivitis take longer to develop in this group. In the survey of Child Dental Health in England and Wales in 1973, 39 per cent of five year olds had plaque present in their mouths, 72 per cent had dental caries, but only 26 per cent had significant gingivitis (Todd, 1975).

In gingivitis, the gums become reddened and swollen in areas adjacent to plaque accumulation; the interdental papillae are often the first to show these changes. There is also a loss of the normal stippled appearance, and with further inflammation the gingival tissues become friable and may bleed with minimal trauma, e.g. toothbrushing.

More extensive periodontal inflammation with loss of bony support for the teeth is fortunately much less common in childhood. In one study, fewer than one per cent of normal 13–15 year old children were found to be affected (Blankenstein, Murray and Lind, 1978). However, in some handicapped and chronically sick children, gingival and periodontal disease may be particularly marked. Such children frequently have very poor oral hygiene and show extensive gingivitis in response to high plaque levels. Children with reduced resistance to infection, such as those with Down's syndrome, or cyclic neutropaenia, may exhibit marked gingivitis with early loss of periodontal support in the presence of relatively small amounts of plaque.

Epileptic children may develop considerable gingival enlargement in response to phenytoin (Epanutin) therapy in the presence of dental plaque. In many of these cases, gingival inflammation and hyperplasia may be prevented or controlled by extremely meticulous oral hygiene. In some cases of phenytoin gingival hyperplasia, however, a change of anticonvulsant therapy may be the only practicable way of achieving complete resolution. Severe gingivitis with extensive swelling, bleeding or ulceration may be a presenting symptom of childhood leukaemia, particularly in the acute monocytic or myelocytic varieties. The sudden onset of a severe gingivitis of this type should alert suspicion as to the possible grave underlying condition.

Prevention of gingivitis

The only effective method presently available to prevent gingivitis is regular and adequate plaque removal. Before teeth erupt, an infant's mouth may be wiped gently with a moistened cotton bud, but once the primary teeth have fully erupted they should be carefully cleaned with a small infant-sized toothbrush. To begin with, toothpaste is not required, but with the full eruption of the primary dentition at 2½–3 years, a small amount of a fluoride containing paste makes brushing more pleasant and effective and has a caries preventive effect.

All accessible surfaces of all teeth should be cleaned systematically. This approach is more important than using a particular technique or method as far as children are concerned. As the child gets older, slightly larger junior-sized brushes may be used, but short headed, multitufted and straight handled brushes are the best for reaching all tooth surfaces. Teeth should be brushed twice a day, with one of the brushings being performed before the child is put to sleep for the night.

Parents should be responsible for either cleaning or supervising the cleaning of their children's teeth at least once a day until six to seven years of age, since younger children are rarely able to undertake this activity effectively by themselves.

DENTAL TREATMENT FOR CHILDREN

Regular attendance at the dentist is a major part of the oral care for children. Not only is it important for the earliest diagnosis and best treatment of disorders, but also to reinforce dental health advice.

Ideally, children should attend the dentist before any disease has occurred – preferably between the ages of two and three years. This enables preventive methods and ideas to be introduced where necessary and the child given a gentle introduction to dental care. In contrast to this, children who are first taken to the dentist with toothache may have a psychologically and physically traumatic introduction to treatment which may colour their attitude to future dental visits for many years. The frequency of visits may vary, depending on the child's oral health and on parental attitude. The take-up of dental care is well known to be lowest in children from families in social classes IV and V, where the need for care is greatest. General practitioners should encourage mothers in these socio-economic groups to secure regular dental care for their children. In Britain, the terms of the National Health Service allow up to three check-up visits a year free of charge for children up to the age of 16 years.

For children over three years of age, it is possible to provide restorative care and simple extractions with minimal discomfort by the routine use of local anaesthetics. Very young or mentally handicapped children may be unable to tolerate the loss of facial sensation, but there are few normal children for whom this technique is unsuitable. Many children fear dental visits because of a previous painful experience. Others are fearful of all types of medical care or they may have a parent or sibling who is afraid of dental treatment. Most of these children will be managed by sympathy and kindness and a gentle introduction to the simple forms of treatment under local anaesthesia. In some cases, however, treatment is either urgently required, or is too extensive to allow this approach. For these children it may be necessary to provide initial treatment under general anaesthesia.

Orally administered sedatives annd tranquillisers have extremely variable results, especially in very young or apprehensive children, and their value for paediatric dentistry is doubtful. Some older children may be helped by the use of nitrous oxide/oxygen sedation, so-called relative analgesia, but both this technique and the use of general anaesthesia require adequate facilities if they are to be safely employed.

Dental treatment requiring antibiotic cover

The most common indication for antibiotic cover in the dental treatment of children is the presence of congenital or acquired heart disease. The aim is to reduce the risk of infective endocarditis. The need for cover is dependent on the severity of the cardiac disease and on the type of dental treatment to be undertaken. The differing risks and indications have been described by Jordan (1979). It is suggested that antibiotic cover is unnecessary in conditions which are unlikely to develop endocarditis. These include ostium secundum atrial septal defect, uncomplicated transposition, Eisenmenger syndrome, myocardial disease without mitral regurgitation and paroxysmal supraventricular tachycardia. In patients where there is a liability to endocarditis, but in which damage is unlikely to be severe, antibiotic cover is recommended for scaling involving the gum margin, extractions and treatments of the dental pulp, but not for routine fillings. This second category includes patients with pulmonary stenosis, Fallot's tetralogy, patent ductus arteriosus, coarctation of the aorta and a Blalock or Waterston's shunt.

In the third category are conditions liable to endocarditis and in which damage is likely to be severe. It is recommended that antibiotic cover be used for extractions, pulp treatments and fillings or scalings that are likely to involve the gum margin in these patients. This group of diseases include aortic stenosis or regurgitation, bicuspid aortic valve, mitral regurgitation, ostium primum atrial septal defect, subaortic stenosis and hypertrophic obstructive cardiomyopathy. Where an antibiotic cover is indicated, penicillin G is the first drug of choice, the dose relating to the age of the child. The best pre-operative route is intramuscular and this should always be used for patients in the third group listed above. One method is to give crystalline penicillin one hour preoperatively and then oral penicillin V six hourly for three days following. Patients in the second group listed above and who are likely to be upset by an intramuscular injection may be given an oral antibiotic such as amoxycillin with a loading dose two hours preoperatively and then six hourly for three days.

Antibiotic cover with penicillin is contra-indicated in patients who are on long term penicillin therapy, those who have been given penicillin within the previous four weeks and those with true hypersensitivity to the drug. Suitable alternatives are cephaloridine i.m. or i.v. (except for those with penicillin hypersensitivity) with erythromycin for follow up, streptomycin by injection for four days, intravenous vancomycin or oral erythromycin in full dose (Jordan, 1979). However, the first priority in the dental care of all children with cardiac disease is to prevent dental disease by all practicable means. This will not only reduce the need for antibiotic cover but also eliminate the risk from the disease.

COMMON DENTAL EMERGENCIES

Pain and swelling of dental origin

Many children with extensive dental disease appear to have suffered little or no discomfort, but dental caries with subsequent pulp and periapical inflammation is capable of producing severe facial pain and swelling. Initially the pain from dental caries occurs momentarily in response to sweet, hot or cold stimuli, but with increasing pulp involvement it becomes constant and severe.

Following pulp death, pain may subside temporarily, but it returns with abscess formation and with the spread of infection to surrounding tissues. With involvement of the supporting structures, the tooth may become raised in its socket, mobile and tender to palpation. Further spread of infection usually results in dento-alveolar abscess formation, possibly a cellulitis and invariably a regional lymphadenitis. The associated facial swelling may be acute in onset and marked in extent, its site being dependent on the anatomical relations of the root apices. Thus, swellings associated with lower molars may extend downwards into the neck, whereas infected maxillary teeth may produce swellings extending upwards in to the maxillary sinus and periorbital tissues.

All children with pain and/or swelling thought to be of dental origin should be seen by a dentist as soon as possible. In the early stages, removal of decay and restoration of the tooth may be possible. Once the surrounding tissues are involved, dental treatment becomes a matter of urgency. Where suppuration occurs, surgical drainage must be established and the cause removed. Extraction of the tooth is often sufficient to do both. A more conservative approach may be drainage through the root canal. In severe cases surgical incision may also be required.

Antibiotic therapy is principally indicated for cases with an associated spreading cellulitis or where dental treatment is unavoidably delayed due to some intercurrent illness, e.g. measles. There is little need for antibiotics when the dental infection is well localised in an otherwise healthy child. The antibiotic of choice for infections of this type is penicillin V given orally every six hours for five days. In severe spreading infections, penicillin G should be given i.m. until the condition is brought under control. An alternative antibiotic for children who are hypersensitive to penicillin is oral erythromycin.

Trauma

Children with traumatised teeth should be seen by a dentist as soon as possible and commensurate with the treatment of their other injuries. Young children with traumatised primary incisors may require little immediate treatment. Attempts should not be made to replace avulsed primary teeth in their sockets as this may damage the overlying permanent tooth germs.

The treatment of traumatised permanent teeth (most commonly incisors) is more complex and depends on a number of factors including the extent of dental injury and the state of root development. An avulsed permanent tooth seen immediately after the accident should be washed free of any contamination with sterile saline and replaced in the socket. When the tooth has been on the ground, tetanus immunisation is a wise precaution, and an appropriate oral antibiotic should be provided in all cases. The child should then be referred immediately to a dentist who will splint the tooth in position. Teeth immediately reimplanted in this way may successfully reattach to the socket wall. Avulsed teeth which are reimplanted later than 30 minutes after injury generally undergo root resorption and are finally shed. However, this process may take many years and the tooth may perform a very useful function throughout this period.

REFERENCES

Blankenstein, R., Murray, J.J. & Lind, O.P. (1978) Prevalence of chronic periodontitis in 13–15 year old children. *Journal of Clinical Periodontology*, **5**, 285–292.

CSO (1979) Central Statistical Office: Annual Abstract of Statistics.

Jordan, S.C. (1979) Dental treatment of children with heart disease. *Proceedings of the British Paedodontic Society*, **9**, 13–17.

Lunt, R.C. & Law, D.B. (1974a) A review of the chronology of calcification of deciduous teeth. *Journal of the American Dental Association*, **89**, 599–606.

Lunt, R.C. & Law, D.B. (1974b) A review of the chronology of eruption of deciduous teeth. *Journal of the American Dental Association*, **89**, 872–879.

Murray, J.J. (1976) *Fluorides in Caries Prevention*. Bristol: John Wright.

Roberts, I.F. & Roberts, G.J. (1979) Relation between medicines sweetened with sucrose and dental disease. *British Medical Journal*, **2**, 14–16.

Royal College of Physicians (1976) *Fluorides, Teeth and Health*. London: Pitman Medical.

Scheinin, A. & Makinen, K.K. (1975) Turku sugar studies I–XXI *Acta. odont. Scand*, **33**, 1–348 (Supp. 70)

Small, B.W. & Murray, J.J. (1978) Enamel opacities: prevalence, classifications and aetiological considerations. *Journal of Dentistry*, **6**, 33–42.

Todd, J.E. (1975) Children's Dental Health in England and Wales 1973. London: HMSO.

Whittle, J.G. & Downer, M.C. (1979) Dental Health and treatment needs of Birmingham and Salford schoolchildren. *British Dental Journal*, **147**, 67–71.

Winter, G.B. (1980) Problems involved with the use of comforters. *International Dental Journal*, **30**, 28–38.

Winter, G.B. & Simpkiss, M.J. (1974) Hypertrichosis with hereditary gingival hyperplasia. *Archives of the Diseases of Childhood*, **49**, 394–399.

Winter, G.B. & Brook, A.H. (1975) Enamel hypoplasia and anomalies of enamel. Dental Clinics of North America, **19**, 3–24.

Winter, G.B., Rule, D.C., Mailer, G.P., James, P.M.C. & Gordon, P.H. (1971) The prevalence of dental caries in pre-school children aged 1–4 years. *British Dental Journal*, **130**, 271–277; 434–436

Witkop, C.J. & Sauk, J.J. (1976) Heritable defects of enamel. In Stewart, R.E. & Prescott, G.H. (eds) Oral Facial Genetics. St. Louis: Mosby.

34

Prescribing for infants and children

Tom Davies

'Doctors who treat the symptoms tend to give a prescription; doctors who treat the patient are more likely to offer guidance' Apley (1978).

Since the War, there has been a very rapid increase in knowledge, which has made the prescribing of medicines for infants and children increasingly difficult, but also increasingly important in view of the vast numbers of new drugs appearing every year. The average general practitioner may expect to have on his practice list one quarter of his patients under the age of sixteen. From the second Morbidity Survey of General Practice, the annual consultation rate in 1971–72 for children under five was 3.6 consultations per child per year and 1.9 consultations per child per year in the 5 to 15 age group (Table 1.15). These figures may well be conservative; indeed consultation rates of eight per year have been reported for children under the age of one (Fry, 1966), and overall rates of five to six per child per year up to the age of fifteen (Sussex and Watson, 1971). The majority of these consultations were for upper respiratory tract infections, and over ten per cent were for cases of diarrhoea and vomiting. Howie (1979) states that prescriptions are issued at some 65 to 70 per cent of all consultations; therefore general practitioners, on average, are issuing at least 6–7 prescriptions a day in the paediatric age group.

Cleary (1976) in her study of prescribing in general practice, among a cohort of 116 doctors, found that for children under 15 penicillin accounted for one quarter of all prescriptions, of which the broad spectrum ampicillin was by far the most popular (see Table 34.1). Cough linctuses and expectorants and anti-histamines were the next most commonly prescribed. More recently figures of prescribing for children under five years in a single practice showed that 33 per cent of the prescriptions were for antibiotics, and 31 per cent were for cough linctuses and anti-histamines (Grace and Goulds, 1980).

The high prescribing of tetracyclines reported by Cleary, which accounted for nearly six per cent of total drugs supplied in an age group for which their hazards had been well known for years, seems to reflect a delay before doctors alter their prescribing habits. Perhaps this has now ended, for in the more recent study of Catford (1980), there were no prescriptions for tetracyclines found in the under 16 age group. However, he found more modern drugs, especially those used in the treatment of diarrhoea, had been prescribed by up to 15 per cent of his study doctors to an age group below that recommended by the manufacturers on their information sheets. This he considered potentially hazardous. He also found that 10 per cent of the doctors studied prescribed tricyclic anti-depressants for children under the age of five. There have been surprisingly few studies to evaluate the quality of prescribing in children, and certainly more attention should be paid to this.

Table 34.1 Prescribing repertoire of cohort doctors for children under 15 (Cleary, 1976). 15 688 prescriptions of 116 doctors

	Percentage
Penicillins	25.4
Cough suppressants/expectorants	13.46
Anti-histamines	8.10
Tetracyclines	5.94
Ear, nose, oropharynx	4.91
Skin corticosteroids	4.51
Anti pyretic analgesics	3.29
Other antibiotics	2.59
Individual forms etc	2.32
Bronchodilators	2.08
Anti diarrhoeals	2.05
Skin sedatives etc.	2.00
Skin antibacterials	1.82
Ear, nose, oropharynx-corticosteroids	1.40
Eye antibiotics	1.40
Total	81.27

MODES OF ADMINISTRATION

Drugs can be given sublingually, orally, rectally or by injection. Injections may be given intradermally, subcutaneously, intramuscularly or intravenously or very rarely intraperitoneally or intrathecally. Drops may be placed in the eyes, nose or ears and an increasing number of drugs may be given by inhalation into the respiratory tract. By far the majority of drugs are given orally for obvious convenience, in liquid form for infants and children, but for any drug prescribed, the prescriber should be aware of the pharmacokinetics of that drug – namely the factors affecting absorption, distribution, metabolism, and excretion.

Absorption

Irrespective of the route chosen, three factors are important in determining how a drug is absorbed from its site of administration, namely:

1. formulation of drug (e.g. tablet or capsule, liquid or solid, suppository or aerosol)
2. solubility in the tissue in which it is placed
3. blood flow through that tissue.

By and large there is no difference between healthy children and adults in the way drugs are absorbed from the gastrointestinal tract, but there are some notable exceptions, namely the slower absorption of ampicillin and cloxacillin in the infant compared to later childhood and adulthood. Food interferes with the absorption of cloxacillin, phenoxymethyl penicillin, and erythromycin and therefore these drugs are best taken on an empty stomach (see Table 34.2); by contrast, nitrofurantoin can cause severe nausea unless taken with meals and has been shown to be better absorbed with food. Comparatively few data sheets say whether the product should be taken with food or on an empty stomach.

Intramuscular absorption is generally quicker than by the oral route but this is not universally true. One particular drug to note is Diazepam (Valium) which is less quickly absorbed intramuscularly than by other routes, as the drug binds to muscle proteins and indeed may be ineffective when a rapid effect is required, e.g. in status epilepticus (Agurell, 1975).

Table 34.2 Drug absorption and food

Drugs best absorbed on an empty stomach at least one hour before food (total absorption probably reduced by food)	
Cephalexin	
Erythromycin	The estolate less than the base and stearate
Lincomycin	
Penicillins	Phenoxymethyl penicillin, ampicillin, amoxycillin, (flu)cloxacillin
Rifampicin	
Tetracyclines	Unsuitable under age of 11
Drugs whose absorption is probably only delayed by concurrent administration of food	
Aspirin	
Barbiturates	
Digoxin	
Paracetamol	
Probably many others	

The most rapid route for absorption is intravenous, but this is rarely practicable or desirable in general paediatric practice (see Table 34.3). The rectal route can give a very rapid absorption because of the rich blood and lymph supply, and unionised, lipid soluble substances are readily absorbed. A suppository (often dosage is only half the adult dose) may not be appropriate, but a solution given by syringe (accurately measured) per rectum can be rapidly absorbed and Diazepam given this way will rapidly take effect.

In general practice the oral route is by far the most common, for obvious reasons. Drugs are given mostly in a syrup form, which is unfortunate, as there is a higher incidence of dental caries in children who have been taking syrup medicines regularly (Roberts, 1979; see also Ch. 33).

Distribution

There are great differences between the various proportions of total body water and extracellular water in infants, children and adults. At three months the total body water is 73 per cent of the total body weight, falling to 59 per cent at one year and approximately 55 per cent of the total body weight in the adult. Similarly, extracellular water falls from 33 per cent of the total body weight at three months to 28 per cent at one year and 20 per cent in the adult.

Water-soluble drugs disperse freely through the extracellular space to reach the site of action and therefore the drug concentration at the reception is inversely proportional to the size of this compartment. A similar dose of a drug per body weight produces higher concentrations in the older child (with the smaller relative extracellular volume) compared to the infant and younger child. In dehydrated states the drug levels are therefore increased, and in uraemic states drug levels are decreased.

Drugs are carried in the blood in two forms: (a) free in solution, pharmacologically active, diffusible and available for metabolism and excretion, and (b) bound (to protein molecules), inert pharmacologically. This factor is important when drugs compete for protein binding sites, or in cases of hypoalbuminuria. Important drugs, largely bound to proteins, are the penicillins, sulphonamides, barbiturates and salicylates.

Metabolism

Drug metabolism occurs mainly in the liver, though also in other organs such as the intestinal wall and lung. In the immature infant, despite the relatively larger liver mass, several enzyme systems may be immature and therefore adversely affect the way in which the body can metabolize certain drugs. The amount and kind of drug metabolizing enzymes are genetically determined, and the rate of drug metabolism varies by as much as a fac-

Table 34.3 Summary of major routes of administration

Route	*Advantage*	*Disadvantage*
Oral	Convenience	Absorption variable, particularly in relation to food Some drugs not absorbed (streptomycin) Some drugs destroyed (insulin, penicillin) Syrup vehicle bad for teeth
Intramuscular	Mostly reliable absorption but notable exceptions (diazepam, phenytoin)	Not suitable for self administration Psychological effects on child Painful
Intravenous	Immediate effect with predictable blood levels Only route for some irritant anti-cancer drugs	Difficult in very small children Intra-arterial injection and overdosage potentially hazardous
Subcutaneous	Reliable action May be self-administered (insulin)	Painful for some preparations
Rectal	Self-administration possible When vomiting or swallowing difficult For uncooperative child	Psychological Dosage of suppositories may be unsuitable Rectal inflammation with repeated use
Inhalation	Rapidly taken up and eliminated High level concentration within the bronchi	Special apparatus and techniques required Drug must be non-irritant Possible overdosage

tor of 10 or more for some drugs. Bilirubin, if displaced from the protein binding sites by various drugs (see above), cannot be readily metabolized and may result in kernicterus in the very small infant. Enzyme induction, whereby a drug after being given for a few days may induce an increase in endoplasmic drug metabolizing enzyme activity, may be used clinically in certain circumstances to aid the elimination of a substance (e.g. phenobarbitone to help to conjugate bilirubin by inducing hepatic glucoronyl transferase). Drugs which are metabolized faster in children than in adults and hence give a lower ratio of plasma level to dose, include the anti-convulsants, phenytoin, phenobarbitone and ethosuximide. Twice the weight-related adult dose is frequently required in children in order to achieve plasma levels similar to those in adults.

Excretion

The kidney is the most important means of excreting drugs, whether altered or unaltered. The glomerular filtration rate of the infant does not reach that of the adult until about five months and drugs excreted by that route (e.g. digoxin, gentamycin) are therefore excreted more slowly and have longer half-lives in the infant under five months. Renal tubular secretion (important for penicillin) equals that of the adult at about seven months, so the half-life of penicillin is longer in the infant under that age. Any child with renal impairment must be prescribed for with the greatest caution, as the plasma half-life of certain drugs given to uraemic patients may be increased from 0.5 hours to as long as 23 hours (penicillin G).

DOSAGE

Infants and children do not behave like a little adults, though for years it was customary to calculate the paediatric dosage according to the weight of the child, and the formula of Clark is still applied occasionally. This states $\frac{\textit{weight of child}}{70}$ (kg) = fraction of the adult dose. However for infants these doses may be two to three times too small. As long ago as 1914 Drayer and Walker, by means of relating dosage to the surface area of the child calculated by a nomogram, were able to produce doses in a formula of milligrams per square metre, but this proved to be a very cumbersome procedure and did not have widespread favour. Catzel (1974) prescribes by the percentage method with the doses being worked out initially by surface area, and by this method one can determine dosage either by weight or by age in the child of average build. For greater accuracy weight can be used, but allowances should be made for the obese child (with relatively smaller extracellular fluid volume), and probably the ideal body body weight should still be used.

Age in years	*Weight in kg*	*Percentage of adult dose*
Adult	70	100
12	40	75
7	23	50
1	10	25

For in-between ages and weights, approximations suffice in the majority of cases. It should be remembered, as Catzel points out, that greater accuracy is rarely required and that the scheme should only be regarded as relevant for starting doses, because all doses should be altered if necessary according to the response of the patient. For infants under the age of one year Catzel suggests:

Age	*Weight in kg*	*Percentage of adult dose*
1 year	10	25
4 months	6.5	20
2 months	4.5	15
2 weeks	3.5	12.5

Under two weeks special problems arise for reasons stated before, and the doses of drugs required fall steeply, but it is not safe to make any generalisation concerning dosage, which should always be looked up for the particular drug at the time.

The introduction of the 5 ml measure has been an important advance but it is to be regretted that there is no consistent relationship in the amount of the drug to be found between the liquid and tablet form. Catzel (1976) proposes with irrefutable logic that it would be advantageous to all if there were to be a fixed ratio between solid and liquid forms, and he proposes that the amount of a drug on a 5 ml spoon should equal one quarter of the adult dose.

By applying his percentages, 5 ml then would be the appropriate dosage for a one year old, 10 ml for a seven year old, 15 ml for a twelve year old and 20 ml for an adult. The use of the 5 ml spoon would best be replaced by a graduated dropper or plastic measuring vessel (as in hospital), allowing for greater accuracy in dosage between these ages and also for infants. With this scheme, 4 ml would then be the dosage for a four month baby and 3 ml for a two month baby.

PRINCIPLES OF PRESCRIBING

Doctors, and general practitioners in particular, have often been criticised for too readily prescribing for almost every complaint. This is said to reinforce the myth that modern medicine is all-powerful and reduces the self reliance of the patient, which in its turn increases demands on already stretched resources, so that the patient returns expecting further treatment. In certain circumstances, the prescriber may be doing the patient a disservice, e.g. antibiotics in the treatment of diarrhoea may well prolong the acute illness, and the risks of adverse reactions, or overdosage should never be minimised. Indeed, adverse reactions, which almost certainly are not fully identified, have been reported as occurring in up to 17 per cent of all children on drugs (Whyte and Greenson, 1977). Adverse reactions occur more readily when more than one drug is used and when more serious illnesses are treated; see Table 34.4.

Ideally, before prescribing any drug, the prescriber should be asking himself the following questions – modified from Herxheimer's list (1976):

a. *Need.* Is the drug really needed? What would happen if no drug is used?
b. *Aim.* What is to be achieved with the drug? How and when will it become effective?
c. *Observation.* Who will judge if the aim has been achieved?
d. *Administration.* How will it be administered: route,

Table 34.4 Most frequently observed adverse drug reactions and their likely causes (Rylance, 1979)

System	*Manifestation*	*Likely drugs*
Gastrointestinal	Nausea/vomiting	Most drugs
	Diarrhoea	Ampicillin
	Monilial infection	Ampicillin
	Mouth ulcers	Vincristine
	Gastric bleeding	Aspirin
	Stained teeth	Tetracycline
Cutaneous	Macular/papular rash	Ampicillin, cotrimoxazole, phenytoin
	Urticaria	Penicillin Aspirin
	Alopecia	Vincristine Cyclophosphamide
	Cushingoid facies	Prednisolone
Neurological or muscular	Drowsiness	Phenobarbitone Antihistamines
	Ataxia	Phenytoin Carbamazepine (Tetretol)
	Dystonia	Metoclopromide Prochlorperazine
	Hyperkinesis	Phenobarbitone
Haematological	Bone marrow depression	Cytotoxic agents Chloramphenicol
	Megaloblastic anaemia	Cotrimoxazole Phenytoin

dosage, frequency of administration? How long should it be given for? The fewer the doses and shorter the course the better.
e. *Alternatives*. What alternative drugs are there? Is the drug chosen the simplest, safest and possibly the cheapest drug available?
f. *Elimination*. How is the drug to be eliminated? Will the child's illness modify this?
g. *Side effects*. What undesirable effects may occur? Are they acceptable, how may they be minimized?
h. *Interactions*. Are there other drugs, foods or activities which the child should avoid whilst receiving the drug?
i. *Patient's ideas*. What does the parent (and, if old enough, the child) know about the drug? Does he remember what he has been told? Is the drug palatable? Will the child take the drug? Will this dosage be strictly adhered to?

In a recent study, only ten per cent of patients considered penicillin a drug; 25 per cent thought it should be used to treat the common cold and 50 per cent thought it an appropriate treatment for diarrhoea (Jones, 1979). No assumptions should ever be made. The treatment of the cause must have priority over the treatment of symptoms. A small repertoire of drugs enables a doctor to become more aware of the side effects, and the way a drug works. Never hesitate to look up anything that one is uncertain about. The *Alder Hey Book of Children's Doses* is an excellent 40 page booklet which contains information about everything a general practitioner needs to know in this field. There is no place for 'guessing' the dosage. Dosages stated in hospital letters, often about drugs that the general practitioner may not be familiar with, should always be checked and never taken 'on trust'. If in doubt, the hospital pharmacist should be contacted for further information.

Every practice should develop and implement a policy about prescribing. If opportunity is taken in the consultation to reassure the parent and child that the child with an upper respiratory tract infection has a clear chest and is not suffering from pneumonia, and that the child with diarrhoea and vomiting is not dehydrated, unnecessary prescribing of potent medicines can be avoided. This reassurance may well be all that the parent seeks. Time taken explaining simple measures for what are very often self limiting conditions, may well save further unnecessary worry for the parent, and indeed may well save further appointments.

When the prescription is issued, the parent and the child as soon as he is old enough, should be encouraged to take as an intelligent interest in the exercise as possible. Ample explanation about what is and is not expected from the drug, and clear instructions about the dosage, frequency of administration, and for how long should be stated. The drug should be limited for use by the person for whom it was prescribed, and should be kept in a safe place out of the way of the child (by law, this must now be stated on each bottle or other container issued).

If the medicine is unfinished the parents should be advised to discard it after a set time. Childproof containers, compulsory for certain drugs sold 'over the counter', are a help in reducing potential poisoning (see Ch. 24).

What can be done to improve compliance? Charney (1967) has shown that faith in and familiarity with the prescribing doctor, and the parent's awareness of the seriousness of the child's illness, is important. Other factors include the doctor's relationship with his patients, reducing the number of drugs which he prescribes and reducing the frequency of administration (Porter, 1969). Written instructions or the use of a calendar chart may help.

When writing the prescription, the name and age should always be clearly written (as a safeguard) and instructions for administration made clear – 'as directed' or 'as before' should never be used. Patient instruction labels, pre-printed stuck on the bottle, advising how the drug should be given, are a tremendous help.

Be not the first by whom the new is tried, nor yet the last to lay the old aside. Pope's advice in 1711 can readily be applied to prescribing today, as can Hippocrates' *First do not harm.*

Great efforts should be made to keep abreast of developments, but one should strive to keep one's prescribing repertoire to a minimum, and try to anticipate potential hazards. If the doctor is careful and caring then hopefully there should never be cause to apply to his patients Matthew Prior's famous couplet, written three centuries ago:

Cured yesterday of my disease
I died last night of my physician

REFERENCES

Agurell, S. *et al* (1975) Plasma levels of diazepam. *Epilepsia*, **16**, 277–283.

Alder Hey Book of Children's doses. 3rd edn. Available from Pharmacy Office, Alder Hey Children's Hospital, Eaton Road, Liverpool L12 2AP.

Apley, J. (1978) *The Child with Abdominal Pain*, 2nd edn, p. 107. Oxford: Blackwell Scientific.

Catford J.C. (1980) Quality of prescribing for children in general practice. *British Medical Journal*, **1**, 1435–7.

Catzel, P. (1974) *The Paediatric Prescriber*, 4th edn. Oxford: Blackwell Scientific.

Catzel P. (1976) Problems in paediatric prescribing. *Practitioner*, **217**, 396–402.

Charney E. *et al* (1967) How well do patients take oral penicillin? *Paediatrics*, **40**, p. 188

Cleary J. (1976) Chapter 6, Prescribing in General Practice, supplement No. 1 Vol. 26. *Journal of the Royal College of General Practitioners*

Editorial B M J (1980) Drug administration and food. *British Medical Journal*, **1**, 289.

Fry J. (1966) Profiles of Disease p. 24.

Grace J.F. & Goulds R.K. (1980) An examination of the prescribed therapeutic experience of five-year-olds in general practice. *Journal of the Royal College of General Practitioners*, **30**, 529–532.

Herxheimer A. (1976) Towards parity for therapeutics in clinical teaching. *Lancet*, **2**, 1186.

Howie J.G.R. (1979) Prescribing Trends in General Practice. 2nd Edition, p. 148. Royal College of General Practitioners.

Jones D.R. (1979) Drugs and prescribing: what the patient thinks. *Journal of the Royal College of General Practitioners*, **29**, 417.

Pope, A. (1711) *Essays in Criticism.*

Porter A.M.W. (1969) Drug defaulting in general practice. *British Medical Journal*, **1**, 218.

Roberts I.F. & Roberts G.J. (1979) Relation between medicine sweetened with sucrose and dental disease. *British Medical Journal*, **1**, 14–16.

Rylance G. (1979) Adverse drug reactions. *British Journal of Hospital Medicine.*

Sussex M.R. & Watson W. (1971) Sociology in Medicine. London, O.V.P.

Whyte J. & Greenson E. (1977) Drug usage and adverse drug reactions in paediatric patients. *Acta Paediatrica Scandinavia*, **66**, 767.

PART FIVE

Clinical care in long-term disorders

35

Congenital heart disease

Geoffrey Sykes

The incidence of rheumatic heart disease is definitely on the downgrade. Improved social conditions, and the free use of antibiotics in the treatment of upper respiratory tract infections may have much to do with this. Conversely, congenital heart disease may appear to be on the increase, but this is doubtful. There is no doubt that improved standards of child health care, particularly the routine screening of infants and young children, have revealed many children with signs suggestive of congenital heart disease. The majority of infants born in hospital today are examined before discharge, particular attention being paid to examination of the heart, palpation of the femoral pulses and a search for other signs of congenital heart disease. It should be clearly understood, however, that a small but significant number of children with serious defects have no signs or symptoms of disease in early life and despite routine screening are missed. The wise general practitioner will, therefore, always be on the lookout for previously unsuspected congenital heart disease.

If the concept of the primary care team in general practice is developed further, then 'primary screening' of all children in the practice may become one of its responsibilities. Ancillary staff and health visitors may be trained to do much of this work, for example some measurements in developmental screening, audiometry and so forth, but screening of the cardiovascular system is one of the tasks that can be undertaken only by general practitioners in the team. A good understanding of management of early signs, and symptoms, is likely to become increasingly important to the general practitioner in future.

The growth of high technology medicine in recent decades has been accompanied by a parallel improvement in the diagnosis and treatment of congenital heart disease. Its study and treatment has been a major growth point in paediatrics since pioneers such as Blalock and Taussig showed how surgery could revolutionise the prognosis of severely affected children. Surgical correction of quite severe disorders in the first few days of life is now commonplace. Of the 2500 children undergoing major heart operations annually in Britain, about half are less than one year old.

Congenital heart disease by its very nature is a distortion of normal embryological growth; the permutations of this are limitless. Year by year the literature increases at a frightening pace. The infinite variety of rare syndromes and minor variations of the more common forms of congenital heart disease need not concern the general practitioner. He will be reassured to know that it is quite possible to care successfully for the affected child with very little detailed knowledge of this complex, rapidly expanding field.

There are three important areas in which the general practitioner makes a contribution to the care of these children:

1. Early diagnosis and screening.
2. General management of the child, and his worried parents.
3. Long-term care of the severely handicapped child.

This chapter will attempt to cover, very briefly, some of the more practical aspects of management of children with congenital heart disease with the above objectives in view. It will omit many aspects which would be of only limited interest and are far better dealt with in the many excellent reference books and monographs on the subject.

INCIDENCE AND AETIOLOGY

Parents of affected children, mothers particularly, often have guilt feelings. Care should be taken to explain that they are not to blame, even in the rare instances where the disorder is hereditary. The first questions the parents of an affected child will ask are 'How did it happen?' and then 'What are the risks of it happening again?'. The general practitioner should be able to answer these important questions in simple terms, which parents can understand. Some basic statistics and appreciation of causative factors are, therefore, essential.

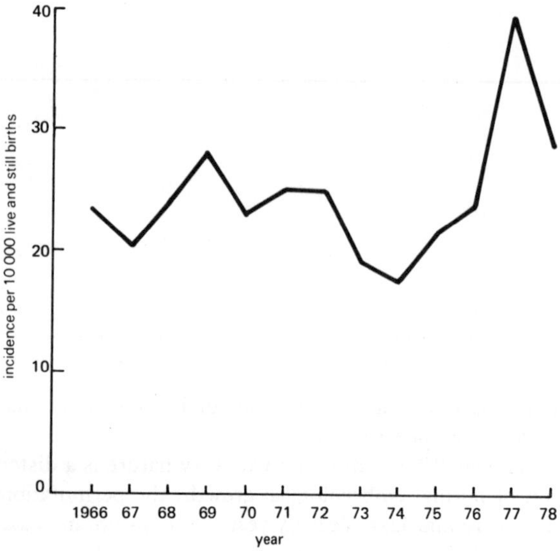

Fig. 35.1 Heart and great vessel defects: incidence per 10 000 live and still births in Northern Ireland, 1968–1978. Source: *BMJ* 1980, 2, 1380

The incidence of significant congenital heart disease has been estimated at between seven and eight per thousand births. There is, however, a heavy death rate in the first month of life of about 30 per cent, and a further 10 per cent of children die before they are one year old. It seems reasonable to suppose, therefore, that a general practitioner with between two and three thousand patients will have between eight and fifteen patients, of all ages, affected by congenital heart disease. There is however a great variation in incidence from country to country, from region to region, and from year to year, as recent estimates from Northern Ireland show (Fig. 35.1).

It is possible that as treatment by open heart surgery improves for gross abnormalities, particularly those of the great vessels, the mortality in early life will drop. The number of survivors is thus likely to increase, and many of these children and their parents will need a great deal of advice, support and encouragement from family doctors if they are to live a normal or near normal life, and not be unduly restricted. Of the children who die, it should be remembered that many have multiple defects involving other systems which are incompatible with life.

The eight common congenital heart defects which account for about 85 per cent of all cases are tabulated below in order of incidence (Table 35.1).

Boys are more prone to suffer from aortic stenosis, coarctation of the aorta, transposition of the great arteries, and tetralogy of Fallot. Girls are slightly more prone to develop patent ductus arteriosis, and atrial septal defects.

Approximately 13 per cent of patients with one congenital heart defect will have an additional cardiac defect. Between 10 and 15 per cent of patients with cardiac defects will have another non-cardiac deformity (Campbell, 1965).

Parents of children with congenital heart disease may occasionally suffer from a defect themselves. The most likely are atrial septal defect and patent ductus arteriosis (Jordan and Scott, 1973).

Death rates in childhood from congenital heart disease are listed in Table 35.2. The numbers have dropped greatly in recent years.

Several writers have expressed concern about the future; survivors of surgery with serious defects may pass on defective genes to their progeny. Others are alarmed about the prospects of intermarriage between those attending cardiothoracic centres. The offspring of such outpatient romances will be awaited with interest!

Heredity

Heredity plays a small part in the aetiology of congenital heart disease. Brothers and sisters of those affected are three or four times more likely to have a heart lesion than the general population. The risk to siblings is approximately between one in 25 and one in 30 with patent ductus arteriosus, and up to one in 100 with other forms of congenital heart disease. Abnormal chromosomes are sometimes associated with congenital heart disease, particularly in mongolism, Turner's syn-

Table 35.1 Incidence of common congenital heart defects

Defect	*Incidence (percentage of all lesions)*
Ventricular septal defect	25
Patent ductus arteriosis	12
Atrial septal defect	10
Pulmonary stenosis	10
Aortic stenosis (including bicuspid valves)	7
Coarctation of the aorta	7
Tetralogy of Fallot	7
Transposition of the great arteries	7

Table 35.2 Deaths from congenital heart disease in children under 15 years old, England and Wales, 1978. Deaths rates per million population. Source: OPCS Child Mortality Statistics, Series DH3

Defect	*Number of deaths* *Males*	*Females*
All defects	521	415
Ventricular septal defect	101	82
Valvular anomalies	80	64
Transposition of the great arteries	61	42
Tetralogy of Fallot	50	42
Atrial septal defect	26	42
Coarctation of the aorta	34	18
Patent ductus arteriosus	19	23
Pulmonary stenosis	17	22
All other defects	133	90

drome, 13/15 trisomy, 18 trisomy, and the 'cri du chat' syndrome. In Marfan's syndrome which is inherited as a Mendelian dominant, atrial septal defect may be due to a mutant gene. Several workers have reported this defect occurring in successive generations of one family.

I have cared for a family in which there were four children with aortic stenosis; in addition an aunt and two cousins were affected. I have also seen a family in which nearly all the children suffered from patent ductus arteriosis; uncles, aunts, and cousins who had emigrated to Australia suffered a high incidence of the same defect.

Other factors

There are many factors of which we are still ignorant. There is the multifactoral hypothesis of McKusick, to which those interested may care to refer (McKusick, 1964). I think we all are aware of the dangers of maternal rubella. Other forms of intrauterine virus infection, viz. influenza, and the Coxsackie B virus, are suspect but not yet proven causes of congenital heart disease.

CONGENITAL HEART DISEASE IN THE NEWBORN AND IN EARLY INFANCY

General practitioners who are involved in the staffing of maternity units, and those general practitioners who still indulge in the ancient art of domiciliary midwifery, will find they are often the 'doctor of first contact' of neonates suffering from congenital heart disease. It is essential to refer suspected infants without delay if effective treatment is to be given. If the baby later proves to be normal, little harm will have been done. Small size is no longer a barrier to curative surgery. Neonates can now be operated on successfully using cardiopulmonary bypass techniques. It is therefore vital that general practitioner obstetricians should be able to spot serious congenital heart disease early, before heart failure and acidosis makes surgical correction more difficult. A few hours delay can make all the difference between success and failure. It is essential to avoid hypothermia when moving these babies. They should be wrapped in foil or cotton wool and transferred quickly by ambulance, in a heated incubator. Cold acidotic babies should be given intravenous bicarbonate to correct acidosis: 4–10 ml of 8.4 per cent sodium bicarbonate slowly into the umbilical vein via a catheter. Inspired guesses as to the degree of acidosis are probably not within the realms of general practitioner medicine, but the above dosage will not do any harm, before the infant is sent on his way.

Alarm signals in neonates

At risk groups

Infants with affected siblings, or a family history of congenital heart disease. Pre-term infants. Infants of diabetic mothers. Infants having other congenital abnormalities. Infants with one umbilical artery (can be associated with renal and cardiovascular anomalies, but by no means always). Light for dates babies.

Heart murmurs

These may be transient, especially in preterm infants. In some infants the fetal circulation persists to some degree for a few hours or days after birth. In very small infants the ductus arteriosus does not always close instantly and for several days a systolic ejection murmur can be heard over the pulmonary outflow tract. This can lead to transient heart failure in very premature, low birth weight babies, but the condition usually corrects itself after a few weeks. Whilst the presence of a murmur cannot be ignored, severely affected infants may not have a murmur. There are more subtle and ominous signs which should be looked for. Ausculcation of the heart alone is not enough; the total condition of the infant should be assessed, it is more telling.

The murmurless heart

One of the greatest problems in deciding whether heart disease is present or not, is the large number of lesions which do not produce a murmur in early childhood. Luckily most of these are rare, with the exception of transposition of the great vessels, and coarctation of the aorta.

Cyanosis

Babies with cyanotic congenital heart disease are nearly always blue from birth. This is due to one of three mechanisms:

1. *Right to left shunt* of substantial amounts of blood,

from whatever cause. The commonest cause of this type of shunt is the tetralogy of Fallot.

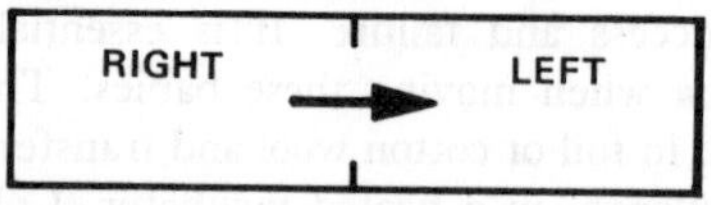

2. *Reversal of flow in a left to right shunt.* If pressure in the left side falls due to heart failure and pressure in the right side rises, reversal of flow results with consequent cyanosis. Straining, coughing, or crying which cause a temporary increase intrapulmonary pressure, can lead to transient cyanosis due to shunt reversal. The consequent and sudden increase in right sided pressure results in the squirting of large quantities of venous blood through a large IVSD or AVSD or PDA. These are the commonest causes of a left to right shunt.

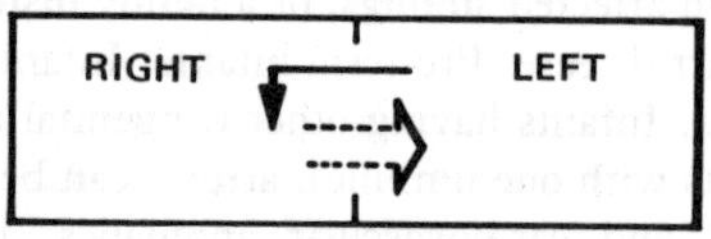

3. *Cyanosis due to poor diffusion of oxygen in the lungs.* For example in pulmonary oedema, pulmonary hypertension or decreased pulmonary blood flow.

Pitfalls in assessing cyanosis

Cyanosis, if associated with a murmur, or if aggravated by crying, coughing, or feeds, and if of the type which is relieved by oxygen, is likely to be significant. It is important to stress, however, that severely cyanosed infants may obtain no relief from oxygen and they may *not* have a murmur.

Cyanosis due to the respiratory distress syndrome or other secondary lung disease is seldom present in the first few hours of birth. Remember, however, that pneumothorax and diaphragmatic hernia can cause cyanosis from birth.

Blue extremities are quite common after delivery, particularly in cool rooms, and do not necessarily mean the child has a congenital heart lesion. If there has been delay with delivery of the shoulders, or the cord has been tightly round the neck, there may be traumatic asphyxia of the head and face. The accompanying cyanosis does not disappear on finger pressure, and should present no problems to the experienced doctor.

Polycythaemia due to delayed clamping of the cord can be a cause of harmless cyanosis after birth and presents a difficulty, but often when the infant screams the cyanosis clears, as the peripheral circulation is no longer stagnant. Babies who have dark skins may appear to be cyanosed around the lips, but careful inspection of the mucous membranes, nail beds and nipples will show that this is not so.

Remember that a slightly cyanosed infant with rapid respiration and a tachycardia may have no audible murmur, and yet be in early heart failure with serious, operable congenital heart disease.

HEART FAILURE IN NEONATES

As a group general practitioners will only rarely see heart failure in a baby, but they should remain alert to the possibility.

The presence of a murmur is not very helpful, as this may occur in relatively minor congenital heart lesions. There may be no cyanosis, no murmur, and yet the child may have serious congenital heart disease, and be already in early heart failure. The most useful signs are:

1. Tachycardia of over 160 per minute when the infant is at rest. (Paroxysmal tachycardia of 240–300 per minute is not uncommon in infancy – see later.)

2. A respiratory rate consistently over 60 per minute when the child is resting (particularly in a full term infant).

3. Liver enlargement. If a large firm liver can be felt more than two centimetres below the costal margin, serious consideration should be given to the possibility of heart failure. This is an important physical sign often missed by the uninitiated, or those who do not see many infants in heart failure. Yet this sign is a familiar everyday feature in general practice, seen in adult heart failure.

4. Excessive weight gain. If a weak, poorly feeding infant gains more than an ounce a day, one should suspect fluid retention due to heart failure. Look for pitting oedema; press firmly on the anterior tibial surface for one minute and observe.

5. Signs in the lungs. The picture of acute left or right heart failure so familiar in an older age group can be seen in an affected infant, although superficially the signs are those of congestive heart failure. Bronchospasm, dry cough, and moist sounds over the whole lung fields are not always due to infection. Heart failure in this age group is unlikely to respond to medical treatment except in the short term. The temptation to persist with this should be resisted. If surgical treatment is to be effective, early referral and assessment are vital. Sadly, many of these infants still cannot be helped by surgical treatment.

To summarise, in early infancy the general practitioner need not concern himself with the type of lesion. It is sufficient for him to have established the fact of an unexplained tachycardia, cyanosis, or suspicion of heart failure, and to arrange immediate safe transport of the infant to the most suitable centre for further investigation and assessment. Successful correction of quite severe abnormalities in the first few days of life is now feasible, due to the continuing improvement of surgical techniques in open heart surgery.

IMPORTANT POINTERS TO CONGENITAL HEART DISEASE IN OLDER CHILDREN

Although the basic principles of examination of the cardiovascular system in children are the same as in adults, there are one or two important differences which are perhaps worth mentioning. Minor degrees of cyanosis may not be evident at rest, but appear only on exertion or when the child is feeding or crying. A malar flush with minimal cyanosis may occasionally give a lead to the existence of underlying disease. In my experience by the time finger clubbing, stunting of growth, squatting after exertion etc. becomes obvious the diagnosis has usually been made. Perhaps in some darker children this is not altogether true, as pigmentation may conceal cyanosis.

Every doctor examining children should try to remember to feel the femoral pulses. Once or twice in a clinical lifetime he or she will be rewarded by finding that they are absent or diminished, and be able to make a diagnosis of coarctation of the aorta without much difficulty.

Blood pressure readings in young children are difficult and time consuming to obtain in general practice. They are also difficult to interpret. To obtain accurate values special sizes of sphygmomanometer cuff are required for each age group. The pressure rises slowly through infancy and childhood, approaching young adult levels about the age of ten years. The 'flush method' is useful in differentiating between the pressure in the upper and lower limbs, e.g. in coarctation of the aorta. (For details, see the description in Forfar and Arneil's *Textbook of Paediatrics*.) Always use the right arm and right leg because a high coarctation may interfere with pressures on the left side.

The apex beat

This should be about ½ inch (1.25 cm) outside the nipple line and normally is easily felt in older children. Moderate hypertrophy of the right ventricle can often be felt with the flat of the hand as a small 'flicking thrust'; it is hard to describe but somehow feels different from that of the normal child. Greater degrees of hypertrophy will easily be felt and seen; they cause progressive chest deformity which should be obvious, particularly over the lower sternum. Thrills in thin children are well felt, particularly in the suprasternal notch and over the pulmonary and aortic outflow tracts. Pulsations of the great vessels of the neck can, occasionally, produce a thrill if they are partly compressed in a normal child.

Heart sounds

Splitting of the first sound is fairly common in children. This is particularly noticeable in nervous, excited children and in those who are feverish or anaemic. Splitting of the second sound is accentuated during deep respiration, and during expiration the splitting is diminished or not heard. 'Fixed splitting' of the second sound, or 'parodoxical splitting', i.e. accentuation during expiration, is abnormal. I think everyone knows that sinus arrhythmia is marked in children, and this should hold no mystery for present day general practitioners. A third heart sound is often easy to hear shortly after the second sound, and may simulate a diastolic murmur. I personally have never found this a difficulty.

Functional murmurs. These are very common in healthy children, and are frequently the cause of much anxiety and confusion.

'Innocent' systolic murmurs. Identification of the innocent systolic murmur remains a major problem, one of the most common and difficult situations in this field which the general practitioner has to face. The murmur is usually early systolic and soft in character, frequently heard most clearly between the sternal border and the apex beat in the fourth or fifth left intercostal space. These murmurs are often heard when the family doctor visits an excited or apprehensive child with a fever. They disappear when the fever has subsided; sometimes they disappear with a change of posture.

Late systolic murmurs. The 'floppy valve syndrome', possibly a *form fruste* of Marfan's syndrome, has been reviewed in a leading article in the *British Medical Journal* and may not be altogether innocent (*BMJ*, 1975). Occasionally, the systolic ejection murmur over the aortic outflow tract in aortic stenosis may be propagated down towards the apex. If the apical area only is auscultated then the unwary doctor may assume this is an innocent systolic murmur, with disastrous consequences.

Innocent mid-systolic murmurs over the pulmonary outflow tract. These are usually early or mid-systolic murmurs over the second left interspace. I find it difficult to distinguish them from mild degrees of pulmonary stenosis without full investigation and assessment.

Diastolic murmurs. A diastolic murmur by itself is never innocent.

Venous hums. A venous hum is a low pitched continuous sound heard beneath the inner ends of either or both of the clavicles, and over the great vessels of the neck. Unlike the continuous 'machinery murmur' of PDA it disappears if the jugular vein is gently compressed. It is nearly always abolished if the child lies down flat.

When dealing with parents, be truthful whenever possible. Most experienced paediatricians would hesitate to label a murmur innocent until it has been fully investigated. I think it would be foolhardy for the average general practitioner to assume that any murmur was innocent until it had been thoroughly assessed and proved otherwise. Parents must be informed, because sooner or later their child will be seen by another doctor, for example, when on holiday, at the school clinic, or by an anaesthetist. They may then assume that the family doctor, who originally heard the murmur and kept quiet about it, was an incompetent fool.

THE EIGHT COMMON DEFECTS

Detailed description of the defects is not possible within the confines of this chapter; brief facts which may be of practical value and help in the management of congenital heart disease in general practice are outlined below.

Ventricular septal defect

This is by far the most common form of congenital heart disease, accounting for one quarter of all cases. About 35 per cent of them close spontaneously, particularly the small and medium size defects. Frequently closure occurs in the first year of life, but clinically many of these children seem to become normal within two decades. This is probably because of differential growth rates within the heart. The defect becomes 'functionally small'; in other words it has no physiological significance and the murmur can no longer be heard. Large ventricular septal defects, of course, lead to pulmonary hypertension and eventual death from heart failure in early adult life unless they can be closed. The optimum age to attempt surgical closure is about one year of age, providing heart failure can be controlled in the meantime. There is a trend to even earlier operation in some centres. The long term followup and assessment of these children, which includes talking to their parents, with their problems and anxieties, is an important if time-consuming part of their management by both paediatrician and general practitioner.

Patent ductus arteriosis

This lesion is twice as common in girls as boys. It is the commonest heart lesion to result from rubella in early pregnancy. The ductus usually closes about 15 hours after birth, but it may remain open for a few days and give rise to a transient murmur in the pulmonary area. Spontaneous closure is rare after the first few weeks of life. During the first few months of life a systolic murmur may be heard; the characteristic to and fro machinery murmur comes later. The treatment of choice is closure of the uncomplicated ductus as soon as it is diagnosed, irrespective of the patient's age. Bacterial endocarditis is a real risk in these patients, greater than that of operation.

Atrial septal defects

70 per cent of these are of the ostium secundum type. There are often no symptoms or signs of disease in childhood; in many cases trouble does not develop until the third decade. Pregnancy may cause heart failure in previously unsuspected cases. Later, pulmonary hypertension develops due to an increased pulmonary blood flow. Ostium secundum defects can be closed using open heart surgery, in suitable cases. The optimum age is between 5 and 14 years. Recently attempts have been made to close ostium secundum defects with an umbrella-like device which is threaded through the femoral vein and inferior vena cava into the atria. Two Decron diaphragms then seal the defect from either side as the 'umbrellas' are opened. If this device is successful, more radical surgical correction may be avoided.

Ostium primus defects are more sinister than ostium secundum defects as they occur lower down the atrial septum in more vital territory. Children with these defects need careful and close supervision. If the mitral or tricuspid valves are involved there may be mitral incompetence or tricuspid regurgitation. The sudden onset of congestive heart failure commonly occurs with little warning. Paroxysmal tachycardia may be associated with these defects, due to involvement of the conducting tissue.

Pulmonary stenosis

This may occur at the level of the valve, or of the infundibulum. Those affected may have little or no cyanosis, particularly at rest. Severely affected infants usually have marked cyanosis. Older children with significant disease usually have a thrill over the pulmonary outflow tract as well as a systolic ejection murmur. Surgical treatment consists of attempts at valvulotomy or infundibular resection, if the condition is sufficiently severe.

Aortic stenosis

The most important thing to know about aortic stenosis is that the children with it can drop dead suddenly after severe exertion. It may be associated with coarctation of the aorta or patent ductus arteriosis. Bicuspid aortic valves may have associated stenosis, but not always so. Those liable to sudden death are likely to have an enlarged heart and systolic ejection thrill over the aortic outflow tract, as well as a systolic murmur carried into the great vessels of the neck. This is *not* always so; the lesion may limit coronary blood flow, without much left ventricular hypertrophy. These lesions are frequently symptomless and the signs are minimal and easily missed. Unless a murmur or thrill is heard over the aortic outflow tract the diagnosis may not be suspected. Children and parents should be told of the risks of severe exertion in competitive games, swimming, football etc., until full assessment has been undertaken. Treatment is by operation using open heart surgery, either by valvotomy or by replacement with an artificial valve. Bacterial endocarditis is a real risk and can make the stenosis worse, and cause incompetence to develop as a further complication.

Coarctation of the aorta

If the femoral pulses are absent, diagnosis is relatively simple. In some cases the femoral pulses are reduced and delayed in relation to the brachial pulse. Systolic pressure in the arms is higher than in the legs, the diastolic pressure may be the same in both arms and legs. Later there is increased pulsation in the suprasternal notch, and the left ventricular pulsation may be forceful. X-ray changes of notching of the ribs by the collateral circulation are seldom present before the child reaches six years of age. Mild cases need no treatment apart from routine advice regarding prophylaxis against bacterial endocarditis. More severe cases undergo resection of the coarcted segment when they are six or seven years old.

Tetralogy of Fallot

After the first year of life this is the commonest cyanotic lesion. Not all 'Fallots' are obvious in early infancy, in that they may not yet be cyanosed or show signs of a right to left shunt. They may be a normal colour at rest, and develop cyanosis or cyanotic attacks only after exertion, coughing, crying or feeding. Sudden exertion may produce rapid cyanosis with unconsciousness, which is occasionally fatal. The child may appear very well between attacks, with only a heart murmur.

In older children, 'squatting attacks' are almost always due to Fallot's tetralogy. The classical picture of the older severely affected child with finger clubbing, congested and suffused eyes and cheeks is I think well known. There is usually a systolic thrill and murmur to be heard over the pulmonary outflow tract; they are frequently polycythaemic. 'Fallots' generally restrict their exercise automatically but parents should be warned, in severe cases, of the hidden dangers of severe exertion. Whilst awaiting surgical treatment, propranolol may be useful in the prophylaxis of cyanotic attacks, and it may also be useful in terminating these attacks. Digoxin should not be used to control cyanotic attacks. In general, 'Fallots' do not go into cardiac failure. There is, therefore, no indication to use digoxin in this condition; indeed, digoxin is thought to be dangerous because increased contraction of heart muscle narrows the already restricted outflow tract from the right ventricle. Most general practitioners carry morphine in their bags; they are less likely to have intravenous propanolol to hand. Morphia can be used in an emergency to control severe sudden attacks of cyanosis.

Eventually, nearly all children require surgical treatment for this condition. Severely affected infants may be treated with palliative operations until they are large enough to undergo complete correction. This procedure, done under open heart surgery using cardiac pulmonary bypass techniques, can offer good results in a high percentage of patients.

Transposition of the great vessels

This is the second most common cyanotic lesion. The term 'transposition' means the aorta and the pulmonary artery have changed places. The degree to which this takes place and the number of associated abnormalities are legion, and the general practitioner need know little about these. What is important for the general practitioner/obstetrician in particular to know and be aware of is that this is *a serious murmurless heart defect*. It is important to diagnose the uncomplicated case in the first two days of life; it is worth reiterating *do not sit on a cyanosed baby at this stage*.

If these children survive they can be treated by the balloon septostomy. A balloon catheter is passed through the foramen ovale into the left atrium. The balloon is filled with a radio opaque dye and jerked forcibly back through the foramen so as to rupture the atrial septum around the foramen. This is done several times; the results though variable can be quite good. The procedure is not without risk, and is often only palliative, as is the Blalock-Hanlon operation. Older survivors then undergo a Mustard operation or some similar corrective procedure.

The techniques of surgical correction of transposition are improving all the time, and the outlook for these children is likely to improve steadily in the future. In some series, workers claim a 50 per cent success rate. Many survivors of the procedure can expect to live a normal life.

In those where the long term outlook is poor, supportive treatment with digoxin and diuretics is needed until they die. Oxygen is of little use except as a placebo for the parents.

MANAGEMENT OF SOME SPECIFIC CONDITIONS

Infective endocarditis

Although general practitioners will rarely see a case of infective endocarditis, all will know of its association with congenital heart lesions. Those most likely to develop endocarditis are IVSD, PDA, coarctation of the aorta, lesions of the mitral valve, and particularly lesions of bicuspid aortic valves.

The disease is rare below the age of two. The source of infection is usually from sepsis in teeth, nose, or tonsils. The signs are well known: fever, malaise, anaemia, the spleen may be enlarged, and there may be finger and toe clubbing. Embolic phenomena such as splinter haemorrhages beneath the fingernails may occur. Unexplained fever in a child with congenital heart disease should be regarded as being due to infective endocarditis until proved otherwise. Seek the help of a paediatrician early; do not delay. The outlook is good with early diagnosis and adequate treatment.

Prophylaxis. Parents should be encouraged to maintain a high standard of dental hygiene in their children. The risks of infected teeth should be spelled out to them in detail. It should be impressed upon them that any operation particularly on the teeth or upper respiratory tract should only be undertaken under an antibiotic cover. The ideal method of prophylaxis, for example, before dental extraction is a large intramuscular injection of antibiotic one hour before the operation, followed by three days of oral treatment. This may not always be practical, in which case oral treatment should start the night before the operation. An earlier preoperative start to treatment is undesirable, because theoretically it may allow the growth of a small colony of resistant organisms on a valve. When penicillin has been used in the immediate past, it may be wise to use an alternative antibiotic such as cephaloridine. It is less well known that when operations on the genitourinary system or gut are contemplated, antibiotics active against gram-negative organisms should also be given.

Paroxysmal tachycardia

When the rate exceeds 210 or to be more practical when it is uncountable, paroxysmal tachycardia should always be suspected. Older children differ little from adults with this condition; it is worth mentioning that attacks of paroxysmal tachycardia are not uncommon in the first year of life. They are often described as 'grey attacks' or 'white attacks', and have to be considered in the differential diagnosis of the 'queer does' that frequently seem to occur in the infants of anxious mothers, with which we are all so familiar. Prolonged attacks can produce the clinical picture previously described in neonatal heart failure, and occasionally result in death. Severe acute continuous attacks respond to DC defibrillation, IV propanolol, or procaine amide, following hospitalisation. Further attacks are usually prevented by continuous administration of digoxin for 12 months, after which time the majority seem to cease spontaneously.

Congenital heart block

A rate usually less than 70 per minute in infants. This disorder may occur alone, but in babies is usually associated with a defect of the conducting tissues, or following surgical correction of, for example, transposition. A pacemaker may help if there are Stokes-Adams attacks.

Primary endocardial fibroelastosis

A rare condition which warrants mention because it is seldom diagnosed before terminal heart failure results in an early death, within the first few years of life. Frequently the child presents with bronchiolitis or bronchopneumonia following an acute URTI, and dies inexplicably of heart failure. Usually apart from gross cardiomegaly there are no abnormal signs until failure supervenes. Other children in the family may be affected.

THE GENERAL PRACTITIONER'S ROLE

Most paediatricians in district general hospitals will agree that they have not the sophisticated resources, nor the time to devote to the detailed diagnosis and treatment of severely affected children with congenital heart disease. This work is increasingly the province of paediatricians with a special interest in paediatric cardiology, working in Regional Cardiothoracic Centres.

If the general practitioner is wise he will turn for help to the local consultant paediatricians with whom he should have a good working relationship, rather than refer his patient directly to a special centre, except perhaps in rare instances when dealing with desperately ill neonates. Quite apart from such considerations as the most effective use of scarce expensive resources and the weighing of the risks of angiocardiography and cardiac catheterisation, the long term care of these children is likely to be shared between the local paediatrician and the family doctor.

The general practitioner's role is quite different from that of the paediatric cardiologist. In the unfamiliar and often awe inspiring atmosphere of a cardiac unit, frightened parents forget to ask vital questions, or are so overwhelmed by the situation that they cannot remember all that has been said. In the more relaxed and familiar setting of general practice these matters can be discussed more easily and in 'small doses'. Many quite intelligent parents need several 'seminars' before they can fully understand the situation as it affects their child. It is thus in the continuing care of the child in the community within the family, general practice complements and supplements the work of the hospital paediatrician and paediatric cardiologist.

As we have seen, the incidence of congenital heart disease in general practice is low, and only a few children will prove to have significant lesions. Yet paradoxically the GP will spend a great deal of time with children who eventually will prove to have innocent murmurs or lesions that do not have any serious effect on the child's life and health.

Experienced GPs will agree that certain key words, and expressions, are extremely emotive to patients and their relatives; they have to be used with great care. 'Angina', 'pneumonia', and 'tumour' spring readily to mind. The words 'congenital heart disease', 'hole in the heart' and 'blue baby' in a similar way should be used with a great deal of circumspection, when talking to parents. Once the words have been mentioned the GP is committed to devoting a considerable amount of time to discussing and explaining the condition. Heart disease in the lay mind equates with 'weak heart', 'strokes', 'coronary thrombosis' and 'sudden death'. The only experience many parents have of congenital heart disease is of a dramatic television documentary, a feature film, or newspaper article, in which major cardiothoracic surgery is the central feature of the entertainment; quite frequently the child dies at the end of it, for unfortunately only life threatening disease is newsworthy. The uninitiated have no way of knowing that only the minority of children are so severely affected.

'Neighbourhood experience' of congenital heart disease is equally dramatic. The cyanosed child in a wheelchair in a village street or shopping area is remembered; his eventual 'disappearance' is noted. The great number of less severely affected children, and those who are treated successfully by surgery, go unrecognised.

Good communication between hospital, general practitioner and the school doctor or community physician is vitally important. They should, if at all possible, tell the same tale; the inevitable overlapping of advice should be as uncontroversial as possible. Parents should be reassured with as much optimism as is compatible with the truth. They should be told, except in rare instances, that there is no danger of heart attacks, or sudden death, and that the child will be able to live a relatively normal life in most instances.

Some parents seem adept at misinterpreting other doctors' remarks. We all at some time make ill-advised comments. The GP will occasionally have to do some pretty fast and persuasive talking, in effect to as we say in Yorkshire 'keep t'band in t'nick'.* The reassurance of parents and the building up of confidence and trust in the care of their child is needed not simply to prevent shattered egos and loss of professional pride but to prevent the child 'going on circuit' and perhaps becoming a cardiac invalid. Frightened or desperate parents may be only too ready to hawk their child round a number of cardiothoracic centres both here and abroad. With some very ill children this cannot always be prevented, but usually, in my opinion, it leads to disaster and an early death. Well meant but misguided efforts of local groups to raise money to send children abroad for major heart surgery are remembered by parents. They need reassurance that their child will be able to receive all the treatment he requires in this country. Often parents have no idea of the high quality of services available locally. Perhaps we as general practitioners should do more to inform our patients about the work of our hospital colleagues in this field.

Occasionally one will be aghast to find a loud murmur in an older, apparently quite healthy child, who was previously not suspected of having a congenital heart lesion. It is important to explain to parents how a child that has been previously screened and found to be 'normal' can have suffered from congenital heart disease without any signs or symptoms. It is important to explain how this state of affairs can arise and not be due to negligence of a colleague.

It is permissible, even at the first consultation, to be mildly optimistic with murmurs and suggest that many children who have heart murmurs grow out of them as they get older. This gives the parents some hope and is, in fact, true of a large proportion of children with the commonest form of congenital heart disease, ventricular septal defect. It is helpful to explain to parents that like coughs, murmurs come in all shapes and sizes. Just as not all coughs are due to serious lung diseases such as TB or pneumonia, so not all murmurs are due to fatal or disabling heart disease.

To summarise then, the good general practitioner will devote himself to the role of medical adviser in the sense that Lindsey Batten meant when he gave his James Mackenzie lecture in 1960. The GP will need to advise the child and his parents on a vast range of factors and problems associated with the child's disability. Counselling and continuing care will be his major functions.

Continuing care

When dealing with these children our first duty is to help the child to grow up in the best possible way, emotionally, physically, and socially, that is compatible with his or her disability. The hospital doctor is principally concerned with accurate diagnosis and treatment of the lesion. The general practitioner's remit is much wider, and covers a much longer period of time, extending into adolescence and adult life. He has to optimise the quality of the child's life by preventing over-protection by his parents on the one hand, and the taking of undue risks on the other.

Knowledge of the family background, parental attitudes and intelligence, are invaluable in this respect. The child must be educated in the most suitable manner; education should always be slanted towards a job which can be tackled when school is over. Parents will ask a thousand and one questions: can the child go swimming? join in games? go climbing? parachuting? go abroad on school trips? on holidays? and so forth. With patience and perseverence many of these children can

* Old Yorkshire saying which relates to the smooth running of the spinning wheel

Table 35.3 Some useful drugs and doses. Note: all dosages are given in milligrams, not micrograms

Name of drug	*Route*	*Times daily*	*Birth to 2 weeks*	*2 weeks to 12 months*	*1 year*	*7 years*	*Adult*	*Comments*
Digoxin	Oral	×2	0.005 mg/kg 0.007 mg/kg Digitalising dose once or twice	0.005 mg/kg	0.05 mg	0.125 mg	0.25 mg	Lanoxin drops B.W. & Co. Stable, accurate dosage in infants and young children. Lanoxin PG tabs 0.625 mg
Frusemide	Oral	B.D. alt. days	5–10 mg		20 mg	40 mg	80 mg	Suspension is unstable. O.K. in hospital. No good in GP. Use Chlorthiazide
Clorthiazide	Oral	×1	125 mg Prems – 62.5 mg	125 mg	250 mg	500 mg	1000 mg	Better for use at home than Frusemide, as it is more stable
Tab Pot. Effervesc. B.P.C. 1 tab = 6.5 mmol/kg	Oral	×3	Dissolve 1 tab in 10 ml give 1 ml/kg	1 ml/kg	1 tab	2 tabs	4 tabs	Contains no chloride. Continued use may lead to hypochloraemic alkalosis
Propanolol	Oral or IV	×3	–	1 mg/kg	10 mg	20 mg	40 mg	Dose may be doubled IV in Fallots etc.
Allopurinol	Oral	×3	–	5 mg/kg	50 mg	100 mg	200 mg	To control iatrogenic gout from diuretics. Also in polycythaemia
Morphine sulphate	IM/SC	×3	0.15 mg/kg	0.2 mg/kg	2 mg	4 mg	8–15 mg	Avoid under 2 weeks and in premature
Methadone HCl Linctus	Oral	×4	Dilute linctus methadone BP 2 mg = 5 ml. 1 volume to 7 volumes of water		Children under 10 5 ml (0.25 mg) 4 hrly Children over 10 10 ml (0.5 mg) 4 hrly		5 ml = 2 mg of adult linctus	Linct. heroin is better. Useful in terminal care

be steered through adolescence into reasonably normal lives, and much cardiac invalidism can be prevented.

The severely handicapped child at home

Other chapters in this book will deal more adequately with this problem which is not peculiar to children with congenital heart disease. No one will disagree that where circumstances permit, these children, often in terminal heart failure, should be cared for at home. In dealing with this situation general practitioners will feel on much safer ground, as in most respects the problems are the same as those involved in managing patients in an older age group with cardiorespiratory failure due to emphysema, bronchitis, or heart failure.

The same drugs are used, the same iatrogenic problems occur; only the dosage is different, and I have included a chart of useful drugs for reference (Table 35.3). Note that the dosages in the table are in milligrams. Microgram dosages of digoxin are increasingly used for neonates, and everyone involved should ensure there is no confusion. A mistake can have fatal consequences.

These children are prone to acute chest infections, and need frequent help with antibiotics as well as digoxin, diuretics, and potassium supplements. Polycythaemic children even suffer from a high serum uric acid and may need allopurinol. A ready supply of oxygen with reserve cylinders is important; it can pose problems with over use by anxious parents. Often it is of little or no value, except to give the parents something to do in acute attacks of dyspnoea and cyanosis. The resources of the community nursing services and the social services need mobilising. A home teacher, and night attendance are important.

The lives of members of the family of a severely affected child are often very restricted. No holidays, the constant threat of death, the demands of healthy siblings, economic loss if mother cannot work. The stress falls particularly on the mother of the child, not only in the emotional sense but in sheer physical demand. No days off or nights off for mum; the most she can hope for is a split shift. Apart from mobilising nursing, social support and relatives, voluntary helpers should be sought to give her some relief. Those who wish to collect money and send the child abroad for unrealistic surgery should be encouraged to 'sit in' and give parents some time away together, and prevent breakdown of the marriage.

Admission to hospital for reassessment can usually be planned to coincide with a short holiday for the family. Paediatricians are always willing to do this in the summer months, when demand on paediatric beds is a little lighter.

REFERENCES

Batten, L.W. (1960) *The Medical Adviser*. The James McKenzie Lecture, RCGP. The Medical Recording Service Foundation (Ref. 60–25), Kitts Croft, Writtle, Chelmsford.

BMJ Editorial (1975) So-called innocent systolic murmurs. *British Medical Journal*, **1**, 229.

Campbell, M. (1965) Causes of malformation of the heart. *British Medical Journal*, **2**, 895.

Jordan, S.C. & Scott, O. (1981) *Heart Disease in Paediatrics*, 2nd edn. London: Butterworth.
Concise, readable, suitable compact reference book for general practitioners and trainees.

McKusick, V.A. (1964) A genetical view of cardio-vascular disease. The Lewis A. Conner Memorial Lecture. *Circulation*, **30**, 326.

Shinebourne, E.A. & Anderson, R.H. (1980) Current Paediatric Cardiology. Oxford: Oxford University Press.

36

Rheumatism and allied disorders

Tom Stewart

Few of these childhood conditions are seen more than rarely in the average general practitioner's working lifetime. However, as with all prolonged illness, the family doctor is the central figure in the therapeutic team, giving help, support and understanding to the young patient and his family. Although the hospital consultant will provide the specialist advice, the general practitioner needs to have a reasonable knowledge of the subject nonetheless.

RHEUMATIC FEVER (ACUTE RHEUMATISM)

Rheumatic fever is principally a disease of school age children, rare under the age of two years, and a first attack is very uncommon after the age of 40 years. Its importance lies in the ultimate outcome of the accompanying carditis. The incidence and mortality have fallen dramatically since the second world war, in large part due to reduced virulence of the group A beta-haemolytic streptococcus and the generally improved standard of living in Europe and North America. One series, in 1963, showed an incidence of between 0.8 and 4.5 cases per 1000 population, with no new cases seen in the last three years (Hodgkin, 1978). The death rate from chronic rheumatic heart disease has not fallen as markedly, however. Whereas environment plays a significant part, heredity does not appear to do so.

The disease is preceded by a streptococcal upper respiratory infection, which may pass unnoticed in up to 50 per cent of children. The latent period lasts from one to four weeks during which time an antibody-antigen reaction, particularly involving heart muscle, is set up. This results in the typical focal inflammatory reaction, the Aschoff node, found in the heart muscle, the pericardium, the heart valves and elsewhere. The damage to the valves is caused by subsequent necrosis and fibrosis.

The disease begins either insidiously or acutely with fever, malaise and joint pains. The pains are migratory, flitting from one joint to another but involving mainly knees, ankles, elbows and wrists. The joint signs may be minimal or they may be red, hot, swollen and very painful on movement. The degree of joint involvement gives no indication of the severity of the carditis.

In at least 70 per cent of children the heart is definitely involved. Signs of carditis include tachycardia, harsh systolic murmur, diastolic murmur, pericarditis, cardiomegaly and rheumatic nodules. These appear over the knuckles and extensor surfaces, are about five millimetres in diameter and are similar, histologically, to Aschoff nodes. Skin rashes similar to erythema multiforme may appear in about ten per cent of cases. Erythema nodosum is not a sign of the disease, however. In severe cases heart failure may ensue, although in children oedema may be absent. The failure at this acute stage is due not to valvular disease, but to myocarditis.

The commonest electrocardiographic change is prolongation of the P-R interval, as the earliest inflammatory changes take place in the region of the atrioventricular node. The laboratory findings include raised erythrocyte sedimentation rate, hypochromic anaemia, leucocytosis and, frequently, raised antistreptolysin 0 titre.

The disease must be differentiated from juvenile rheumatoid arthritis, acute septic arthritis, tuberculous arthritis, poliomyelitis, haemophiliac arthritis, acute leukaemia, congential heart disease and benign limb pains. Cardiac involvement rarely, if ever, occurs in these conditions.

Treatment consists of rest, salicylates and penicillin. Unnecessary restrictions should not be placed on the child in bed unless there is definite evidence of carditis and all but the severe cases may be cared for at home, provided the conditions and support are adequate. Salicylates probably do not prevent the onset of carditis or subsequent heart damage, but they do seem to reduce the rheumatic activity and relieve pain. Soluble aspirin should be used with care where there is obvious heart damage already, but otherwise in doses of about 120 mg/kg body weight per day. A lookout should be kept for signs of toxicity. Erythromycin, rather than tetracycline, should be given to penicillin sensitive children. Although the final outcome is not known, corticosteroids should be used for about four to six weeks in those children with definite carditis. Digoxin and diuretics are indicated if heart failure occurs. In general, drug treatment should continue until all rheumatic activity has ceased.

The risk of developing rheumatic fever after a streptococcal infection varies from nought to five per cent in the general population, but is ten times greater in those who have already had one attack. Recurrences are commoner in younger children, in the years immediately after an attack and in those with multiple attacks.

Prevention of the first attack is hardly practicable, but a ten day course of oral penicillin or erythromycin should nonetheless be given for an attack of proven streptococcal respiratory infection. Prevention of subsequent attacks should, ideally, involve taking a daily antibiotic until at least the age of 25 or so, but this may well not be acceptable to the teenager.

RHEUMATIC (SYDENHAM'S) CHOREA

The incidence of this condition may be 0.3 per 1000 population. It usually occurs about eight weeks after an attack of rheumatic fever or streptococcal sore throat and may last from four to 12 weeks and occasionally up to two years.

Rheumatic meningoencephalitis occurs clinically more commonly in the 10 to 15 year old age group and girls are more often affected. The condition is easily recognised by the typical rapid but essentially non-repetitive gestures, bizarre unilateral facial grimacing and the dinner fork shape at the wrist as a result of muscle hypotonia. Ataxia may be present in severe cases. The importance of the condition lies in the fact that rheumatic heart disease may develop later in the absence of other clinical manifestations of rheumatic fever. In addition, personality problems may present many years later, suggesting possible brain damage.

The erythrocyte sedimentation rate and antistreptolysin 0 titre may be normal.

Treatment consists of sedation, with bed rest in the early stages. Drug therapy should be continued as long as irritability persists. The danger of later heart disease makes the use of prophylactic penicillin or other antibiotic advisable for some years.

HENOCH-SCHONLEIN PURPURA

This condition was probably first described by William Heberden and is also known as anaphylactoid purpura. The cause is unknown but it is probably an allergic response, giving rise to widespread vasculitic disease, the commonest being thought by many to be to the toxin of the beta-haemolytic streptococcus. Others argue that the evidence is not clear-cut enough but that a wide variety of agents, including insect bites, may be responsible.

The characteristic rash affecting typically the lower legs, feet, buttocks and knees occurs usually between the ages of two and 15 years. It also may affect the arms and hands, but rarely the trunk. The initial papules are not unlike erythema multiforme but rapidly progress to become purpuric and may coalesce or vesiculate. Urticaria may appear elsewhere. The disease may be characterised by relapses and remissions, often presenting with abdominal symptoms consisting of pain, gastrointestinal bleeding or intussusception. In 60 to 70 per cent of cases there may be inflammation, usually without effusion, involving one or more joints. These pains do not migrate as in rheumatic fever and there is no permanent damage.

Almost half the affected children have renal involvement with haematuria and proteinuria. Permanent renal damage may be a feature, although this is less common in the younger child.

The erythrocyte sedimentation rate is raised, Hess's test may be positive, but the platelet count is normal and the antistreptolysin 0 titre may be raised in about 30 per cent of cases.

There is no proven effective treatment but salicylates, antihistamines and antibiotics are often used. Stronger analgesics may be needed for the occasionally distressingly severe abdominal pain. Corticosteroids should be tried in severe cases, but the results are usually disappointing. Rest in the early stages, if oedema is present, is indicated. Iron is recommended to correct any anaemia and surgery will be needed in some cases of intussusception.

JUVENILE RHEUMATOID ARTHRITIS

Although polyarthritis in childhood had been described some years before, it was not until 1897 that Sir George Frederick Still, whilst working as a registrar at Great Ormond Street, published his well known account of the disease. He postulated that it differed from adult rheumatoid arthritis in that lymph node enlargement and splenomegaly formed an invariable feature in children. Most clinicians nowadays believe that Still's disease is the juvenile form of rheumatoid arthritis.

Ansell's and Bywaters' is the definition generally accepted. They stipulate that:

1. the disease must begin before the age of 16 years
2. there should be inflammatory involvement of four or more joints for a minimum of three months
3. if less than four joints are involved biopsy of the

synovial membrane should show histological changes compatible with rheumatoid arthritis
4. other causes of arthritis should be excluded.

Little information concerning the incidence is available, but a figure of four cases per 1000 population has been quoted in the United States.

The aetiology is unknown and genetic factors play no role in the development of the disease. It starts more commonly between the ages of three and five years, is uncommon in the first year of life and the incidence rises to just before puberty. It is slightly more prevalent in girls.

The onset is usually abrupt and is characterised by a high and often swinging fever and generalised joint pains, although sometimes only one joint is affected at first. The polyarthritis then usually settles in the wrists, hands, knees, elbows and ankles which become painful and swollen with shiny overlying skin. The fingers may show characteristic spindling at the interphalangeal joints, whilst in some cases the cervical spine is affected. Joint involvement may be absent at the onset and this together with the monoarticular mode of onset may lead to difficulties in diagnosis. Considerable deformities due to bony growth disturbances and attendant muscle wasting may be seen and there is retardation of general physical development. These bony growth disturbances are a cardinal feature of the disease. Lymphadenopathy is present in all cases and splenomegaly occurs in many. Transient skin manifestations resembling erythema annulare are not uncommon.

The course of the condition is characterised either by relapses and remissions or, less commonly, by an inexorable advance to considerable deformity and growth retardation. At each relapse there is a recurrence of fever and malaise with joint swelling. After each relapse a little more joint disability remains. Contractures tend to form in those joints where effusions are less pronounced, although erosive changes are less common than in the adult variety of the disease. Other differences from the adult type include less evidence of ulnar deviation, more peripheral joint involvement and more frequent hip arthritis leading to eventual bony ankylosis.

Acute and chronic iridocyclitis are the most important complications, necessitating topical corticosteroids and expert ophthalmological supervision. Another not uncommon complication is percarditis which may come on insidiously or acutely. Other cardiac conditions are rarely seen. Subcutaneous nodules, pleural effusions and pneumonitis are sometimes found.

Laboratory investigations usually show a considerably raised neutrophil leucocyte count, a raised erythrocyte sedimentation rate and frequently a positive rheumatoid factor test. The antistreptolysin 0 titre remains normal. Antinuclear factor may be present in older children. Radiological changes include marked osteoporosis, banded rarefaction, premature fusion of the epiphyses, periosteal thickening and soft tissue swelling, compression fractures, and collapse of the cervical vertebrae; but erosions, except in the sacroiliac joints, are a rare feature.

The diagnosis is differentiated according to the way the disease presents. Where fever is the principal finding, meningitis and acute leukaemia should be excluded. When monoarticular arthritis is the main feature, osteochondritis, trauma, tuberculous or septic arthritis, gout or haemarthrosis should be eliminated as causes. When the presentation is that of a moderately ill child with a limp, the differential diagnosis should include synovitis, slipped epiphyses, osteomyelitis, bone tumours and bony deformities.

Management of the condition should involve supervision by the district nurse and the health visitor. Treatment consists of initial rest, relief of weight bearing joints, intermittent splinting of the smaller joints and gentle physiotherapy, but only if pain is absent. Drug treatment differs from that used in the adult variety of the disease in that salicylates should be used with caution in doses of 80–120 mg/kg body weight daily. D-penicillamine may be helpful in children with resistant disease but great care must be taken to monitor renal and bone marrow function and sensitivity reactions. Corticosteroids may be used if these measures fail but a careful watch must be kept for the development of further osteoporosis, growth retardation, Cushingoid features and overwhelming infection. Giving the drug on alternate days may reduce the incidence of some of these complications. The anti-malarials, phenacetin or phenylbutazone should not be used although other anti-inflammatory drugs, especially the newer ones in more palatable suspension form, may be tried. General measures to maintain the child's health, such as the correction of any anaemia and attention to diet, should be taken. Because the prognosis in juvenile rheumatoid arthritis is so much better than in the adult form, a more conservative approach to surgery should be adopted, although joint replacement has a place where destruction of weight bearing ones has occurred.

In some children the disease may persist for some years. The prognosis is better if the disease starts before the age of ten years, and significantly poorer if the age of onset is later and the active phase is prolonged.

ANKYLOSING SPONDYLITIS

Although primarily a disease of young adulthood and early middle age, ankylosing spondylitis may begin as early as five years of age. Males are more commonly affected.

In about half the children affected, the first sign may be peripheral joint involvement. The shoulders, hips, knees and ankles may be involved as well as the dorsilumbar spine and sacroiliac joints. Pain is often transient, asymmetrical, worse at night and relieved by movement. Unlike juvenile rheumatoid arthritis the lower spine is involved first. Interference with chest movements due to involvement of the thoracic spine occurs early in the disease. Rheumatoid nodules are usually absent, as are joint effusions, but malaise, fever, anorexia and growth retardation may occur. Loss of dorsilumbar spine mobility is a typical feature.

There are no specific laboratory findings. The erythrocyte sedimentation rate is raised, rheumatoid factor tests are usually negative and there may be anaemia. Characteristic changes in the sacroiliac joints and dorsilumbar vertebrae are seen radiologically. These may take several years to appear.

Treatment consists of pain relief, usually by soluble aspirin, and physiotherapy to maintain mobility, good chest movements and satisfactory posture. The disease may arrest at any stage or the entire spine may become progressively ankylosed with total loss of flexibility.

HAEMOPHILIAC ARTHRITIS

This disease tends to occur in severely affected children early in life. The usual pattern is of an acutely painful, hot, tender and swollen joint. The repeated episodes of intra-articular bleeding which can occur spontaneously or as a result of even minimal trauma are to blame and may eventually produce degenerative changes, osteoporosis, muscle atrophy and a fixed unusable joint.

Radiological changes include subchondral bone cyst formation, 'squaring' of the patella, epiphyseal changes and severe osteoporosis.

Treatment consists of stopping the bleeding as quickly as possible and immobilising the joint in the optimum position until this is achieved. Analgesics, but not aspirin or other drugs interfering with platelet function, should be given. Subsequently gentle mobilisation or traction may be used and corrective surgery may ultimately be needed, taking suitable precautions. These children will need to be admitted to hospital. Prevention of trauma should be an important aspect of care.

ACUTE LEUKAEMIA

This condition may present in a way similar to juvenile rheumatoid arthritis and should always be suspected in a child under five years of age who presents with fever and migratory joint pains with swelling. Secondary infection of joints in these children is common. Arthritis rarely occurs in chronic leukaemia. See further, Chapter 32.

SICKLE CELL DISEASE

This should be suspected in any black child presenting with aseptic necrosis of an epiphysis. See further, Chapter 32.

PROGRESSIVE SYSTEMIC SCLEROSIS (SCLERODERMA)

Although principally a disease of middle age, it can occur in childhood. It is characterised by diffuse sclerotic lesions of the skin, heart, muscle, gastrointestinal tract and kidneys. It may also occur in a localised form as morphoea, localised scleroderma and linear scleroderma. The prognosis in children is variable. Treatment is generally unsatisfactory.

DERMATOMYOSITIS

This rare disease is usually seen in the later decades of life, but may occur in childhood. It is an inflammatory condition affecting the skin, subcutaneous tissue and muscle. The symptoms include malaise, fever and muscle tenderness. A violaceous rash with erythema develops on the face followed by malar oedema. The muscles and skin become thickened and have a solid feel.

Corticosteroids are the treatment of choice, but few children respond dramatically. The prognosis is very poor; 50 per cent of children are dead within two years from cardiac failure, infection or gastrointestinal perforation. The prognosis improves slightly if the child survives the acute phase but the skin and muscles atrophy and contractures may develop.

POLYARTERITIS NODOSA

This disease is rare in childhood; the average practitioner may see only one adult case in 10 years. The lesions result from ischaemia due to vascular thrombosis and subsequent necrosis of the arterial walls, and may be widespread. Renal damage is common and lesions may occur in the skin, heart and major vessels.

Corticosteroids may be helpful and immunosuppressive agents have been used in adults. The disease is usually fatal.

DISSEMINATED LUPUS ERYTHEMATOSUS

The onset of this rare disease is gradual with a characteristic butterfly rash over the bridge of the nose and face, accompained by fever and joint pains. Polyarthritis, nephritis, pleurisy, peritonitis and pericarditis may occur. Central nervous system involvement may be dramatic.

The disease is recognised in the laboratory by the almost invariable presence of the LE cell in the blood and positive tests for antinuclear factor. Sensitivity to a specific drug may be a cause. Treatment is not altogether satisfactory and should consist of corticosteroids with or without azathioprine or other immunosuppressive drugs.

REFERENCES

Ansell, B.M. & Bywaters, E.G.L. (1959) Prognosis in Still's disease. *Bulletin on Rheumatic Diseases*, **9**, 189.

Boyle, A.J. & Buchanan, W.W. (1971) *Clinical Rheumatology*. Oxford: Blackwell Scientific.

Hodgkin, G.K.H. (1978) *Towards Earlier Diagnosis*, 4th edn. Edinburgh: Churchill Livingstone

Neale, A.V. (1964) Juvenile rheumatism: clinical, environmental, social, and nutritional factors in its epidemiology. In *The Advancement of Child Health*, pp. 123–152. London: Athlone Press.

Schaller, J.G., Wedgwood, R.J. & Wannamaker, L.W. (1979) Rheumatic Diseases of Childhood. In Vaughan V.C. III, McKay, R.J. jnr & Behrman, R.E. (eds) *Nelson Textbook of Paediatrics*, 11th edn, pp. 651–695. Philadelphia: Saunders.

Shanks, R.A. (1978) Collagen or connective tissue diseases. In Forfar, J.O. & Arneil, G.C. (eds) *Textbook of Paediatrics*, 2nd edn. Edinburgh: Churchill Livingstone.

Still, G.F. (1897) On a form of chronic joint disease in children. *Medico-chirurgical Transactions*, **80**, 47.

37

Asthma and bronchitis

Ian Gregg

INTRODUCTION

Asthma and bronchitis in childhood differ in several respects from the forms which they take in adults. Before discussing their aetiology and management in children, certain general aspects of the two conditions need to be considered.

Several problems arise in any discussion of asthma and bronchitis. There is still much ignorance over the pathogenesis of both conditions which is reflected in uncertainties concerning their management. Widely held preconceptions have been repeated in countless review articles and this sophistry has perpetuated notions which lack any scientific validity.

Much of our present confusion derives from an inability to define asthma or bronchitis with precision, while other terms whose use is unavoidable in discussion of their pathogenesis, notably allergy and infection, have also defied precise definition. Insistence upon the need to use terms with as great a degree of exactitude as possible is not the exercise of sheer pedantry which many regard it. An indiscriminate usage of terms engenders confusion of thought and misunderstanding in communication and also has important practical implications in clinical management and epidemiological research.

This chapter will concern itself with principles, rather than attempting to provide a description of those clinical features and aspects of management which should be sufficiently familiar to require no repetition here. Consideration of the problems inherent in defining asthma and bronchitis will proceed to an outline of what is known about their pathogenesis: only then will it be possible to discuss problems of diagnosis and management on a rational basis.

PROBLEMS OF DEFINITION

Aetiological factors

The most satisfactory way to define a disease is by reference to a specific causal factor which is readily identifiable. Thus, measles can be defined as an infection by the measles virus which uniquely is capable of causing the disease. Similarly, tuberculosis (despite the widely different forms in which it may present) is readily definable on the basis of infection by the tubercle bacillus.

It is now clear that many factors are capable of provoking those episodes of disordered breathing which clinicians denote by the term 'asthma'. However, none is common to every patient with asthma, while in many patients no causal factors whatever can be identified. Therefore, it is impossible to define asthma on an aetiological basis.

A similar situation obtains in the case of bronchitis. Though acute episodes are generally regarded as being of infective origin, non-infective agents can give rise to an identical condition. In chronic bronchitis of adulthood, several factors are believed to play a causal role in pathogenesis, yet none has been shown to be specific and thus capable of serving as a criterion for definition.

Histo-pathological criteria

Certain diseases can be defined by reference to a specific pathological reaction which characterises them. For instance, myeloid leukaemia and sarcoidosis are definable by haematological and histological criteria. No specific pathological criteria are characteristic of asthma or bronchitis (leaving aside the practical difficulties of identifying them in living patients), hence neither condition can be defined on a pathological basis.

Biochemical and hormonal abnormalities

Another means of defining a disease is by reference to over- or under-activity of an identifiable biochemical or hormonal factor. Phenylketonuria, vitamin B_{12} deficiency anaemia and hyperthyroidism are all readily definable on this basis. Although asthma is almost certainly a disorder of specific chemical mediators, not enough is yet known about these to provide a means of definition.

Descriptive definitions

Because of the problems enumerated above, it is only possible at present to define asthma and bronchitis in a descriptive manner. This has entailed the selection of a single characteristic which is invariably found in each condition. Unfortunately, those chosen to define asthma and bronchitis are not exclusive to them but occur in other respiratory disorders. The situation is analogous to that which would arise if hypothyroidism had to be defined by reference to one of its clinical features, all of which occur in other diseases.

MEANINGS OF TERMS

Asthma

Few diseases have proved to be so difficult to define as asthma (Gross, 1980). The definition which has received greatest acceptance is that proposed by Scadding (1963): 'a disease characterised by variable dyspnoea due to widespread narrowing of peripheral airways in the lungs and varying either spontaneously or as the result of treatment'.

Clearly, this definition could be applied either to *episodes* or to a *constitutional state*. The difference between these two senses of the term is evident from the following statements:

'The patient had asthma frequently during his childhood'
(i.e. episodes)
'Beta-blocking agents are contra-indicated in asthmatics'
(i.e. constitutional state)
'Asthma and allergy are frequently associated'
(i.e. episodes or constitutional state)

There is now general agreement that the cardinal criterion of asthma is variable obstruction to airflow in the bronchi. However, the application of this criterion immediately presents problems, since variable airflow obstruction occurs in certain clinical situations which are not generally regarded as asthma. Among the most common of these are episodes of 'wheezy bronchitis' in children who never wheeze except when they have a respiratory infection. Yet, if asthma is defined on the basis of variable airflow obstruction, there is no justification for making a distinction between it and wheezy bronchitis, since the underlying physiological disorder is common to them both.

While the definition of any disease does not necessarily prove to be equally satisfactory for both clinical practice and epidemiological purposes, lack of precision in the definition of asthma is responsible for problems which are of concern to clinicians and epidemiologists alike. Thus, estimates of its prevalence in childhood vary enormously, depending upon what position is adopted over its definition. For instance, the prevalence of 'typical' asthma in childhood has been reported by many studies to be between two and seven per cent, whereas studies which included children with recurrent 'wheezy bronchitis' have reported far higher figures, ranging from 15 to 20 per cent (Gregg, 1977a).

Bronchitis

Bronchitis literally means inflammation of the bronchi. The term is generally understood to imply an infective origin, but inflammation of the bronchi can be due to non-infective causes and, as will be seen, it is an important component of asthma.

It is usual to qualify the term bronchitis by the addition of the words 'acute', 'recurrent' or 'chronic'. This chapter will be concerned mainly with its acute and recurrent forms, since chronic bronchitis, in the sense that the term is applied to adults, rarely occurs in childhood. Nevertheless, inclusion of chronic bronchitis in this chapter is justified by the findings of recent studies which suggest that asthma and bronchitis in childhood may often be antecedents of chronic bronchitis in adulthood (Holland *et al*, 1969; Colley *et al*, 1973).

The CIBA Symposium (1959) defined chronic bronchitis as follows: ' a condition of subjects with chronic or recurrent excessive mucous secretion in the bronchial tree'. Thus, the clinical criterion chosen for defining chronic bronchitis is persistent or recurrent expectoration. Although this rarely occurs in children (and if it does, it should suggest the possibility of cystic fibrosis or bronchiectasis), persistent expectoration in adults is a common symptom of many other diseases besides chronic bronchitis.

Subsequently, the Medical Research Council (1965) suggested that chronic bronchitis, when it is accompanied by persistent airflow obstruction, should be termed chronic *obstructive* bronchitis.

Infection

Surprisingly, there is no generally accepted definition of infection. It is conventionally regarded as a clinical illness caused by a micro-organism. Yet it is clear that a micro-organism may cause detectable changes in a host without causing symptomatic illness, the term 'subclinical infection' often being used to describe this situation.

In this chapter the term 'infection' will be used in the following sense: 'the relationship of a micro-organism to its host which induces an identifiable reaction in the latter, regardless whether this is perceived as a clincial illness'.

Understandably, discussion of infection tends to focus attention upon the role of the micro-organism since this is the ultimate cause of the events which ensue. However, the host's defences are equally important in determining the outcome of infection, which can be conceived as a resultant of the interaction of the pathogenic properties of the micro-organism and the competence of the host's defences. If the latter confer complete protection, there will be no clinical evidence of infection, the only proof of its having occurred being a rise in the level of antibodies. If the host's defences fail to prevent replication of the micro-organism to the point at which it causes noxious effects, a clincially recognisable illness will occur. If the response of the host's defences is excessive, the clinical features of the illness may transcend those caused directly by the micro-organism.

Allergy

Few terms have given rise to so much confusion. Fundamentally, allergy is an abnormal immunological response to provocation by an antigen. Its essential nature is hypersensitivity but there is no clear distinction between this and 'normal' immunological mechanisms, including those which confer protection against infection.

The term allergy is often used, incorrectly, to denote one particular form of hypersensitivity whose basis is the excessive production of immunoglobulin E (IgE) antibody. This attaches to the surface of mast cells and, if it reacts with its specific antigen, it causes the cells to disrupt and to release various chemical mediators. This is the basis of the immediate flare and weal reaction of a positive skin test. When an antigen unites with IgE on the surfaces of mast cells in the bronchi, the mediators released give rise to muscle constriction or mucosal inflammation or both.

Hypersensitivity due to IgE antibody is termed type 1 or immediate and is the commonest form of allergy associated with disease, of which hay fever and other forms of allergic rhinitis are the most familiar clinical expressions. The term 'atopy' is used to describe a constitutional liability to develop type 1 hypersensitivity to common environmental antigens as a result of an ordinary degree of exposure to them. While many patients with asthma can be shown by skin tests to be atopic, it should not be concluded that the hypersensitivities which they display are necessarily the cause of their asthma.

Other forms of hypersensitivity, which do not depend upon mast cells or IgE, are known to cause disease but it is uncertain how important they are in the pathogenesis of asthma or bronchitis.

THE PATHOPHYSIOLOGICAL BASIS OF ASTHMA AND BRONCHITIS

Asthma

Direct knowledge of the changes in the bronchi which occur in asthma can be derived only from post-mortem findings. Clearly, these may be far from representative of the situation obtaining in less severe asthma. Our limited understanding of the pathophysiological changes occurring in acute attacks or in persistent asthma is based upon animal experiments, bronchoscopic findings and cytological examination of sputum or biopsy specimens. Another informative means of studying the behaviour of the bronchi is to observe their response to various forms of provocation and different pharmacological agents by measuring changes in airflow obstruction.

Two processes, occurring independently or in combination, are responsible for airflow obstruction in asthma. These are constriction of the smooth muscle in the bronchial walls and an inflammatory reaction in the bronchial mucosa, consisting of oedema and intraluminal exudation (which may eventually progress to 'plugging' within the airways). The relative contributions which muscle constriction and inflammation make to airflow obstruction in a given patient vary according to circumstances. As will be seen, the distinction between these two components is of cardinal importance in the management of asthma.

Bronchitis

The pathological features of acute bronchitis are an inflammatory reaction of the bronchial mucosa and hypersecretion of mucus. There are important structural and functional differences between large bronchi (which together with the larynx and trachea comprise the middle respiratory tract) and small bronchi and bronchioles. Inflammation in the larger airways (apart from croup) causes minimal obstruction to airflow, whereas in small airways it may cause considerable obstruction, this being the basis of 'wheezy bronchitis'.

In chronic bronchitis in adulthood there is hypertrophy and hyperplasia of mucus-secreting glands in the large airways and a proliferation of goblet cells throughout the respiratory tract as far as terminal bronchioles. However, these changes are not, per se, responsible for disability, this being due to structural damage or obliteration of small airways which causes permanent, irreversible airflow obstruction. That form of chronic bronchitis in which these abnormalities occur is denoted by the term 'chronic obstructive bronchitis'. In childhood similar changes occur in cystic fibrosis.

AIRFLOW OBSTRUCTION

As we have seen, variable airflow obstruction is the fundamental abnormality of function in asthma. It also occurs in acute bronchitis if inflammation extends into the smaller airways. In contrast, airflow obstruction in chronic obstructive bronchitis is irreversible, being caused by structural damage of the airways or (in emphysema) of the lung parenchyma.

In adults, asthma and chronic obstructive bronchitis commonly co-exist, in which case the obstruction will have both reversible and irreversible components. There are good reasons for believing that structural changes in the bronchi, leading to irreversible obstruction, occur in certain circumstances in patients with asthma, particularly if inflammation or plugging have persisted over a long period. This would explain the finding of irreversible obstruction in a small proportion of adolescents who have had severe, persistent asthma throughout their childhood.

Differentiation of reversible from irreversible obstruction is often far from easy, particularly when both components are present. The most important source of difficulty is the fact that reversible obstruction does not always respond to bronchodilator agents, a situation which can conveniently be denoted by the term 'refractory'.

The word 'bronchospasm' should be discarded since it suggests that muscle constriction is the principal or even the sole condition causing airflow obstruction in asthma. As we shall see, inflammatory changes are far more important in severe or life-threatening asthma. It is also undesirable to use this term to denote the findings elicited by auscultation, since it is impossible to distinguish between sounds generated by muscle constriction and those caused by inflammatory changes or irreversible obstruction.

Refractory obstruction

If airflow obstruction does not respond to a bronchodilator and there are grounds for believing it to be refractory rather than irreversible, the inference can be made that it is caused by mucosal inflammation which may have progressed to plugging.

Identification of refractory obstruction is of great importance in the management of asthma. Its implications with regard to the pathological processes responsible for it must be taken into account in deciding what measures are required for its relief.

Assessment and evaluation of airflow obstruction

The salient clincial manifestation of airflow obstruction, whether it be reversible or irreversible, is wheeze. However, both doctors and patients use this term in an indiscriminate manner to denote either what is perceived as abnormal respiration or the sounds which are caused by breathing through obstructed airways. Further confusion is apt to occur because often parents use the term to refer to the rattling sounds caused by excess mucus in the larger airways. It is preferable, therefore, to restrict the use of the term to describe the physical sign, elicited by auscultation, of a prolonged, high-pitched sound which is enhanced by forced expiration. A better term for denoting the symptom of disordered respiration in asthma is tightness of breathing.

The loudness or other characteristics of wheeze detected during ausculation are an unreliable and sometimes very misleading guide to severity of obstruction. Accurate assessment of the latter can be made only by instruments such as the Wright peak flow meter or the recently introduced Mini-Wright meter, both of which measure peak expiratory flow (PEF). This test can easily be performed by most children over the age of four or five years.

By observing whether and by how much PEF improves after inhaling a bronchodilator aerosol, it is possible to assess what proportion of the total obstruction is readily reversible. A small improvement suggests that any residual obstruction is refractory or irreversible. Proof of its being refractory depends upon the eventual return of PEF to normal, either spontaneously or after a course of corticosteroids.

CAUSAL FACTORS IN ASTHMA

It used to be conventional to classify asthma as allergic, infective or psychological. Such a classification may be permissible for denoting *episodes* of asthma but it is patently absurd to classify the disease itself in this manner. A large number of other factors are now recognised to be capable of provoking attacks and only rarely is a single factor responsible for every attack suffered by an individual.

Furthermore, this outmoded classification suggests that a given patient would never have asthma were it not for the operation of one or other of these factors. Since asthma occurs in only a minority of persons who are afflicted by allergy or psychological stress, and since it is a universal experience to suffer periodic respiratory infection, it is clear that none of these factors alone can be responsible for the constitutional state of asthma.

When considering the pathogenesis of asthma, three separate yet interdependent aspects must be distinguished (Gregg, 1977). These are: its *inception* – the establishment of a constitutional state in which the bronchi are liable to undergo narrowing, ie. the development of hyperreactivity: its *persistence* over the course of time: and its *provocation*, clinically expressed as episodic or continuous airflow obstruction.

Inception

It has long been recognised that asthma tends to run in families. Studies of the family histories of asthmatic patients have shown clearly that there is a strong genetic predisposition to the disease. Yet, the fact that there is not complete concordance for asthma in monozygotic twins (Edfors-Lubs, 1971) suggests that some as yet unidentified environmental factor is required to convert genetic predisposition into the constitutional state of asthma. Fortuitous encounter with such a factor would readily explain the large differences between patients in their age of onset of asthma. However, it is difficult to conceive of an environmental factor which did not affect simultaneously both of a pair of monozygotic twins. In one study of two pairs of discordant monozygotic twins, it was found that in each case the asthmatic twin had had a respiratory infection in early childhood which the other had escaped (Falliers *et al*, 1971).

It is well recognised that the prevalence of asthma and recurrent wheezy bronchitis is higher in boys than in girls. A recent genetic study has shown that there is no demonstrable genetic basis for this difference (Sibbald, 1980). Therefore, some other factor, which determines the inception of asthma or enhances the likelihood of its being provoked by enviromental stimuli, must act preferentially in boys. Many studies have shown that boys are more susceptible to respiratory infection and this might be the factor responsible for their higher incidence of wheezy bronchitis and asthma.

Respiratory syncytial (RS) virus commonly infects infants and young children and it has been postulated that bronchiolitis caused by this virus might be responsible for the inception of asthma. However, only a very small proportion of all children with asthma give a history of bronchiolitis in infancy. Although retrospective studies have found that about 50 per cent of infants who have had acute bronchiolitis subsequently develop a liability to wheeze and in about 25 per cent a diagnosis of asthma is eventually made (Rooney and Williams, 1971), this is not proof that bronchiolitis was responsible for the inception of asthma. An alternative interpretation might be that in certain infants who would have eventually developed asthma in any case, some defect of their host defences determined their susceptibility to bronchiolitis when they were infected by RS virus.

Epidemiological evidence suggests that the inception of asthma is influenced by some factor associated with modern, urbanised lifestyles. The prevalence of asthma is very low in isolated, primitive societies (Anderson, 1974; Gregg, 1977), but the adoption of Western living habits by migrants from such communities has been shown to lead to an increased incidence (Weinberg *et al*, 1977; Waite *et al*, 1980). There is also evidence which supports the impression of many clinicians in Western countries that the incidence of asthma has increased over the last quarter-century.

Several factors inherent in Westernised lifestyles have exerted a progressively greater influence over this time-span but have had, as yet, little impact upon primitive societies. Among these are a decline in breast-feeding, immunisation programmes in early childhood (which, particularly in the case of pertussis, may have other immunological effects than conferring protection) and the allegedly greater stress associated with modern, urbanised societies. However, there is a good deal of evidence against any of these having been responsible for an increased inception-rate of asthma.

One other factor has had a progressively greater influence in Western countries since the last World War. This is the use of additives in food as colouring agents or preservatives. Of the very large number used, tartrazine, benzoic acid and sulphur dioxide are well recognised to be capable of provoking acute airflow obstruction in certain asthmatics when taken in relatively high doses (Freedman, 1977). The underlying mechanism is not allergic hypersensitivity but direct interference of chemical mediators. It is possible that the chronic ingestion of additives in very small dosage might cause persistent asthma either directly or indirectly by rendering the bronchi hyperreactive to other provocative stimuli.

It is probable that other host factors than an inherited predisposition play an important role in the inception of asthma. It is well recognised that asthma and atopy are frequently associated, especially in children. The findings of a recent genetic study suggest that they are inherited independently but that an inherited predisposition to atopy enchances the probability that an inherited predisposition to asthma will become manifest clinically (Sibbald *et al*, 1980).

Persistence

The factors responsible for persistence of the constitutional state of asthma, once this has been established, are not understood, nor is it known what determines the tendency of many children to grow out of asthma. It is likely that the same factor(s) responsible for its inception continue to operate, thus maintaining and reinforcing hyperreactivity of the bronchi. In some patients an attack of asthma appears to enhance hyperreactivity for several weeks thereafter, thereby rendering them more susceptible to any provocative factor which they encounter. Hence, in such patients asthma can be conceived as a self-perpetuating condition.

Not only is there evidence that the incidence of asthma in Western countries has increased over the last twenty or thirty years, but many clinicians are convinced that it now occurs in a serious form more frequently than in the past. In Britain the rate of admissions to hospital in children with asthma more than doubled between the years 1958 and 1973 (Anderson, 1978).

The phenomenon of growing out of asthma must be due either to a cessation of the factor(s) responsible for its persistence or to the development of some protective mechanism. This is further discussed in a later section of this chapter.

Provocation

Until recently, concepts of the pathogenesis of asthma

have been based mainly upon observations of the circumstances under which acute attacks occur. The commonest factors recognised to provoke asthma are exposure to allergens, respiratory infection, emotional disturbance, physical exertion and certain drugs.

Allergy

Asthma occurring in an atopic subject is generally referred to as 'extrinsic'. Unfortunately, this term is often used to imply that every attack of asthma in an atopic subject is caused by type 1 hypersensitivity to an antigen. It is now known that in at least 15 per cent of normal children who have never had asthma nor any other atopic condition such as hay fever, skin tests will give unequivocally positive reactions to housedust mite or pollen (Horn and Gregg, 1973; Godfrey and Griffiths, 1976). Therefore, the term extrinsic should be restricted to those children in whom there is clear, circumstantial evidence of provocation by exposure to an antigen.

The most common antigens recognised to provoke asthma in children are the housedust mite and the dander of cats, horses and other fur-covered animals. In young children, hypersensitivity to grass pollen is a less frequent cause of asthma than of hay fever. It is noteworthy that the onset of hay fever commonly occurs at the same age as that when children tend to cease having asthma.

Recently, it has been shown that in some patients a single exposure to an antigen may be followed by a succession of nocturnal attacks over the course of the next few days (Davies *et al*, 1976; Siracusa *et al*, 1978). It is not known what is the mechanism responsible, nor in what proportion of adults or children it occurs, but clearly this phenomenon may make it difficult to identify a causal association between recurrent asthma and allergic provocation.

The association of atopy with asthma is commonly found in children, positive skin tests being given by about 90 per cent of asthmatic children (Horn and Gregg, 1973). In the remainder, who give wholly negative skin tests, asthma is termed 'intrinsic'. This form, which is relatively much more common in adults, tends to be persistent and usually is less amenable to treatment by bronchodilators than extrinsic asthma.

Infection

Acute viral infection of the smaller bronchi is a common cause of airflow obstruction, particularly during childhood. Such episodes are generally referred to as 'wheezy bronchitis' and they occur not only in children who are regarded as having asthma but also in other children, in whom wheeze is never observed except in association with respiratory infection.

Williams and McNicol (1969) have been foremost among those who believe that there is no justification for distinguishing between asthma and wheezy bronchitis. However, although the physiological disorder of airflow obstruction is common to both conditions, their own findings and those of the author and his colleagues (Gregg, 1975; Horn *et al*, 1979) suggest that children with unequivocal asthma (whether or not they have episodes of wheezy bronchitis) differ in several respects from children who have recurrent wheezy bronchitis but never wheeze under other circumstances. Chief of these are a higher prevalence of positive skin tests in children with asthma and their capacity to react to a wide variety of allergic and other stimuli, including exercise. However, it is impossible to draw a clear distinction between the two groups of children, since some children with recurrent wheezy bronchitis later develop the liability to wheeze when provoked by other factors besides infection and then come to be regarded as having asthma. The findings of a recent study of the genetic basis of asthma and wheezy bronchitis suggest that children with either condition share a common genetic defect (Sibbald *et al*, 1980b).

Other provocative factors

Psychological stress is widely believed to be a frequent and important provocative cause of attacks. Excitement, fear and other emotional reactions are undoubtedly capable of inducing acute airflow obstruction. Luparello *et al*, (1968) have shown that suggestion is capable of provoking asthmatic attacks in some patients. Nevertheless, the importance of psychological factors as a cause of asthma has been exaggerated. Of much greater importance are the psychological reactions which occur as a result of having asthma and these are discussed in a later section.

Physical exertion, particularly when this involves running or jumping, is a frequent cause of acute asthmatic reactions. For reasons which are not clear, swimming and cycling are much less prone to provoke these. Crying can induce asthma, probably by hyperventilation.

REMISSION OF ASTHMA

It is inconceivable that growing out of asthma is due merely to a cessation of exposure to provocative factors, since the likelihood of encountering antigens or viral infection persists throughout life. Therefore, it would seem more probable that prolonged remission is attributable to the development of some protective mechanism which prevents those environmental factors, which formerly provoked attacks, from still being able to do so. The fall in incidence of wheezy bronchitis with increasing age could be explained on this basis since, as children grow older, their host defences mature and they acquire a progressively wider immunity to the large number of species and serotypes of respiratory viruses (Gregg, 1975; Horn *et al*, 1979).

IS ASTHMA A SINGLE ENTITY?

The striking differences between patients in the form which their disease may take and in the factors which provoke it raise the question whether asthma is a single entity or a group of conditions sharing the common pathophysiological disorder of variable airflow obstruction.

The greatest contrasts are to be seen between the truly extrinsic and intrinsic forms. The former is typically episodic and attacks are generally easily reversed by bronchodilators; intrinsic asthma tends to be unremitting and airflow obstruction is refractory. The majority of patients have some features of both these polar extremes. Moreover, the expression of asthma in an individual patient does not necessarily conform to a consistent pattern but varies according to different circumstances and over the course of time.

Genetic studies suggest that predisposition to asthma (and wheezy bronchitis) depends upon a single inherited factor. However, the likelihood that it will be expressed and the clinical form it takes are determined by other inherited factors, particularly atopy (Sibbald *et al*, 1980a & b), and by environmental influences.

CAUSAL FACTORS IN ACUTE BRONCHITIS

Viral infection is the most common cause of acute bronchitis in children whether or not this is accompanied by wheeze. Primary or secondary bacterial infection is uncommon, except in children with pre-existing lung disease (notably cystic fibrosis and bronchiectasis).

Wheezy bronchitis

The typical course of events leading to an episode of wheezy bronchitis has been described by countless mothers as a 'cold which goes onto the chest' and within a day or so is followed by cough and wheezing. The accuracy of this observation has now been amply confirmed, many studies having shown that viral infection of the upper respiratory tract is usually the initial event in wheezy bronchitis (Horn *et al*, 1979). Rhinoviruses (Ch. 19) are numerically the most important agents associated with wheezy bronchitis (Gregg, 1969; Minor *et al*, 1974a; Horn *et al*, 1979), probably because of their large number of serotypes against which cross-immunity does not apparently occur (Minor *et al*, 1974b).

In the majority of children, of course, viral infection of the respiratory tract is not complicated by bronchitis, let alone by wheeze. It would seem that in some children with asthma and in those other children who wheeze only with infection, some defect of their host defences fails to prevent infection from extending into the lower respiratory tract. A study of sputum expectorated with the aid of physiotherapy during episodes of wheezy bronchitis has confirmed the presence of viral infection in the bronchi (Horn *et al*, 1979). Not only does the ensuing inflammatory response itself cause airflow obstruction but it probably gives rise to the release of mediators which cause muscle constriction and prolong the inflammatory response. A heightened degree of hyperreactivity usually persists beyond the time required by host defences to eliminate the infection (Gregg, 1975).

The role of secondary bacterial infection in wheezy bronchitis remains uncertain. No study has produced evidence that it occurs at all commonly even when antibiotics are withheld. However, this may be a reflection of the inexactitude of bacteriological techniques which may be unable to detect minor degrees of infection. It is possible that even a minor and undetectable degree of bacterial infection – particularly by *H. influenzae* – can cause some form of immunological reaction which enhances bronchial hyperreactivity.

GENERAL PRINCIPLES OF MANAGEMENT OF ASTHMA

The principal objective in the management of asthma is to relieve airflow obstruction: this must take priority over the attempt to counteract supposedly causal factors.

On the other hand, identification of causal factors and measures to counteract these are clearly important in prevention and long-term management. Intensity and frequency of exposure to allergens can be reduced to some extent by control of house dust and, where practicable, by avoidance of other allergens. By means of sodium cromoglycate it is possible to prevent asthma being provoked by allergens and also by exercise.

Anti-asthmatic therapy

The drugs available for the treatment of asthma can conveniently be classified as *palliative*, *preventive* or *suppressive*, although clearly there is some overlap between them.

Palliative

This category comprises bronchodilator agents whose action is to reduce existing airflow obstruction, principally by their relief of muscle constriction. There are three different types of bronchodilator – adrenoreceptor stimulants (sympathomimetic), derivatives of methylxathine which prevent the degradation of cyclic AMP, and anticholinergic agents (parasympatholytic). All have relatively short actions, lasting only a few hours.

Preventive
In children, sodium cromoglycate has proved to be of great value for preventing exercise-induced asthma and, when taken as maintenance therapy, for reducing the frequency and severity of attacks caused by exposure to antigens. Its mode of action is still not fully understood.

The only other form of preventive treatment is hyposensitisation (desensitisation), its object being to stimulate the production of blocking antibodies which prevent the contact of antigens with IgE attached to mast-cells.

Suppressive
Corticosteroids are the only treatment capable of suppressing persistent mucosal inflammation and plugging and hence of relieving refractory obstruction. There is little doubt that this is their principal action, but Shenfield *et al* (1975) have suggested that they also act by restoring the sensitivity of bronchial muscle to bronchodilators: even if this is the case, it is probably of relatively small importance.

Clinical assessment as a guide to treatment
Whatever treatment is prescribed, it should have a clear purpose. This can be decided only after careful assessment of a large number of factors. Questions that the GP should ask himself are listed in Table 37.1.

The most important items of assessment are the severity of airflow obstruction and its components. In younger children this has to be based entirely on clinical findings, but in children over the age of five years measurement of PEF is mandatory. Observed values of PEF should be compared with predicted normal values of children of corresponding height. Nomograms for this purpose, based on the findings of Godfrey *et al* (1970), are available from Clement Clarke International Ltd, Harlow, who manufacture the Mini-Wright meter.

In long term managment serial measurements of PEF are essential and the observed values should be compared with the highest value previously achieved by the child, making allowance for the increase in PEF which occurs with growth.

Table 37.1 Questions which should be asked in the clinical assessment of asthma

Present state	Is airflow obstruction present now? If so: how severe is it? how much is readily reversible? is there a refractory component? What circumstances are relevant to the child's present state? Is the child in danger?
Previous history	How frequently have attacks of asthma or wheezy bronchitis occurred in the past? How severe have they been? Have they caused much absence from school? Have they imposed restrictions on play, etc.?
Treatment	What treatment is the child currently receiving or been given previously? How successful has each treatment been? What treatment is appropriate in this particular child?
Long term considerations	Has obstruction persisted during periods of remission? If so: is it readily reversible? *or* is there a refractory component? *or* is there evidence of irreversible obstruction? Has the child's growth been affected by asthma or treatment? What is the child's emotional reaction to having asthma? How much do the parents understand about asthma and its treatment? How intelligent are the parents? Will they prove reliable in supervising treatment and co-operate in follow-up?

Assessment of immediate reversibility can be made by measuring PEF before and after inhalation of a bronchodilator aerosol. Isoprenaline, because of its rapid action, is the most convenient for this test, its effect being detectable within a minute and maximal after about five minutes.

The steps to be taken in assessment of airflow obstruction can be represented in the form of a decision tree (Fig. 37.1).

Education of parents and older children

It is all-important that parents and older children should have a clear understanding of the nature of asthma and the purpose, correct use and possible dangers of whatever treatment has been prescribed. Parents must be encouraged to share responsibility in management and they should know the indications for giving treatment on their own initiative. The better their understanding, the greater will be the benefits of treatment, while the liability to severe attacks will be reduced.

TREATMENT OF ACUTE ATTACKS OF ASTHMA AND WHEEZY BRONCHITIS

The steps to be taken in the management of acute attacks of asthma are shown as a decision tree in Figure 37.2.

The first essential is to assess the severity of obstruction. Assessment usually has to be based on clinical findings, since a GP is unlikely to have a peak flow meter if he is visiting a child at home while, in any case, the child may be too young to perform the test. Therefore, account must be taken of the duration of the attack, any treatment which has already been taken, respiratory and pulse rates, and the degree of impairment as shown by hyperinflation, the use of accessory muscles and indrawing of the intercostal spaces.

Bronchodilatation

The first measure is to give a bronchodilator. This alone may prove effective in relieving the attack. If it fails to do so, it can be inferred that the major cause of obstruction is inflammation or plugging and that other treatment will be required.

If the child has not already used a bronchodilator aerosol during the attack, the doctor should administer this treatment himself. If the child is seen in the practice premises and these are equipped with the means to nebulise a bronchodilator this treatment is generally more effective. Compressors, which rapidly nebulise a bronchodilator, are of great value for the emergency treatment of asthmatic attacks and they are available for a cost of about £40 to £90.

Of bronchodilators which can be given by injection, the choice lies between an adrenoreceptor stimulant and aminophylline. Adrenaline, given by subcutaneous in-

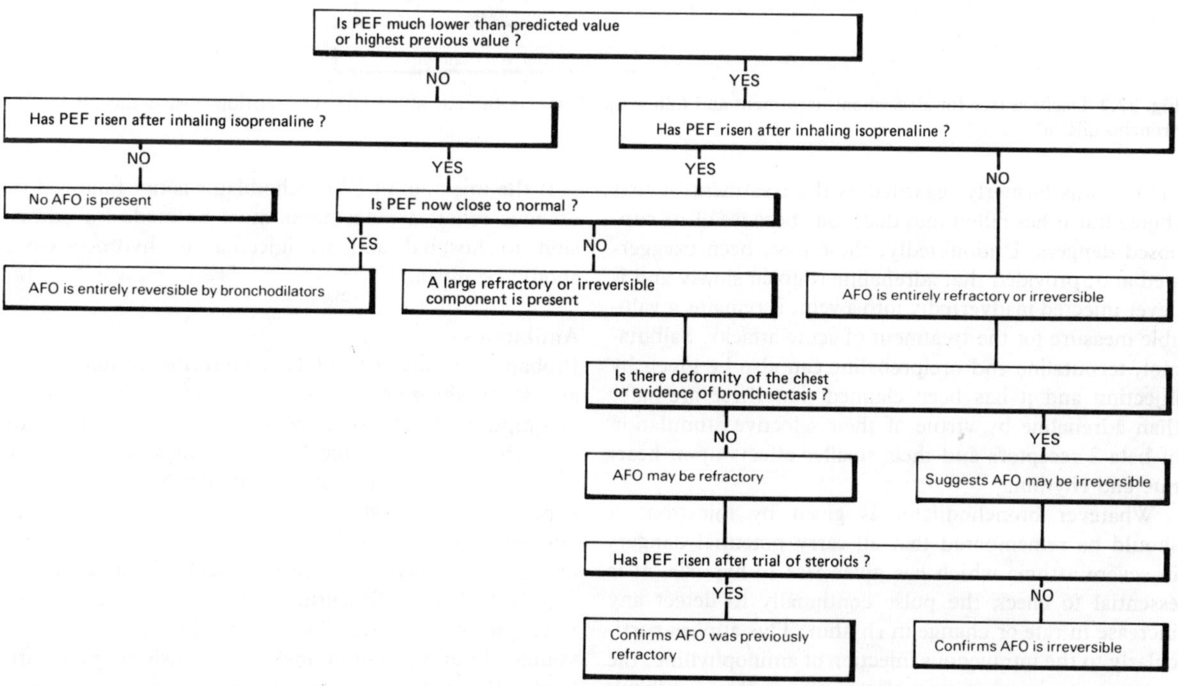

Fig. 37.1 Decision tree to be followed in the assessment of airflow obstruction (AFO = airflow obstruction)

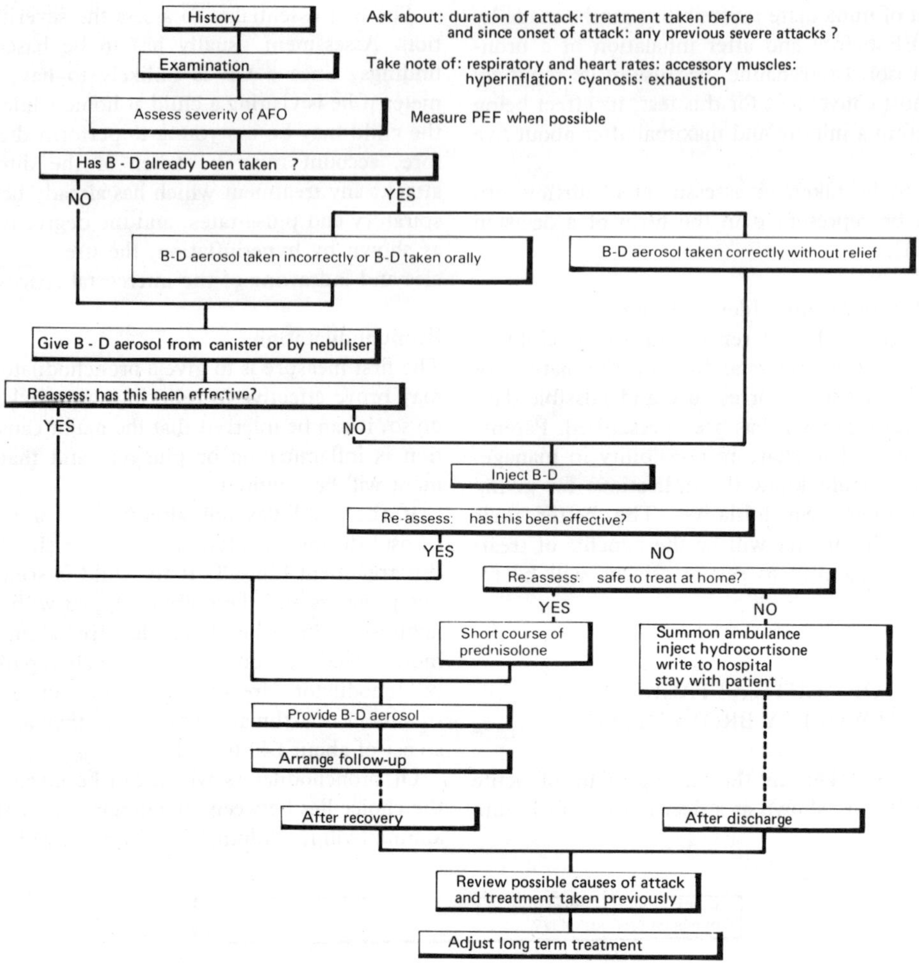

Fig. 37.2 Decision tree for assessment, treatment and follow up of acute asthmatic attacks (AFO = airflow obstruction, B-D = broncho-dilator)

jection, was formerly regarded as the treatment of first choice but it has fallen into disfavour because of its supposed dangers. Undoubtedly, these have been exaggerated and, provided that adrenaline is given slowly and is never injected inadvertedly into a vein, it remains a valuable measure for the treatment of acute attacks. Salbutamol, terbutaline and orciprenaline can also be given by injection and it has been claimed that these are safer than adrenaline by virtue of their selective stimulation of beta-2 receptors and their smaller effects upon heart rate and rhythm.

Whatever bronchodilator is given by injection, it should be remembered that all carry potential dangers in severe asthma which has given rise to hypoxia. It is essential to check the pulse continually to detect any increase in rate or change in rhythm. This applies particularly to the intravenous injection of aminophylline; the necessity to inject it very slowly makes this a difficult procedure in a restless and frightened child.

If the injection of a bronchodilator is not followed by obvious relief, arrangements must be made for admission to hospital and an injection of hydrocortisone should be given.

Antibiotics

Probably the majority of GPs prescribe antibiotics for attacks of wheezy bronchitis. This policy is based on the assumption that these episodes are analagous to acute exacerbations of chronic bronchitis in adults and that baterial infection, if not already present, is liable to supervene. Although, as we have seen, there is little evidence that secondary bacterial infection occurs at all commonly in wheezy bronchitis, it is understandable that the difficulties of diagnosis in general practice, particularly that of recognising pneumonia in young children, should make GPs wish to play safe. Certainly, such complications of bacterial infection as empyema and bronchiectasis occurred more frequently in the pre-antibiotic era than nowadays.

It is often argued that, even if antibiotics may be unnecessary, they do no harm. Although their safety record is so good, there are objections to prescribing them indiscriminately. Not only are there risks of sensitisation and promotion of resistant strains, but the automatic resort to antibiotics often leads to the neglect of other measures, of which the most important is relief of airflow obstruction.

Corticosteroids

In severe attacks of asthma and wheezy bronchitis, airflow obstruction is due mainly to inflammation. Steroids are the only form of treatment which is capable of suppressing this and thereby relieving refractory obstruction.

There is now general acceptance that steroids should be given in any severe attack which has not responded to a bronchodilator given in adequate dosage. This situation requires admission to hospital and, while awaiting the ambulance, an intravenous or intramuscular injection of hydrocortisone (200 mg) should be given.

In less severe attacks which the GP considers it warrantable to treat himself, the use of steroids is controversial. Many paediatricians regard their use in anything less than a life-threatening situation as unjustifiable. Although they seldom offer explicit reasons for such a view, it would appear to originate in the fear that, once a child has begun to take steroids, it may prove impossible to withdraw them and the child is then exposed to the risk of the well-known side effects of prolonged steroid therapy.

The widespread prejudice and fear surrounding the use of steroids in children, not only on the part of paediatricians but also the majority of GPs, has deprived many children of the only form of treatment which could have effectively relieved their attacks and, if given soon enough after their onset, even prevented them.

The introduction of steroid aerosols, which are not absorbed and therefore cause no systemic side-effects, has removed many of the fears of steroid therapy. A steroid aerosol is seldom effective as initial treatment of attacks of asthma, because airflow obstruction prevents its being inhaled sufficiently deeply. It can be substituted for a systemic steroid as soon as the latter has abolished refractory obstruction, generally within two to three days.

A course of prednisolone in a daily dose of 20–30 mg for three or four days causes negligible side-effects and it can be safely repeated several times a year. Recurrent attacks, resulting in considerable interference with schooling, should be treated pre-emptively with a short course of prednisolone, followed by a steroid aerosol as soon as the child can inhale it effectively. It is permissible to give intelligent parents a small supply of prednisolone and to instruct them how to give this on their own initiative at the first sign that their child has a cold which is 'going onto the chest'.

The author has used corticosteroids on many occasions to treat attacks of wheezy bronchitis. So far from having encountered any undesirable consequences, the duration of attacks has been greatly reduced and children have often been able to resume school within two or three days.

Although it is generally considered that steroids interfere with host resistance to infection, it is unnecessary to prescribe antibiotics concurrently, nor is there any evidence that the viral infection which provoked the attack in the first place is enhanced by steroids.

Physiotherapy

The value of a domiciliary physiotherapist attached to a practice for the management of acute attacks of asthma and wheezy bronchitis has been clearly shown (Horn, 1975), but unfortunately few practices have this facility. Therefore, mothers should be taught simple techniques of postural drainage and percussion to promote the clearance of mucus from the bronchi.

Review on recovery

Every severe attack in a patient already receiving treatment for asthma should be regarded as a failure of his or her previous medical care and it calls for a thorough review. Enquiry should be made about possible causative factors and assessment made of the appropriateness or otherwise of the treatment being taken before the attack. Decisions about future long term treatment should be made in the light of all the evidence. Instruction must also be given about measures to be taken at the first onset of any future attacks.

LONG TERM MANAGEMENT

Some children have only occasional attacks and merely require treatment on an *ad hoc* basis. It is often possible to identify the circumstances which provoke attacks and sometimes it is possible to avoid these – for instance, contact with animals. Children subject to exercise-induced asthma should take sodium cromoglycate a few minutes before games, which usually provides protection for at least an hour. A bronchodilator aerosol should be provided which parents can use for relieving occasional attacks provoked by exposure to allergens. The management of children whose attacks are provoked solely by infection has already been discussed.

The majority of children have frequent attacks over the course of several years and some are never entirely free of airflow obstruction. Measurement of PEF during

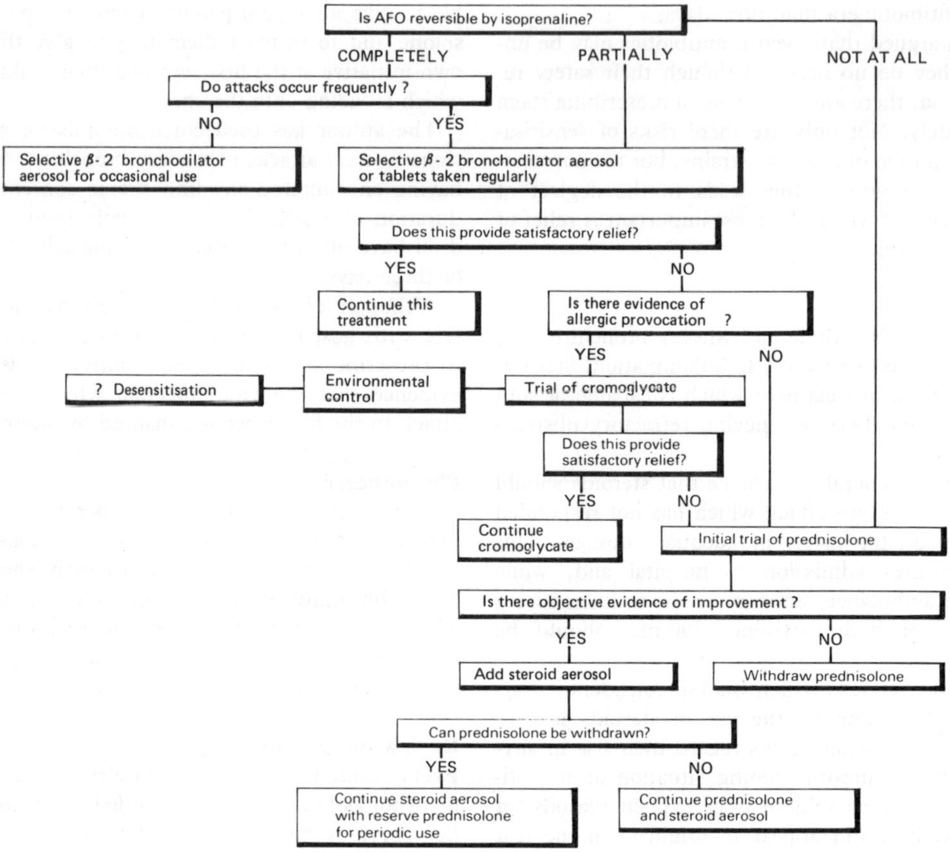

Fig. 37.3 Decision tree for the rational choice of drugs in the long term treatment of asthma (AFO = airflow obstruction)

remission, when wheeze may not be detectable, will identify persistent obstruction.

Children subject to frequent attacks require regular treatment. Its principal aim should be preventive, but because this is sometimes difficult to achieve, palliative treatment with a bronchodilator will be necessary from time to time. In a very small number of children, long term suppressive treatment with steroids is the only measure which can provide freedom from asthma.

The rational use of drugs for the long term management of asthma must be based on the findings at regular reassessment. The essential steps to be taken are illustrated in Figure 37.3.

Preventive treatment

Sodium cromoglycate is unquestionably the most valuable form of preventive treatment in children. The technique of inhalation can be learned by children as young as five years of age. Despite the reservations of some paediatricians, the combination of sodium cromoglycate with isoprenaline (Intal Compound) is of value in some children in preventing reflex bronchoconstriction. Its disadvantage lies in parents becoming confused by the immediate effect of isoprenaline and their consequently believing that the treatment is intended to relieve attacks rather than to provide regular protection.

Hyposensitisation against grass pollen may be effective in preventing asthma in children in whom this is caused solely by exposure to pollen (generally accompanied by symptoms of hay fever). Hyposensitisation against housedust mite may have a limited place in children who not only have a positive skin test to housedust mite but whose asthma appears to be provoked by exposure to it (Warner *et al*, 1978). However, in most children hyposensitisation against housedust mite has been disappointing.

Bronchodilators

In young children bronchodilators can be given only in syrup or tablet form. In older children there is the alternative of inhalation: this has the advantage of avoiding systemic side-effects, since the dose of drug required when it is delivered directly to the bronchi is far smaller than that which has to be taken orally and its speed of action is much greater.

Despite these advantages, many paediatricians condemn the use of inhaled bronchodilators by children. This stems from a fear that they may be used excessively and reflects the alarm caused by the increased mortality in children during the 1960s, for which bronchodilator aerosols were alleged to have been responsible. However, retrospective evidence suggests that the majority of deaths during that epidemic were due to asthma which had become refractory and were not directly caused by excessive dosage of bronchodilators. On this view, patients died *despite*, not because of, their usage of aerosols.

Bronchodilator aerosols can serve as a valuable index of impending danger. If a child needs to use his aerosol more than once in two to three hours and obtains less than his wonted relief, it signifies the development of refractory obstruction and this should be taken as a warning of a potentially dangerous situation. The parents and the child should understand that an increased frequency of taking the aerosol will be unavailing and they should seek medical advice. Had this information been imparted to all patients who were prescribed bronchodilator aerosols in the 1960s, many of the deaths which occurred then might have been avoided.

A new method of inhaling salbutamol has recently been introduced. Capsules, containing single doses of the drug in powder form, are used in a device (termed a Rotahaler) and inhaled in a manner similar to that of sodium cromoglycate. The more deliberate action required to load the rotahaler on each occasion reduces the risk of excessive use.

Sustained-release tablets of salbutamol or theophylline taken at night are valuable in preventing asthma during the early hours of the morning. This commonly occurs when asthma is not fully controlled, and in certain patients it is so pronounced that they have been termed 'morning dippers'.

Long term corticosteroids

If asthma cannot be prevented by sodium cromoglycate and bronchodilators are ineffective in providing more than transient relief, the most likely reason is the development of refractory obstruction. In this situation, corticosteroids must be considered, not only to enable the child to lead a normal life but also to prevent structural changes in the bronchi. These may occur if inflammation is allowed to persist, particularly if it has progressed to plugging.

Gillam *et al* (1970) and McNicol and Williams (1973) examined adolescents with a history of asthma and identified a small proportion who had chest deformity and persistent impairment of respiratory function. McNicol and Williams (1973) commented that often the existence of chronic, severe asthma in these children during their earlier childhood had not been recognised and, significantly, it appeared that the children had tended to make very little complaint. Radiological abnormalities, as well as impaired respiratory function, were found in children who had had severe chronic asthma by Simon *et al* (1973).

Before the introduction of steroid aerosols, the risk of side-effects from long term systemic steroids, of which the most serious are suppression of growth and adrenal function, had to be weighed against those of asthma itself. Apart from the possibility of permanent structural changes in the bronchi, persistent asthma causes suppression of growth and may also give rise to emotional disorder. This dilemma has largely been resolved by steroid aerosols.

Systemic effects are unlikely to occur when steroid aerosols are taken in the conventional dose (400 micrograms daily) or even in higher doses up to 1000 micrograms daily. Their principal limitation is that it is impossible to inhale them sufficiently deeply in the presence of severe obstruction (Gregg, 1975, 1980). Therefore, they are of little value for the treatment of an acute attack and a short, initial course of prednisolone should be given to reverse the obstruction: once this has been achieved, a steroid aerosol can be substituted. It must be appreciated that satisfactory maintenance treatment with a steroid aerosol may be interrupted by an episode of wheezy bronchitis, in which case the child will be temporarily deprived of any protection. In these circumstances, a short course of prednisolone should be given, as described in an earlier section.

In a very small number of children, maintenance treatment with a steroid aerosol is ineffective in suppressing asthma adequately and there is no alternative to long term treatment with prednisolone. Regular follow-up is mandatory and the situation should be continually reviewed with periodic attempts to replace prednisolone by a steroid aerosol. The maintenance dose of prednisolone must be kept at the lowest necessary to suppress asthma and this can only be achieved by serial measurements of PEF.

Systemic steroids given on alternate days are said to cause less suppression of growth and adrenal function than if given daily. Corticotrophin gel avoids the risk of adrenal suppression and it has been claimed to cause less suppression of growth. However, both the gel and the synthetic form of corticotrophin (tetracosactrin) occasionally cause severe reactions and even deaths have been reported. For long term treatment, therefore, prednisolone is to be preferred.

THE INTER-RELATIONSHIP OF THE GP AND HOSPITAL SERVICES

If the concept of primary care has any validity, asthma should be managed by GPs to a much greater extent than is the case at present. Not only should the GP be readily accessible for providing emergency treatment for the seemingly unpredictable attacks which are a characteristic feature of the disease, but it has been shown that preventive care by the GP can reduce the likelihood of their occurrence or at least minimise their severity (Gregg, 1968; Horn, 1975). However, this can only be achieved by continuity of care and education of patients (or parents) about the nature of asthma and the purpose, correct use and possible dangers of whatever treatment is prescribed for them (Gregg, 1977b).

The GP is better placed to provide both these elements of preventive care than an outpatients department or a chest clinic, where patients may see a succession of junior doctors often with little experience of asthma. However, there has been a clear trend for the hospital services to take over the treatment of acute attacks and there seems little doubt that they will increasingly adopt a primary care role in long term management also.

This has largely come about as a consequence of the alarm caused by the epidemic of deaths from asthma during the 1960s. Retrospective enquiries (Fraser *et al*, 1971), disclosed that in many deaths which were regarded as unexpected there had been a failure by patients or relatives and often their GPs to appreciate the seriousness of their attacks. Similar findings emerged from a survey of deaths occurring outside hospital (MacDonald *et al*, 1976).

The belief that a reduction in the present mortality rate from asthma (about 1000 deaths per annum) can be achieved only if every patient is seen without delay has led to the adoption by some hospitals of a self-admission or 'open door' policy. The experience of one such centre suggests that it has succeeded in the saving of lives (Crompton *et al*, 1979).

Those who advocate an extension of this policy will be encouraged by the findings of a recent survey of admission rates of children with asthma, aged 5 to 14 years, between 1970 and 1978 (Anderson *et al*, 1980). During this period admissions increased by 167 per cent but, of much greater significance and concern to GPs, there was a more than fivefold increase in self-referrals – that is, children who were taken directly to hospital without the mediation of their GPs.

These findings lead to the inescapable conclusion that the provision of emergency treatment by many GPs has been unsatisfactory. One can also infer that they reflect a generally poor standard of long term management. Unless the quality of care in general practice is greatly improved, the present trend towards the hospital services will continue and justification for it will come from the preferences of patients themselves.

MANAGEMENT OF PSYCHOLOGICAL ASPECTS

It is all-important that children with asthma should lead as normal lives as possible and every effort must be made to prevent them regarding themselves as invalids or inferior to other children whom they see enjoying activities in which they cannot themselves participate.

There is no doubt that acute attacks of asthma can be provoked by emotional stress. Some children learn to use their asthma as a form of attention-seeking and to manipulate their parents. Only if there are clear grounds for believing that a child or his family are emotionally disturbed should the opinion of a psychiatrist be sought. Unfortunately, the widely held notion of asthma being a psychosomatic disease has led many GPs to regard the majority of asthmatic children as being psychologically disturbed. This belief derives from impressions of a largely anecdotal nature: understandably, a few children who are disturbed are more readily called to mind than the far more numerous asthmatic children whose behaviour is normal.

The findings of several controlled surveys are inconsistent with the proposition that there is any specific association between asthma and psychological abnormality (Graham *et al*, 1967; Zealley *et al*, 1971). In severely asthmatic children, emotional disturbance is often present (McNicol *et al*, 1973) but the fact that its prevalence is similar to that in children with other forms of physical disablement, such as heart disease and orthopaedic conditions, suggests that it has arisen secondarily (Graham *et al*, 1967).

The GP's role is of vital importance in foreseeing and dealing with secondary psychological problems in asthmatic children. Many parents have a great fear of the disease and this is one reason why some doctors hesitate to use the term asthma. Yet, parents themselves often suspect that their child has asthma even though the doctor may never have mentioned it. Therefore, it seems a wiser policy to admit that a child has asthma but to reassure the parents that it need not prove to be the severe, incapacitating and frightening disease that they believe it to be.

A guardedly optimistic prognosis should be given of the likelihood of growing out of asthma and it should be stressed that the treatments now available are usually highly effective. Both the GP and the parents must instil confidence into the child and encourage him to take as full a part as possible in all normal activities.

Never should it be forgotten that the greater the GP's success in preventing asthma and of bringing its attacks under prompt control, the easier will be the child's and his parents' emotional adjustment to the disease.

REFERENCES

Anderson, H.R. (1974) The epidemiological and allergic features of asthma in the New Guinea Highlands. *Clinical Allergy*, **4**, 171.

Anderson, H.R. (1978) Increase in hospitalization for childhood asthma. *Archives of Disease in Childhood*, **53**, 295.

Anderson, H.R., Bailey, P. & West, S. (1980) Trends in the hospital care of acute childhood asthma, 1970–80: a regional study. *British Medical Journal*, **2**, 1191.

CIBA Foundation Guest Symposium (1959) Terminology, definitions and classification of chronic pulmonary emphysema and related conditions. *Thorax*, **14**, 286.

Colley, J.R.T., Douglas, J.W.B. & Reid, D.D. (1973) Respiratory disease in young adults: influence of early childhood lower respiratory tract illness, social class, air pollution and smoking. *British Medical Journal*, **3**, 195.

Crompton, G.K., Grant, I.W.B. & Bloomfield, P. (1979) Edinburgh emergency asthma admission service: report on 10 years experience. *British Medical Journal*, **2**, 1199.

Davies, R.J., Green, M. & Schofield, N.M. (1976). Recurrent nocturnal asthma after exposure to grain dust. *American Review of Respiratory Disease*, **114**, 1011.

Edford-Lubs, M.L. (1971). Allergy in 7000 twin pairs. *Acta Allergologica (Kbh)*, **26**, 249.

Falliers, C.J., Cardoso, R.R. de A., Bane, H.N., Coffey, R. & Middleton, E. (1971). Discordant allergic manifestations in monozygotic twins: genetic identity versus clinical, physiological and biochemical differences. *Journal of Allergy*, **47**, 207.

Fraser, P., Speizer, F.E., Doll, R., Waters, S.D.M. & Mann, N.M. (1971). The circumstances preceding deaths from asthma in young people in 1968–69. *British Journal of Diseases of the Chest*, **65**, 71.

Freedman, B.J. (1977). Asthma induced by sulphur dioxide, benzoate and tartrazine contained in orange drinks. *Clinical Allergy*, **7**, 407.

Gillam, G.L., McNicol, K.N. & Williams, H.E. (1970). Chest deformity, residual airway obstruction and hyperinflation, and growth in children with asthma. II: Significance of chronic chest deformity. *Archives of Disease in Childhood*, **45**, 789.

Godfrey, R.C. & Griffiths, N. (1976). The prevalence of immediate positive skin tests to Dermatophagoides pteronyssinus and grass pollen in school children. *Clinical Allergy*, **6**, 55.

Godfrey, S. (1977). Exercise-induced asthma. In Clark, T.J.H. & Godfrey S. (eds) *Asthma*, ch. 3, p. 56. London: Chapman and Hall.

Godfrey, S. Kamburoff, P.L. & Nairn, J.B. (1970). Spirometry, lung volumes and airway resistance in normal children aged 5–18 years. *British Journal of Diseases of the Chest*, **64**, 15.

Graham, P.J., Rutter, M.L., Yule, W. & Pless, I.B. (1967). Childhood asthma: a psychosomatic disorder? Some epidemiological considerations. *British Journal of Preventive and Social Medicine*, **21**, 78.

Gregg, I. (1968). Longterm corticosteroid treatment of asthma. *British Medical Journal*, **2**, 175.

Gregg, I. (1969). A study of recurrent bronchitis in childhood. *Respiration*, **27**, (Suppl). 133.

Gregg, I. (1975a). The role of viral infection in asthma and bronchitis. In Proudfoot, A.T. (ed.) *Symposium on Viral Disease* p. 82. Royal College of Physicians of Edinburgh.

Gregg, I (1975b). The place of beclomethasone dipropionate aerosol in the treatment of asthma. *Drugs*, **10**, 161.

Gregg, I. (1977a). Epidemiology. In Clark, T.J.H. & Godfrey, S. (eds) *Asthma*, ch. 11, p. 214. London: Chapman and Hall.

Gregg, I. (1977b). The role of the family doctor in management. In Clark, T.J.H. & Godfrey, S. (eds) *Asthma*, ch. 19, p. 395. London: Chapman and Hall.

Gregg, I. (1980). The importance of patient education in the use of inhaled steroids. Chapter 11 in 'Topical steroid treatment for asthma and rhinitis'. p. 137 Edited by N. Mygind and T.J.H. Clark. London: Ballière-Tindall.

Gross, N.J. (1980). What is this thing called love? – or, defining asthma. *American Review of Respiratory Disease*, **121**, 203.

Holland, W.W., Halil, T., Bennett, A.E. & Elliott, A. (1969). Factors influencing the onset of chronic respiratory disease. *British Medical Journal*, **2**, 205.

Horn, M.E.C. (1975). An asthma and bronchitis clinic for children in a general practice. *Update*, **1**, 759.

Horn, M.E.C. and Gregg, I. (1973) The role of viral infection and host factors in asthma and chronic bronchitis. *Chest*, *32*, *suppl*. **4**, 44.

Horn, M.E.C., Brain, E.A., Gregg, I., Inglis, J.M., Yealland, S.J. & Taylor, P. (1979). Respiratory viral infection and wheezy bronchitis in childhood, *Thorax*, **34**, 23.

Horn, M.E.C., Reed, S.E. & Taylor, P. (1979). Role of viruses and bacteria in acute wheezy bronchitis in childhood: a study of sputum. *Archives of Disease in Childhood*, **54**, 587.

Luparello, T., Lyons, H.A., Bleecker, E.R. & McFadden, E.R. (1968). Influences of suggestion on airway reactivity in asthmatic subjects. *Psychosomatic Medicine*, **30**, 819.

Macdonald, J.B., Seaton, A. & Williams, D.A. (1976). Asthma deaths in Cardiff 1963–74: 90 deaths outside hospital. *British Medical Journal*, **1**, 1493.

McNicol, K.N. & Williams, H.E. (1973a). Spectrum of asthma in children I: Clinical and physiological components. *British Medical Journal*, **4**, 7.

McNicol, K.N., Williams, H.E., Allan, J. & McAndrew, I. (1973b). Spectrum of asthma in children III: psychological and social components. *British Medical Journal*, **4**, 16.

Medical Research Council (1965). Definition and classification of chronic bronchitis for clinical and epidemiological purposes. *Lancet*, **1**, 775.

Minor, T.E., Dick, E.C., De Meo, A.N., Ouellette, J.J., Cohen, M. & Reed, C.E. (1974a). Viruses as precipitants of asthmatic attacks in children. *Journal of the American Medical Association*, **227**, 292.

Minor, T.E., Dick, E.C., Peterson, J.A. & Docherty, D.E. (1974b). Failure of naturally acquired rhinovirus infections to produce temporal immunity to heterologous serotypes. *Infection and Immunity*, **10**, 1192.

Rooney, J.C. & Williams, H.E. (1971). The relationship between proved viral bronchiolitis and subsequent wheezing. *Journal of Pediatrics*, **79**, 744.

Scadding, J.G. (1963). Meaning of diagnostic terms in broncho-pulmonary disease. *British Medical Journal* **2**, 1425.

Shenfield, G.M., Hodson, M.E., Clarke, S.W. & Paterson, J.W. (1975). Interaction of corticosteroids and catecholamines in the treatment of asthma. *Thorax*, **30**, 430.

Sibbald, B. (1980). Genetic basis of sex differences in the prevalence of asthma. *British Journal of Diseases of the Chest*. **74**, 93.

Sibbald, B., Horn, M.E.C., Brain, E.A. & Gregg, I. (1980a) Genetic factors in childhood asthma. *Thorax*, **35**, 671.

Sibbald, B., Horn, M.E.C. & Gregg, I. (1980b). A family study of the genetic basis of asthma and wheezy bronchitis. *Archives of Disease in Childhood*, **55**, 354.

Simon, G., Connolly, N., Littlejohn, D.W. & McAllen, M. (1973). Radiological abnormalities in children with asthma and their relation to the clinical findings and some respiratory function tests. *Thorax*, **28**, 115.

Siracusia, A., Curradi, F. & Abbitti, G. (1978). Recurrent nocturnal asthma due to tolylene di-isocyanate: a case report. *Clinical Allergy*, **8**, 195.

Waite, D.A., Eyles, E.F., Tonkin, S.L. & O'Donnell, T.V. (1980). Asthma prevalence in Tokelauan children in two environments. *Clinical Allergy*, **10**, 71.

Warner, J.O., Price, J.F., Soothill, J.F. & Hey, E.N. (1978). Controlled trial of hyposensitisation to Dermatophagoides pteronyssinus in children with asthma. *Lancet*, **2**, 912.

Weinberg, E.G., Van Niekerk, C.H., Shore, S.C., Heese, H. De V. & Van Schalkwyk, D. (1977). Prevalence of asthma. *Lancet*, **2**, 500.

Williams, H.E & McNicol, K.N. (1969). Prevalence, natural history and relationship of wheezy bronchitis and asthma in children: an epidemiological study. *British Medical Journal*, **4**, 321.

Zealley, A.K., Aitken, R.C.B. & Rosenthal, S.V. (1971). Asthma: a psycho-physiological investigation. *Proceedings of Royal Society of Medicine*, **64**, 825.

Diabetes in childhood

Robert Russell

Diabetes is uncommon in childhood, with a prevalence in the general population of only about 0.2–0.4 per 1000, so that the list of the average general practitioner is likely to include no more than one diabetic under the age of sixteen years. Although it is desirable and most likely that the patient's treatment and management will be supervised at a special hospital clinic, the family doctor will from time to time be called upon to advise on problems which occur, and to treat the patients during acute crises.

The maximum incidence of diabetes in childhood occurs at or shortly before puberty, between eleven and thirteen years; it is rare under five years and exceedingly rare in the first year of life, the sex incidence being approximately equal. The diabetic child does not differ appreciably in mental and physical development from his non-diabetic fellows. However a study of the adult height of 35 young identical twin pairs, of whom one or both had diabetes, shows that of twelve pairs in which one twin developed diabetes before puberty and the other did not, the affected twin was shorter (Tattersall and Pyke, 1973). When both twins developed diabetes or one twin developed diabetes after puberty and the other did not, then there was no significant difference in height.

AETIOLOGY AND EPIDEMIOLOGY

Genetic factors have long been considered important in the aetiology of diabetes, though their mechanisms are ill understood. In a study of 1307 diabetics, 21 per cent were found to have a first degree relative with diabetes, compared with 7.5 per cent among 859 non-diabetic controls (College of General Practitioners, 1965). The difference was much greater in early life than later. Available evidence indicates that genetic factors are significant in the development of diabetes of juvenile onset type in the young, but not nearly as significant in its development in later life. A positive family history is found in 30 to 40 per cent of diabetic patients in Britain, the higher figure being in the young. An epidemiological study of new cases of juvenile diabetes notified to the British Diabetic Association is being undertaken (Gamble, 1974; Bloom, Hayes and Gamble, 1975). A questionnaire providing evidence of social class, family size and age structure, area of residence, urban/rural differences, race, and month of birth is being collected from the same patients, as these are all variable factors which have an influence on the incidence of infectious disease. This has made apparent the seasonal incidence of juvenile onset diabetes, the onset of the disease being commoner during the late autumn and winter than in the summer.

A highly significant excess of diabetics with antibody to Coxsackie B4 virus was found, when compared with controls (Gamble *et al*, 1973). This excess was confined to diabetes in the 10–19 years age group and was not found in the younger patients. Information gained by postal questionnaire of family doctors regarding illnesses in the six months prior to the diagnosis of diabetes in 1663 children showed a significant excess of consultations for mumps, the greatest excess being in the month before onset (Gamble, 1980).

Recent findings of antibodies to islet cells (ICAs) in 60 to 80 per cent of newly diagnosed insulin dependent diabetics have been made. Their greater incidence and longer persistence in patients with other endocrine diseases has been found to be associated with a high incidence of phenotype HLA B8, giving rise to speculation on the possibility of an autoimmune type of diabetes (Bottazza *et al*, 1978).

Histocompatibility antigens of the HLA (Human Lymphocyte Antigen) system are located on chromosome 6 at four major gene subloci (HLA A, B, C and D). Associations between certain genotypes and various medical disorders have been found. The phenotypes B8, Bw15, Dw3 and Dw4 are particularly associated with the incidence of insulin dependent diabetes, but the disease does occur with other phenotypes also. Identical HLA bearing chromosomes (No 6), are inherited by juvenile onset insulin dependent diabetics to a significant degree in families where more than one member suffers from that disease. This is interpreted as showing that some individuals have a genetic predisposition to the disease which may be demonstrated by typing HLAs on the 6th chromosome, (Nerup, 1974). The addition of an evironmental factor, such as a virus infection, in such an individual, may precipitate the overt disease.

CLINICAL PICTURE

The onset of diabetes in the young is usually, but by no means always, acute and the symptoms are severe. Some or all of the classical symptoms of diabetes, thirst, polyuria (sometimes with a return of nocturnal enuresis), pruritus vulvae or balanitis, loss of weight, lassitude and malaise may be present. These symptoms may be accompanied by an acute infection, commonly respiratory. Duration of symptoms at diagnosis is usually only a few weeks (Malins, 1970), but this is by no means invariable and the child may give a history of several months duration; sometimes a single symptom, such as loss of weight or a return of nocturnal enuresis, may be the only one presented. A few patients will present in ketoacidosis or precoma.

The only notable physical sign which is commonly present at diagnosis is that the child is usually underweight for age and height, and may show some signs of wasting. Slight to moderate hepatomegaly is frequently present but responds to control of the diabetes (White, 1960). The signs of acidosis—flushed face, hyperpnoea and smell of acetone in the breath, together with those of dehydration—dry tongue and loss of skin elasticity, will be added if severe ketosis is present. The differential diagnosis of severe infection, such as pneumonia, gastroenteritis or of the acute abdominal emergency will occasionally arise in the very young and if severe ketoacidosis is present. The demonstration of glycosuria and of hyperglycaemia will establish the diagnosis of diabetes. Urine testing will frequently reveal mild ketonuria, and if ketoacidosis is present slight proteinuria, both disappearing rapidly after treatment of the diabetes. Complications of diabetes are seldom present at diagnosis in the diabetic child.

TREATMENT

One must aim for control of the diabetes within the framework of a full and active life, both socially and educationally, together with normal growth and development. Control of the diabetes is primarily the prevention of ketoacidosis and the relief of symptoms, without provoking frequent or severe attacks of hypoglycaemia. There is of necessity considerable compromise in the treatment, as rigid control of diet in particular is likely to cause resentment and precipitate emotional stresses between parent and child. Since the peak incidence of childhood diabetes coincides with early puberty, these problems, if allowed to develop, may be considerable. Unrestricted freedom however, commonly leads to inadequate control and the danger of severe ketoacidosis with frequent hospital admission and its attendant emotional trauma.

It has in the past been impossible to produce any satisfactory evidence that good biochemical control of diabetes had any influence on the incidence of the microvascular complications, retinopathy, neuropathy and nephropathy in diabetics, or of the peripheral vascular and cardiovascular disease to which many of these young diabetics will eventually succumb. In recent years evidence that poor control does contribute toward microvascular complications has been provided. A retrospective Belgian study (Pirart, 1977), following 4398 diabetics over 25 years demonstrated that the only factor which correlated with the development of microangiopathy was the duration and severity of hyperglycaemia, and that increasing hyperglycaemia was associated with a high frequency of severe and progressive forms of diabetic retinopathy.

A prospective trial comparing the effect of single daily injections of a long acting insulin with multiple injections of shorter acting insulins, showed that those patients receiving multiple injections had better biochemical control and developed fewer retinal microaneurysms over a four year period (Tchobroutsky, 1978).

Almost all children with diabetes need insulin from diagnosis onwards. There are a few children whose diabetes is initially mild and in whom the diagnosis is established very early, perhaps by a diabetic relative, who are able to be controlled initially on diet only, or diet plus some form of oral treatment. However these patients are few and far between and need insulin treatment before many weeks or months have elapsed.

Opinions vary upon whether the patient should be admitted to hospital or attend frequently as an outpatient to achieve initial control of his diabetes. Those who favour hospital admission for all cases maintain that the child can be educated intensively in diet, injection technique, urine testing etc., and experience hypoglycaemia while being kept physically active in the ward under observation for only a few days. Others favour most of their patients being controlled at home in their customary environment, with frequent outpatient attendances for assessment, advice, and adjustment of diet and dosage, together with home visits by clinic health visitors to give support and advice, the district nurse administering the insulin until the patient has been taught to inject himself. There are no doubt convincing arguments to support both schools; my own experience is of outpatient control except when the severity of symptoms or presence of ketoacidosis necessitate admission.

Diet

The cornerstone of all diabetic treatment is diet. Requirements for normal physical development must be borne in mind when advising the child and his parents, particularly during the growing period. There must therefore be an adequate calorie, protein and vitamin content in the prescribed diet. It is customary to allow unrestricted protein and fat, with a controlled quantity of carbohydrate. Only if the child is unduly obese is fat restricted. During childhood, dietary control must be fairly flexible because of variations in the requirements due to growth and widely varying patterns of physical activity.

Carbohydrate is prescribed in 10 g. portions, it being more satisfactory to assess these portions or to use household measures than to weigh them.

Diabetes in the first year of life is treated with the usual babies diet, together with one or two doses of insulin daily. Between one and five years of age the dietary carbohydrate content is increased gradually from about 120 g to 150 g daily, and the increase is continued up to about 250 g daily by the time of onset of physical maturity (Oakley *et al*, 1968). After adolescence it is often possible to reduce the daily carbohydrate to below 200 g.

After infancy the carbohydrate intake is apportioned over the day with the major allowance at the three main meals and smaller buffers between meals and before bedtime to minimise the risk of hypoglycaemic attacks before meals and during the night. A diet containing 150 g of carbohydrate could be divided into three 40 g portions at breakfast, lunch and tea, leaving three 10 g portions to be taken mid-morning, mid-afternoon and at bedtime. A larger mid-morning snack is usually necessary if a short acting insulin is given before breakfast, and similarly a larger bedtime snack would be necessary with a long acting insulin given before breakfast or a shorter acting insulin given before tea. It may sometimes be necessary to wake the child during the late evening to have a snack of milk and biscuits, to avoid hypoglycaemic attacks before morning. School meals are on the whole acceptable, though it is probably more satisfactory if the child is able to return home for meals, particularly in the earlier school years. Additional carbohydrate must be taken before games are played or any unusually vigorous exercise taken; 20 g of carbohydrate is a suitable quantity but sometimes this may need to be considerably exceeded.

The child's diet must be varied as much as possible to avoid boredom and likelihood of rebellion; similarly if the child has a large appetite, then his hunger must be satisfied. It is important that the diabetic child's diet should not differ appreciably from the rest of the family, and his meals need not differ very much in composition, though usually the carbohydrate content will be necessarily less. Most children miss sweets and some concentrated carbohydrate foods to which they have been used, and will resent not having them. Ice cream as part of their diet may be allowed occasionally, though puddings should be avoided if possible, and cheese or fresh fruit substituted. This enables school meals to be satisfactory, providing the co-operation of teaching and catering staff are sought and obtained.

Children should be encouraged to eat, and parents to provide, wholemeal bread instead of white bread, and regular high fibre vegetables in the diet. Guar gum containing foods are not widely obtainable and are unpalatable. These foods tend to moderate the post prandial glucose peaks which occur.

Foods suitable for diabetics such as specially prepared jams, sweets and chocolates are available; it is better however to reserve these for special occasions, rather than to allow unrestricted use.

If the child should suffer a gastrointestinal upset or intercurrent illness accompanied by vomiting, the necessary carbohydrate may be provided in liquid form. Ribena (10 g in 15 ml), or Lucozade (10 g in 60 ml), are well known porprietary preparations which are well tolerated. Both are rapidly absorbed and their glucose content is rapidly available, so that to give small quantities frequently, for example 20 g every two hours, is a suitable method of administration.

Adolescents in particular frequently resent dietary restrictions, and their co-operation and trust must be gained if success in their management is to be achieved. They must be persuaded that regularity of diet is most important and that it is possible for them to lead a full, active, and useful life while still observing this.

Oral drugs

In a very few children the diabetes may at first be mild, and satisfactory control is obtained with the administration of sulphonylurea drugs. This state of affairs however does not persist for long and treatment with insulin becomes necessary. The biguanide drugs (phenformin and metformin) have been used in some patients in conjunction with insulin when variations in blood sugar levels have been wide, in the hope of achieving less variable control and perhaps reducing insulin dosage. Result however have not been encouraging and gastrointestinal upset with these drugs is common. The occurrence of lactic acidosis with phenformin therapy is a strong contraindication to its use.

Insulin

The vast majority of diabetic children require treatment with insulin from diagnosis for the rest of their lives.

In infancy the insulin requirement is seldom above four to eight units daily, rising in young children to 24 units or more (Oakley *et al*, 1973). Thereafter the dose continues to rise until puberty when 60 to 100 units daily is the usual requirement. As the dose increases it is necessary to increase the number of injections from one to two, the first injection continuing to be given before breakfast and the second being introduced before tea. Parents should be warned of the necessity for twice daily injections some time before they are commenced, usually between 10 and 12 years.

With the introduction during the past four years of new highly purified insulins there are now 24 insulin preparations available in this country (see Tables 38.1, 38.2).

Because of their non antigenic properties it is likely

Table 38.1 'Old' insulins

Type	*Origin*	*Duration of action*	*Maximum action after injection*
Short acting			
Soluble insulin	Bovine	8 hours	2 to 4 hours
Nuso insulin	Bovine	8 hours	2 to 4 hours
Medium acting			
Semilente insulin	Porcine	up to 24 hours	4 to 12 hours
Isophane insulin (NPH)	Bovine	up to 24 hours	4 to 12 hours
Globin zinc insulin	Bovine	up to 24 hours	4 to 12 hours
Long acting			
Ultralente insulin	Bovine	up to 30 hours	6 to 12 hours
Lente insulin	Mixed	up to 30 hours	6 to 12 hours
(30 per cent Semilente)			
(70 per cent Ultralente)			
Protamine zinc insulin	Bovine	up to 30 hours	6 to 12 hours

Table 38.2 'New' highly purified insulins

Type	*Origin*	*Equivalent acting 'Old' insulin*
Short acting		
Neusulin	Bovine	
Hypurin neutral	Bovine	Soluble
Actrapid MC	Porcine	Nuso
Leo Neutral	Porcine	
Medium and long acting		
Leo Retard	Porcine	
Neuphane	Bovine	Isophane
Hypurin isophane	Bovine	(NPH)
Semilente MC	Porcine	Semilente
Ultratard MC	Bovine	Ultralente
Lentard MC	Mixed	
Monotard	Porcine	Lente
Neulente	Bovine	
Hypurin protamine zinc	Bovine	Protamine zinc
Insulin mixtures		
Rapitard MC		No equivalent
25 per cent Actrapid	Porcine	
5 per cent Insulin zinc suspension (crystaline)	Bovine	
Leo Mixtard		
30 per cent Leo Neutral	Porcine	
70 per cent Retard	Porcine	
Leo Initard		
50 per cent Leo Neutral	Porcine	
50 per cent Leo Retard	Porcine	

Table 38.3 Some common twice daily insulin regimes

Insulin or insulins in same syringe	*Additional short acting insulin if required*
Soluble b.d. Isophane b.d. Soluble plus isophane b.d.	Soluble
Rapitard MC b.d. Semilente b.d. Semitard MC b.d. Leo Retard b.d. Leo Retard plus Leo Neutral b.d. Mixtard b.d. Initard b.d.	Any short acting insulin of Neutral pH, i.e. Actrapid MC or Leo Neutral
Ultratard plus Actrapid MC b.d.	

that all newly diagnosed young insulin dependent diabetics will be stabilised on highly purified insulin. There does not appear to be any case for the change over of patients satisfactorily controlled on the older insulins to new insulins, except in the case of pregnancy or the presence of insulin fat atrophy.

Soluble insulin and its purified equivalents have the advantage of rapid action in the presence of ketosis (Malins, 1970) and are used in initial stabilisation when ketoacidosis is present. Because of their short duration of action they usually need to be combined with an insulin of intermediate action to control blood glucose levels over twenty four hours with two injections. In the absence of ketoacidosis the child may be started on a morning dose of an intermediate acting insulin, for example, Isophane Insulin or Leo Retard Insulin, or a mixture of short acting and intermediate acting insulins, such as Rapitard or Mixtard Insulins. If Isophane or Retard insulins are used initially, a short acting insulin (Soluble BP with Isophane, Leo Neutral with Retard) may be mixed with them in the syringe if more insulin activity is required in the early part of the day. Similarly, more short acting insulin may be added to the insulin mixtures, though it must be remembered that soluble insulin BP should not be mixed with highly purified insulin as this would nullify their non antigenic property and because of its low pH (see Table 38.3).

In these early stages the control of the child's diabetes is fairly easy, and indeed after initial stabilisation the insulin requirement usually falls, and in a few cases even the smallest dose of insulin provokes hypoglycaemic reactions, and control may be maintained on diet only for several weeks or months. This is the so called 'honeymoon' or 'remission' phase, considered to be due

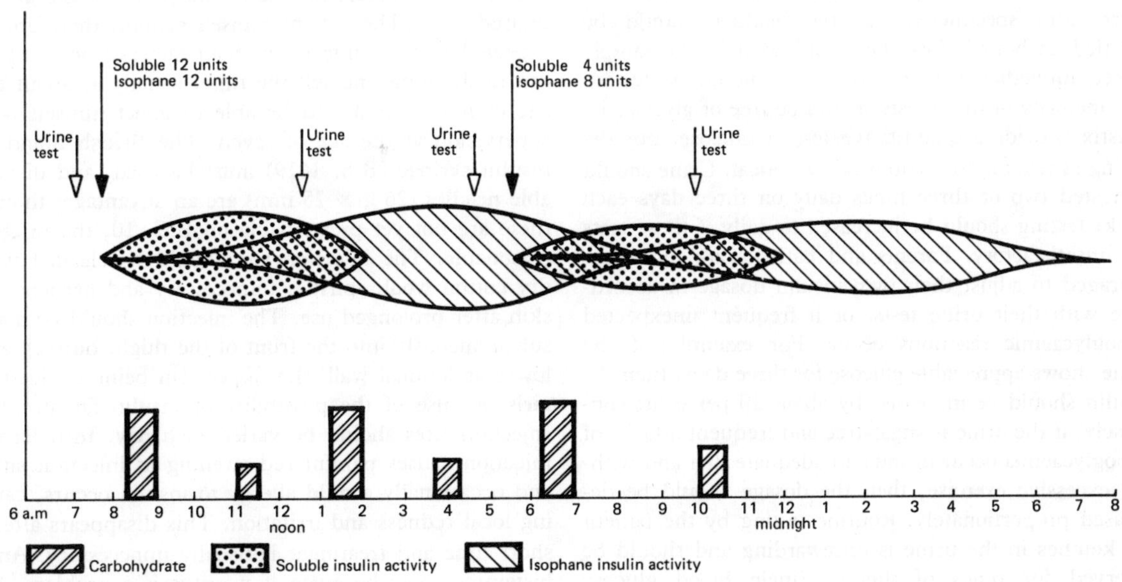

Fig. 38.1 A day on B.D. insulin

to β-cell recovery occurring when the blood glucose is lowered by control of the patients diabetes. It frequently ends abruptly and often coincidently with an infection, insulin being required again. Further remissions do not occur.

When the daily insulin dosage increases to more than about 40 units, twice daily injections become necessary. When the onset of diabetes is over the age of 10 years, twice daily injections should be introduced as soon as possible to avoid possible hostility to their introduction at the more difficult age of puberty. Approximately two thirds of the total daily dose is usually given before breakfast, the remainder before tea. If a mixture of a short acting and an intermediate acting insulin is given, then a relatively larger proportion of short acting insulin is usually required in the morning injection. Hypoglycaemic reactions are most likely to occur at times when insulin is having its maximum effect (Fig. 38.1), and carbohydrate buffer snacks should be planned to avoid these.

ASSESSMENT OF CONTROL

The child's growth and development should be comparable with that of the normal child, and he should feel well and energetic. His weight will be measured at each clinic attendance, and height recorded periodically. The patient and his parents will be taught to test the urine for glucose with clinitest tablets, as a quantitative measurement of glycosuria is necessary; the results of these tests should be recorded in a book. The most convenient specimens of urine to test are those passed before breakfast and before bedtime. These should be short term specimens, i.e. the bladder should be emptied an hour before the meal and then the sample passed immediately before the meal should be tested. The majority of these tests should be free of glycosuria. Diastix provide a quantitative test of glucose, but the timing of reading the strip is fairly critical. Urine should be tested two or three times daily on three days each week, testing should be increased to daily if these tests are unsatisfactory. Parents and patients are to be encouraged to adjust their own insulin dosage in accordance with their urine tests, or if frequent unexpected hypoglycaemic reactions occur. For example, if the urine shows appreciable glucose for three days, then the insulin should be increased by about 20 per cent; conversely, if the urine is sugar-free and frequent attacks of hypoglycaemia occur despite an adequate diet and without excessive exercise, then the dosage should be decreased proportionately. Routine testing by the patient for ketones in the urine is unrewarding and should be reserved for times of illness. Single blood glucose estimations, taken if possible shortly before a meal, should be regarded cautiously, as wide variations are possible within short periods. The overall state of control should, therefore, be assessed by observing all the afore-mentioned factors together.

The recent development of enzyme strip tests for blood sugar estimations (such as Dextrostix and Reflotest), and direct reading meters (Glucocheck or Hypocount) and their high level of acceptability in the young, (Sönksen *et al*, 1978), has focussed interest on home monitoring of blood glucose levels and also illustrated that freedom from glycosuria does not necessarily illustrate good control of blood glucose. Although it seems unlikely that young children would accept frequent finger pricking for home monitoring it would be very helpful in adolescence when control is frequently difficult. If this method were used, preprandial normoglycaemia would be their target. The measurement of the proportion of glycosylated haemoglobin (Hb_{1c}) gives an accurate indication of the degree of blood glucose control which has been maintained during the previous month (Goren, 1978). A level of 10 per cent of haemoglobin A_1 would appear to indicate good mean glucose concentration over the previous four weeks.

INJECTIONS

Injections together with diet cause most apprehension, fear and parental worry in the care of the diabetic child. It is necessary that the technique of measuring the required dosage and injection should be taught to someone preferably the child or parent, who is capable of injecting the correct dosage at the proper place at the desired time. The patient himself cannot, therefore be expected to treat himself without supervision until he can read, count and tell the time, usually at about the age of nine. He should be able to inject himself with supervision at the age of seven. The British Standard insulin syringe (B.S. 1619) must be used, and disposable needles (26 g × 25 mm) are an advantage; though these are not yet prescribable on E.C. 10, the price is reasonable. The injection site should be cleaned with dry cotton wool; spirit is unnecessary and hardens the skin after prolonged use. The injection should be made subcutaneously into the front of the thigh, buttock and lower abdominal wall, the upper arm being avoided in girls because of the possibility of insulin fat atrophy. Injection sites should be varied each day. Intradermal injection causes painful red swelling at injection sites, and occasionally a mild allergy to insulin occurs, causing local redness and irritation. This disappears after a short time and treatment is usually unnecessary. Antihistamines may be given if pruritus is a problem. Insulin fat atrophy, an unsightly disappearance of subcutaneous fat at injection sites, is common, occurring in about a quarter of diabetic children with an equal sex incidence before puberty. The cause is unknown but the condition does improve in time. Reputedly, fat atrophy does not occur with highly purified insulins. Repeated injections into the same site may result in 'tumour' formation. These are fatty lumps which may interfere with insulin absorbtion, so that hypoglycaemia may occur when a fresh site is used.

The apprehensive child may be helped by the use of a Palmer automatic injector which inserts the needle and prevents hesitation in making the injection, or a hypoguard which is simpler and only assists in inserting the needle (Grant, 1976).

HYPOGLYCAEMIA

If diabetes is to be adequately controlled with insulin, then occasional attacks of hypoglycaemia are inevitable. Low blood sugar levels appear to be rather better tolerated in children than adults. Symptoms of hypoglycaemia vary from those in adults. Nausea, vomiting and headache are common, paraesthesia of lips and tongue uncommon. Irritability and naughtiness in the young child may be caused by hypoglycaemia, but care should be exercised lest the child is feigning symptoms to get his own way or to obtain sweets. When the diagnosis of hypoglycaemia is in doubt Dextrostix gives a quick, and at lower levels accurate, measurement of blood glucose.

The risk of hypoglycaemia should be minimised by the insistence on snacks between meals and extra food before exercise. Sugar must be carried at all times and should be taken if suggestive symptoms occur. If the attack progresses to unconciousness, with the child pale and sweating with swallowing impossible, 20 ml of 50 per cent Dextrose solution should be administered intravenously; usually this is rapidly effective. Glucagon 1 mg may be given subcutaneously or intramuscularly and will often raise the level of consciousness sufficiently for oral glucose to be taken. With patients who have frequent attacks of hypoglycaemia with little warning, the parents should be given a supply of glucagon to administer when necessary.

Hyperglycaemia occurring as a reaction to overtreatment with insulin has been described (Somogyi, 1959); the mechanism is attributed to hypoglycaemia stimulating the excessive production of adrenaline and corticosteroids, which raise blood sugar. This is most frequently encountered in the form of heavy morning glycosuria following undiagnosed nocturnal hypoglycaemia. In this instance, reduction rather than increase of insulin dosage results in decreasing glycosuria.

INTERCURRENT ILLNESS AND KETOSIS

If the patient is poorly controlled glycosuria will increase and ketones will appear in the urine; this occurs more rapidly in the presence of infection. All too frequently when a child is admitted to hospital in ketoacidosis, insulin has been omitted because of fear of hypoglycaemia when the patient has been unable to eat or has been vomiting. Infection increases the insulin requirement and this should preferably be given as soluble insulin. It is a good principle to keep some soluble insulin in the patient's home even if it is not part of his normal regime. When an infection occurs or persistent heavy glycosuria is present, the frequency of urine tests should be increased to four times daily, and ketonuria assessed with Ketostix. If vomiting is a problem or food is refused, the required carbohydrate should be given in liquid form. Extra insulin is administered, depending on urine tests. If glycosuria exceeds one per cent on clinitest before breakfast, then two to eight extra units of soluble insulin (depending on total dose) should be given. A similar regime should be instituted before the evening meal, introducing an extra injection if the child is on once daily insulin. Frequent visiting of the patient will be necessary, and if vomiting is persistent and continues for more than about six hours, or if signs of ketoacidosis present, then urgent hospital admission should be sought. Any infection present must be treated energetically.

Late complications such as retinopathy, nephropathy and neuropathy are rare and do not constitute a problem in the care of the diabetic child. True diabetic cataract does occur uncommonly in childhood, reputedly usually following a period of poor diabetic control and early in the disease. I have personal experience of a case where the reverse appeared to be true; bilateral cataracts occurred following a series of low blood glucose recordings at a clinic, followed by dramatic clearing of lens opacity and improvement in visual acuity after reduction in insulin dosage.

RELATIONSHIPS AND RESPONSIBILITIES

The family remains the primary social unit in our society and the parents must accept and bear the major share of responsibility for the welfare and care of their child. Parental attitudes have a profound influence upon the child's diabetic management. Overprotection against self injection and an obsessional attitude to diet are to be discouraged, and self reliance and independence encouraged. If the child is failing to make appropriate progress because of this, or because of lack of understanding or failure in communication on the part of the parents, then a short holiday at one of the camps for diabetic children (Shinebourne and Hargreave, 1968) organised by the British Diabetic Association and open to all diabetic children from six to 17 years of age will help them learn about injections and diet, and help promote independence. When the home circumstances are a considerable problem then a period spent at a hostel for diabetic children may be required (Carne, 1975). Children live at these hostels during term, attend schools in the vicinity of the hostels, and return home for school holidays.

Fortunately, most children have good competent parents who manage their child only with periodic help and advice from the diabetic clinic or their general practitioner. Telephone advice properly given and used can often help in correcting early deviations from good control. Health visitors specially trained in diabetes are being increasingly used by many clinics, and are able to advise both in the clinic and in the patient's own home. Patients are advised to join the British Diabetic Association, 3–6 Alfred Place, London WC1E 7EE, and also its local branch if there is one nearby. Here they will meet more experienced families and be able to discuss domestic problems informally. The Association also publishes much useful diabetic literature for patients, including cookery books and carbohydrate exchange lists used in most clinics. Some branches have formed parents' groups who are available to advise less experienced parents (Farquhar, 1975).

The staff of the child's school should be informed of his diabetes, preferably by the parents, and advised of the necessity to recognise the signs of hypoglycaemia and how to treat it; they should ensure that meals and snacks are taken, and know the importance of an extra snack if the child is detained for punishment after school. Smoking should be strongly discouraged because the increased liability of diabetics to vascular disease, and because once started the habit tends to persist. As adolescence approaches the patient more frequently tends to comply poorly with his dietary restrictions, and he occasionally becomes hostile and rebellious or apathetic about his condition. These reactions usually conceal unspoken fears of the future concerning careers, marriage and infertility, and fears of late diabetic complications. Urine tests and indeed specimens may be fraudulent, and insulin injections resented or even refused. These episodes require skill and patient management; the GP with his knowledge of the whole family is advantageously situated to help effectively in such situations.

The medical care of the child with diabetes must be shared between the diabetic clinic with its specialised knowledge and facilities, and the GP with his first hand knowledge of the child's total environment and his primary care in acute episodes.

The present expectation of life of a diabetic child at age 10 under the best management is of the order of 40 years (Godber, 1974). Whether or not this will be improved upon as our knowledge and resources increase, only time will show, but of one thing there can be no doubt. The pattern of care built up during the early months and years after diagnosis is of immense importance, for the child is taught techniques and set standards of management which may influence greatly his future morbidity and happiness. Herein lies the crux of the general practitioner's responsibility towards his young patient with diabetes.

REFERENCES

Bloom, A., Hayes, T.M. & Gamble, D.R. (1975) Register of newly-diagnosed diabetic children. *British Medical Journal*, **3**, 580–583.

Bottazzo, G.F., Cudworth, A.G. , Moul, D.J., Doniach, D. & Festenstein, H. (1978) Evidence for a primary autoimmune type of diabetes mellitus. *British Medical Journal*, **2**, 1253.

Carne, S. (1975) Diabetes in children. *Proceedings of the Royal Society of Medicine*, **68**, 277.

College of General Practitioners (1965) The family history of diabetes. *British Medical Journal*, **1**, 960.

Farquhar, J.W. (1975) *Notes for the Guidance of Parents of Diabetic Children*, 2nd edn, p. 34. Edinburgh: Churchill Livingstone.

Gamble, D.R., Taylor, K.W. & Cumming, H. (1973) Coxsackie viruses and diabetes mellitus. *British Medical Journal*, **4**, 260.

Gamble , D.R. (1974) Epidemiological and virological observations on juvenile diabetes. *Postgraduate Medical Journal*, **50** (Suppl. 3), 538.

Gamble D.R. (1980) Relation of antecedent illness to development of diabetes in children. *British Medical Journal*, **281**, 99.

Godber, G. (1974) The Health of the School Child 1971–71, p.3. London: HMSO.

Goren B., Rubenstein A.H., Rochman H., Tanegas, and Horwitz D.L., (1977). Haemoglobin A_1: an indicator of the metabolic control of diabetic patients. *Lancet*, **2**, 734.

Grant, D.B. (1976) Management of the diabetic child. *Journal of Maternal and Child Health*, **1**, no. 5, 2–8.

Malins, J.M. (1970) The treatment of diabetes mellitus in childhood. *The Practitioner*, **204**, 157.

Nerup J. (1974) HL-A antigens and diabetes mellitus, *Lancet*, **2**, 864.

Oakley, W.G., Pyke , D.A. & Taylor, K.W. (1968) Clinical Diabetes and its Biochemical Basis. 1st edn, chap. 23, p.599. Oxford and Endinburgh: Blackwell Scientific Publications.

Pirart J., (1977). Diabetes mellitus and its degenerative complications: A prospective study of 4,400 patients observed between 1947 and 1973 (in three parts). *Diabete et Metabolisme*, **3**, 97, 173 and 245.

Shinbourne, E. & Hargreave, F.E. (1968) Medically supervised holidays for diabetic children. *Lancet*, **1**, 911.
Somogyi, M. (1959) Exacerbation of diabetes by excess insulin action. *American Journal of Medicine*, **26**, 169.
Sönksen P.H. , Judd S.L., and Lowy C. (1978) Home monitoring of blood glucose. *Lancet*, **1**, 729.
Tattersall R.B. & Pyke, D.A. (1973) Growth in diabetic children: studies in identical twins. *Lancet*, **2**, 838.
Tchobroutsky G. (1978) Relation of diabetic control to development of microvascular complications. *Diabetologia*, **15**, 143.
White, P. (1960) Childhood diabetes, its course, and influence on the second and third generations. *Diabetes*, **9**, 345.

39

Epilepsy in infancy and childhood

Peter McWilliam

Epilepsy is a common disorder of great antiquity. References to it appear in the Bible ('falling sickness') and many famous historical characters are said to have suffered from it, e.g. Julius Caesar.

Epilepsy has no succinct yet all embracing definition but is regarded as a symptom of cerebral dysfunction, and whilst there are many useful descriptions and classifications of the different types of manifestation (sometimes called the 'Epilepsies') these must never be regarded as disease entities. The traditional classification into symptomatic (i.e. associated with structural CNS change or metabolic abnormality) and idiopathic (i.e. apparently without such abnormality) is useful but perhaps 'origin as yet unknown' could usefully replace 'idiopathic'.

Children with epilepsy have special needs. There are age specific manifestations and the often profound effect of epilepsy on growth and development, education, family life and pre-employment training requires special care and consideration over long periods of time.

There is a good deal of interchange between the terms 'fits', 'convulsions' and 'seizures' and generally they correctly merit the adjective 'epileptic'. However, a child is correctly diagnosed as having epilepsy only if there is a continuing tendency to suffer from such manifestations. That is, epilepsy is never correctly diagnosed on the basis of one epileptic fit or seizure.

The GP has an important and varied role to play in the total management of childhood epilepsy. First of all, he must help to prevent new cases developing by identifying the known associated factors and taking appropriate preventive measures. Then he must recognise the potentially sinister, yet sometimes apparently innocuous manifestations of the rare and severe forms so that the children may be promptly referred for accurate assessment so as to aid proper family counselling. Finally he must help all the children under his care who suffer from epilepsy to enjoy the maximum quality of life consistent with their handicap.

Emphasis in this chapter will be on the clinical aspects of epilepsy in infants and children, especially as they present to the GP, rather than on the niceties of seizure classification.

INCIDENCE AND PREVALENCE

Epilepsy is neither a disease entity nor a notifiable condition. Unfortunately it is still associated with much unwarranted prejudice, which leads to concealment, thus making difficult the collation of accurate figures. Estimates in the United Kingdom give the approximate figure of one in 200 as suffering from epilepsy in the population overall – i.e. roughly 12 cases of epilepsy (of all ages) per 'average' G P list. It is considered that a significant number of the 5000 new cases of epilepsy which develop each year in the United Kingdom could be prevented. The incidence of all types of epilepsy in school children is of the order of eight per 1000, whilst the overall frequency of convulsions (from all sources) is thought to be 12 per 1000 in neonates and 50 per 1000 in the toddler age groups (Brown, 1973; Brett, 1973; Rutter, Graham and Yule, 1970; Ross *et al*, 1980).

GENETICS

When the epilepsy is part of a recognised and established genetic disorder, the expected risks apply. Epiloia (Tuberose Sclerosis) is one such disorder. It is a dominant condition so that the risk of affected offspring is 50 per cent. The clinical features include epilepsy, skin manifestations, eye, nail and heart defects and usually progressive mental deterioration. The epilepsy may take the form of infantile spasms or tonic/clonic or other seizures in older children. One affected child will alert the doctor to the risk of the condition appearing in siblings but since there is variable penetrance of the gene, it does not necessarily follow that all affected children will be incapacitated to the same degree. Thus one affected child may have all the components of the syndrome, whereas another may develop only insignificant skin pigmentation. Phenylketonuria is an example of an autosomal recessive condition where the risks are one in four. Again the manifestations of the associated epilepsy may be infantile spasms or major epilepsy in older children.

Other recessive conditions exist which have epilepsy as part of their clinical pattern, for example, the muco polysaccharidoses, but these are so rare as to preclude effective counselling. All the foregoing conditions are examples of 'symptomatic' epilepsy but a less clearly defined genetic factor is thought to exist in the so called 'idiopathic' epilepsy. This is usually referred to as a 'familial tendency' and is recognised in some variations of photosensitive epilepsy and especially in the febrile convulsions of early childhood. The existence of these varieties of epilepsy should alert the GP to anticipate their emergence in siblings, especially the febrile convulsions when the risk in some families may be as high as one in three.

AETIOLOGY

A correctly functioning nervous system depends on the well ordered electrical rhythms of neuronal activity, which depend in turn on finely adjusted cellular biochemistry. A convulsion or other epileptic manifestation is thought to occur when there is a sudden disorganised discharge of electrical activity across the brain which spreads along existing anatomical pathways so as to produce the observed phenomena. It is well known that there are many varieties of CNS insults (mechanical, electrical, inflammatory and biochemical), any one, or any combination of which, may produce an epileptic manifestation in any individual if the insult or stimulus is sufficiently great. The tendency of different individuals to react to these stimuli in such a way as to produce an epileptic manifestation varies considerably and is thought to be due to the individual adjustment of inhibitory or controlling mechanisms, usually biochemical. This leads to the 'convulsive threshold' concept, which may be genetically determined but cannot as yet be quantified.

The immaturity of the infantile brain and the abundance of potential insults in the perinatal and neonatal periods explain the greater incidence of convulsive disorders in the early weeks of life. A study of the aetiology of neonatal and infantile convulsions indicates how some of these may be prevented. Some of the commoner causes are as follows:

Hypoglycaemia

This is common in the dysmature or 'light for dates' babies seen in placental insufficiency states. It is a well-recognised cause of early neonatal convulsions, cerebral damage and chronic epilepsy. It can also occur as a result of brain damage. Infants of mothers with diabetes mellitus are also at risk from hypoglycaemia. The 'light for dates' baby should be anticipated during antenatal care and the confinement arranged in a hospital with a special care baby unit. The same applies for mothers with diabetes mellitus. Prompt feeding, preferably with breast milk should be offered to all babies.

Hypocalcaemia

This usually occurs after the fifth day of life in artificially fed infants. The convulsions produced are tetanic and the usual cause is thought to be due to the homeostatic attempts of the infantile para-thyroid glands being overwhelmed because of the reciprocal depression of the serum calcium due to the high phosphate content of the artificial milk. Though not as damaging as the convulsions due to hypoglycaemia, they are frightening and usually unnecessary. They can be prevented by breast feeding and can be treated by giving calcium supplements. There may be an associated magnesium deficiency (for which there may be several causes) and this must be suspected if the response to calcium supplementation is disappointing.

Sometimes hypocalcaemia may be associated with hypoglycaemia and evidence of cerebral damage.

Asphyxia

Asphyxia and consequent cerebral anoxia is a potent cause of neonatal convulsions, cerebral damage and (amongst other things) chronic epilepsy. Good ante natal and obstetric care with early referral to an obstetric unit of suspected abnormalities is needed.

Infection

Intra uterine infection e.g. rubella, cytomegalovirus infection and toxoplasmosis can result in a 'burnt out' encephalitic form of brain damage which may produce convulsions soon after birth and later.

Meningitis (viral and bacterial) is a dangerous condition which often produces brain damage and epilepsy. It should be considered in all babies and young children who are unwell for no readily apparent or otherwise explainable cause, e.g. pyelitis or bronchopneumonia, especially if they present with their first convulsion. Umbilical cord sepsis, giving rise to E. Coli septicaemia and Listeria monocytogenes infection from an organism infecting the female genital tract, are well known causes of neonatal meningitis. Clinicians should have a high index of suspicion of meningitis in dealing with ill babies, bearing in mind that fever, tense fontanelle and neck stiffness are very often absent. Referral for diagnostic lumbar puncture is necessary and the empirical use of antibiotics is deplored.

Infantile gastro enteritis may produce fluid and electrolyte disturbances leading to hypernatraemic dehydration, in which the plasma sodium level will be greater than 150 m ml/l. Under these circumstances, brain shrinkage may occur, causing traction on and rupture of cerebral blood vessels, producing bleeding and other cerebral damage, often leading to epilepsy, spastic lesions and poor intelligence.

Sometimes mothers may unwittingly produce hypernatraemia by making the artificial feeds unnecessarily concentrated. The increased sodium in the feeds produces thirst (and it is thought, dehydration headache) which produces crying and irritability. The mother may interpret this as hunger and offer more feeds. Clear fluids between feeds and proper feeding advice are required. The rehydration of hypernatraemic babies requires special care and is best done in hospital.

Injury

Trauma, apart from and in addition to, that from obstetric causes, produces brain damage and convulsions. After severe head injuries in children, the appearance of convulsions within the first week is of special prognostic significance (Jennett, 1969, 1972). Non accidental injury, in the battered baby syndrome is now well recognised and cerebral damage may be present with no outward sign of injury. Guthkelch (1971) has drawn attention to the causation of subdural haematomata and cerebral damage in babies and young children by vigorous shaking, producing shearing injuries to meningeal vessels. Occasionally, these injuries have been unwittingly produced by parents shaking children with coughing paroxysms of pertussis in the mistaken belief that this affords relief. Also, in severe pertussis, the paroxysms themselves may produce traumatic cerebral petechiae, which can be epileptogenic.

Fever

Fever is a common precipitant of convulsions which will be considered later.

Metabolic causes

Many inborn errors of metabolism produce toxic chemicals leading to convulsions and cerebral damage. Kernicterus is much less common now that Rh incompatability is better understood and managed but it still occasionally occurs. Phenylketonuria has already been mentioned and there are many more metabolic conditions.

Pyridoxine (B6) deficiency may cause infantile convulsions and intra-uterine convulsions have been ascribed to this cause. Convulsions due to secondary pyridoxine deficiency caused by the action of other drugs e.g. Isoniazid have been recorded. In managing the new born babies of drug addicted mothers or alcoholic mothers, withdrawal convulsions should be anticipated and various types of poisonings have convulsions as part of their clinical picture, as for example, in lead poisoning.

Degenerative neurological disease

Diseases such as Tay Sach's Disease, Huntington's Chorea and Epiloia (Tuberose Sclerosis) are but three of those which have epilepsy as part of their total pattern of clinical manifestations.

DIAGNOSIS

Epilepsy is a clinical diagnosis and great care and circumspection should be exercised in making it. It must be clearly differentiated from masturbation, vaso vagal faints (which, if severe, may have some tonic/clonic movements), night terrors, benign paroxysmal vertigo, and in older children, migraine or collapse due to cardiac arrhythmias or heart block.

Many children referred to hospital with a diagnosis of epilepsy do not have it (Jeavons, 1977). One must be keenly aware of the implications of an erroneous diagnosis of epilepsy. Eye witness accounts from teachers, and cub/scout or brownie/guide leaders can usefully supplement the evidence of parents who may be too upset or otherwise unable to give adequate histories. Many doctors have proformas which they invite the parents to complete and there is much to commend the idea of Jeavons (1978) of the doctor having a repertoire of typical fit patterns which he personally demonstrates to the parents.

Occasionally, even experienced observers find the diagnosis of epileptic convulsions in babies very difficult. A grand mal type of tonic/clonic seizure is very rare and the more usual fragmented seizure may be difficult to recognise. In very small babies convulsive movements may be better appreciated by light palpation rather than by inspection. Other neonatal convulsive movements may take the form of barely perceptible eye ball movements, minor facial twitching or alteration in respiratory rate. Occasionally there can be real difficulty in differentiating a neonatal convulsion from an apnoeic attack.

THE GRAND MAL OR MAJOR, TONIC/CLONIC SEIZURE

These may be like those noticed in adults with many of the features of aura, cry, generalised convulsions, tongue biting and incontinence, etc., and are followed sometimes by automatism and sleep. Retrograde amnesia may be present and the child may know nothing of the attack until he is 'coming round', as distinct from a vaso vagal faint. The post epileptic confusional state is not always appreciated by parents and teachers and special care is often required so far as hazards like fire and road traffic are concerned. Todd's palsy, a transient hemiparesis lasting up to 36 hours may follow. This is not to be confused with the acute infantile hemiplegia syndrome (thought to be due to middle cerebral artery occlusion) which results in a long generalised convulsion, coma, residual permanent hemiplegia and chronic epilepsy.

Whilst fit patterns vary enormously between children, they are usually constant and unique in each child and it is helpful if older children can carry a card indicating the usual duration and other salient features of their attacks.

If the major seizure does not stop as anticipated and continues for more than 20 minutes or if there are recurrent major seizures with no return to consciousness (as distinct from serial fits in which the child recovers consciousness between attacks) then the dangerous and potentially fatal condition of status epilepticus exists.

STATUS EPILEPTICUS

In this frightening condition the brain has increased metabolic demands and there are varying degrees of airways obstruction; hence the risk of cumulative and permanent anoxic cerebral damage leading to mental sub-normality. Hyperpyrexia, aspiration pneumonia and exhaustion are likely and, if the condition is prolonged, death from a combination of these may ensue Thus it is urgently necessary to secure control with the utmost speed.

The commonest cause of status epilepticus is the abrupt cessation of anticonvulsant therapy, although some children (and adults) may be 'status only' cases and these patients require special long term follow up. 'Lone status epilepticus' may occur in older children or adolescents who may later develop a cerebral tumour (Rowan and Scott, 1970).

FOCAL ATTACKS

These may occur in children as well as adults and may comprise an aura, unilateral convulsive movements of the limbs or part of the face of variable duration, disturbances of sensation and varying degrees of impairment of consciousness – ranging from slight confusion or inattention to coma. Any combination of these features may then progress to a generalised convulsive seizure. The 'aura' or warning usually precedes convulsive movements and denotes the start of the electrical disturbance and although a child may be able to describe the aura accurately and in detail after the fit, sometimes he may be prevented by fear or apprehension from 'taking cover' at the time. There may be a Jacksonian 'march of events' as is occasionally noted in adults. Study of the focal fit pattern may provide useful localizing information and focal discharges in sensory areas of the brain may produce focal sensory seizures. Information about these may not be volunteered by the child so that appropriate enquiries should be made, age and intelligence permitting.

A separate syndrome occurring in otherwise healthy children and called benign focal (or Rolandic) epilepsy of childhood is now recognised. The features comprise nocturnal seizures, salivation, drooling, facial twitching, and inability to speak, rather than loss of consciousness. There are characteristic EEG correlates in the form of spike foci in the Rolandic areas, which disappear, with the seizures, in the second decade of life.

PSYCHOMOTOR, UNCINATE OR TEMPORAL LOBE ATTACKS

These are a specific type of focal epileptic attack of special importance in childhood and adolescence. They may take many bizarre forms and occasionally may be considered by quite experienced observers to be hysterical or malingering episodes. Sudden, unexplained, unusual or inappropriate behaviour, especially if associated with mumbling, confusion, fumbling with clothing, lip smacking or chewing movements, with a return to normal behaviour in a short time are typical. A major seizure supervening gives a clue to the epileptic nature of the disturbance. Also the stereotyped repetitive nature of the manifestations indicate the likelihood of epilepsy. Sometimes inappropriate laughing or crying may occur.

Unprovoked outbursts of rage, perhaps accompanied by flushing and later followed by confusion may also occur as manifestations of temporal lobe epilepsy, but care should be exercised in affixing a label of epilepsy or of 'epileptic equivalent', if outbursts of rage or temper tantrums are the only abnormality noted, as these may occur in emotionally disturbed children in whom there is no evidence of epilepsy or any other organic brain disorder.

Temporal lobe epilepsy should be suspected when there are recurrent primitive gut symptoms, e.g. 'stomach turning over and rising' and in cases where confusion is associated with loud borborygmi. Occasionally fear may be a feature of this type of epilepsy as in the case of a small child who always runs to his mother in fright at the commencement of an epileptic attack. Any persistent complaint of some aberration of sensations mediated by the temporal lobe e.g. sound, taste, smell etc., should alert the doctor to the diagnosis of possible temporal lobe epilepsy, as in the following example:

Stephen was a bright little five-year-old who had had several admissions to hospital in generalised status epilepticus. A temporal lobe lesion was suspected, despite negative clinical, radiological and specialised electrophysiological (sleep EEG recording) examinations because of his recurrent complaint of 'smoke going up his nose'. About a year after the onset of his attacks he was found to have developed papilloedema and soon afterwards a temporal lobe tumour – possibly an ependynoma – was resected.

Other epileptogenic structural lesions affecting the temporal lobe are abscesses and more commonly the various non-progressive lesions, including scarring and slcerosis from anoxia (often from earlier convulsions) post inflammatory state, trauma and congenital malformations. In children however temporal lobe foci can come and go in the absence of structural changes.

Yet another manifestation of this form of epilepsy is the absence seizure which consists of a brief episode of lightly impaired consciousness, or confusion, after which the child resumes his former activity. This is often confused with petit mal epilepsy.

PETIT MAL EPILEPSY

This tends to be over diagnosed. Just as 'all that wheezes isn't asthma' and 'all that waddles isn't dystrophy', all absence seizures are not petit mal! The distinction is more than academic, for petit mal is almost always idiopathic, whereas, as noted earlier, absence seizures due to temporal lobe epilepsy may, in some instances, be amenable to surgery. Also the two types of absence seizure require different drug therapy. Petit mal absences usually last for under a minute but may occur many times per day – often over a hundred. After them the child resumes his former activity. Thus, the fork poised in mid air is transferred to the mouth and the interrupted conversation is resumed. That is, 'the world has passed on a bit'! Rhythmic blinking of the eyes and or eyelids at a frequency of three per second, sometimes accompanied by slight nodding of the head may occur, but by no means always, leading to diagnostic difficulty and delay. Children with this condition may be considered to be disobedient or inattentive at home and at school and it is not unknown for the correct diagnosis to be made by the psychiatrist at a child guidance clinic.

A simple provocative diagnostic test which is easily carried out in the surgery or clinic is to get the child to hyper-ventilate for a timed two minute period, usually by blowing a piece of paper held near his face. This washes out the alveolar CO_2 and induces a temporary state of relative alkalosis, which activates latent convulsive tendencies. An EEG examination however with the demonstration of the characteristic three per second spike and wave discharge in all channels is essential for and pathognomonic of the diagnosis of petit mal. An EEG examination may occasionally reveal the existence of the three per second spike and wave discharge when even on careful clinical observation of the child, there is no visible evidence of an absence seizure. The child may have unsuspected impaired attention. This is the condition of sub-clinical petit mal seizure discharge and is an exception to the rule that epilepsy is always a clinical diagnosis.

Although petit mal is less dramatic and less physically dangerous than grand mal, its effect on the childs' road safety is obvious and the effect on his school work can be devastating, especially since there is evidence that children with petit mal have a brief period of retrograde amnesia associated with the seizures (Ounsted *et al*, 1963).

Petit mal is essentially a condition of the school child and should be considered in any child who is under-achieving in school, for no apparent reason. It is only very occasionally seen in adults. Usually the attacks cease in adolescence, but they may be replaced by other sorts of attacks. Sometimes petit mal status is seen and occasionally grand mal and petit mal co-exist.

The unfortunate tendency to use 'petit mal' as a collective diagnosis for all minor seizures which are not grand mal, is wildly inaccurate and is to be deplored.

INFANTILE SPASMS

Many eponyms and descriptive terms exist for this condition, e.g. West's syndrome, EMIH, BNS, etc., and this is a rare but age specific variety of paediatric epilepsy, usually affecting children in the first year of life.

Typically, there is a sudden onset in a young infant of recurrent seizures or spasms or short rapid episodes in which the child may suddenly curl up and shoot out his arms or flex his trunk and thighs (jack-knife convulsion) or he may extend his trunk or display the salaam posture. If sitting he may be flung forwards suddenly, so that his head may strike his feet. Relaxation follows after the spasm but many spasms may occur in succession throughout the day. Occasionally the limbs on one side may be involved, suggesting a focal lesion. The spasm may be accompanied by a short giggle or a short cry, which may lead to the erroneous diagnosis of 'colic' or even intussusception. In a very young baby the initial attack may be confused with the Moro or startle reflex. The fingers extend in the Moro reflex and usually flex in a convulsive seizure. Coincidental with the onset of the spasms is the abrupt cessation of the exhibition of previously acquired developmental skills or even regression of these, which the mother may volunteer: 'He hasn't smiled since these turns started, doctor.'

This is a devastating condition, not only on account of the distressing number of spasms, whose sinister nature may be disregarded or not fully appreciated, but for the inexorable mental deterioration which very often follows. Early diagnosis and treatment are extremely important and if this condition is suspected urgent referral to a paediatric unit is mandatory. There is usually a typical EEG pattern called 'hypsarrhythmia', because of the chaotic pattern of disorganised cortical electrical activity with large amplitude spikes and slow waves ('hyps' means mountains). The syndrome is usually known as infantile spasms, hypsarrhythmia and mental retardation and is really epilepsy in miniature, being classically divided into 'symptomatic' and 'idiopathic'.

In the former group are infants who have suffered a perinatal insult, inborn error of metabolism, degenerative disease, congenital malformation of the CNS, or an encephalitic episode – perhaps following an immunisation procedure. The idiopathic or cryptogenic groups have no such associated lesions although in the case of tuberose sclerosis, the diagnostic skin lesions may not become obvious until several months after the onset of the spasms so that these cases, which are really sympatomatic initially appear to be cryptogenic.

The condition will 'burn out' after several weeks or months with the cessation of the spasms and the disappearance of the typical EEG pattern, but leaving the mental retardation. When one sees mentally retarded children for the first time (e.g. for assessment), it is worth enquiring about spasms earlier in life.

The *Aicardi syndrome* is related in that it presents with infantile spasms but, only girls are affected and the EEG pattern often shows asynchronous 'suppression burst' activity instead of hypsarrhyhmia. There are gross CNS skeletal and eye abnormalities and life expectation is poor. Although rare, this condition may be diagnosed largely on clinical grounds (there are characteristic retinal lacunae which are traversed by blood vessels) and an accurate, albeit gloomy diagnosis can be made.

The *Lennox syndrome* affects older children (1–6 years) and may be known as petit mal variant, or myoclonic astatic epilepsy. The EEG findings are those of irregular spike and wave complexes of approximately two per second, with absences confusion tonic/clonic fits and mental subnormality. The causes are varied, treatment is disappointing and difficult and the outlook is poor.

There is some overlap of the Lennox syndrome and infantile spasms and they may be considered to be manifestations of the same type of childhood epilepsy, modified according to the age of the child. Since they denote severe cerebral dysfunction and usually have a gloomy prognosis, it is essential from a family counselling point of view that they be recognised and referred for diagnostic evaluation as soon as possible.

FEBRILE CONVULSIONS

These are very common, affecting children between the ages of six months and approximately four years, and are less benign than was originally supposed. They are distinct from fever-precipitated epilepsy such as occurs in older children and adults.

Because of a febrile illness, due to a common cause, e.g. tonsillitis, pyelitis or otitis media, a child may already have exhibited delirium and hallucinations. The sudden onset of a generalised epileptic seizure can then occur which can be very frightening to the parents, especially at night. There may be a family history and the same child may have similar convulsions with further febrile illnesses whilst remaining in this age group. The features of the syndrome are generalised tonic/clonic seizure with unconsciousness lasting 15 minutes or less, with no detectable CNS abnormality and a normal inter-seizure EEG recording – after the disappearance of the post-ictal EEG disturbance. Occasionally an apparent febrile convulsion (according to the above criteria) progresses into generalised status epilepticus lasting for 30 minutes or more, and Ounsted, Lindsay and Norman (1966) have indicated the relationship between such prolonged convulsions and the development of mesial temporal sclerosis with the subsequent development of temporal lobe epilepsy. Intelligent management of febrile convulsions is important in the prophylaxis of temporal lobe epilepsy.

MYOCLONIC EPILEPSY

Sudden involuntary incoordinated jerking affecting individual muscles or groups of muscles constitutes myoclonus.

This can arise at spinal level or it can be synchronous with a cerebral dysrhythmia and become myoclonic epilepsy with EEG changes and some (usually slight) disturbance of consciousness. Myoclonic epilepsy in children may be associated with other convulsions and these may be features, together with dementia, of a progressive degenerative or metabolic disease, e.g. subacute sclerosing panencephalitis – a rare complication of measles – or some of the storage diseases.

True myoclonic epilepsy of childhood, as described by Harper (1967) is a rare but distinct form of childhood epilepsy, unassociated with other features, affecting children between three and seven years and having its own characteristic EEG features. Typically there is a negative family history and although response to therapy is disappointing there is a tendency to spontaneous improvement with time.

Myoclonic epilepsy of whatever variety is a very distressing condition as the childs' facial scars and haematomata of scalp testify. Sudden, massive, violent muscular contractions result in the child being flung to the ground without warning. These attacks are socially embarrassing, especially at meal times. An object held in the child's hand at the commencement of an attack may be thrown some distance and the transitional states from sleeping to waking and vice versa are common times for these attacks. Breakfast is their worst meal. There is no warning, impairment of consciousness is momentary and usually minimal although occasionally attacks may occur in rapid succession. Sorbo rubber 'crash helmets' or riding hats help to minimise injuries to the head and scalp and soft plastic table-ware is helpful, especially at breakfast time.

REFLEX EPILEPSY

Generalised epileptic seizures may be precipitated by specific sensory stimuli, especially auditory and visual. Perhaps the commonest in children and adolescents are the flicker sensitive seizures of which television epilepsy is a well known example. Typically these children have a tendency to sit with their faces just in front of the television screen and even if the set is correctly adjusted, the movement of the lines composing the picture may precipitate a seizure. An EEG is necessary taken whilst the child is looking directly at a stroboscopic light in order to distinguish true flicker seizures from coincidental epileptic fits either arising spontaneously or emotionally precipitated.

Flicker seizures may also occur in discotheques and on visits to the seaside when the child looks directly at reflected sunlight from a choppy sea. Occasionally children may induce their own flicker seizures by interposing an outstretched hand moving from side to side, between their eyes and the sun.

MANAGEMENT OF THE CHILD WITH EPILEPSY AND THE FAMILY

'Doctor, I thought he was dying,' is a phrase not infrequently used by parents in describing their child's first seizure, especially if complicating a pre-existing illness. Although they may deal competently with this and subsequent seizures, the unpleasant memory of the first seizure tends to remain for a long time and understandably, contributes to over-protection to the eventual detriment of the child, his siblings and the family generally. By inviting discussion of the difficulties experienced by the parents, the GP can make a very worthwhile contribution to the stability of the family. He must of course be prepared for his efforts to be bedevilled by ignorance, prejudice and the decorticate regurgitation by friends and neighbours of careless and unkindly remarks which even now inevitably follow the use of the word 'epilepsy'.

Individual assessment of risks, realistically reviewed at frequent intervals rather than the imposition of arbitrary blanket embargoes on all the things children like to do, should determine the childs' activities. 'Activity is the best anticonvulsant' may be an overstatement but there is no doubt that pleasurable well motivated activity makes for good seizure control, a happy well-adjusted child, and prevents the development of secondary psychological handicaps. Sports like football, basketball, cricket and athletics should be freely encouraged even in children with poor seizure control, but one can understand reservations about boxing. Pending better seizure control however, horse-riding, cycling on busy roads and the use of wall bars and climbing frames should be discouraged. Swimming is permissible even though there is incomplete seizure control, providing the child can be supervised on a one to one basis, by a competent swimmer in the water, who is prepared to life-save if necessary. Later, this close degree of supervision can be gradually relaxed as seizure control improves but it would be inadvisable in this highly litigious age to allow swimming in school groups under the nominal supervision of one teacher until the child has been seizure free for at least one year and preferably two, even though he may still be on anticonvulsant therapy.

Regular hours and meals, the avoidance of extreme hunger and fatigue, constipation and dietetic or alcoholic excess together with regularity of taking prescribed rational medication, all help to secure good seizure control. Perhaps it could be reiterated that the commonest cause of status epilepticus is the sudden withdrawal of anticonvulsant therapy.

MANAGEMENT OF SEIZURES

Ideally a child having a fit for the first time should be referred to hospital for investigation. In an acute illness this will often include a lumbar puncture because of the risk of menigitis presenting with fits.

Care of a child in a major seizure is limited to protecting him from the hazards of traffic and water, both during the attack and in the often confused post ictal state.

If the fit is prolonged then attempts must be made to keep the child on his side and wipe away the froth from his mouth so as to help his airway.

It is useless to try and restrain the convulsing limbs as torn muscles and ligaments and even bony fractures may result. The traditional manouvre of attempting to force a padded spoon or similar article between the clenched teeth in order to prevent the tongue from being bitten, is to be discouraged. The richly vascular tongue soon heals whereas teeth may be broken or even dislodged or inhaled (especially first dentition teeth) with the possibility of pulmonary collapse or lung abscess. Parents should be told how to recognise status epilepticus, and pending the arrival of medical aid, they should employ the measures outlined above and try and cool the patient. They should not put on extra clothing.

If medical aid is not immediately forthcoming, then a 999 ambulance call is justified. If the GP can suck out the secretion, insert an airway and administer an anticonvulsant drug other than orally, so much the better. It is urgently necessary to stop the convulsions as soon as possible because of the risk of anoxic brain damage and all that is thereby implied. If the child is transferred to hospital the GP should notify the nature, dose, time and route of administration of any drug given.

Febrile convulsions should be anticipated and febrile children at risk should be physically cooled by undressing, guarded electric fans and antipyretic drugs such as aspirin. Tepid sponging can also be employed but care must be taken not to produce shivering as the temperature may then rise! The oral administration of the usual anticonvulsant drugs is of no value since effective blood levels are not achieved sufficiently quickly. Where children are prone to febrile convulsions, intelligent parents could be instructed in the administration of rectal diazepam (prophylactically and therapeutically) and a supply of ampoules of the drug and disposable syringes made available (see below).

The debate continues as to the advisability of putting children prone to febrile convulsions on continuous prophylactic therapy for their 'risk years' (NIH Consensus, 1980). At present it seems reasonable to do so if a child has had two or more episodes, with a positive family history and the first attack occurring either before the age of thirteen months or between thirteen and thirty months (Lennox Buchthal, 1973). More recently in Wales, Wallace and Aldridge Smith (1980) have demonstrated the equally successful prophylaxis of febrile convulsions using daily Phenobarbitone (4–5 mg/kg), or daily Valproic acid, (20–30 mg/kg). Valproic acid appeared the drug of choice (see below).

Usually television epilepsy can be treated without drugs. The child should view the screen from a distance of at least two metres, either in an illuminated room or with an illuminated table lamp on the set (preferably colour rather than black and white) in order to diminish the contrast. Should it be necessary for the child to approach the set, then one eye should be firmly occluded with the palm of one hand, for there is good experimental evidence that this greatly reduces the amount of seizure discharge (Jeavons and Harding, 1972). Should a drug ever be required in the management of this condition, then sodium valproate is the one of choice (BMJ Editorial, 1977). Polaroid sunglasses should be worn on visits to the seaside.

DRUG THERAPY

Unless there are very special reasons to the contrary, it is hoped that all children with convulsive disorders will have the investigations, assessment and the commencement of any indicated drug therapy at appropriate hospital level as envisaged in the Reid report, 'People with Epilepsy' (1969).

In this way some of the very small number of children likely to benefit from neurosurgery will be identified. Between out-patient reviews it is hoped that the G P will provide interested supervision. Such consultations are necessary for discussion of individual problems, clinical examination for the detection of new physical signs (especially for the early signs of untoward drug reaction) as well as for the issuing of prescriptions for the anti-convulsant drugs. The 'mail order' method, whereby repeat prescriptions for these drugs are issued and the child not seen for a long time – often years – is to be deplored. Optimal rational drug therapy of children with epilepsy is vital to their quality of life.

Drug metabolism in infants and young children differs from that in adults in many ways (Ch. 34). Children are thought to metabolize drugs quicker than adults (Richens, 1975), and as Illingworth (1973) has pointed out factors such as acidosis, dehydration and activity affect children to a greater degree than adults.

During the last few years, largely due to the availability of methods for measuring serum levels of anticonvulsant drugs, our knowledge has increased greatly concerning the interaction between anticonvulsants and between anticonvulsants and other drugs. Although most of the work has been done on healthy adult volunteers it seems reasonable to suppose that (subject to the differences in drug metabolism between adults and children discussed earlier) the results are largely applicable to children.

Commonly used anticonvulsants like phenobarbitone, primidone, phenytoin and carbamazepine have the capacity of inducing the activity of liver enzyme systems. Often this results in the increased metabolism and excretion of anticonvulsants and other drugs, and consequent falls in therapeutically effective serum levels.

Steroid metabolism is accelerated by these anticonvulsants which may account for the poor response to dexamethazone, for example for children with asthma and epilepsy, and for the failure of the contraceptive pill in girls with epilepsy. The treatment of concurrent fungal infections with griseofulvin may be similarly disappointing. In the case of sulthiame however the reverse may happen when prescribed with phenytoin. Phenytoin metabolism may be inhibited, with the rise of phenytoin serum levels and the production of toxic signs or even an increased number of fits.

Vitamin D metabolism is increased by anticonvulsant induced liver enzyme activity and anticonvulsant rickets in children or osteomalacia in adults are now recognised.

It is thought that children with epilepsy on the commoner anticonvulsant drugs have a greater incidence of bony fractures perhaps due to their frequent falls in fits and to defective mineralisation of their bones because of the mechanism just described. In controlled studies in Denmark, Christiansen and his colleagues (1975) have indicated the possible benefit of concurrent prophylactic Vitamin D and anticonvulsant therapy. Folate deficiency, which has long been recognised – in varying degrees – as an accompaniment of prolonged anticonvulsant therapy could be due to liver enzyme induction and it has also been postulated that the same mechanism may be responsible for the depletion of Vitamin K dependent clotting factors in the babies of mothers taking anticonvulsants, with the consequent production of spontaneous – often cerebral – haemorrhages in their new born babies.

Anticonvulsant drugs are now considered to be 'probable' teratogenic drugs and malformations are significantly more common in the offspring of mothers with epilepsy taking anticonvulsants in pregnancy than in the general population or in the offspring of mothers with epilepsy not taking anticonvulsant drugs (Smithells, 1978). Clinically indicated anticonvulsant therapy clearly must be continued in pregnancy – or even increased – and since it has been postulated that a folic acid deficiency state may be involved in the teratogenic action of these drugs, it seems sensible to commence folic acid supplements very early in pregnancy (Richens, 1978). An increased incidence of cleft palate, minor correctable peripheral skeletal defects (such as syndactyly or polydactyly) and the correctable forms of congenital cardiac lesions (ductus arteriosus and coarctation of the aorta) born to pregnant mothers taking phenytoin has been noted (Speidel and Meadow, 1972).

Principles of anticonvulsant therapy

Maximal seizure control with minimal or no untoward effects should be the aim. Regularity of administration of prescribed medication, with adjustment of dosages due to changes in weight, are important. The traditional thrice daily administration, previously decided on clinical grounds has now been replaced by once or twice daily administration, as a result of a better appreciation of the plasma half life concentration of the drugs made possible by the development of techniques for measuring anticonvulsant serum levels.

In recent work, for example, Corvanis and Jeavons (1980) advocate single daily doses – at night – with sodium valproate and other anticonvulsants, with the exception of carbamazepine which requires twice daily administration. It is now thought best to commence therapy with a small dose and in the absence of side effects quickly increase to an average dose, having regard to the child's body weight, in order to establish effective blood levels as soon as possible. This is especially true of primidone, where, occasionally, only one very small dose will produce extreme and prolonged drowsiness. Similarly, unacceptable dizziness may accompany other than small initial dosages of carbamazepine.

In view of the new knowledge of drug interactions, the current aim, whenever possible, is to stabilize the child on one drug, or two at the most. The dose of the single drug should be increased until there is good seizure control or unacceptable side effects supervene. Before being considered ineffective, the drug should be given in full therapeutic dosages for up to a month. If it proves to be unsatisfactory therapeutically, then another drug should be substituted. This is best accomplished by starting the new drug in small dosages and increasing these quickly with the patient under close supervision until the second drug is in the therapeutic range for about a week, before withdrawing the first drug gradually. Where the first drug has caused acute toxic signs then it should be withdrawn more quickly and the second drug started as indicated above.

When discontinuation of anticonvulsant therapy is advised by hospital, usually after a period of two or three seizure free years and there being no contraindication (e.g. incipient puberty or subclinical seizure discharge), this should be implemented gradually and progressively over several months.

Diabetes mellitus and epilepsy are two conditions which commonly become uncontrolled with puberty. If a child has been seizure free and reduction of anticonvulsant therapy is indicated, it would be wise to defer this until adolescence is well established, if there are signs of early puberty. Before leaving therapy, perhaps mention should be made of other methods of treating epilepsy. For practical purposes at the present time, this concerns the various diets. Ketogenic diets – composed largely of fats and medium chain triglyceride diets – are used in some cases as an adjunct to drug therapy or alone, where there has been a disappointing response to the treatment of severe epilepsy by anticonvulsant drugs. These diets require expert supervision from hospital paediatric and dietetric departments.

Safety in prescribing

The GP should never write a prescription for an anticonvulsant drug for a child, even on the written advice of a consultant, without being aware of its mode of action, rate and method of excretion, contraindications and side effects, interaction with other drugs and dosage. Errors in typing and at other stages in the transmission of information are all too easy and call for con-

Table 39.1 Drug treatment of status epilepticus

Drug	*Dose (mg/kg)*	*Route*	*Directions*
Diazepam	0.25–1.0	IV	Slow IV injection which may be repeated if necessary in 30 min. Contra indicated in children with diabetes mellitus or other types of disordered carbohydrate metabolism. Do not give if paraldehyde or barbiturates administered parenterally in the same episode of status unless resuscitative measures are to hand, because of respiratory depression McMorris and McWilliam (1969)
Diazepam	0.25–1.0	Rectally	Undiluted parenteral preparation administered rectally using a disposable polystyrene syringe lubricated with usual rectal lubricating jelly or bland household soap. Buttocks then strapped together. Preliminary rectal examination and manual evacuation of faeces if indicated. (Status epilepticus often noted in children with epilepsy, who are constipated.) Considered to be a safe and effective procedure. Should be administered early in the status. Care should be taken if the child is receiving prophylactic barbiturate therapy. Selected parents may be trained to use this mode of therapy both therapeutically and prophylactically, to prevent febrile convulsions. May be repeated in 30 min. For further details see Knudsen (1979) and Wallace (1978)
Clonazepam	0.01–0.09	IV	Requires to be reconstituted. 1 mgm clonazepam in 1 ml solvent with an ampoule containing 1 ml water for injection. Infants and young children in status epilepticus should have 0.25 mgm by slow IV injection and repeated at intervals of 30 secs until the convulsion ceases. For further details see Congdon and Forsythe (1980)
Phenytoin	5	IM or IV	Requires to be reconstituted before use. (Freeze dried preparation and diluent.) Slow injection which may be repeated in 30 min
Paraldehyde	0.1–0.2	IM	Bolus dose IV injection not advised. Give by deep IM injection, preferably in upper outer quadrant of buttock. Risk of abscess formation and damage to nerve trunks. Must be fresh and correctly stored in a cool dark place – otherwise oxidation to acetic acid occurs. Use in polystyrene syringes not advised although polypropylene syringes may be used

Table 39.2 Common anticonvulsant drugs

Drug	*Daily dose (mg/kg)*	*Type of seizure for which the drug is indicated*	*Comment*
Phenytoin	5–8	Major and focal	Usual first choice. Narrow margin between therapeutic and toxic doses. Gum hypertrophy common. Watch for ataxia, nystagmus, hirsutes (irreversible) and glandular fever like illness with rash and lymphadenopathy. Megaloblastic anaemia and permanent cerebellar damage may occur rarely. Toxic doses may actually increase the number of fits
Phenobarbitone	5–8	Major and focal some neonatal seizures	Less popular than before. Poor but fairly safe anticonvulsant. Causes irritability in young children and drowsiness and behaviour difficulties in older children
Primidone	5–15	Major, focal and temporal lobe	A barbiturate derivative. Use very cautiously at first, with very small doses because of the initial extreme drowsiness. Avoid combination with other barbiturates
Carbamazepine	20–30	Major, focal and especially temporal lobe	Very useful drug. May help 'mood'. Watch for extra pyramidal signs, erythematous and light sensitive eruptions. Blood dyscrasias are rare. Commence therapy with small doses because of initial dizziness
Sulthiame	10–15	Major and temporal lobe	Hyperpnoea occasionally noted with theoretical precipitation of associated petit mal seizures. Paraesthesia of extremities and crystalluria may occur. Tendency to inhibit the metabolism of concurrently prescribed phenytoin with the production of phenytoin toxicity. A sulphonamide derivative
Nitrazepam	0.5	Myoclonic and infantile spasms	Lethargy and feeding difficulties in babies may occur
Ethosuximide	20–60	Petit mal only	Drug of choice for many years. May precipitate latent grand mal seizures. Rarely ataxia and leucopenia may occur
Troxidone	20–60	Petit mal only	First effective drug for petit mal. Not much used now. May precipitate latent grand mal. Glare phenomena, agranulocytosis and nephrotic syndrome may occur

Table 39.2 Continued

Drug	*Daily dose (mg/kg)*	*Type of seizure for which the drug is indicated*	*Comment*
Sodium valproate	20–30	Petit mal, especially Ethosuximide resistant. Major seizure, flicker epilepsy and prophylaxis of febrile convulsion where indicated	Relatively new in UK but many years of continental use. May cause temporary loss of hair, affect the appetite – and rarely cause thrombocytopaenia and/or hepatotoxicity. Probably idiosyncratic rather than dose-related. Monitoring of platelets and liver function advised for children on long term therapy. See Ware and Millward Sadler (1980)
Triclofos syrup	20–50	Neonatal and infantile seizures. Serial grand mal seizures	Tolerated better than chloralhydrate. Often successful in preventing serial major seizures from progressing to status epilepticus
Clonazepam	0.5–1 (infants) 1–3 children up to 5 3–6 children from 5–12 years N.B. These are total daily dosages which may be divided	Neonatal seizures, tonic/clonic seizure, myclonic epilepsy, focal seizures	Commence therapy with low doses (i.e. 0.5 mgm/day for children and 0.25 mgm/day for infants and small children and then progressively increase dosages, within the appropriate age range until a clinical response is obtained. Watch for somnolence, hypotonia, incoordination and excessive salivation.
Acetazolamide	5–10	Mild forms of petit mal useful adjunct to other anticonvulsants	Not an anticonvulsant as such, but a diuretic. Helpful in premenstrual exacerbation of fits but thought to potentiate the action of other anticonvulsants by lowering cerebral pH. A sulphonamide derivative; crystalluria and rarely thromboycytopoenia may occur
ACTH Prednisolone		Infantile spasms	Use under hospital direction

stant vigilance. The GP cannot be expected to carry all the information in his head, but it should be available at his elbow in the consulting room and he should not be ashamed to refer to the BNF and other works of reference when necessary, even in front of the mother and child. The mother and when old enough, the child, should be instructed carefully and precisely on dosage and of the dangers of not keeping strictly to the dosage prescribed. Drugs should be kept in locked receptacles when young children are at risk in the house. There should be an established routine in the surgery for the issue of repeat prescriptions, with close control by the GP who should ensure that he is seeing the child frequently enough to ensure complete surveillance. It is helpful if school children taking anticonvulsant drugs can carry a card giving details of therapy and the address of the issuing hospital and the GP. See Tables 39.1 and 39.2 for further details of anticonvulsant drugs.

EDUCATION

Children with epilepsy are educationally vulnerable in ways which may not be readily apparent, even if their control of overt seizures appears good. Thus detailed enquiries about a childs' school progress from parents, teachers and from colleagues in community medicine, together with perusal of school reports, should form an important part of the total management of these children.

Apart from the practical long term consideration of any child with a chronic handicap being optimally educationally equipped so that he can become self supporting, it should be appreciated that educational failure and under achievement at school are potent causes of frustration, ridicule and inevitably behaviour problems. It will just not do for a child to sit at a desk and 'give no trouble'. He must be totally and actively involved in the full life of the school.

It is recognised that a child with epilepsy can be free from overt seizures and alleged to have an IQ within the normal range yet do badly in school: some of the causes are as follows:

1. The child may be having sub clinical seizure discharges – as discussed earlier – which diminish his intellectual performance. Familiar tasks may be performed quite well but he may have difficulty in coping with more complicated ones (Holdsworth and Whitmore, 1974).

2. A verbally biased intelligence test like the Terman Merrill, may produce a spuriously high IQ score – especially in a child from an articulate family, by concealing difficulties in perception, caused by selective structural brain damage as in temporal lobe lesions or sub clinical seizure discharge in areas of the brain which deal with the reception, processing and appreciation of sensory information. A comprehensive psychometric assessment in a child with epilepsy who is under-achieving is therefore mandatory, so that appropriate teaching programmes may be devised.

3. Drug therapy per se may be responsible for poor school performance. Hutt et al (1968) have shown that decision making and other tasks in paced situations may be impaired by phenobarbitone at therapeutic, i.e. non toxic blood levels. Also, Stores (1975) has drawn attention to the subtle and selective ways in which some anticonvulsant drugs, especially phenobarbitone, phenytoin and sulthiame can sometimes affect learning processes. Holdsworth and Whitmore (1974) studied children with epilepsy attending ordinary schools. They found that only a third of the children were making wholly satisfactory progress, half were performing indifferently or below average, a sixth were falling appreciably behind and a fifth presented serious behaviour problems.

Residential placement is indicated for children who by reason of their epilepsy are failing to make progress in non residential schools or whose epilepsy is causing significant disruption in the school.

Whilst understanding the initial reluctance of some parents to consider such placement where recommended by a paediatrician and specialist in community medicine (child health), the GP can do a great service to the child by encouraging the parents to accept the offer. Once placement is recommended the sooner it is implemented the better. In a modern boarding school environment, with frequent home contacts, the child will have investigation and treatment of his epilepsy, maybe involving such up to date techniques as long term ambulatory EEG monitoring (using an invisible portable apparatus) with superimposition of the tracing on a closed circuit TV screen picture, thus correlating the EEG pattern and the appearances of the child. At the same time education is carried out in smaller classes, where self pacing techniques and fractionation of the information to be presented in the lessons are used. If indicated, the children are then referred to nearby neurological or neurosurgical departments. Rehabilitation is the aim of these establishments and many children are sufficiently fortunate to return home with their epilepsy controlled, having had remedial education, so that they may attend their appropriate local school.

No account of epilepsy should fail to mention the British Epilepsy Association which exists to improve the lot of all people with this condition and membership is open to all who are sympathetic to its aims. It is actively concerned with children and its activities range from sponsoring research to practical advice with regard to employment and holidays. There is a vigorous and comprehensive education programme, designed to disseminate reliable information about epilepsy to all sections of the community. Membership of the Association is wholeheartedly recommended to parents of children with epilepsy and to GPs. Further information and help can be obtained from the Secretary, The British Epilepsy Association, Crowthorne House, New Workingham Road, Workingham, Berkshire RG11 2AY, (STD 034 46) 3122.

REFERENCES

BMJ Editorial (1977) Management of childhood epilepsy. *British Medical Journal*, **1**, 986.

Brett, E.M. (1973) Epilepsy in Childhood. *British Journal of Hospital Medicine*, **9**, 177.

Brown, J.K. (1973) Convulsions in the Newborn Period. *Developmental Medicine & Child Neurology*, **15**, 823.

Christiansen, C., Rodbro, P. & Thoger Neilson, C. (1975) Iatrogenic Osteomalacia in Epileptic Children. *Acta Paediatrica Scandinavia*, **64**, 219.

Congdon, P.J. & Forsythe, W.I. (1980) Intravenous Clonazepam in the Treatment of Status Epilepticus in Children. *Epilepsia*, **21**, 97.

Corvanis A. & Jeavons P.M. (1980) Once daily Sodium Valproate in the Treatment of Epilepsy. *Developmental Medicine & Child Neurology*, **22**, No.2 202.

Guthkelch A.N. (1971) Whiplash Injuries and Subdural Haematoma. *British Medical Journal*, **2**, 430.

Harper J.R. (1968) True Myoclonic Epilepsy in Childhood. *Archives of Disease in Childhood*, **43**, 28.

Holdsworth L. & Whitmore T.K. (1974) A study of Children with Epilepsy Attending Ordinary Schools. *Developmental Medicine & Child Neurology*, **16**, 746.

Hutt S.J., Jackson P.M., Belsham A. & Higgins G. (1968) Perceptual Motor Behaviour in Relation to Blood Phenobarbitone Level: A Preliminary Report. *Developmental Medicine & Child Neurology*, **10**, 626.

Illingworth R.S. (1973) Drug Dosage for Children. *Prescribers Journal D.H.S.S. Volume 13 No 6*, 124.

Jeavons P.M. (1977) Choice of Drug Therapy in Epilepsy. *The Practitioner*, Volume **219**, 542.

Jeavons P.M. (1978) The Practical Management of Epilepsy *Update*, Volume 10, No 3. 269.

Jeavons P.M. & Harding G.F.A. (1970) Television Epilepsy. *Lancet*, **2**, 926.

Jennett W.B. (1969) Early Traumatic Epilepsy Definition and Identity. *Lancet*, **1**, 1023.

Jennett W.B. (1972) Head Injuries in Children. *Developmental Medicine & Child Neurology*, **14**, 137.

Knudsen F.U. (1979) Rectal Administration of Diazepam in Solution in the Acute Treatment of Convulsions in Infants and Children. *Archives of Diseases in Childhood*, **54**, 855.

Lennox Buchthal M.A. (1973) Febrile Convulsions A Reappraisal *Electro encephalography & Clinical Neurophysiology Suppl*, **32**.

McMorris S. & McWilliam P.K.A. (1969) Status Epilepticus in Infants & Young Children Treated with Parenteral Diazepam. *Archives of Diseases in Childhood*, **44**, 604.

NIH Consensus (1980) Febrile seizures: long-term management of children with fever-associated seizures. *British Medical Journal*, **2**, 277–279.

Ounsted C., Hutt S.J. & Lee D. (1963) The Retrograde Amnesia of Petit Mal. *Lancet*, **1**, 671.

Ounsted C., Lindsay J. & Norman R. (1966) Biological Factors in Temporal Lobe Epilepsy. In Clinics in Developmental Medicine, Spastics Society London: Heinemann.

Reid Report (1969) People with Epilepsy. D.H.S.S. London: H.M.S.O.

Richens A. (1975) Drug Interaction in Epilepsy. *Developmental Medicine & Child Neurology*, **17**, 94.

Richens A. (1978) Choice of Drugs in Epilepsy. Prescribers Journal D.H.S.S. H.M.S.O. London **18**, No 6 126.

Ross E.M., Peckham Catherine, West P. & Butler N. (1980) Epilepsy in Childhood: Findings from the National Child Development Study. *British Medical Journal*, **1**, 207–210.

Rowan A.J., & Scott D.F. (1970) Major Status Epilepticus. *Acte Neurologia Scandinavica*, **46**, 573.

Rutter M., Graham P. & Yule W. (1970) A Neuropsychiatric Study in Childhood. In Clinics in Developmental Medicine London: Heinemann

Smithells, R.W. (1978) Drugs, Infections and Congenital Abnormalities. *Archives of Disease in Childhood*, **53**, 2, 93.

Speidel B.D. & Meadow S.R. (1972) Maternal Epilepsy and Abnormalities of the Foetus and Newborn. *Lancet*, **2**, 8, 39.

Stores G. (1978) Behavioural Effects of Anti Epileptic Drugs. *Developmental Medicine & Child Neurology*, **17**, 647.

Wallace S.J. (1978) Febrile Convulsions and Epilepsy in Childhood. *Medical News*, **10**, No 41, 15.

Wallace S.J. & Aldridge Smith J. (1980) Successful Prophylaxis Against Febrile Convulsions with Valproic Acid and Phenobarbitone. *British Medical Journal*, **280**, 383.

Ware, S. & Millward-Sadler, G.I. (1980) Sodium valproate and liver disease. *Lancet*, **2**, 110.

40

Deafness in childhood

John Tuke

The family doctor's special relationship with his patient and his understanding of the deaf child's personal environment render him the ideal person to oversee and guide his development. Quality of care in medical, social and educational terms dictates the alternatives of disaster or success for this child's life. Late diagnosis, inadequate support and poor educational facilities lead to a future with unintelligible speech, absence of social and academic skills, emotional disturbance and dismal job prospects. Early suspicion, precise diagnosis and understanding help for the family can lead to near-normal speech and communication. Amplification of sound, making use of every scrap of residual hearing, together with the teaching methods now available, can enable the deaf child to take his place in society as a literate and whole personality, expressing himself through the normally understood media. All this depends upon the early application of modern teaching methods, initially through home tuition and sustained throughout his school years.

The tactful family doctor can play an important part in ensuring the provision of all these ingredients for success, though often he is required merely to observe with approval. There will be occasions, however, when his co-ordinating capacity will be invaluable in ensuring that his patient receives the best service available. He also carries the key to early detection and diagnosis. Failure to discover the deaf child early, leaves the door shut to all other assistance. In order to benefit from the help now obtainable, we must aim at the detection of congenital hearing loss by nine months of age. The majority of children suffering from severe deafness are still not discovered until their third or fourth year, (BATD, 1977; Upfold, 1978). The reduction of this timelag should now be engaging the attention of us all.

At least one child in every thousand is born profoundly deaf. It has been estimated that as many as 20 per cent of school entrants show some hearing impairment if only unilateral, most of these being of a conductive type associated with the common ENT problems found in that age group. In the National Child Development Study some five per cent of seven year olds showed a degree of hearing impairment, and four years later in the same group 1.2 per cent had some significant loss (NCDS, 1969, 1974). These children with partial and temporary hearing loss are educationally at a disadvantage, and certainly merit medical treatment (see Ch. 18).

The concept of 'at risk' observation registers proved counter-productive but whilst all infants and children should be screened for deafness, there is certainly a group who are generally liable to be born with this handicap and they deserve special consideration from those responsible for infant surveillance. This group includes infants in the following categories:

1. Family history of deafness.
2. Perinatal hypoxia.
3. Low birth weight.
4. Hyperbilirubinaemia – for example due to rhesus incompatibility.
5. Cerebral palsy and central nervous system underdevelopment.
6. Maternal rubella in pregnancy.

Intra-uterine rubella may be responsible for a large number of cases of congenital sensory deafness. Of 112 profoundly deaf children under four years of age, 61 had rubella antibodies compared with 7.1 per cent in a control group. In the same study this disease was thought to be the cause of deafness in 82 of 139 children of six months to seven years of age. In 60 of these children hearing loss was the only rubella defect noted. (Gumpel *et al*, 1971). In the light of these findings the incidence of congenital deafness may fall during the next 10 years as a result of the current programme, which aims to immunise all schoolgirls against this virus infection.

Post-natal illnesses carrying a high risk of subsequent deafness are meningitis and encephalitis. All infants in these high risk categories require special observation and merit repeat hearing tests. The first suspicion of deafness usually arises in the parents (Lawson, 1980).

Reassurance of the mother anxious about her infant's hearing, requires the scientific positive evidence of repeated and properly performed hearing tests. The relative rarity of severe congenital deafness may lead to complacency, resulting in easy optimistic encouragement with subsequent disaster. An unusually quiet and contented baby or excessive monotonous crying can both suggest hearing impairment. Failure to startle to sudden noise and a lack of response to mother's voice are obvious but frequently missed early signs.

The early detection of hearing loss is vitally important because the first eighteen months of life appear to be a critical period for reception of sound stimulation and a time during which the child is 'ready to hear', rather parallel to the first few weeks of life during which he is 'ready to swim'. Once past, this intense receptivity is not repeated. During the second year of life the infant is 'ready to speak'.

Diagnosis before 12 months of age is of such consequence that an understanding of the methods used is necessary for all those responsible for monitoring the development of infants and children. The actual procedures for hearing testing will usually be performed by health visitors or community nurses, but the doctor involved with his own practice child health clinic or the clinical medical officer in an area health authority clinic will need to be reassured of the validity of such test results by critical observation of the technique used in the light of his own knowledge.

Whereas in 87 per cent of 210 Health Districts in England, Wales and Northern Ireland, all infants are hearing tested by health visitors, many must pass this test who subsequently prove to be profoundly deaf (Health Visitors Association Survey, 1977). Some 72 per cent of these health visitors have received special training, usually a two day course. There appears to be some lack of uniformity in this training and in the provision of refresher courses. In many areas no re-training is provided and in most, the health visitors themselves do not receive hearing tests, though normal hearing is important for adequate interpretation of tests.

Over the speech range of sound frequencies, approximately 250 Hz to 8000 Hz, hearing loss may involve predominantly more or less of the various low or high frequencies. The commonly used charts display hearing loss in decibels – db. It is normally accepted that ability to detect pure tones up to 20 decibels over the 400 Hz to 4000 Hz range constitutes normal hearing for speech. This would be expressed on the chart as shown, meaning that the child hears these sounds at a minimum intensity of 20 db or in other words has a 20 db hearing loss. A mild hearing loss of 20 to 30 db evenly distributed over this frequency range is often found in acquired conductive deafness, due for example to otitis media or 'glue ear' and will cause some difficulty in discrimination of speech even if only unilateral (Fig. 40.1). The more severe congenital 'nerve' deafness usually involves predominantly the high frequencies (Fig. 40.2).

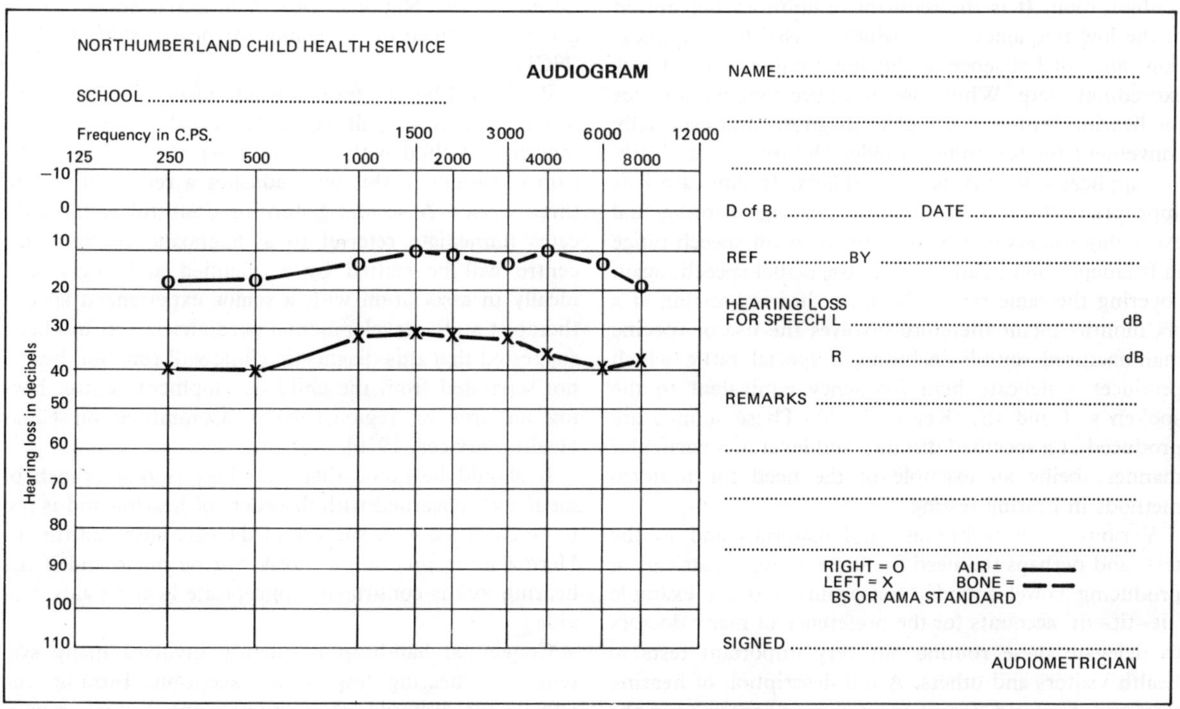

Fig. 40.1 This child's school progress had deteriorated over the previous three months

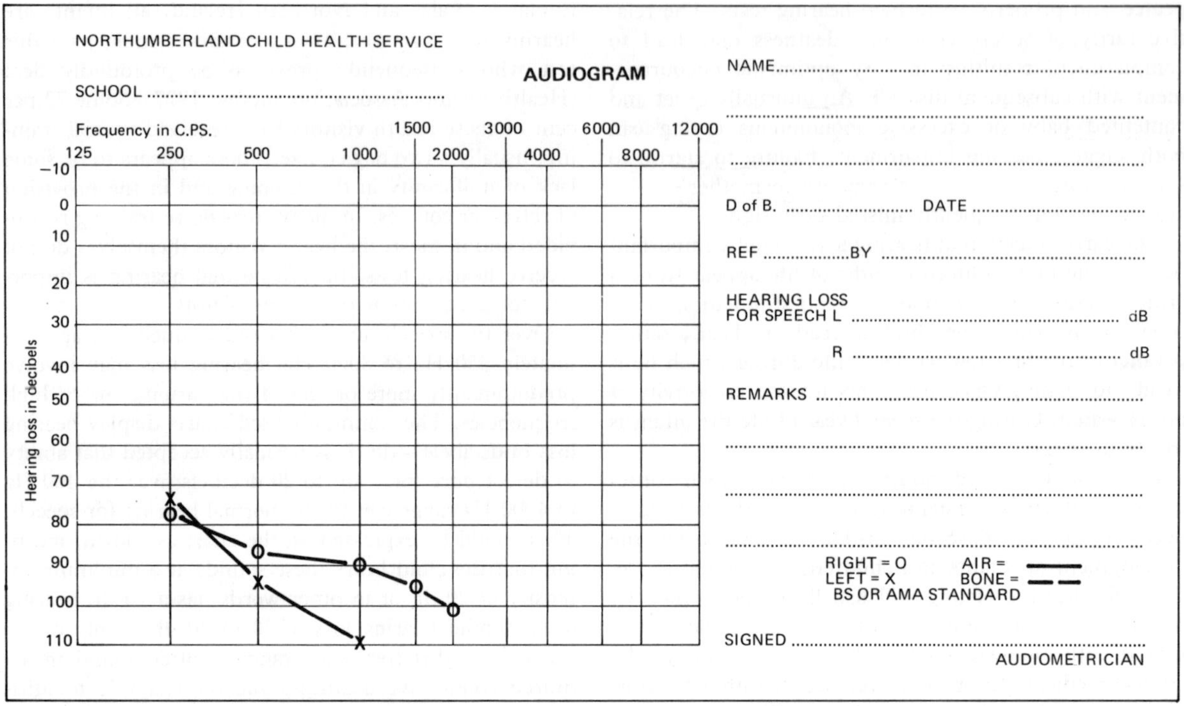

Fig. 40.2 Severe congenital deafness with some residual low frequency hearing detected at 9 months screening examination

The potential for speech development depends upon the degree of hearing loss rather than the audiogram configuration. It is the remnant of auditory perception in the low frequency range which is used for amplification, and total absence of this low frequency residue is exceedingly rare. Whilst use of a pure tone audiometer for hearing testing is useful in diagnosis and especially convenient for screening in older children, it is clearly not applicable to infants and toddlers. In any case it is appropriate to test an infant's hearing using actual every-day sounds which cover the relevant speech range in frequency and in addition, to use actual speech, again covering the same range. Adequate hearing testing of a six months infant therefore involves the use of specific manufactured sounds including a special rattle which produces a delicate high frequency equivalent to the spoken s, f and sh, (Kemp, 1976). These sounds are produced at a specified distance and level in a particular manner, being an example of the need for uniform methods in hearing testing.

Various other techniques and materials add to the test, and perhaps the need for some minor theatricals in producing vowel sounds, consonants and for example 'tit–tit–tit' accounts for the preference of many doctors to delegate these routine but very important tests to health visitors and others. A full description of hearing tests suitable for different age groups is contained in the *Manual for Stycar Hearing Tests* by Mary Sheridan (1976). This comprehensive booklet is provided with the Stycar equipment. A brief policy document produced by the National Deaf Children's Society gives general guidance on screening for deafness in children (NCDS, 1980).

Performed by two trained health visitors in quiet conditions the tests will certainly reveal a six to nine months old child with hearing impairment. Any suspicion of failure in this test indicates a repeat in two to three weeks. A second failure or doubtful result indicates immediate referral to a diagnostic centre. This centre will be staffed by a qualified audiologist and ideally in association with a senior experienced speech therapist and a developmental paediatrician. It has been suggested that this diagnostic clinic will function best if not separated from the child development centre, having an area or regional basis (Committee on Child Health Services, 1976).

It should be noted that audiology is that branch of medicine concerned with disorders of hearing and is not to be confused with surgery of the ear, nose and throat. Here a more precise diagnosis will be made and if the hearing loss is confirmed, appropriate hearing aids provided.

Congenital handicap frequently involves many systems and hearing loss is no exception. Intra-uterine rubella for example, may produce intellectual impairment, visual disorders, motor and other problems. It is therefore important to avoid treating the hearing loss in isolation without overall assessment. Hence the need for readily available opinions from psychologist, developmental paediatrician and ENT surgeon. A multiple handicapped child may require the additional diagnostic facilities of electrical response audiometry including electro-cochleography, brain stem auditory electric response and post auricular muscle response. In a mentally retarded child such techniques can be especially helpful in diagnosis. Only certain specialised centres can offer these facilities.

Detection of hearing loss in the older child is simpler to perform and will not be detailed here. These tests will normally be carried out at two years of age, in the first school year and subsequently at least every two years whilst at school. At two years of age the responsibility will lie with the child health clinic and testing usually forms part of a birthday examination. Speech delay at this time will always give rise to suspicion of hearing loss, though this may be only partial or unilateral. The hearing tests are designed to display these defects. It is important to ensure that once a diagnosis of permanent deafness has been made, a full account is entered in the general practitioner's case record. Some form of tagging of the record is also desirable.

A diagnosis of congenital deafness having been established in the audiology clinic, a home tutor for the deaf will commence visits forthwith. This teacher is primarily concerned with development of communication abilities and speech but will also help the parents to develop their own skills in offering their child the maximum stimulation through other senses and through hearing aids. There is an increasing awareness of the need for specially trained social workers and it is at this point, shortly after diagnosis, that their support will be of maximum value. The National Deaf Childrens' Society can offer help to the family, for example by introducing experienced parents with a similar problem. Parents repeatedly speak of the need for support, especially in the months following diagnosis. In areas having an adequate number of home tutors, this support has hitherto been supplied by them. Families express gratitude for the dedicated help given by the home teacher for the deaf but an increase in the number of social workers with their special expertise will answer the dissatisfaction frequently expressed regarding lack of information about equipment, financial aids available, educational toys and self help groups.

We have seen that early diagnosis should very quickly lead to medical assistance, counselling and special teaching methods. The latter will be home based. This teacher will work closely with the audiologist, health visitor and social worker, when available.

The terms manualism and oralism represent the extremes in the basic methods of teaching deaf children. They refer to the use of sign language and conversely the development of natural speech. Communication by means of manual signs alone has virtually disappeared in Great Britain and there is a strong movement towards vocal speech methods. Various systems have developed, using differing proportions of these systems. Enthusiasts in each camp can produce convincing arguments in their favour and further research is needed to establish the most effective methods. A system of oralism where some residual hearing allows the use of hearing aids, enables the child to remain in a normal school with the assistance of a special unit for the hearing-impaired. The great advantage is the more natural socialisation with hearing children. However, a more concentrated system in a special school for deaf children using both oral and sign systems, can achieve excellent communication. The obvious disadvantage is the relative isolation and the tendency to encourage the concept of handicap in the child's environment.

The whole subject of teaching methodology is under review. The system described here relates to many areas in the United Kingdom. At present there are at least 480 units for partially hearing children attached to ordinary schools. The pre-school child with a specific hearing loss will normally attend a nursery group with a unit for hearing-impaired children but will join the main-stream in the school for many activities. He will not be taught sign language but will 'listen' with his residual hearing and will become a skilled lip reader. He will have the advantage of hearing and producing normal language with the help of electronic equipment such as the Sonic Aid stereophonic transmitter/receiver, allowing teacher to pupil communication on a radio basis. This system gives the child freedom of movement and incorporates frequency control whereby his personal transmission is matched to his audiogram profile.

As his education progresses the deaf child will attend similar special units, but always within normal schools. He will usually spend a reducing period of his day in this unit and on reaching his GCE period may attend only occasionally, having now developed communication skills approaching those of his friends with normal hearing. The teaching staff employed in these departments have specialised training and qualifications and will be in close touch with the child's parents and his audiologist.

The young person with a handicap requires particular assistance when nearing school leaving age. In some areas therefore the 15 year old with hearing loss will be the subject of a 'school leavers' panel'. This system proves supportive and effective in finding suitable employment or further educational prospects and deserves to be more widespread. The panel meets twice during the subject's penultimate school year and his final year. It is attended by teaching staff, educational psychologist, school medical officer and the youth employment officer with special responsibility for the handicapped. The subject's parents are also invited. Some young people discussed at these meetings require little assistance, having achieved adequate language development and with good academic prospects.

As always in medical practice, one hears such a satisfying result without complacency. What action ought we to be taking to prevent the future deafness of those young people exposed to sustained levels of sound above 100 db in discotheques (BMJ Editorial, 1970; Swain, 1974)?

REFERENCES

British Medical Journal Editorial (1970) Music causing deafness. *British Medical Journal*, **2**, 127.

British Association for Teachers of the Deaf (1977) Association Evidence to the Royal Commission on the National Health Service.

Committee on Child Health Services (1976) *Fit for the Future*. Court report. London: HMSO.

Gregory, (1976) *The Deaf Child and his Family*. London: Allen and Unwin.

Gumpel, S.M., Dudgeon, J.A. *et al* (1971) Congenital Perceptive Deafness; Role of Intrauterine Rubella. *British Medical Journal*, **2**, 300.

Kemp, D. (1976) The Nuffield Rattle. *Journal of the British Society of Audiology*.

Lawson, G.R. *et al* (1980) A Survey of Deaf Children in Northumberland. Awaiting publication.

National Deaf Children's Society (1980) The Screening of Hearing Impaired Children. NDCS, 45 Hereford Road, London.

Sheridan, M.D. (1976) *Manual for the stycar hearing tests*. Slough: NFER.

Swain, M.S. (1974) Discotheque Deafness. *British Medical Journal*, **4**, 532.

Upfold, J. (1979) *Medical Journal of Australia*, **2**, 507.

41

Visual disorders in childhood

Philip Whitfield

When considering visual disorders in childhood it is necessary to understand some general principles. At birth neither the retina nor the visual cortex is fully functioning and normal visual experience is necessary for visual acuity to develop. A baby with congenital cataracts will therefore require early surgery if permanent and irreversible visual handicap is to be avoided. The acuity of a newly squinting eye may be lost in a few weeks. Young babies are interested in near objects, such as their own fingers and their mother's face, and can fixate and follow objects from birth. Any visual deprivation may have a lasting effect during these early critical days, so every effort must be made to detect defects early, to correct them as soon as possible, and to make maximum use of all residual vision.

Children will be unaware of visual defects until they are old enough to compare experiences with their contemporaries. The routine testing of all babies and young children is therefore essential if defects are to be discovered early enough to respond to treatment. Particular attention should be given to those at special risk: very small babies, especially those given oxygen at birth; babies whose mothers contracted infections during pregnancy; children with other physical or mental handicaps; and babies born into families with a history of visual defects.

Deaf children need keen eyesight to interpret lip movements and facial expressions; their vision should be carefully tested at regular intervals throughout childhood, to make sure that they are able to learn from visual stimuli. Mentally handicapped children derive benefit from progressive training in visual perception and visual communication.

Many general practitioners are now experienced in checking the visual competence of babies and young children, or they work with health visitors who are themselves specially trained and experienced. They should review regularly the arrangements for testing the children in their practices, insisting upon a high standard of competence in themselves and others.

The eyesight of all babies should be checked at a very early age to see whether they follow a light or a hanging ball, at about 12 inches, and whether the pupils react. By six months most babies will observe a pellet on a flat surface and may approach it with the hand. Matching tests are useful for older children, until they can manage Snellen's types. The matching tests may first be carried out using miniature toys, and later with Stycar five-letter or seven-letter cards. The child matches with his finger on a card the letter being shown. The use of a dark screen with a ball on a stick may be more convenient in general practice than the rolling balls test. Important though these early tests are, there is no point in attempting to correlate them with visual acuity as expressed in terms of Snellen's types.

Failure to pass a simple screening test should never be interpreted as an actual visual defect unless this has been confirmed by an ophthalmologist or ophthalmic optician. Specialist help should always be sought if any doubt exists. It should be possible to satisfy oneself that a child has normal vision by the time he has reached the age of two years.

Expert testing of vision and eye movements should be part of the general assessment of all children with actual or potential handicap of any kind. Handicaps are so often multiple. General practitioners should always make sure that handicapped children in their care do in fact receive competent visual assessment by appropriate experts at suitable intervals.

REFRACTIVE DISORDERS

Optical abnormalities, including hypermetropia and astigmatism, are inherited conditions. It is important to detect the severer forms in early childhood; particularly hypermetropia, which predisposes to squint. If one of the parents has such a condition it should be looked for in the child. Ophthalmologists are generally glad to see children at the age of two years whose parents have themselves worn glasses from an early age. Uncorrected refractive errors may have a serious effect upon visual development.

Optical anomalies do not change much as the eye develops, except in those children who develop myopia later on, usually after the age of six years. Screening the visual acuity of children at school entry is essential, using Snellen's types, or Stycar tests if necessary. Children in primary schools should be tested annually. In secondary schools testing on alternate years should be sufficient, provided no children are missed.

This testing is usually undertaken by school nurses, not always under entirely satisfactory conditions. The Keystone apparatus has certain advantages, but children who fail should be re-tested on ordinary Snellen's cards before they are referred for an ophthalmic opinion.

The standard Snellen chart consists of block capital letters without serifs. It should be used at six metres (20 ft), or three metres if looked at through a mirror. The acuity is indicated by the last complete line that can be read. The card should be on a level with the child's eye, in a good light, and free from glare. The eyes should be tested together first, then separately with the other eye occluded without pressure on the eye-ball.

Dr Mary Sheridan, using Stycar material under good conditions, obtained a normal distant vision of 6/4.5 in each eye, in a high proportion of children. She therefore considered that a visual acuity of 6/9 should be considered sub-optimal. However, under normal school conditions a visual acuity of less than 6/9 in either eye, or a discrepancy in the acuity between the two eyes, is usually the standard accepted as an indication for further testing.

The parents of children who fail these screening tests should be informed that their child appears to require sight-testing and they should be asked to take him to their general practitioner or to an ophthalmic optician. A child under the age of seven years should be referred by the general practitioner to an ophthalmologist in the first instance. Some health authorities run school eye clinics for children who have failed screening tests. These are becoming increasingly difficult to staff and so peripheral consultant units, conveniently situated, may be set up to avoid long journeys and waiting times for parents and children. General practitioners should ensure that children with disorders which may require prompt treatment to prevent visual deterioration do not have to contend with long waiting lists.

School nurses should be able to check that all children who fail screening tests are in fact further investigated. They should also be able to obtain the result of such an investigation.

A near vision test card with print of standard size should always be used at the end of a school entry vision test. Impairment of near vision may be due to hypermetropia or to astigmatism. Astigmatism is seldom important in children unless associated with a squint. In the absence of a squint hypermetropes do not usually require glasses either.

Myopic children may need re-testing as often as twice a year for a while. Changes in their error of refraction are unpredictable. They may deteriorate rapidly until their late teens. The ocular changes which cause myopia are a long eye-ball and failure of the cornea and lens curvature to compensate for this. These characteristics cannot be influenced by treatment. Myopic children tend to do well at school work and this should be encouraged. The condition is not made worse by reading.

Good cooperation between general practices and community child health services is essential if all children are to be properly screened at the appropriate ages, with further investigation of those who fail the screening tests and effective follow-up of all those who are referred to consultant units. Unless there is a fool-proof system for checking attendances and for the follow-up of defaulters, some children (particularly the socially disadvantaged who need these services most) will be missed, to the detriment of their education and sometimes with serious and permanent damage to their eyesight. Provisions for visual screening of children vary widely in their effectiveness throughout the UK. In each practice, the general practitioners and health visitors should review together from time to time the adequacy of this service in their locality, and take steps to improve it when necessary. Community child health services are supplementary to general practitioners services and in no sense a substitute for them. It is therefore part of a general practitioner's duty to his patients to see that these supplementary services are fully appreciated and used and that they are of a high standard.

ORTHOPTISTS

Orthoptists spend much of their time working with children. They analyse eye movements and field of vision defects, and also undertake precise testing of vision.

It is helpful if health visitors and school nurses concerned with the testing of children can receive training from orthoptists in the use of visual screening equipment. This avoids the unnecessary referral of many 'false positives'. Orthoptists can be very helpful in the investigation of children who appear to have squints or who fail visual screening tests. Unfortunately there are at present too few of them to fulfil these functions adequately. More use might be made of the orthoptic training which ophthalmic opticians now receive. General practitioners wishing to do the best for their young patients should refer them to specialists who have impartial appreciation of the value of glasses and a good knowledge of developmental ophthalmology.

SQUINT

Squint is a failure of the visual axis of one eye to be directed to an object being fixed by the other eye. Squint may be constant or intermittent; it may be concomitant, when the angle of squint is the same whichever eye is being used for fixation; or inconcomitant, when the angle of squint is greater during fixation by the affected eye. Squint may be right-sided, left-sided, or alternating; it may be convergent or divergent.

The achievement of binocular vision is a gradually acquired characteristic. Binocular visual reflexes may fail to develop or they may be disrupted once they have been established. Double vision is due to the stimulation of different parts of the retina by the same object; confusion is caused by two different objects stimulating the same area of the retina. Suppression follows, the visual cortex actively neglecting the image from the squinting eye. This suppression soon becomes permanent, and then amblyopia has developed.

Attention should always be paid to a mother's suspicion that her child has a squint. Examine the positions of the reflection of a distant light on the cornea of each eye. The reflections should lie in identical parts of the cornea. This will help to distinguish a true squint from the apparent convergent squint of a child with well-marked epicanthic folds.

The cover test is also useful. Rapidly cover each eye in turn with the hand while the child fixes a distant object, such as the spot of light from a pencil torch or a small toy on a stick. There will be no movement of either eye during the test if there is no squint. Repeat the test to tire the fusion correction.

A squint may be associated with an organic lesion such as cataract, retinoblastoma, or retinal dystrophy of some kind; or there may be a lesion of the afferent visual pathways, such as a craniopharyngioma. Visual acuity should therefore always be tested. A vertical element in a squint may show itself by the child tilting his head to compensate. A constant squint, no matter how young the child, requires urgent investigation. An inconstant squint should be referred if still present at the age of six months.

All children with squints must wear the glasses provided for them. This is part of the treatment, not merely a substitute for surgery. The same applies to the patching of the non-squinting eye, to compel the squinting eye to work.

After surgery the originally defective eye may still have much less than full vision but the cosmetic appearance is important. Also, the child will probably have a potentially useful eye should anything go wrong with the better one. Children with multiple handicaps should have their squint attended to at the time most appropriate from the point of view of their general development, otherwise the treatment may hold up their general progress.

COLOUR VISION

Colour defectiveness is an X-linked recessive trait. Complete absence of colour vision is extremely rare. Some degree of colour defectiveness occurs in eight per cent of males and 0.4 per cent of females. The defects are due to the absence or deficiency of photopigments in the retinal receptor cells, the cones. Of the eight per cent males most have red-green colour defects, complete in about half the cases. Defect of the third primary colour, blue, is rare.

The various screening tests are more likely to be accurate if carried out on children over the age of five years. It is reasonable to undertake colour vision screening at the same time as screening for visual acuity at school entry, but usually the testing is not done until the child goes to secondary school, when it is undertaken by school nurses. Ishihara plates are made up of dots on a background of different coloured tints. They will detect the whole range of colour defects. Children who do not recognise their numbers may be asked to trace the coloured lines with a dry paint brush. Teaching aids usually avoid colours which might be confusing to a colour-defective child, but it may be helpful for a teacher to know at an early stage.

General practitioners are not always informed when defects of colour vision are detected at routine school screening tests, but it is to be hoped that as cooperation develops such passing-on of information will become routine. If only as a back-up facility, every general practice should possess a set of Ishihara plates as part of its basic equipment. When detected, colour vision defects should be carefully recorded in the child's case notes.

The sooner a colour vision defect has been detected the easier it is to divert the youngster from preparing for an unsuitable occupation, such as air-line pilot, locomotive driver, fabric designer, naval deck personnel, or possibly electrician. If in doubt, a child may be referred to the local Employment Medical Adviser for testing with the materials actually used in industry, such as colour-coded electric wires.

EDUCATING VISUALLY HANDICAPPED CHILDREN

Children who have had sight in only one eye since infancy suffer no serious disability, provided that the remaining eye is normal.

Difficulty in reading is obviously a handicap in education, more so than poor distance vision. Reading difficulties usually become particularly serious at about seven years of age, when the ability to read small print fluently becomes imperative.

Visually handicapped children should if possible be brought up in their own homes, with the advice and support of special teachers, social workers, and field workers of the voluntary organisations. They should be encouraged to lead as normal a life as possible. Their parents and family will require every possible help in a very difficult task. A certain amount of vision is usually present and much can often be made of quite small amounts. The visual limitations can often be overcome to a remarkable degree. Only children with additional handicaps or with serious social disadvantages should require residential care.

Advisory teachers for the visually handicapped should be consulted as soon as a serious disability is recognised. There is no point in waiting until the diagnosis has been fully established, nor until it is possible to register the child as blind or partially-sighted. A specially trained teacher can give invaluable help from a very early age, sometimes using magnifiers and other low visual aids. The child's general practitioner should make sure that such help is available and is being used.

There is no clear distinction between blindness and partial-sightedness. The latter term usually refers to persons with a visual acuity of less than 6/24 in both eyes. Such children certainly require special educational methods. Blindness usually means a visual acuity of 3/60 or less, and by definition prevents people from undertaking any work for which eyesight is required.

The decision about the special educational requirements of a visually handicapped child will be made by the education authorities, in the light of ophthalmic and other reports, and bearing in mind many factors to do with the child's intelligence and social background. The sooner an advisory teacher comes to know the child and his home, the easier it is to plan suitable education for him and to enable him to achieve his full potential.

Many children with severe visual handicaps make steady educational progress, using braille literature and equipment, recorded material, and a variety of other aids and apparatus. Some kind of further education is highly desirable. Some are able to take advantage of University courses. There are a good many careers which visually handicapped persons may be able to follow; and many lead full lives in every sense.

It is evident that children with severe visual handicaps have many needs and therefore should be the concern of a number of people with different professional skills. Their investigation and assessment should be carried out in association with a child development centre, where these different professions are represented. Where there is no identifiable child development centre, there should be working arrangements established between the different branches of the medical, nursing, educational and remedial professions, to ensure that the child and his family and teachers receive clearly presented and coordinated support and advice.

GENETIC COUNSELLING

The possible risk to future generations must always be borne in mind in relation to visually handicapping conditions. The situation should be carefully explained to each young person individually, certainly before leaving school. Some will need reassurance about unexpressed and groundless fears. It is worth remembering that inherited visual disorders generally become apparent at about the same age in succeeding generations. General practitioners should make sure that their patients receive reliable advice in terms which they can understand.

OTHER OCULAR CONDITIONS

Some of the conditions about to be mentioned are rare ones which will seldom, if ever, be encountered in general practice; but it is important not to allow one's differential diagnosis to become too restricted.

Congenital cataracts may be due to factors operating during intrauterine life, such as maternal rubella. This may be associated with Down's syndrome or other congenital abnormalities. The development of cataracts in infancy may be associated with biochemical abnormalities, such as galactosaemia, or with the long-term administration of steroids. Congenital cataracts do well if they are operated upon early, if they are bilateral; if unilateral the outlook is poor. Surgical treatment should usually start when the baby is about three months old.

Lacrimation in a white, painless eye in infancy is due to delayed canalisation of the nasolacrimal duct. It has usually cleared by the age of nine months. Mechanical probing requires a general anaesthetic and should be avoided if possible. If there is associated infection, local antibiotic ointment or drops may be necessary.

Coloboma of the iris is a congenital absence of a section due to failure of fusion of embryonic tissue. It should be treated with respect in case the defect extends into the retina and choroid.

Congenital ptosis requires treatment only if the eyelid covers the pupil.

Congenital glaucoma (buphthalmos) is a rare condition except in families with a marked predisposition. It is usually unilateral and due to a failure of separation of the iris and cornea, producing obstruction to the flow of aqueous humour at the angle of the anterior chamber. The baby is irritable and photophobic. The condition is often curable, especially in the first year of life, but it is easily missed.

Retinitis pigmentosa is usually inherited as a recessive genetic characteristic and may be associated with obesity, mental retardation, hypogonadism and polydactyly (Laurence-Moon-Biedl syndrome). The disorder usually appears in childhood, starting with night-blindness and progressively contracting visual fields. There are punctate black areas in the retinae. The general practitioner's aquaintance with the family history of his patients may assist early diagnosis.

Retinoblastoma is a tumour of undifferentiated embryonic cells in the retina. Where there is a strong family history, babies should be screened for this condition at birth, and subsequently at regular intervals. In suitable cases, the eye may be saved by prompt treatment at specialised units. Several siblings may be similarly afflicted. In unscreened children the symptoms are usually obvious by six or seven years of age. It may be possible to see a yellow reflex through the pupil. Excision of the eye should then be carried out without delay. If only one eye is affected a watch must be kept on the other one for many years. The siblings must also be examined by an ophthalmologist at regular intervals.

Non-accidental injury is a cause of some optic abnormalities, particularly associated with retinal haemorrhage. Ophthalmic examination is therefore essential in all suspected cases.

In some infants blindness is present from birth as a result of *primary optic atrophy* of unknown origin. *Secondary optic atrophy* may be associated with hydrocephalus or any other cause of raised intraocular pressure.

Some visual defects in young children are difficult to elucidate. Examination under anaesthesia may be necessary, using highly specialised techniques. General practitioners should not hesitate to refer to an ophthalmologist any young child whose eyesight is in doubt.

Prevalence

The National Child Development Study examined nearly 16 000 children born in one week in March 1958. At the age of seven years, 97 per cent of the children tested had optimal or near-optimal vision in their better eye, and 92 per cent achieved this with both eyes; 2.6 per cent had a moderate and 0.9 per cent had a severe (6/24 or worse) visual defect in their better eye. Six per cent of the total sample had been prescribed glasses. 85 per cent of these achieved optimal or near-optimal vision in their better eye after correction. It is therefore recommended that children wearing glasses should be put in front of the class if possible.

When followed-up at the age of sixteen years, 75 per cent of the children had normal visual acuity in both eyes, and for near vision 85 per cent. Eighteen per cent had glasses prescribed for current use, but one-third of these did not have their glasses with them when examined. Twenty per cent of the children who had been prescribed glasses had normal, or almost normal, distant vision. Nearly half of those not using their glasses fell into this category. Not surprisingly, adolescents do not usually welcome glasses if they have fairly normal distant vision. At this age eight per cent had an unaided visual acuity of 6/24 or worse in one or other eye. Five per cent had an unaided visual acuity of 6/18 or 6/12. Two per cent had very poor unaided near vision in the left eye and the same proportion in the right eye.

In the NCD Study a definite squint was present in over three per cent of the seven year olds. It was one of the commoner physical defects noted in the Study, and frequently it was associated with poor visual acuity. Nearly 60 per cent of the children of this age who had been prescribed glasses had past or present squints. The condition was commoner in children in poor socio-economic circumstances. At the age of 16 years a squint had been corrected by operation in two per cent of the children.

In a recent study in Hampshire 84 per 100 000 children born between 1st September 1959 and 31st August 1975 were found to have moderately or severely impaired vision, likely to disadvantage their educational progress at some stage. About half of these had been registered as blind or partially-sighted at the time of the study. The diagnosis was not always clear, but the commoner causes were various congenital anomalies including cataract, unexplained optic atrophy or retinal dystrophy, nystagmus, high myopia, albinism and injury. There were eleven cases (three per 100 000 children aged 0–16 years) of congenital glaucoma and six cases (1.6 per 100 000) of retrolental fibroplasia. Two cases of retinitis pigmentosa were reported.

This degree of visual handicap was commonly associated with the following conditions in order of frequency: mental handicap (21.1 per cent), cerebral palsy, hydrocephalus, defective hearing, maternal rubella, cerebral tumour, Down's syndrome, epilepsy, and the sequel of meningitis or encephalitis.

Congenital malformation is therefore the commonest cause of severe visual disability in the United Kingdom. In the world population trachoma is the commonest single cause of blindness, followed by onchocerciasis (river blindness), and measles in association with malnutrition.

Voluntary organisations for children with visual defects are listed at the end of this book. Practitioners should strongly encourage parents to join them, as the children benefit enormously.

Registration

In order to qualify for the statutory welfare services for blind or partially-sighted persons registration is necessary. The form has to be completed by a consultant ophthalmologist for the social services department.

REFERENCES

Gardiner, P.A. (1979) *ABC of Ophthalmology (BMJ)*.

Ingram, R.M. (1973) The role of the school eye clinic in modern ophthalmology. *British Medical Journal*, **1**, 278, 2, 548.

MacLellan, A.V. & Haker, P. (1979) Mobile orthoptic service for primary screening of visual disorder in young children. *British Medical Journal*, **1**, 994–995.

Peckham, C.S., Gardiner, P.A. & Tibbenham, A.D. (1978) Vision Screening in Children Tested at 7, 11 and 16 Years. *British Medical Journal*, **1**, 1312–1314.

Sheridan, M.D. (1974) *Children's* Developmental Progress from Birth to Five Years In: *Developmental Medicine and Child Neurology*, ch. 16, p. 189. Windsor: NFER.

Taylor, D. (1978) Assessment of Visual Function in Young Children: An Overview. *Clinical Paediatrics*, **17**, 226–232.

Tibbenhan, A.D., Peckham, C.S. & Gardiner, P.A. (1979) Vision Screening of Adolescents and Their Use of Glasses. *British Medical Journal*, **1**, 1111–1112.

Weale, R.A. (1978) Left Eye, Right Eye. *Lancet*, **1**, 548–549.

42

The clinical care of handicapped children

Denis Pereira Gray

The clinical care of handicapped children is one of the most challenging and interesting aspects of modern family practice, one that has been relatively little explored, and a field in which there is enormous potential for the future.

DEFINITIONS

The word 'care' is used here in the sense defined in the *Oxford Dictionary* (1964) 'feel concern or interest for or about, e.g. children'. Similarly the broadest use of the word 'child' is employed to include the whole pre-adult phase of development, that is birth to adolescence inclusive. From the general practitioner's point of view the most useful definition of 'handicap' is that of the American Public Health Association: 'a child who is hindered from achieving his full physical, mental, and social potentialities'. This identifies in one sentence the child's future potential and the three key elements of care: physical care, emotional care, and social care.

The prevalence of children handicapped as defined in my own practice is 5.0 per cent of the children under the age of 18.

CLINICAL CARE

The phases of the clinical care provided by a general practitioner for handicapped children consist of successive stages of suspecting, detecting, assessing, explaining, managing, and preventing the handicap. These stages can be considered in relation to the main functions of the GP in the United Kingdom which are: to provide primary care, family care, continuity of care, domiciliary care, and above all whole-person care.

SUSPECTING THE HANDICAP

Suspecting the handicap is a difficult role because it depends on an attitude of mind, a way of thinking in probabilities rather than in certainties. The concept of children being 'at risk' is crucial but it does require the ability to organise information, and to co-ordinate and co-operate with colleagues and attached staff, especially health visitors.

Sheridan (1969) has produced a useful classification of factors which should arouse the suspicion of handicap. She divides these into: Group 1, those with a family history, Group 2, those with prenatal factors, Group 3, those with natal factors, Group 4, post-natal factors, and Group 5, children showing what she calls 'developmental warning signals'.

Family history

Family histories are of crucial importance to family doctors and there are several handicapping conditions which are known to be familial such as, in the organic field, congenital deafness, epilepsy, squints, and congenital dislocation of the hip, and, in the emotional field, anxiety state, and some forms of psychosis.

There is another group of rarer recessively transmitted metabolic disorders, the commonest of which is diabetes, and one of the best known of which is phenylketonuria, which are now being detected increasingly by screening.

Prenatal factors

Many of the prenatal factors occur in pregnancy; for example, toxaemia and antepartum haemorrhage may impair placental function and are associated with fetal abnormalities. Similarly, high maternal age and maternal diabetes are known to be unfavourable factors in a pregnancy.

The thalidomide disaster has shocked the world into realising the vital importance of drugs administered in pregnancy, but many more examples will doubtless be discovered. The use of ionizing radiations suggests that antenatal X-rays may increase the chance of leukaemia subsequently developing in childhood and it has taken many years for the profession to discover that the use of oestrogens in pregnancy may be associated with the development of cervical cancer in adolescent girls. King

(1975) has already carried out one of the first surveys of this in Britain, checking the records in his general practice. The avoidance of handicapping conditions by good antenatal care is discussed further in Chapter 9.

Natal factors

Natal factors should be noted by whoever is responsible for the birth. One of the great advantages in the past of the family doctor being actively involved in both obstetrics and child care was that he was often able to do this work himself. This is happening less often nowadays and therefore there is a correspondingly greater need for full obstetric records to be sent to general practitioners by hospital departments. The Apgar scoring system is widely accepted and should be recorded for all births and it is also helpful to count routinely the umbilical blood vessels as an abnormality raises the suspicion of internal congenital abnormality. The exact birth weight should be recorded as well as the degree of maturity, as the small-for-dates baby is now recognised as being at risk and to differ from the premature. See further, Chapter 26.

Postnatal factors

Postnatal factors associated with handicapping usually consist of either injuries or infections. Serious infections such as meningitis need to be particularly recorded, but undoubtedly many of the so-called benign infectious diseases, such as measles and mumps, can be associated with handicapping conditions such as deafness.

Developmental warning signals

Sheridan's final category, the 'warning signals', depends on the doctors having adequate knowledge of normal child development and deep understanding of the range of normality. Indeed, general practitioners active in child development work are largely responsible for defining the boundaries of normality.

Sheridan has usefully summarised the work by saying that it is the doctor's job to see that all children can 'see, hear, walk, and talk satisfactorily'.

DETECTING THE HANDICAP

Detection does not necessarily mean that the handicap is permanent. It may well be possible to eliminate the handicap and, for example, a congenitally dislocated hip should no longer result in a child becoming handicapped, as effective treatment is now available if it is detected in time.

In a series of 80 handicapped children examined in general practice I found that 70 out of the 80 were detected clinically, and so it appears that complex equipment is required for the identification of only a minority of handicaps. As Hunter said in the eighteenth century the main requirements for diagnosis are: an observant eye, an attentive ear, an experienced hand, and an open mind. Routine examination at birth should be carried out by the clinician responsible for the care, who will still often be the family doctor himself. The examination has been described fully by Hooper (1975).

Brimblecombe and Lightwood (1953) have recorded that the most frequent major handicaps are talipes (4.4 per thousand), cardiac abnormalities (4.1), spina bifida (3), hydrocephalus (2.6), anencephalus (2), cleft palate or lip (1.9), mongolism (1.7) and congenital dislocation of the hip (0.7). All these can be detected clinically by a general practitioner. The incidence of neurological handicaps is falling dramatically with modern antenatal care.

ASSESSING THE HANDICAP

The process of suspecting and detecting a handicap in a child is common to all doctors. The GP's approach is similar to that of his hospital colleagues and is predominantly scientific. However, after the handicap has been suspected and detected, the next step is assessment and, if detection is a science, then assessment is an art.

The main contribution to assessment by the general practitioner lies in measurement of the repercussions of handicap against the background of a particular child in a particular family in a particular home at a particular time. The child in other words will be considered within a framework which inevitably includes his siblings, his parents, and his home.

The emphasis in general practice is inevitably more concerned with function than with structure, and with prognosis rather than with pathology. This so-called 'whole person' approach is what is now referred to in general practice as the 'holistic concept of child care'.

Because this assessment is concerned with physical assessment, psychological assessment, and social assessment, and the interrelationship of the three, I described it in 1969 as being a 'three-dimensional assessment'. This analogy emphasises these three dimensions or aspects of care and helps to underline the solidarity of the doctor/patient relationship.

The physical assessment will, of course, follow the traditional orthodox approach to medicine, including such factors as aetiology, investigation, differential diagnosis, treatment, and prognosis. The psychological assessment will include the emotional factors both in aetiology and occurring within the family as a whole, and the social assessment will include the need for changes in the child's environment or social situation including special schools, school transport, supporting services of all kinds and discussing the problem of the impact of the handicap in school and on future employment and marriage. It goes without saying that in all three dimensions of assessment the general practitioner co-operates fully with paediatric colleagues in hospital and at special assessment centres, with other members of the practice team, and with workers in the voluntary and statutory social services.

EXPLAINING THE HANDICAP

There is no agreement among doctors about who should explain the handicap to the parents. There are, however, some theoretical reasons why it is best done by the family practitioner.

First of all, there may be several different doctors involved. Secondly, general practitioners have special skills in adapting their language to the patient's needs and may be well aware of the unhappy significance of certain phrases. Next, the GP is likely to have the longest relationship with the patients, to have known them before the handicap was detected, and is likely to have continuing care of the child in the long-term future. Finally, in some circumstances home visits may be the best place for talking to parents and family doctors are most experienced at working in patients' homes.

The golden rule is that adequate time must be allowed for this work, the importance and significance of which to the patient has probably been underestimated in the past. The news that a child is handicapped is one of the greatest problems any parents may have to bear. It is essential that they are given plenty of time to talk about what this news means to them. Furthermore it is never possible to achieve this satisfactorily in any single consultation. A series of talks according to the severity of the handicap are always needed. It is important to appreciate that many of the fears of patients in relation to particular handicaps are not necessarily founded on scientific fact, as it may be possible to relieve parental anxiety substantially through discussion. The emotional tension, however, tends to be high and it has been said that the general practitioner has to act, as it were, as a lightning conductor, picking up and carrying safely to earth excessive nervous tension generated in such patients.

Parental reaction

The reaction of parents to the news that their child is handicapped has been studied in general practice and has been analysed. It consists of three phases: first the phase of surprise, followed by the phase of emotion which may be turned outwards to form resentment or inwards to form guilt, and, thirdly, the phase of adjustment or maladjustment.

The initial phase of surprise is usually fairly short lasting and may consist of a series of questions such as 'Is it really true, why has it happened?' The emotional reaction to the presence of the handicap itself, however, may be one of the most severe reactions seen in general practice. Anger and resentment are common emotions and it is a good working rule in general practice that the care of the parents is not complete until anger has been identified and allowed to be expressed. This may be particularly disturbing for doctors as the object of the anger is often themselves or a colleague. This should be regarded as common if not inevitable because doctors and nurses are so involved in the care of pregnancy and children.

Guilt, which can be regarded as anger turned inwards, may be either rational or irrational. As doctors can now increasingly tell one parent of their genetic responsibility, so it is increasingly common for that parent to become burdened by guilt.

The final phase of parental reaction is either adjustment or maladjustment. Adjustment can be regarded as the stage of coming to terms with the handicap, and when the family unit as a whole is stable GPs can then predict with a high degree of probability the future behaviour of children and those around them. Maladjustment, on the other hand, represents an unfavourable parental reaction and usually consists of the perpetuation of either resentment or guilt, and there may be serious consequences for both the parent and the child, and also for other members of the family. Such family behaviour is characterised by sudden and impulsive decisions which may be both unpredictable and unwise.

One useful analogy is to regard the parents of handicapped children as being like those who have been bereaved. The concept is that such parents are, as it were, bereaved of the death of an ideal, the ideal being the parental hope of perfection in the off-spring, and the usual hopes and aspirations of the child's success. This analogy has practical use in general practice in that it sets the scene for the process of explaining and emphasising not only the severity and sequence of events but also the time scale over which they may develop. As in the case of bereavement the family often needs to see the four seasons round before adaptation occurs.

MANAGING THE HANDICAP

One of the first decisions that needs to be taken, after the parents have been informed, is to discuss with them the wisdom of referral to another doctor, usually a consultant paediatrician. This is normally the case and in my series only three out of 80 handicapped children had not been referred.

The very substantial advances in paediatrics and its related disciplines in recent years mean that specialist paediatricians may be able to bring to children with handicaps much care which was not available in the past. It is important for the primary doctor to identify in his mind what he is seeking from the hospital services, what skills they have to offer, and what is his own role before, during and after referral (Pless and Pinkerton, 1975).

Difficulties arise because of the ambivalent feelings between the two branches of the profession which can at times impair the total care received by the handicapped child and his family. The feelings between the two kinds of doctor will tend to get in the way of good coordination and communication, and, for example, Drysdale (1969) is quoted in the *British Medical Journal* at a symposium on handicapped children as saying 'The family doctor should not get too involved with the parents. He should leave it to one of the expert team'. While the very anonymity of the last five words is revealing, this view does seem to deny the role the family doctor has.

However, it is helpful to remember that many of the leading paediatricians appreciate the opportunities and potential of general practice. For example, Holt (1965) from the Institute of Child Health in London has stressed the importance of the handicapped child's environment, and in effect recommended paediatricians to follow current attitudes and developments in general practice: 'Bedside clinical teaching led to great advances in medicine and paediatrics, but in paediatrics now the need is to go further and study the child in his environment. This will lead to many advances, and the paediatrician who is willing to emancipate himself from the sick child in the hospital bed will find a fruitful field for his study'.

It is useful to remember that some of the most modern paediatric units are now designed so that the hospital staff wear ordinary clothes, where children are seen with toys around them and with their own parents and a deliberate attempt is made to keep the room 'as much like home as possible'. All these conditions are, of course, always available to general practitioners who, perhaps have taken them rather for granted in the past and have not always appreciated their great natural advantages.

The role for GPs should be complementary and not antagonistic to consultants, and certainly continues long after referral. It is a good working principle for the GP to continue to see parents regularly after they have been referred to hospital and thus make it clear that he is not in any way rejecting them and is still available to help them with long-term difficulties.

Management in general practice includes two main components: family care and continuity of care.

Family care

As the discoveries in the behavioural sciences have increasingly influenced sociologists, educationalists, and doctors, so behaviour in human groups has been better understood.

An ordinary family is, of course, itself a human group and family doctors thus have the longest tradition of all of working with groups of people. Doctors can gain information through verbal communication from members of the family to the doctor, and much information can also be gleaned by careful observation of non-verbal communication within the family.

One of the first and most important consequences of stress in the family such as the presence of a handicapped child is the distortion which occurs in the relationships between the members of the family itself. The most common reaction is in the mother/handicapped child relationship, but other common relationships are the marital relationship, the sibling relationship, and the relationship between the parents and unaffected children.

These effects are so common and so important that it is a valuable concept to consider the whole family as the focus of care rather than just the handicapped child. This has been the approach in the present chapter, and the subject is discussed further in Chapter 50.

One of the basic techniques of obtaining information about families is to see several members of the family simultaneously. In this way a family doctor may be able to identify behaviour which could not be seen in any other way. All members of a family group, of course, behave more naturally at home than in the doctor's consulting room, and home visits still have a valuable part to play in assessment and reassessment of progress.

One of the commonest reactions is for the parent, usually the mother, to be over-protective. Usually the strength of this reaction is related inversely to the number of children in the family, being most intense when a handicap occurs in an only child. The significance for the child is that his development may be restricted in physical, emotional, and social terms, if he is not provided with appropriate external stimuli.

Amongst the common resources which the GP has available to counter overprotection are firstly, explaining and interpreting it to the parent – a task much easier to describe than to perform. Secondly, efforts should be made to enable the child to meet and mix with his peers. This can often be done through playgroups, special schools, or clubs, or even arranging for exchange visits. Thirdly, it is often possible to direct the mother's attention in other directions, most commonly in general practice by encouraging part-time work.

Handicapped children present problems to their families often about decisions as to whether or not to restrict the child in some activity. Should a spastic be allowed to go horse-riding? Should an epileptic cycle to school? Three principles apply in the clinical management of such decisions in general practice. First, each child should be assessed individually in line with the old maxim that 'in general practice there are no diseases – only sick people'. Secondly, each individual restriction should be carefully considered. It is so easy to be always 'on the safe side' and say 'no'. Thirdly, the doctor should progressively transfer the power of decision making to the family, making it clear that he is there to help and advise.

Taking difficult decisions is one of the ways in which groups mature – and handicapped families are no exception. The danger for the doctor is that he slips into his traditional authoritarian role and he should instead act as a guide leaving the family progressively to take decisions themselves and accept the corresponding responsibility.

Such work is time-consuming and illustrates another general principle of the care of handicapped children, that such management can be more challenging intellectually and emotionally than diagnosis, and may form as much as 75 per cent of the work in general practice.

Management is always more difficult for the family doctor because he is dealing not with a docile, institutional patient, but with a whole family group. A family which, moreover, may be living in its own, often unsuitable, home, and may hold strong and often undesirable ideas about life in general and children, whether handicapped or not, in particular. The GP's role is thus to deal with people and not with cases, and with groups of people on their own terms and in their own homes.

These conditions affect the doctors who work with them. They lead to a greater flexibility of thought, a tendency to compromise on the less essential, and a greater understanding of the patient's point of view. Family doctors thus show a readiness to cut the coat of management according to the cloth of family potential.

The keystone of family group behaviour usually rests on the twin pillars of the parental attitudes. Whatever any doctor advises, the care a handicapped child usually receives depends upon the parents' attitudes and behaviour. These attitudes and behaviour are therefore worthy of study and in some research in 1969 the results tabulated overleaf were obtained (Table 42.1).

I suggest that these five parental reactions occur more often in families with handicapped children. Why should this be so? Three of the reactions, moving house, transferring from one doctor to another, and marital disharmony, can be considered together. They represent some form of change. In short, these parents tend to change their house, their doctor, or their spouse. This group of behavioural responses can be regarded as an attempt, conscious or subconscious, to change the environment.

When these five reactions are considered in relation to the families it is found that some may be either appropriate or inappropriate, according to the individual circumstances. All five occur together in only a minority of families, but in the series of handicapped children there was a clustering, so that many of the features occurred in a small group of handicapped families. It is suggested that these are the families with maladjusted parents.

One maladjustment index is shown opposite (Table 42.2). A score of five points or more is usually associated with parental maladjustment. Scores of ten points or more indicate severe maladjustment.

In summary, sustained abnormal emotional tension is the commonest single finding in the handicapped group

Table 42.1 Comparison of behaviour in handicapped families and controls. From Gray, D.J. Pereira (1971) The care of the handicapped child in general practice. *Transactions of the Hunterian Society*

Observation	*80 Handicapped*	*80 Controls*
1. Limitation of family size		
a. No younger sibling	41	20
b. Only child	10	4
2. Moving house	23	15
a. Total number of moves	40	15
b. Recurrent (= more than 3) moves	5	0
3. Transfer from GP in same area	12	6
a. Double transfer	1	0
b. Parental transfer (either parent)	2	0
4. Severe marital disharmony	12	4
a. Referral to marriage guidance	5	0
b. Divorce/separation	7	4
5. Parental psychological disorders	42	32
Referral to psychiatrist	9	5

Table 42.2 A maladjustment index. From Gray, D.J. Pereira (1971) The care of the handicapped child in general practice. *Transactions of the Hunterian Society*

Criterion	*Points*
1. Voluntary limitation of family size	(Score zero if on medical advice)
a. No younger sibling	1
b. The handicapped child is an 'only'	2
2. Change of address	1 per change
3. Transfer from general practitioner in same area	2 per transfer
4. Marital disharmony	
a. General practitioner referral to marriage guidance or equivalent	2
b. Separation or divorce	3
5. Parental psychological illness (either parent)	3
Referral to psychiatrist	4

Interpretation: a total score of 5 or more suggests maladjustment, and 10 or more suggests severe maladjustment

as a whole and in the maladjusted group of parents. Perhaps the key to the first four behavioural reactions described above lies in the fifth.

Continuity of care

Providing medical care on a continuing basis is one of the general practitioner's great responsibilities and rewards in dealing with the handicapped family. It can be regarded as providing the longitudinal perspective over time, whereas caring for the handicapped child in the setting of his own brothers, sisters, and parents (family care) can be regarded as giving a horizontal perspective.

The doctor/patient relationship has been intensively studied in general practice during the last 25 years (Balint, 1964; Browne and Freeling, 1967). The first and most obvious variable is the duration of the relationship. Although there is increasing mobility of patients, especially in big cities, in a provincial city like Exeter I have found that half of all the known handicapped children in the practice and half of all a group of controls had received absolute continuity of general practitioner care, i.e. had been born in the practice and remained with it up to the point of the survey.

Contrary to the old music hall quip that doctors bury their mistakes, general practitioners continue to meet theirs on many different occasions for many different reasons for many years. In other words continuity constitutes a form of evaluation of previous care. It is therefore a discipline, a discipline of consequences. Continuity of care provides a backcloth before which the GP acts out his many other roles. Often in the background, it impinges on almost all the other aspects of care the handicapped child receives. Thus the stage of assessment, for example, ceases to have a once-and-for-all quality and becomes a stage of continuous reassessment.

PREVENTING THE HANDICAP

Since the Oxford Dictionary defines 'care' as 'being concerned with', caring for the handicapped must include seeking to prevent the disability. The prevention of illness or disability can be regarded as the supreme triumph of the doctor.

The general practitioner has six roles in preventing handicap in children:

1. Treating adequately and completely conditions which otherwise might progress to handicap, for example, rheumatic fever.

2. By the detection of conditions which, while not handicapping at that time would, through their own natural history, progress to handicap if left untreated, for example, congenital dislocation of the hip.

3. The general practitioner can often prevent situations in which the child might be at risk. Much of the modern management of antenatal care is designed to prevent the fetus and subsequently the child suffering (see Ch. 9). Similarly, all the specific immunisations are now given to healthy children with a view to prevent the disease and hence also the incidence of handicapping complications, for example, the prevention of measles also prevents the complications of measles (see Ch. 11).

4. Preventing the birth of handicapped children. It is now possible under the 1967 Abortion Act for general practitioners to recommend a termination of pregnancy when there is an expectation of the child being severely handicapped. The commonest condition is, 'There is a substantial risk that if the child were born it would suffer such physical and mental abnormalities as to be seriously handicapped' (*Abortion Act*, 1967). The commonest indication in general practice is the infection of the mother with rubella during the first 15 weeks of

pregnancy. However, amniocentesis is now becoming increasingly available to general practitioners through special centres, and in the future is going to be used more for the detection of mongolism. A range of tests has also been developed for the detection and assessment of neurological disorders of the fetus in early pregnancy (Ch. 9). The parents can then be offered the option of late termination of the pregancy.

5. Preventing pregnancies which might lead to handicapped children. There is evidence that handicapped children both in the physical and psychological sense, are more common in unwanted pregnancies. As more effective contraception is being made available through general practice the number of such unwanted pregnancies and children should fall, and it is hoped the number of handicapped children is likely to fall disproportionately in the future.

6. Preventing a marriage. Very rarely general practitioners may be consulted about the wisdom of a marriage when two relatives are concerned. It is known that marriages between close relatives are more likely to produce handicapped children and this information may occasionally influence a young couple.

In these six roles the general practitioner's preventive influence is removed progressively further from the actual existence of the handicapped child.

ACKNOWLEDGEMENTS

I would like to thank my wife without whose help this work could not have been done. I am most grateful to the Editor of the *Transactions of the Hunterian Society* for permission to quote from my Hunterian Society Gold Medal Essay of 1969. I would also like to thank Mrs Margaret Topham for typing the manuscript.

REFERENCES

Drysdale, C.F. (1969) *British Medical Journal*, **2**, 167.
Gray, D.J. Pereira (1970) *Transactions of the Hunterian Society*, **28**, 121–175.
Holt, K. (1966) *Proceedings of the Royal Society of Medicine*, **59**, 139.
Hooper, P.D. (1975) The examination of the newborn. In Hart, C. (ed.) *Screening in General Practice*. Edinburgh: Churchill Livingstone.
King, R.L. (1975) *Journal of the Royal College of General Practitioners*, **25**, 252–54.
Lightwood, R. & Brimblecombe, F.S.W. (1963) *Sick Children*, 8th edn, p.97.
Pless, I.B. & Pinkerton, P. (1975) *Chronic Childhood Disorder: Promoting Patterns of Adjustment*. London: Kimpton.
Sheridan, M.D. (1962) *Monthly Bulletin of the Ministry of Health Laboratory Service*, **21**, 238.
Sheridan, M.D. (1969) *Health Trends*, August, **6**.

PART SIX

Essays in family care

43

The sick family

Geoffrey Smerdon

A sick child is often the presenting symptom of sickness in the family. What is this sickness?

DEFINITION

A family is more than the sum of its parts, nor are its members necessarily connected by ties of blood or marriage but by the intimacy of the relationships between them. These can only be sustained by the acceptance of a system of values and the maintenance of communications with sufficient feed-back to enable members to adjust their mutual needs. Because of this intimacy the non-verbal channels of communication are more important than the verbal, and will usually be heeded when conflicting messages are being received.

The health of a family is measured by its capacity to foster the development and growth of its members as individuals without sacrificing its own stability. It is the frustration of these processes of change, which are the life-cycle of the family, that constitutes sickness within it.

RECOGNITION

Every family – like every person – has problems, but these are mostly resolved inside the home. When the healing resources of the family are inadequate the pressures may overflow into the community, and generate displaced or blocked signals which are the physical signs of sickness for which we must look.

These signs are inappropriate behaviour, shown by our patients or induced by them in others. This may be seen in the home, at school or work, and in social life, but it is reflected in the consulting room and in any interface between patient and doctor such as messages, receptionists and nursing staff. It may be repeated by others, and though we must not discuss patients we are free to listen.

Because illness is still seen by the public as primarily physical, emotional pressures in the family will often distort the presentation of organic illness, or present in physical terms with no organic component. We frequently see minor illness in a child complicated by mother's anxieties, which in turn may be a displacement of anxieties or criticisms from elsewhere, such as a ny.

In an unstable family anxieties may be passed from one member to another, gaining in volume as they are passed through each member, until eventually we are presented with an inflationary spiral of rising hysteria. Blocked signals are less easily recognized, but what is not said is often more important than what is. Here outside information and non-verbal signs may help us and we must be diligent in pursuing them. They are not accidental but will be found to lead on to matters which the family is not able to discuss with itself, much less with the doctor. When the family is extremely rigid in resisting change and the feedback is ignored signals may become progressively deviant until they appear in a disguised – and often bizarre – form, focussed on a scapegoat for the family.

Between the wars the first health centre claimed to have defined the unit of living: not the individual but the family (Pearse and Crocker, 1943). The illness behaviour of patients over many years when carefully recorded and analysed establishes that the family must indeed be looked upon as a unit in itself with its own disorders, disease and pathogenesis (Huygen, 1978). It follows that no understanding of a patient can be adequate until the medical records of his family have been examined, and this manoeuvre will often reveal what was previously hidden. It will also usually reveal alarming gaps in our knowledge of the family's origins, history, composition, communications, viewpoints and expectations, which as family doctors we need to remedy.

ACTION

Patients frequently incite their doctors to intervene in family conflicts by 'having a word' with third parties.

This is seldom effective and the addition of the doctor's authority does not make the patient's solution – which he was unable to apply himself – any more valid for others. It is particularly difficult to help a disturbed child directly who is usually quite overwhelmed by the status of the doctor and the restrictions of his practice.

Doctors new to general practice and trained in the precision of natural science applied to physical disease find the vagaries of human behaviour difficult to handle. They are used to thinking from cause to effect with the aim of establishing a diagnosis with which to understand, and hopefully influence, events. However the reciprocal, and often circular, nature of interaction in the family is such that disordered communication is often self-perpetuating even when the original 'cause' has ceased to operate. Here, rather than a diagnosis, an assessment is needed of what is happening in the here and now. In this situation our long training in organic medicine is inappropriate, indeed it may even have discouraged us from bringing our basic social skills to our work. The detailed analysis of consultations by the use of audio-tapes has established the extent of the problem, and has suggested ways out of it (Byrne and Long, 1976).

Traditionally the doctor-patient relationship is seen as a one to one, individual, personal contract. The use of reassurance and support, for so long the only techniques generally used for emotional problems, has during the past twenty-five years been increasingly widened by an understanding of the function of the doctor as a therapeutic agent in his own right (Balint, 1957). However the mode in which he deploys himself is not only very restricted but is becoming even more so as the proportion of home visits to consultations decreases (Gray, 1978) and as his accessibility is reduced by more partners, more staff, and the increasing use of appointments and special clinics in the surgery.

The primary care team, though diluting contacts, has extended the range of skills available. Psycho-social problems are often taken over by the health visitor and in a few practices social workers and councillors may work on the premises. Such a team, welcome as it is, is little more than a summation of its members. The advent of co-therapy for sexual problems, where two professionals working together multiply their skills, has opened up a new dimension.

Similar innovations have developed at the patient's end of the transaction. Marriage and sexual difficulties – two major dysfunctional communications in the family – are now treated as a relationship between a pair and requiring a joint approach.

Contacts between people become more demanding as they become more personal but they also become more rewarding, which is the incentive for us to become involved with our patients' problems. The extent to which we can become involved – because our friends, our family, our hobbies, and those who supply our needs all live within the community of our patients – is frequently a source of alarm to those new to these complexities, but it is also a source of strength and certainly our patients value such involvement.

These same circumstances place us well to practice family therapy. Our availability in the community by day and night, our mobility between consulting room and home, our resources at the centre of the primary care team, and the relationships we already have with the family are valuable assets. To deploy them the general practitioner needs to break away from the model he is used to: a person to person exchange in the consulting room.

If the family is seen as a constantly adjusting transactional system, each part depending on all the others, it becomes evident that treatment needs to be aimed at the whole rather than at the component parts, or at one part of the system by pressure upon another (Walrond-Skinner, 1976). If the primary care team can work together as a small group this will provide both a therapeutic function and training and support for its members.

FUTURE

The scope of general practice has for many years been challenged by the expertise of adjacent disciplines. Many of our responsibilities have been whittled away, but ground lost can be regained as we have demonstrated with family planning and antenatal and well baby clinics. We shall be failing the needs of our patients and the expectations of society if we do not equip ourselves to discharge such a central part of our task as the care of the whole family.

Health cannot be studied by examining disease. We in general practice have our own controls in those families whose children grow into stable and effective adults, equipped to live and work with others, and able to transmit these qualities to those around them and to future generations (Howells, 1965).

REFERENCES

Balint, M. (1957) *The Doctor, his Patient and the Illness.* London: Pitman.

Byrne, P.S. & Long, B.E.L. (1976) *Doctors Talking to Patients.* London: H.M.S.O.

Gray, D.J.P. (1978) *Journal of the Royal College of General Practitioners.* **28**, 6–17.

Howells, J.G. (1965) Organization of child psychiatric services. In Howells, J.G. (ed.) *Modern Perspectives in Child Psychiatry*. Edinburgh: Oliver and Boyd.

Huygen, F.J.A. (1978) *Family Medicine*. Nijmegan: Dekker Van de Vegt.

Pearse, I.H. & Crocker, L.H. (1943) *The Peckham Experiment.* London: Allen and Unwin.

Walrond–Skinner, S. (1976) *Family Therapy*. London: Routledge and Kegan Paul.

44

Poverty and child health

Bernice Tanner

There are few general practitioners who should be surprised or startled by the grim medical facts on childhood poverty. The misery, handicap and repeated illnesses of our poorest children never seem to diminish substantially. This may account for the part doctors played in drafting our early Victorian factory acts and the enrolment of physicians in the field of public and community health.

In the study of poverty, objectives and disciplines are important. They exemplify our shift in attitude about poverty. The classic work of Rowntree in 1893–1899 rested on the investigation of primary and secondary poverty (Rowntree, 1913). Primary poverty for him was where total earnings were insufficient to obtain the minimum necessities of life. Secondary poverty affected families 'whose total earnings would be sufficient for the maintenance of merely physical efficiency were it not that some other portion of them is used by other expenditure either useful or wasteful'. The latter form of poverty is one which in its broadest meaning would involve the general practitioner because it involves poverty related to human illness. The findings of Rowntree

Table 44.1 Numbers living in poverty 1974–1976, in thousands (Great Britain)

Year	Incomes below supplementary benefit level					
	Above pensionable age		*Below pensionable age*		*Total*	
	families	persons	families	persons	families	persons
1974	450	550	470	860	920	1410
1975	590	750	560	1280	1150	2030
1976	700	870	650	1410	1350	2280
Year	**on SB or below SB level**					
	Above pensionable age		*Below pensionable age*		*Total*	
	families	persons	families	persons	families	persons
1974	2260	2680	1190	2450	3450	5130
1975	2270	2720	1370	3080	3640	5800
1976	2360	2820	1600	3550	3960	6370
Year	**On SB or below SB level + incomes less than 40% above SB level**					
	Above pensionable age		*Below pensionable age*		*Total*	
	families	persons	families	persons	families	persons
1974	4160	5400	1960	4990	6120	10 390
1975	4270	5590	2730	8070	7000	13 660
1976	4590	6000	3270	8870	7860	14 870

	Children		
	Below SB	On SB or below	On SB or below or less than 40% above SB
1974	260	1000	2250
1975	410	1220	3170
1976	500	1460	3900

Source: House of Commons Hansard, 22 November 1976; 1 August 1978; 28 February 1978; 3 August 1978

have been the traditional way of describing the poverty line.

In recent years, the concept of poverty has changed. This is largely due to social theorists like Peter Townsend who look at poverty as a state of *relative deprivation* (Townsend, 1980). He defines it as a 'lack of resources necessary to permit participation in the activities, customs and diets approved by our society'. The resources of people must therefore be examined not merely in 'cash earnings' but from a wider perspective. In an age of instant general communication the attitudes of patients to lack of amenities is far more intolerant. The over-crowding of homes, lack of space and play facilities, poor heating, inadequate toilets and unhygienic conditions are now a well-known picture of our deprived areas.

The extent of poverty in the British Isles is thought by many to be serious and worsening. If one accepts that poverty is a state of relative deprivation, the DHSS statistics can show that 14 million people or 26 per cent of the nation are living in a state of poverty (CPAG, 1980). Broadly, this is arrived at by calculating the numbers of traditional families, single parents, old age pensioners, single people and unemployed living below supplementary benefit level, on supplementary benefit, or within 40 per cent of the poverty line as defined by supplementary benefit. In 1976 there were 5 860 000 children living in relative poverty (Table 44.1).

The rising numbers of children living at poverty level can be seen by checking those entitled to free school meals (see Table 44.2).

In 1973 six per cent of all households were overcrowded and 23 per cent of all large families lived in inadequate space, that is with more than 1.5 persons per room. 75 per cent of these children lived in urban inner areas.

In the last thirty years there has been an accumulation of statistical data about the effects of poor income on the health of our children. The *National Child Development Survey* was mounted in England, Scotland and Wales from a sample of 17 000 children born in a particular week in March 1958 (Davie *et al*, 1972). It studied the social and obstetric factors associated with still-birth and death in early infancy. These children were then followed up so that their social, physical and educational development could be monitored. This was done in 1965 when they were seven years old; in 1969 during their last year at primary school and in 1974 when they were 16. Other studies in Newcastle, the Isle of Wight and London have amplified and corroborated a good deal of their findings.

All national surveys in child health use the social classification adopted by the registrar general for census purposes (Table 44.3). It has been modified from time to time but the basic framework is determined by the

Table 44.2 Numbers receiving free school meals (England and Wales)

October each year	*Numbers (thousands)*
1956	216
1960	247
1966	330
1970	627
1971	805
1972	850
1973	795
1974	750
1975	784
1976	839
1977	997
1978*	1159

*provisional
Source: House of Commons Hansard, 26 October 1977, vol 936, col 826; Department of Education and Science and Welsh Office

Table 44.3 Social class. The Registrar General's definitions

I	Professional occupations, e.g. doctors, lawyers	
II	Intermediate occupations (managerial and lower professional), e.g. teachers, managers	
III	Skilled occupations, often divided into:	
	III N Non-manual,	e.g. clerks, shop assistants
	III M Manual,	e.g. bricklayers, coal miners below ground
IV	Partly skilled occupations, e.g. bus conducters, postmen	
V	Unskilled occupations, e.g. general labourers, porters	
Unclassified:	the armed forces, students, those about whom there is no information, those whose occupations do not fit into the classification	

occupation of the parents, usually the father, unless it specifically includes the single parent group.

For the doctor this is a convenient way of measuring some aspect of the child's environment which must determine in part later development. Although little is said about heredity in some of the studies the doctor must assume that heredity and environment interact in every individual to produce the mature human being.

USE OF SERVICES AMONG THE POOR

The cycle of deprivation begins before birth. Although some of the most lethal and adverse perinatal effects can be modified by clinical attention, e.g. breech birth, prolonged delay in establishing respiration, etc., social conditions continue to exert a major role. Use of our modern facilities and health services provided by the hospital, general practitioner and community health services have a bad take-up by the poor people of class IV and V. The most deprived use the services least and get worst attention.

Examples of poor take-up are numerous and have been investigated extensively (Wedge and Prosser, 1973). Where good ante-natal care was provided 70 per cent of class IV and V mothers had not attended an ante-natal clinic by week 15, compared with 42 per cent of other groups. Vaccination, immunization, ante-natal and post-natal supervision, uptake of vitamins were also badly utilized. Surveys of dental clinics, chiropody and family planning units also revealed poor attendance (Cartwright and O'Brien, 1976).

The use of the general practitioner by groups IV and V is also depressing. Surgery attendances are frequent but consultations are shorter. There are scanty enquiries about the nature of illness; prescription costs per item are lower and compliance less. Hospital consultations confirmed a similarly poor use of services. While most people wanted the consultant to say whether or not they were ill, only 24 per cent of semi-skilled or unskilled patients wanted to know any details. Saddest of all is the evidence that the community-based health visitor who is oriented and trained to detect need was found to concentrate services more readily and easily on the well-off.

Contact with the psychiatrist is also less for the most needy group (Brown *et al*, 1973, 1975) . This is almost predictable. Brown has shown within the London conurbation that a main cause for depressive illness in working class mothers is not only the large number of stressful events but their increased vulnerability after the event. This is due to the fact that the working class housewife gets less support after stress than her middle class counterpart. They communicate poorly with their general practitioner, and also are referred less to psychiatric care. The need for more pervasive health eduction in the surgeries and possibly for the use of financial incentives for antenatal attendances, as in France, are often suggested as antidotes to the poor take-up of class IV and V mothers. In all surveys smok-

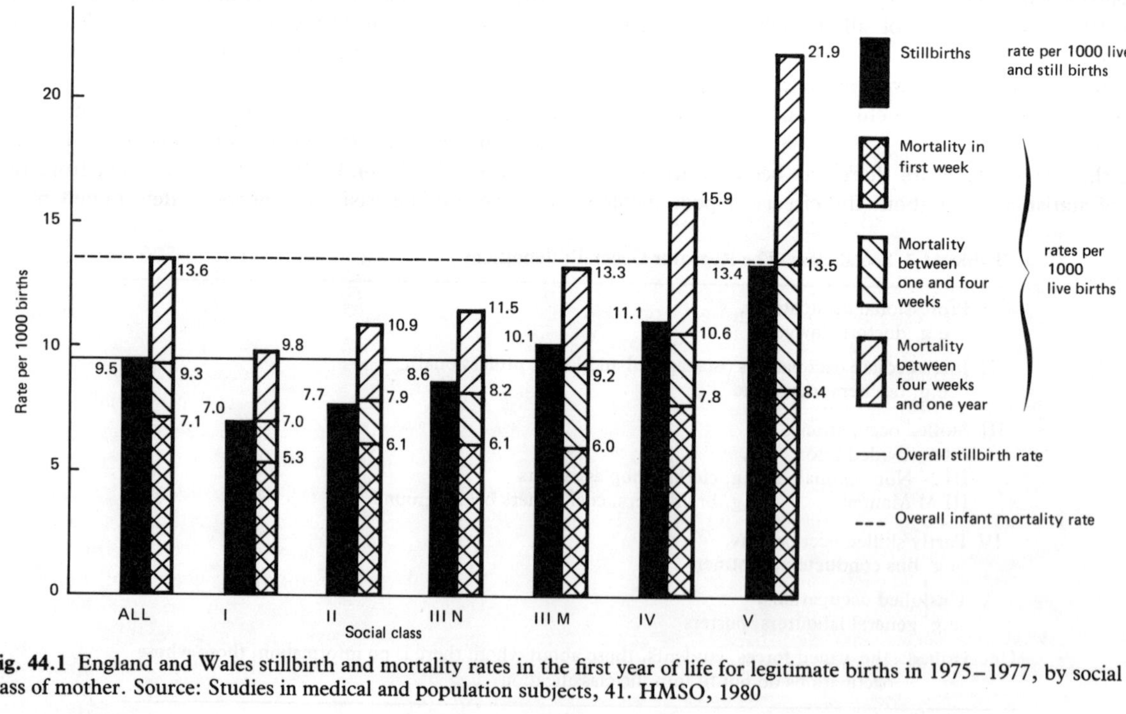

Fig. 44.1 England and Wales stillbirth and mortality rates in the first year of life for legitimate births in 1975–1977, by social class of mother. Source: Studies in medical and population subjects, 41. HMSO, 1980

ing habits, large families, and shorter periods between pregnancies all show a high correlation with poverty, handicap and death.

The perinatal mortality survey shows the class vulnerability (Macfarlane, 1979). In the statistics of averages variations are often hidden. Although the average perinatal mortality in 1977 was stated to be 15.2 per 1000 live births, classes IV and V actually had rates as high as 17.6 and 20.6 per 1000 live births (see Fig. 9.4, p. 74). The postneonatal mortality for the years 1975–7 showed an even greater divergence, being nearly twice the national average for babies in class V families, whose death rate for this period of life was three times the rate for babies in class I families (Fig. 44.1).

HANDICAP AND POVERTY

Poverty always compounds handicap (Younghusband *et al*, 1970). If the term handicap is used loosely this statement might be questioned, but if it is defined as Younghusband has suggested, the word has a specific meaning. She calls it a defect or disability which for a 'substantial period can permanently retard, distress and otherwise affect normal growth, development of adjustment to life'. For the doctor trained in traditional medicine *a defect* is a demonstrable and objective condition which can cause bodily or mental abnormality. *A disability* is the functional impairment associated with defect. Handicap must be assessed in social terms and not confused with demonstrable defect.

At one extreme it has been shown that when a severe congenital defect is accepted by the home and family, there may be less handicap than when the child is poorly cared for. This was true in thalidomide victims, where some children did better than others because their homes were more helpful (Davie, 1975). Handicap from brain damage can also be modified or at least contained when appropriate help is available. Similarly, less spectacular defects like deafness, poor vision and enuresis may reveal differences in handicap which are related to surrounding environment. The effects of physical illness, intellectual retardation, educational backwardness and psychiatric disorders are always related to the amount of familial and communal support obtainable.

Physical illness producing handicap

The general practitioner is the doctor most involved with acute illness both minor and severe. The range and frequency of illness seen at GP consultation has been well tabulated by the RCGP (Court, 1976). Infectious illness and respiratory complaints comprise 39 per cent of all consultations for children. Skin complaints (10.1 per cent), accidents (5.8 per cent), preventive procedures (9.9 per cent), and ill-defined symptoms, possibly behavioural (12.7 per cent), are the other problems mainly seen. The prevalence of respiratory complaints is always increased where social conditions are poor. Coughs, colds, sore throats, bronchitis and ear infections are statistically more common among poorer children. Hospitals corroborate the increased incidence of pneumonia from class IV and V homes. The only exception to this is the higher incidence of allergic asthma and hay fever to be found in children of non-manual families.

The other group of hospital-general practitioner treated illnesses like diabetes, epilepsy, metabolic disorders, heart disease, cystic fibrosis, malabsorption syndromes and leukaemia are not as a rule social class related. Dental caries may be defined as a disease of civilization and is not confined to any one social class. However the use of dental hygiene and dental care has more take-up in the better off groups of our society. But the handicap from all of these acute and chronic illnesses is more severe in poor families and homes. Poor school attendance after an acute illness is positively connected with large families, overcrowding and the other stigmata of adverse socio-economic conditions.

Accidental injury has increased in the last 20 years. It is thought that this is due to more overcrowding, inadequate parental vigilance and the disruption of communal life so that neighbours cannot act as parent substitutes. There is a marked social class variation in childhood road traffic accidents, with heavy loading to the detriment of the more deprived children (Jackson, 1978). Homes are now more unsafe than roads; that is, they are a common source of accident (Ch. 24). Burns, scalds, poisonings and tissue injuries are statistically more prevalent in conditions where homes are poor.

Non-accidental injury (NAI) is another problem, social related, whose gravity is becoming more acknowledged (Kempe *et al*, 1962). It is reckoned that NAI is now the fourth most common cause of death in the first five years of life and in 1976 affected 5000 children in England alone.

Developmental defect and disability

As the general practitioner becomes more involved with developmental surveillance and screening, defects and disabilities will be the subject of more surgery consultations. The social dimension of these liabilities may be recorded in general practitioner notes on an even larger scale. At one end of the spectrum, although the severe congenital defects are not looked after by the family doctor, the family doctor may be asked to cooperate with the community handicap team and therefore become involved in the care of a disabled child.

Patients with a poor obstetric history are likely to produce low birthweight infants who may have an increased incidence of congenital deafness, mental subnormality and cerebral palsy. Dr Gerald Neligan pioneered the Newcastle survey whch studied a three year cohort of 14 000 infant survivors of the first month of life in 1960–1962 (Neligan, 1974). The poor obstetric history which they looked at included apnoea, clinical asphyxia, cardiac distress of the fetus and premature labour. The analysis and significance of social and medical factors in children with brain damage was one of the objects of the Newcastle study. The brain damage ranged from the severe and easily recognisable types like paraplegia and quadriplegia, to those with lesser degrees of impairment.

The survey recorded the gestation period and intrauterine growth in order to measure biological and nutritional factors in brain damage. But they found that social factors were far more important than other perinatal factors in the degree of handicap from brain damage (see also Ch. 10). For example, social factors such as large families, housing, poor mothering and little space between pregnancies had a significant effect on intelligence. IQ scores estimated by non-verbal testing showed that in children with similar brain damage there was greater disparity related to social class at the age of ten than at age five. In fact neurologically handicapped children of classes I and II had a three-fold advantage over children of manual workers.

At the other end of the scale the more common defects encountered in the world of general practice are those related to vision, hearing, speech and bladder control. The figures for prevalence of partially sighted children are inaccurate as the condition is not notifiable. But squint and refractive error found in the routine checks done in the *National Child Development Survey* showed that these were the most common developmental defects and that the recognition and treatment were worst in class IV and V children. The strong correlation between squint and clumsiness is again a contribution to handicap (Davie *et al*, 1972). The chances of these children doing well at school, or aquiring skilled job training is substantially diminished. The cycle of poverty is reinforced.

Notifiable deafness has not been analysed. But deafness due to congenital defect is positively correlated to low birthweight and occurs more often in class IV and V children. Intermittent deafness associated with recurrent respiratory and middle ear infections is more prevalent in poor children. This again will have a crippling effect on verbal skills, education and future job training.

Poor speech and verbal development is a major handicap in our society although never as spectacular as, for instance, cerebral palsy. But for many people it is the great class divider. Analysis of vocabulary, sentence length and ability to communicate with comprehensibility are altered where speech development is delayed. Speech delay is present more often in homes with emotional stress and maladjustment. There is also a definite class bias in the incidence of stammer and stutter. Although the attendance at speech therapy clinics is divided equally between children of all social classes, the need for attendance has been found to be greater in poor children.

Enuresis is a handicap often taken care of by the general practitioner. At the age of five years it can affect 18 per cent of children but by the age of 15 only 2 per cent of adolescents suffer this disability. Analysis of bed-wetters reveals a greater proportion in large families with older mothers living in poor social adjustment. These factors correlate positively with social class, family size, or both.

Physical growth and the social dimension

The study of physical growth and the regular recording of height is becoming a standard procedure in surgeries, community clinics and paediatric outpatients. There is a greater understanding about the many factors which influence the final height of an individual. Among these factors, the social circumstance is important.

The quality and quantity of diet found in poor children from large families, is associated with a corresponding alteration in lack of growth in height and weight (Tanner, 1962). There is a slower rate of growth in height in children of large families resulting in short stature at the age of six which persists through the age of ten and probably into adult life (Acheson, 1960). There can be a significant retardation of growth (about ¼ inch) in a year in children following an acute illness like bronchitis and pneumonia of not more than a few weeks. Retardation of height growth is also more positively correlated with food expenditure than alteration in weight. Any failure of growth in height below the third centile, or falling velocity over a period, calls for investigation.

The rates of growth of children have now been recorded in detail in many countries of the world. Class differences in growth and final height are found in USA, Britain and most capitalist and communist countries as well as the countries of the third world. Only in Scandinavia have growth rates become the same for all classes of people, and that only recently. If class divisions are related to prevalence of illness, family expenditure on food, housing amenities, conditions of work and incidence of handicap, the height of our children makes a very strong social comment. The Newsom Committee found a relationship between reading scores, height and weight (Tanner, 1962).

Diet

Nutritional problems in the poor are subtle in their

manifestations. Undernutrition and faulty nutrition may affect weight, height and general behaviour. Malnutrition is rarely found in the British Isles.

Undernutrition of the mother has both immediate and long-term implications for the health of the infant (Edwards *et al*; 1979; *BMJ* Editorial, 1980). The optimum growth and development of the baby is related to the nutritional state of the mother not only during but for many years before pregnancy (Fisch *et al*, 1975).

All height and weight measurements should be recorded on charts which serve to compare them with the percentile standards for the population. This is easily done in the surgery or assessment clinic. These records show not only where the child stands vis-a-vis others but if done at regular intervals in the same child, how that person is growing in relation to his peers.

The calorie and iron intake of children living on supplementary benefit incomes where there are more than four children or with a single parent are insufficient. The intake has been estimated at 72 to 80 per cent of the average recommended amount (Nelson and Naismith, 1979). Supplementary benefit income is insufficient to buy adequate food and it is possible nutritional intervention may become indicated for this group of children.

The long-term effects of dietary inadequacy may be felt throughout adolescence and adult life. Insufficient caloric intake is conducive to lethargy and poor educational performance. Cheaper types of diet that use badly processed and too refined foods may lead to a greater incidence of constipation, appendicitis and other bowel disturbances.

Education handicap

Wherever educational opportunity is limited, from whatever the cause, life becomes socially more difficult, possibly self destructive and contributes to the cycle of poverty. Physical illness, with its poor school attendance, developmental disabilities, particularly the visual-auditory group, and congenital defect take their toll upon educational enhancement.

On the environmental side, educational retardation is directly related to poor housing amenities. In England today, household mobility is common to all classes but the house move is less destructive to the non-manual groups. Even where facilities like kitchens and inside bathrooms are improved, the children of manual workers, skilled, semi-skilled and unskilled often go into environmentally poor conditions. The housing estate has not been a successful replacement for terraced communities despite better plumbing. There is often lack of play space, loss of the granny as well as other kin, and an absent working mother. With tower blocks, the problems are even greater.

For the very poorest, it has been shown that where even cheaper housing exists, the slum places will be let to the worst off. Among the immigrant community, 25 per cent of all coloured households have poor amenities as compared with 6 per cent of the white population. And although class divisions within coloured immigrants are largely the same as those of the rest of the population, the differences between the West Indian households and those of other coloured people are more marked than between coloured and white (see further, Ch. 48).

Reading attainment shows a direct correlation between overcrowding and basic amenities, with a two to three month retardation in reading age (Fig. 44.2). Arithmetic attainment shows a similar but not so obvious relationship (Fig. 44.3). Many surveys demons-

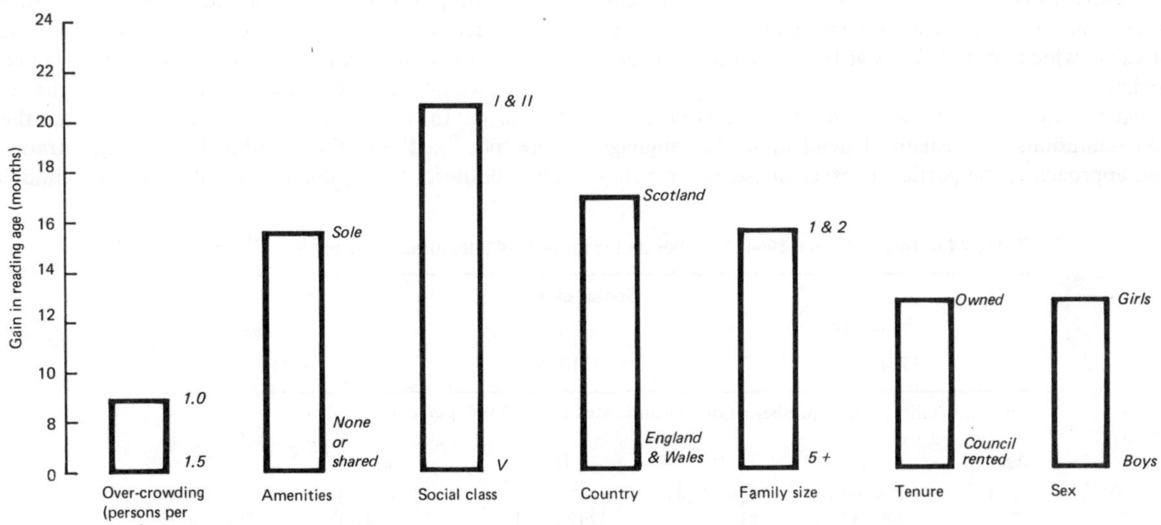

Fig. 44.2 Overcrowding, lack of amenities, and reading attainment at the age of seven

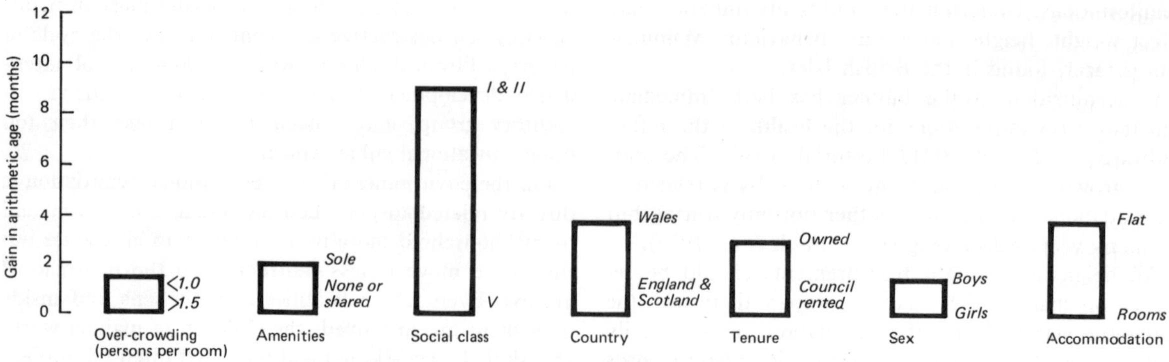

Fig. 44.3 Overcrowding, lack of amenities, and arithmetic attainment at the age of seven

trate that intellectual retardation without any recognizable neurological defect is related to adverse socio-economic conditions. Reading retardation is more complex in that there are some biological factors involved, and the effect on this of economic hardship is not as direct as it is upon intellectual retardation.

Social mobility in generations has been studied (Rutter *et al*, 1970). The grandchildren of a group of grandfathers of a particular social class chosen by occupation, were studied for intellectual and reading retardation. Poorer performances of the grandchildren were correlated with family size, type of housing, occupation of parent and position of the child in the family. Other poor performance factors were related to frequent illnesses and poor obstetric history.

Behaviour defect

It is commonly assumed that there will be a relationship between behavioural abnormalities and social class (Fogelman, 1976). This in fact is not the case in Britain. Results of studies are complex and point to other areas of cause which are not necessarily purely economic and social.

Psychiatric abnormalities have many classifications and definitions will usually depend upon the language and approach of the particular psychiatrists and psychologists. The major study by Rutter, of children in the Isle of Wight divides psychiatric disorders by diagnostic groups into neurotic, conductive, mixed conductive and neurotic, enuretic, hyperkinetic and psychotic. They were further divided into sub-classifications. The disorders were diagnosed in essentially descriptive or phenomenological terms.

Where general psychiatric disorder could be demonstrated, there was frequently poorer IQ performance and some reading retardation. Neurotic, antisocial and delinquent symptoms were part of larger and wider psychiatric disturbances such as anxiety, obsessiveness, hypochondriasis and other sub-classifications. Neurotic children were often eldest children and sometimes came from smaller families. Antisocial behaviour was shown in children of larger families. Some deviant behaviour was more common in manual skilled working families. Conduct disorders ranging from antisocial acts to truancy, bullying, stealing and delinquency were slightly more common where children had to share a bedroom and sometimes a bed. But there was a sad class relationship in some behaviour which would not be noticed by and would not necessarily be disturbing for the rest of society. In the very poor the boys often felt that they were 'not liked' and they exhibited poor concentration. The bullies, the violent and destructive children

Table 44.4 Infant deaths, 1964. Number and rates per 1000 legitimate live births

Social class		
I and II	*III*	*IV and V*
1714 (12.8)	7110 (17.2)	4131 (20.8)

Child mortality, 1964 (number of deaths and rates per 100 000 per year)

Age	I	II	III	IV	V
1–4	436 (69.0)	1329 (73.4)	6147 (88.7)	7324 (93.3)	1521 (154.0)
5–9	209 (32.8)	818 (35.1)	3242 (41.1)	1234 (41.4)	744 (66.6)
10–14	173 (29.6)	823 (28.8)	2771 (31.3)	1091 (30.3)	555 (41.4)

appeared to be greater in number in the children of skilled manual families.

In the National Child Development Survey, children of the semi-skilled and unskilled were less settled in their plans at the age of 16 (Fogelman 1976). Teachers and families had little influence on their work training and their peer group was the most determining factor. Like their younger group they continued the pattern of feeling isolated and not liked. At school they felt that they were not good at work and their chances for moving out into skilled jobs were very slight.

Death

The grim statistics in the perinatal and infant mortality surveys continue into the older age groups. Accident, violence, poisoning and pneumonia continue to be class related (Court, 1976). (See Table 44.4).

REFERENCES

Acheson, R.M. (1960) Effects of Nutrition and Disease on Human Growth. In: Tanner, J.M. *Human Growth*. London: Pergamon.

BMJ Editorial (1980) Pregnancy and the underweight woman. *British Medical Journal*, **1**, 1154.

Brown, G. Harris, T.O. & Peto, J. (1973) Life Events and Psychiatric Disorder. *Psychological Medicine*, **3**.

Brown, G. *et al* (1975) Social Class and Psychiatric Disturbance among Women in an Urban Population. *Sociology*, **9**.

Cartwright, A. & O'Brien, M. (1976) Social Class Variation in Health Care and in Nature of GP Consultations. *Sociological Review Monograph*, **22**.

Court, S.D.M. (1976) *Report of Committee of Child Health Services*. London: HMSO.

CPAG (1980) Child Poverty Action Group. *Poverty*. Macklin St, London

Davie, R., Butler, N. & Goldstein, H. (1972) *From birth to seven* Report on National Child Development Study

Davie, R. (1975) *Children and Families with Special Needs*. University College, Cardiff.

Edwards, L.E. et al (1979) Pregnancy in the underweight woman. Course, outcome, and growth patterns of the infant. *American Journal of Obstetrics and Gynaecology*, **135**, 297.

Fish, R.O. et al (1975) Obesity and leanness at birth and their relationship to body habits in later childhood. *Paediatrics*, **56**, 521.

Fogelman, K. (1976) *Britain's Sixteen Year Olds*. National Children's Bureau Report.

Jackson, R.H. (1978) Archives of Disease in Childhood 53, 807.

Kempe, C.H. et al (1962) The Battered Baby Syndrome. *Journal of the American Medical Association*, **181**.

MacFarlane, A. (1979) Social Class Variation in Perinatal Mortality. *Journal of Maternal and Child Health*, **4**, 9.

Neligan, G., Prudham, D. & Steiner, H. (1974) *The Formative Years*. Nuffield Provincial Hospitals Trust. OUP.

Nelson, M., & Naismith, D.J. (1979) *Journal of Human Nutrition*, **33**.

Rowntree, B., & Seebohm (1913) *Poverty, a Study of Town Life*, 2nd edn. London: Nelson.

Rutter, M., Tizard, J. & Whitmore, K. (1970) *Education, Health and Behaviour*. London: Longman.

Tanner, J.M. (1962) *Growth at Adolescence*. Oxford: Blackwell.

Townsend, P. (1980) *Poverty in the United Kingdom. A Survey of Household Resources and Standards of Living*. Harmondsworth: Penguin.

Wedge, P. & Prosser, H. (1973) *Born to fail*. Arrow.

Younghusband, E. et al (1970) *Living with Handicap*. National Bureau for Cooperation in Child Care.

45

Behaviour problems in childhood

Norman Cook

Two recent continental investigations have suggested that childless marriages may be happier than others, and certainly happier than had previously been thought. Be that as it may, there is no doubt that today's young parents, most of whom were members of small families, can find the behaviour (often normal) of their children a source of uncertainty and unhappiness.

The legendary Dr Spock with an insight deserving the highest admiration has suggested that the mother in the recent past has had too much advice from every sort of medium – advice which often conflicted with and lowered her confidence in her natural instincts. For advice there has been in plenty. Since the end of World War II, we have had a child-centred society with a lot of attention paid to child development and behaviour. With a falling birthrate and disillusion with the results of more permissive child rearing methods, the pendulum is already beginning to swing back, to create more problems for the future. Behavioural problems of childhood are difficult to classify, and do not therefore lend themselves easily to statistical evaluation, but some idea of their frequency of presentation to general practitioners can be obtained from published morbidity statistics (Table 45.1).

In the past, local authority infant welfare clinics have been the main centres of advice for minor behavioural problems, but the general practitioner must inevitably take over their work in time. With the assistance of an attached health visitor, he should be well qualified for the task with his knowledge of the local social mores, the family and the home environment.

As in other fields of general practice, supply creates demand, and the doctor sympathetic to parents with behaviour problems will get more requests for help than one who is not. This interest may be advertised by the setting aside of one or two afternoons per week for a well-baby clinic (infant welfare, child development, call it what you like, but it is essentially a time and place when mother and doctor can feel free of the pressure of a waiting queue and a feeling that the doctor's time may be wasted).

It is convenient to divide behaviour problems into those commonly met with in the pre-school ages, and those following school entry – a major event in any child's life which itself may cause or expose some behaviour abnormalities, but which (thankfully) also cures others. In the first period, problems are best considered in a clinic setting such as described above, when a good attached health visitor can give invaluable help.

The child of school age must be brought into the decision making and arrangements must be made to interview the parent out of his earshot and also to interview the child away from his parents. The father may have to be interviewed and also the child's teacher, if only by

Table 45.1 Episode frequency of some symptoms and disorders reported to selected general practices in England and Wales in 1970–71. From *Morbidity Statistics from General Practice* (1974) HMSO

Symptom or disorder	*Episodes per 1000 patients*		
	All ages	*Ages 0–4*	*Ages 5–14*
Insomnia	9.6	13.5	1.7
Enuresis	2.5	5.9	11.2
Tension headache	4.9	0.5	1.7
Migraine	8.1	0.6	4.5
Anxiety neurosis	38.1	2.0	4.6
Physical disorders, presumably psychogenic	19.7	1.8	6.1
Constipation	7.5	13.6	4.8
Anorexia	0.8	2.9	0.9

telephone. All this can be very time consuming as a difficult case is going to require many sessions, and a busy GP may have to make the decision as to whether he is dealing with a simple, perhaps self-limiting condition amenable to simple advice and reassurance, or whether the time factor makes it imperative to refer the child to a child psychiatrist.

It is a saddening and salutatory experience sometimes to look back through an adolescent's notes and discover that in some patients' life styles there is a fearful appearance of inevitability. The feeding problem of two months becomes the food refusal of two years, the constipation of five, the cyclical vomiting of seven, the migraine of thirteen, and possibly the duodenal ulcer of adult life. Before one gives up in despair, one should reflect that it was a *patient*, or even better, an *individual* of three months who had a feeding problem and later grew into an individual who refused food at two years.

Did I help that individual at three months and two years in any way, or was the end result inevitable? So often we shall never know, but we know that the attempt must be made, as in making the attempt at least some sympathy and support is being offered to the parents. Then there is always the thought that many behaviour problems, like most paediatric illnesses, will end in spontaneous recovery.

THE PRE-SCHOOL YEARS

As the baby develops from the original helpless creature having all his wants immediately supplied, he gradually becomes aware of an expanding universe of relations, friends and strangers and also of the whole exterior world. Many normal babies go through a normal stage of shrinking back and clinging to their mothers ('He won't go to anyone now and I can't leave him with anybody'). With sympathetic handling this stage passes as the baby gains in security and his curiosity spurs him on to explore the outside world.

Somewhere between the ages of eighteen months and three years the toddler will discover that there are certain methods by which he can gain additional attention. Every mother of a toddler soon learns that there are three things that she cannot make her child do. She cannot make him eat, sleep or use his bowels to order; all she can do is create the loving, stable climate that makes the child desire her approval and dislike her disapproval.

So what can we do to help the parents of a child who demands attention with screaming fits, refusal to eat, refusal to sleep, or who loads his rectum to the extent that he suffers from continual dirty pants? We have to sympathise and explain, a form of medical treatment that can be so difficult, requiring time, an appreciation of the understanding of the parents and a gauging of the art of the possible for a family in an impossible situation.

Explanations must be concrete. If you want the mother to show more attention to the child, she must be told real everyday ways in which it must be done and also how it must not be done. How giving attention to the child is not the same as giving way to him.

'Attention' means setting aside time to talk to and (very important) time to listen to the child. It means time for the child apart from that given to his brothers and sisters. It does not mean the provision of expensive toys, bought with the proceeds of the mother's earnings. Whilst simple explanation and modification of the family programme may produce excellent results, especially if father can be brought in as a therapist, sometimes deeper problems emerge.

A mother of four admitted to me that she loved babies, but could not bring herself to cuddle or show physical affection with her older children, yet she had one little girl who positively yearned for it. Then it came out that the mother had never been cuddled herself in a disturbed childhood, and much deeper psychotherapy was required.

Temper tantrums

Judging by the questions mothers ask at playgroup get-togethers, this is one of the commonest problems in the pre-school age group. It needs an audience, is designed to command attention, and is a certain type of child's reaction to frustration and betrays a deficient training in the ability to cope with obstruction.

The child usually shouts and screams rather than cries, lies on the floor and kicks, using all his muscles in a tornado of frustration. There can be a danger of injury when a child bangs his head repeatedly on the floor. The child should be put where he is unlikely to harm himself and deprived of any possible audience. When it is all over, the incident should not be referred to again, but love and attention should be given for more sociably acceptable behaviour.

Every child tries a temper tantrum or other means of gaining attention at some time or other, and if laid on in the correct place, such as a crowded bus or a supermarket for example, it can be very effective. If the parents remain calm, showing a minimum of reaction, the behaviour fades out, whereas overt parental distress and anxiety will reinforce the behaviour, making it more and more difficult to stop. It is more likely to occur when there is inconsistent disciplinary control, or when several adults are in the home. The worst thing to happen is for the parent to try to avoid a similar situation arising in the future by allowing the child his own way. To cope with frustration is all part of growing up.

A more worrying phenomenon is the breath-holding

attack which may complicate a temper tantrum or be in itself a child's reaction to frustration. Unconsciousness or very rarely even death may complicate an attack. The rare severe outcome should not be mentioned to the mother, but unlike the temper tantrum an attack should be ended as soon as possible by a sudden sharp stimulation such as a shake, a slap or cold water on the face. The situation of excitement or frustration which produces the attack enables it to be differentiated from any form of epilepsy. In doubtful cases, especially with frequent attacks, an electroencephalogram or specialist opinion will be required.

In the older child, temper tantrums give way to aggressive behaviour and the 'terror of the playgroup' phenomenon. Such a child may find this a method of gaining attention, or he may be a hyperkinetic child unable to get rid of his surplus energy in more regulated ways. He may come from a strict family or one where physical movement is inhibited, such as living in a tower block of flats. Conversely he may come from a family with variable standards of discipline so that he has not been taught to control his desires. Aggressive attacks occurring at definite intervals with no obvious environmental cause are an indication for an electroencephalogram, especially if there is an abnormal perinatal history.

A mother of an aggressive child will need a great deal of support. If the love bond is still present the outlook is good, but if the child's aggression is a reaction to rejection, the going is long and difficult, with the mother requiring most of the therapeutic effort. In a minor case the child needs plenty of physical activity to use up his energy, and demonstration that he is still loved despite his antisocial behaviour. Whilst individual aggressive acts must be firmly stopped and disapproval shown, it is harder to remember to praise a period when they have been absent.

Eating problems

A problem of increasing frequency today is the trend for over-alimentation of children, with excessive weight gain as a result. This is a problem of the mother and is most likely to happen if the child is premature, underweight or handicapped and the mother overcompensates by feeding excess food to the child.

On the other hand, a poor or apparently poor appetite will cause intense concern, and I have seen many a mother reduced to tears by her child's lack of interest in food. I always tell such mothers that I have never seen a child die of selfinduced starvation yet.

Sometimes there is a history of difficulty with feeds and weaning since birth, but often the child has an apparently normal appetite until, somewhere between the first and second birthday, the baby discovers that if he refuses food he becomes the centre of attention. Mothers frequently feel that missing one or two meals may lead to serious illness in the child, and may need a lot of support to accept the advice of ignoring the child's food refusal but continue to serve up his usual food at meal times only.

A word of warning is necessary. Eating is such an essential activity in the minds of mothers that when it stops mothers seize on it as the most important symptom, and omit to tell the doctor that Johnnie is also complaining of a sore throat or that Mary is complaining that it hurts when she passes urine. So that whilst the doctor's instinctive unspoken reply to the mother's complaint that a child is not eating may be 'He would', or 'How fortunate with food the price it is!', it is essential to examine the child before labelling the case as a behavioural problem.

Sleeping problems

To parents fond of a well ordered existence, it is an unfortunate fact that children vary so considerably in the amount of sleep they require. There are well identified cases of babies who never sleep easily and regularly from birth, and against whom all our medicaments are of no avail.

When the presenting symptom is the complaint that the child will not, or cannot, sleep, we want to know for how long the child has been giving trouble, what part of his sleep is he losing, and if there is any obvious or hidden cause.

When there is a long history, treatment is going to be difficult. The child's sleeping habits may be a reflection of general domestic upset (such as marital disharmony) going on around him. He may be one of the babies mentioned above who seem to need their sleep only in short naps to everyone's inconvenience. A disorganised household may have prevented the establishment of the habit of a regular bedtime. The bedtime ritual of washing, tooth cleaning, story, relaxation leading to sleep may never have been established.

In considering the time of night involved in sleep loss, the simplest problem is the child who cannot go to sleep on being put to bed. Many parents solve this problem by putting the child to bed later and putting up with a later hour of rising, until starting school causes readjustment difficulties. If the child does not suffer from late hours then time will solve the problem. As with other behaviour disorders of childhood, failure to go to sleep may be an attention-seeking device from a child who is visibly and tenaceously fighting off sleep. Failure to go to sleep is the one sleep disorder that may be helped by drugs.

The child who goes to sleep only to wake up two or three hours later full of energy and eager to play is a great problem and parents of such a child have basically two choices – to love 'em or leave 'em. To take the child into bed with them is a treatment advocated with enthusiasm by a distinguished paediatrician (H. Jolly). My only criticism of the advice is that most of the mothers who consult me on the subject say that they have already tried it!

Many mothers will admit that they just could not in any circumstances leave the child to cry. A determined return of the child to bed after making sure that the child is not frightened and that there is some light present with a way of communication to the parent through open doors, can however nip a bad habit in the bud if applied early enough. The parents must be prepared to repeat the performance many times at the beginning for success to be achieved.

For those parents who object to the marital bed being invaded and who cannot leave a child to cry indefinitely, the compromise suggestion of Dr Christopher Green may be of practical help. He suggests that after being left to cry for a period the child should be cuddled, reassured and then put back in its bed. If he cries again, he should be left for a period longer than the first before being cuddled again. This process continues with the child being left for longer and longer periods. Parents who really want to solve this problem must be warned to write off a few nights sleep before peace reigns.

More dramatic is the case of the child who cannot go to sleep or who wakes up in the night with night terrors often associated with nightmares. The present obsession of the entertainment industry with monsters of one kind or another does not help and children with inborn tendencies to fear and anxiety should be protected from them. Many parents do not realise the delayed action effects of such programmes as 'Dr Who', because the child watches the programme with apparent enjoyment and the fear only appears after dark.

Sometimes it is difficult to discover what the child is really afraid of, and what experience has set the symptom in train. It may need many interviews and perhaps recourse to such devices as persuading the child to draw or model what he is afraid of, actions which may have therapeutic value in allowing the child to ventilate the anxiety under controlled conditions.

In practice one resorts sooner or later to the administration of some form of hypnotic, especially if the mother is at the end of her tether. This is perfectly permissible provided one realises that one is only treating the symptom and it is not the sole answer if, for example, there is a basic underlying insecurity or buried fear. The child with difficulty getting to sleep can be helped by the classical syrup of chloral, or by the proprietary preparations of triclofos (Trichloryl) or dichloralphenazone (Welldorm). The child with nervous tension and prebedtime rituals is helped by half a tablet (2.5 mg) of nitrazepam (Mogadon).

These drugs are often useful in suppressing nightmares but are of very limited value in the case of children waking after a few hours sleep as the effect of a bedtime dose has worn off. Drug therapy is effective where a temporary disturbance of habit or a treatable cause is present. Where disturbed nights seem to be a normal part of that child's make-up or there is a deep seated cause of long standing, cessation of medication seems doomed to bring about a relapse or else increasing tolerance of the drug reduces the effect.

Bowel disorders

Diarrhoea

When I look down a child's notes and find that he has had a fair number of attacks of diarrhoea, I think it is time (a) to consult my health visitor about the state of hygiene in the home, and (b) to reflect whether this child is under more tension than he can stand. Of course, there are many causes of chronic and recurrent diarrhoea which must be excluded, but an irritable colon indicating an irritable psyche is a common one. Questioning will usually elicit other signs of tension such as odd pains, and may show a relationship between symptoms and environmental stress such as school plays or examinations etc.

Encopresis and constipation

Being presented with dirty pants or, even worse, finding them hidden in various parts of the house is an experience few parents can accept with equanimity. We can persuade them to accept the wet bed and they may accept that a sleeping child is not responsible for his actions, but in encopresis the apparent deliberate soiling can set up extreme tension between the child and other members of the family.

Dirty pants are often due to an overflow phenomenon caused by chronic constipation. If constipation has been present from birth, it is important to exclude abnormalities of the colon or rectum, but the majority of cases are of psychogenic origin.

Thus we have to treat the child and not his rectum alone. Occasionally, there is a rare case of the child unable to use a lavatory because of its association with some shock experience such as sexual assault or being locked in, but usually encopresis is associated with such factors as sibling jealousy, a desire for attention, lack of security and perhaps, especially, a feeling of rejection. The latter is often due to a breakdown in family relationships, such as a parent leaving home.

Re-establishing a stable family environment or helping a child to readjust to a state that cannot be changed may be a long procedure, taxing the patience of all concerned. In a bad case, with the rectum overloaded, the best thing may be to order an enema. Recurrent enemata with their dramatic drawing of attention to the rectum are undesirable, but if the rectum is emptied at the beginning the symptoms should be relieved, at least for a few days during which an attempt can be made at improving family relationships. If she does not want to find dirty pants in odd places, mother must learn to accept an 'accident' in a matter-of-fact way.

A habit of regular bowel action can be helped by the administration of one of the 'physiological' bowel stimulants such as petrolagar, dioctyl sodium sulphosuccinate (Dioctyl-medo, Normax) and lactulose.

THE SCHOOL YEARS

The child with a pain

A child soon learns that a complaint of pain enables him to get sympathy and attention, so that it is not surprising that a child feeling unhappy, rejected or frustrated should complain of a pain. The little malingerer is usually easily distinguished from the child who has genuine pains of physical or psychogenic origin, by the way his pains occur at convenient times (e.g. 8.45 a.m. on a Monday morning) and disappear when their maintenance is inconvenient (e.g. at 9.30 a.m.). The child who frequently pretends to pain is a problem in itself of course.

More difficult is the child who suffers from real pain, perhaps severe enough for hospital admission under the suspicion of an acute surgical emergency. The commonest sites are the head and the abdomen, with less common complaints in such sites as a joint or joints, the ear or the chest. Sometimes the pain is accompanied by other symptoms such as vomiting or diarrhoea.

The child with a pain is a child with a worry, the nature of which may take some time to elucidate. If the child could explain why he had the pain he would not have it, so investigation may not be easy. In the middle of a busy consulting session, one's heart sinks when mother says the child keeps having headaches, as one realises that theoretically the child might be suffering from any illness in the paediatric textbook and that unless the diagnosis is fairly obvious or the symptoms slight enough to permit a waiting policy, there is nothing for it but to examine the child from top to toe.

The majority of children with headaches and the 'little belly-achers' described so well by Apley (1975) are suffering from tensions, fears and anxieties due to the family tensions that we have considered in the aetiology or another does not help, and children with inborn tenjected after a new birth in the family or after the departure of a parent, may display inward tension with pain, especially if he hears frequent complaints of pain from a parent. School may be the cause of his trouble, especially if the pain only occurs in term time and is absent at the weekend. Marked symptoms are generally due to a more than general dislike of school, and are usually associated with some such factor as bullying, an unsympathetic teacher, an inability to make friends with other children, or (a recent new cause) a feeling of insecurity in children in some modern schools where a lot of work is left to the child to be done on his own to a schedule.

The tranquillisers that are used so often with their parents undoubtedly give satisfactory results with children with psychogenic pain. Valium 2 mg twice or sometimes thrice a day will often relieve symptoms and, where the cause is temporary, there will be rapid resolution. If the child cannot, however, be helped to resolve his tension, he will return with the pain again, perhaps in another part of his anatomy.

Enuresis

The majority of cases of bedwetting seen by the GP are more accurately described as developmental rather than behavioural problems, but nevertheless behaviour problems can be the result as well as the cause of enuresis. Many surveys have shown that about one in ten children are still wetting the bed at the age of five, and one in 20 at the age of ten.

The history is an important guide to management. The child who has always wetted the bed since birth is, in the absence of evidence to the contrary, probably a late developer as far as bladder control is concerned. The child who gained control satisfactorily but then lost it at a later stage may need longer consideration. If the history is short, an organic cause must be excluded, as rarely one meets the urinary infection whose only symptom is enuresis. More likely the relapse was caused by a psychological disturbance, a common example of which is the birth of a new brother or sister. Here bedwetting is often accompanied by other regression symptoms, such as thumb sucking and a desire to be fed.

A child who wets himself in the day but not at night is probably making some sort of protest, or crying for help, and a full psychological investigation is indicated. There are the fairly easily spotted cases where the child wets himself only in school because he does not like the school lavatories. Most of the cases of children above the age of four who wet both by day or night are from homes with unintelligent or socially deprived parents. Very often the family history will reveal one or more siblings with enuresis, and further enquiry may show that one or both parents were also enuretic in childhood. Here any hope of cure lies in a long slog on the part of health visitor, social worker and GP. In the case of a child from a good home, diurnal enuresis (unless there is a fairly quick response to treatment) is an indication for consultant opinion to exclude abnormality of the renal tract.

After taking the history, the child should be examined completely (this is in all the books) to exclude such things as slight spina bifida and other neurological rarities. In practice the GP should be able to look up the results of the child's last developmental or other routine examination to reassure himself that he found nothing suspicious then. A specimen of urine should always be examined by the laboratory, and abnormal findings appropriately followed up.

Having decided that a case belongs to the majority group of simple delayed development, one has to clear the decks for action by ascertaining the attitudes of the child and parents, preferably by seeing each alone. The child will often have been brought to see you as a form of actual or implied punishment and be very ashamed of his affliction. He must be put at his ease and the complaint treated with cheerful optimism. The parent must not be promised miracles, but given a matter of fact explanation of the condition with instructions to praise the child for a dry bed and ignore a wet one.

As in many conditions, the enthusiasm of the doctor is an important therapeutic agent and for this reason, I normally see children at no greater than fortnightly intervals. The child must be *seen* and his progress discussed with him. The practice of sending in for a repeat prescription is bad. Treatment is partly behaviouristic and partly by drugs. The praise-but-no-blame advice to the mother is part of the former, and the issuing of calendars for the child to mark or stick stars on every dry night achieved is another. If such a device is used (and I find them very useful), the child should not be asked to record failures, and should not commence such a record until he has already achieved a basic score of one or two dry nights per week, otherwise he may be faced with having no success at all to show at the next consultation.

Of drugs in common use, by far the most successful are those of the tricyclic group, imipramine (Tofranil) and amitryptyline (Tryptizol). Many hospital paediatricians condemn the use of these drugs as they are justifiably alarmed at the rising death toll in children poisoned by them. There were 27 such deaths in children under 10 in Scotland, England and Wales in the years 1973–77, yet it would be unfortunate to lose a treatment for which so many mothers are grateful. Moreover, it has to be realised that most of the childhood fatalities from these drugs arise from children taking imipramine and amitryptyline prescribed for their parents rather than for themselves. Many enuretics come from disorderly homes and suffer from poor parenting and in these cases a doctor must ask himself if the parents can be trusted with a potentially dangerous drug. In all cases mothers must be warned of special care in the use and storage of the medicine.

Imiprimine 25 mg or amitryptyline 10 mg is given as 5 ml of syrup at night, the dose being increased after a week or two to 10 ml. Later if results are poor, the dose for the older child can be raised to 15 ml. Side effects are unusual; sleepiness the next day, and sometimes behaviour changes, are rarely reported. Occasionally a parent will report an improvement in behaviour, possibly resulting from an alleviation of depression.

Belladonna, ephedrine, amphetamine, propantheline (Probanthine) and hyoscine butylbromide (Buscopan) have all been used in the treatment of enuresis, but they are now considered only in those cases for whom the antidepressants are contraindicated (such as epileptic children). Diazepam (Valium) 2 mg at night will sometimes help the child whose bedwetting seems to be part of a light-sleeping, generally hyperkinetic syndrome.

With tricyclic therapy one often seems to get stuck at a point where the child has one wet bed per week or per fortnight, but one wet bed per week is better than seven. Occasionally, as also in the case of the child who makes no signs of improvement at all, it helps to stop all treatment for a month and start again.

A disadvantage of the tricyclics is that on the cessation of treatment, there may be a dramatic relapse. To prevent this I maintain full dosage until at least a month of dry beds is recorded. Then I reduce the dose by 2.5 ml of the syrup per fortnight, but the patient is prescribed the same volume of medicine as before and not told that he is on a reduced dose until success has been assured. After this relapses usually respond quickly to further courses of treatment.

The alarm-bed is a form of treatment using behaviouristic methods where the child wetting a sheet completes an electrical circuit that sets an alarm bell ringing. This wakes the child who switches off the bell, empties his bladder, resets the device, and puts on a dry sheet. With a well motivated child who is able and willing to cooperate, the treatment is very effective. With an older child (ten and over) who is keen to be dry, one can almost guarantee a fairly rapid cure, and this may be the treatment of choice. It is essential that the GP familiarises himself with the apparatus, so that its proper use can be fully explained to parent and child. For a good description, with diagrams, see Brooks and Mallik (1982). Alarm beds are not so expensive as to be beyond the resources of a group practice, but it would help if the metal gauze sheets were available on prescription. Most local authority clinics will lend them out but there is usually a waiting list.

Not every child will respond to treatment rapidly, but even with the most persistent enuretic there is good cause for optimism in the long term, for the condition rarely persists after puberty.

School phobia

'School phobia' is a term that has come to mean the state in which a child has tremendous fear of going to school for no obvious reason. The term is a bad one as most of the cases are not due to fear of school at all but to fear of leaving the home and/or the mother. School refusal or separation anxiety are better terms. The truant child does not like school but is not usually afraid of it.

Occasionally a child will be reluctant to go to school on account of bullying, being overwhelmed by the massive size of a comprehensive after a small junior school, or for a more bizarre reason such as that of the little girl who could not stand the hymn singing of morning assembly because it reminded her of a funeral of a beloved relative. These 'rational' causes of dislike of attending school are sometimes not definitely mentioned by the child and have to be discovered in private interviews. Usually something can be done to help the child to solve the problem.

The typical case of school phobia can sometimes be anticipated when a child who is known to have had an overprotected upbringing (perhaps an only child or a later child of elderly parents) is suddenly brought up with a multitude of minor ailments that only occur in term time. This is the time to recognise that the doctor's job does not end with excluding organic disease. The mother must be warned that the child's attendance at school must be kept going at all costs, as once a child actually ceases to attend it may take a considerable time, perhaps months or even a year, for attendance to be resumed.

Treatment has to be directed at the causes of the abnormal tight but ambivalent bonds that tie mother and child together, to breaking the bonds and to rehabilitating the child back into the school situation. In a longstanding and difficult case, the parents may need specialist psychiatric help. Sometimes the father is retiring or works away and takes too little interest in the child, so that the child and mother become too bound together. He must do his share in taking the child out from the home and widening interests. Mother may well be imposing an excessive burden of emotion on the child, perhaps projecting frustrations from her own early life on the child.

These children are usually stay-at-homes and efforts have to be made to persuade them to join guides, scouts, clubs etc., and if they are reluctant to do this then efforts must be made to get friends into the house so that the child can be given props for future ventures from the home.

There is little hope of rapid cure of a marked case of school phobia without the wholehearted co-operation of the school head teachers. (This is essential anyway for any GP attempting to cope with the behaviour problems of school children).

In a severe case, a child must be relieved of all pressure to return to school for a time and be provided with a home teacher, and/or regularly supplied work from school, while attempts are made to disentangle and rebuild the parent-child relationship. Some parents have a sort of satisfaction at the child's obvious preference for their company rather than the school. Some on the other hand develop intense frustration and hostility to the inconvenience caused by a child.

Later a 'desensitisation' process can be attempted. The child attends school for morning assembly, perhaps for only the first lesson and then return home. Later attendance reaches morning break, then the dinner hour and finally school attendance becomes full again.

Recently a more aggressive approach has been described in which sufferers from school refusal were physically forced back to school. It is claimed that this procedure (applied with concurrent family psychotherapy) produced quicker and better results. If this work is confirmed then perhaps the point may be conceded to those cynics who maintain that the increase in numbers of school refusal cases of recent years is because, 'They would never have dared to try it on years ago'!

REFERRAL

For various reasons, however experienced the GP will find it necessary to refer some behaviour problems to a psychiatrist. Some children will not improve despite his best endeavours; with some parents he will have such difficulty in establishing sympathy that he will feel it better to let some uninvolved outsider attempt treatment. Some behaviour problems are so dramatic and arouse such high emotion in the parents (such as school refusal and encopresis) that they will be reluctant to accept the fact that treatment may be a long and difficult process, making heavy demands on the parents themselves, from anyone less than a consultant.

We must accept that the very process of referral is a therapeutic action in itself. I have often found parents after referral realising that their child cannot be cured in three days, then return and become much more co-operative in our joint efforts to find a solution.

Behaviour problems can be irritating, time consuming, inconvenient and exasperating, but helping to turn a miserable, unhappy little human being into a cheerful, smiling friend can be one of the great pleasures of general practice.

FURTHER READING

Apley, J. (1975) *The Child with Abdominal Pain*, 2nd edn. Oxford: Blackwell.

Bain, D.J.G. (1975) Prescribing psychotropic drugs for children. *Journal of the Royal College of General Practitioners*, **25**, 49–53.

Blagg, N. (1979) *Behavioural treatment of school refusal*. Thesis, University of London.

Bowlby, J. (1965) *Child Care and the Growth of Love*. Harmondsworth: Penguin.

Brooks, D. & Mallik, N. (1982) *Urology and Renal Medicine*, ch. 13. Library of General Practice. Edinburgh: Churchill Livingstone.

Forfar, J.O., McCrae, W.M. & Wolff, S. (1973) Psychiatric disorders in childhood. In Forfar, J.O. & Arneil, G.C. (eds) *Textbook of Paediatrics*, pp. 1711–1757. Edinburgh: Churchill Livingstone.

Fraser, M.S. (1972) Nocturnal enuresis. *The Practitioner*, **208**, 203–211.

Green, C. (1980) Management Problems of the Toddler. *Journal of Maternal and Child Health*, 64–71.

Jolly, H. (1977) *Book of Child Care*. London: Allen & Unwin.

Powell, B.W. (1972) Sleep disorders in childhood. *The Practitioner*, **208**, 198–202.

Seiler, E.R. (1972) Sleep problems in children. *The Practitioner*, **208**, 271–275.

Wolff, S. (1969) *Children Under Stress*. Harmondsworth: Penguin Books.

The spoilt child

Cyril Josephs

Among the many reasons given to explain a child's abnormal or unusual behaviour, that he is 'spoilt' is one of the most popular. What exactly is meant by 'spoiling a child' is not easy to ascertain. After all, one can spoil a cake or spoil a well-laid out garden, but how does one spoil a living human being, short of killing it? This I would prefer to call 'destroying it'. Spoiling the child nearly always means that he behaves in a way contrary to the wishes of his parents. If only babies and young children could vocalise their thoughts and impressions, we would all learn a lot.

It is axiomatic to state that 'all children are born good' (unless we believe in original sin); it is we grown-ups who make them bad. (I ignore, for the purpose of this essay, the sad case of the child with mental retardation or genetic handicap who cannot be expected to obey the rules.)

'Spoiling' usually means letting a child have his own way. Not only do we assume that we know best – that the child does not know what is good for him – but we will go to enormous lengths to enforce our will on the child. The mother who hears her children making rather more noise than usual in their playroom calls out to her husband in a vexed voice 'Go and see what the children are up to and stop them', before she even knows what they are 'up to'.

So much depends on why we wish to prevent a child having his own way, and even more important on how we hope to achieve this objective. It has always seemed to me that behaviour disorders arise very frequently from parents endeavouring to make their child behave as they want him to, notwithstanding the protestations of the child who will always, unless he is an imbecile, put up some kind of defence against the constant battering and nagging.

FEEDING

The commonest cause of underfeeding is fear of overfeeding. From the earliest infancy we dictate how much food a baby should have, when feeding to satisfaction and on demand would be better, though possibly more demanding of the mother.

It is when the child is a little older that so many troubles start. We are told in countless books that feeding a child is a great art, and difficult to learn. Dire consequences are forecast for those who ignore the vitamin requirements, carbohydrate excesses and calorie needs of the growing child. We grown-ups are allowed to eat what and when we like and seem to survive, but not the child. Food forcing by over-fussy, over-anxious and usually well meaning parents is undoubtedly the commonest cause of food refusal. A life-long hatred of a certain food can usually be traced back to an insistence on its being eaten in childhood. The increasing modern habit of schoolchildren having their dinners at school, where so often a failure to clear the plate results in punishment of some sort or some humiliation, leads to at best a strong dislike of school dinners and at worst a strong dislike of the school. The child subjected to repeated food-forcing (and I have met cases where physical forcing has occurred when the parent, usually the father, will not be outdone) will rapidly resort to defences which include vomiting, abdominal pain, migraine, anxiety, and many other symptoms. The child can become thin, wan, unhappy, pale, anaemic and prey to frequent infections; the very opposite to that which the parents expect from their actions.

On the other hand, it is a delight to meet the robust child who is 'so easy to feed' for he has been allowed to eat what he likes. After all, we grown-ups eat what we like (apart from those unfortunates who are not free agents) and enjoy our food. It is time we learned once and for all that in the matter of feeding children are but young adults.

PARENTAL CONTROL

Often the child's abnormal and aggressive behaviour is put down to lack of parental control. In severe cases of misbehaviour, the child is taken away from his parents and put under control of a local authority who must know how to bring up the child. Whilst it is always the parents who need the controlling in these cases, one has to admit that sometimes it is necessary to remove the child from their control and put him elsewhere, because the parents are too far gone and are beyond help in this matter. So often we find that such parents suffered similar traumas when they were young.

To be worthwhile, parental control should be synonymous with love and affection. Nearly all parents love their children, but there is still an odd hesitancy in expressing this. It is a natural urge and should be freely expressed. Young children are extremely sensitive to love and affection. The more freely this is displayed, the more the child will respond to the parents' wishes. The more the control is exercised by the heavy hand, the nagging tongue and the disapproving look, in an attempt to exact obedience, the more the child will rebel and disobey. I believe that if less use were made of such expressions as 'naughty', 'dirty', 'you're wicked', 'I don't love you now', and if they were replaced by 'good', 'I trust you', 'I love you', 'thank you', 'I'll tell you why you shouldn't do that', the result would be the disappearance of many of the common difficulties.

Correct control does not mean the heaping of love and affection one minute and dire punishments the next. Showering kisses and presents one day in return for half killing him the day before will just not do; it will neither fool the child nor prevent him being confused and apprehensive. I am minded of the young boy who feared each Saturday tea-time because his father, an ardent supporter of his local football club, would be impossible if his team had lost. It interested me that the child feared the worst rather than he looked forward to the best.

PUNISHMENT

This is a very emotive subject and certainly brings out the passion in us. There are those who proudly say that corporal punishment never did any harm, and those who believe one must never hit a child. I am always surprised that we allude to physical punishment as 'good'. We happily talk about giving a 'good smack' or a 'good thrashing', 'six of the best', or even a 'good, sound whipping'. Why, I wonder, are these never 'bad'? On the whole I come down clearly on the side of the non-violent. Children are rendered quite insecure by punishment. It always represents a failure on the part of the parents. Since we are none of us perfect (and whilst perfection is a seemingly laudable objective, it must be somewhat dull to have no failings whatsoever) we must be forgiven the occasional lapse. But it is important to recognise that it is a lapse; it is nothing to be proud of, even if it be a universal failing.

This does not mean that I advocate giving in to a child's every whim. Every child must learn the meaning of 'no'. But the more we explain and the more we set a good example, the less will be the need for correction. The occasional slap will do no great harm to the child; the cold-blooded calculated physical punishment does harm to both parties. The former represents nothing more nor less than a loss of temper on the parents' part; the latter is an expression of a more deep rooted disorder which may need urgent treatment.

Children are so often punished and rebuked for actions which may not be wrong or may have been copied from their parents, or for which they are entirely irresponsible. An old man with incontinence is not punished, yet how often do we hear of a bedwetting child being smacked; both the man and the child would dearly love to be dry.

The mother who brings to the doctor the child who, despite repeated daily good hidings, is unmanageable, is herself likely to be unmanageable. She needs the help. Occasionally, she will suffer from organic illness such as thyrotoxicosis or anaemia or depression. More often the problem will be of parental insecurity and unhappiness; without alleviating these problems there is little hope of improvement for the child.

Fortunately for us, most children are robust enough to survive our attempts at control, even if they less often benefit from them.

EDUCATIONAL STRAIN

A further way in which children can be spoiled during their formative years is by imposing excessive stress on their educational abilities. Parents naturally want their children to have the best possible chance of getting on in the world. Often the underachieved father insists that his son should reach the heights to which he, the father, aspired but never gained. Learning can never be forced. The child, for his part, anxious to please, may well set himself an impossible goal and end as a thoroughly mixed-up and depressed schoolboy or undergraduate. The large number of careers open to young people nowadays makes choice difficult, even with the help of trained career officers. The child of the father who has achieved career satisfaction and high status may have an impossible job emulating his father.

The imposition of extra activities against the child's wishes causes unnecessary stress and friction. I have seen a boy with a rapid type of speech which was almost unintelligible and which caused him untold troubles at school with increasing anxiety symptoms, rapidly and completely cured by barring his overbearing piano teacher from his house and by using the money so saved to buy him fishing tackle. He never was a musician;

neither was his father. But both fished happily together and the boy's performance at school improved immeasurably. Tolerance, guidance and acceptance are the passwords for the parents in these matters. It is important that the child who falls short of our expectations in one way is not allowed to acquire feelings of inferiority and worthlessness; so surely as he does feel a failure, will he fail further.

THE ROLE OF THE FAMILY DOCTOR IN THE TREATMENT OF THE SPOILT CHILD

The family doctor has an important part to play in ironing out these common family problems. He must be a patient listener and whilst recognising the failings of the parents he must be slow to accuse. To win over the parents to his side is not always easy. Sometimes it will be impossible. The views expressed by the doctor will often be unacceptable; we all of us tend to ask advice hoping to hear what we already believe in. Occasionally we might be asked, 'Where did we go wrong?' Even with this *crie du coeur* it can be an uphill struggle. I often find it useful to say 'You have tried your way for X years (X being the age of the child) without success. Please try my way for X weeks and we will see what happens'.

The doctor can often forecast the future juvenile delinquent – a sad prophecy which he will attempt to disprove. In the final analysis I believe that a community gets the number of delinquents it deserves. The more the doctor can restore an attitude of peace and harmony in the home, the more hopeful is the outlook for his young patient.

No child, I believe, is ever spoilt by too much affection. It is time we changed the old proverb to 'Spare the love and spoil the child'.

ACKNOWLEDGEMENT

This essay owes its inspiration to the teaching of the late Professor C.W. Vining, Emeritus Professor of Paediatrics at the University of Leeds, Yorkshire. I was privileged to work with him for several years, and his philosophy of paediatrics has been a constant source of enthusiasm to me.

47

Communication and learning disorders in childhood

Emanuel Tuckman

At the age of four, about six per cent of children have definite retardation of language development and more than ten per cent have speech which is unintelligible. Delay in language development may be due to many physical causes including deafness, infantile autism, cerebral palsy, intellectual handicap, specific developmental language disorder and sociocultural deprivation. Children with such disorders will already have been identified during developmental screening, and general practitioners will be concerned mainly with the young child who seems to be slow in developing speech and language, but who is apparently otherwise normal.

The first essential is to reassess the child to ensure that there are indeed no physical abnormalities, paying particular attention to his hearing responses and his understanding of the world around him. The clues can be obtained from the mother – when he plays with toys, such as cars and dolls, does he treat them as mere objects or does his play show that he understands their function? Does he ever point at objects she names, does he help her with household tasks, and does he do what she tells him? Early developmental landmarks should be checked and an estimate made of the level of speech and language for verbal comprehension, verbal expression, articulation and intelligibility. By the age of two, normal children have a vocabulary of about 200 words, but they show considerable variation in speech production, though less in comprehension. Their words are mostly nouns but pronouns begin to appear and verbs are used to form two-word sentences. Simple instructions are understood and 'inner language' is evidenced in symbolic play.

The general practitioner's knowledge of the sort of words the local children of that age usually use and the range of play materials with which they are familiar is valuable for assessment. He will also be aware of the normal variations of cultural sub-groups who may be living within the community but not necessarily sharing common forms of child-rearing practices. Local environmental factors such as type of housing, overcrowding or absence of play space, may force upon parents methods of control and communication to which they would not normally subscribe.

A child who is simply slow at developing speech needs to be observed from time to time between his second and third birthdays. During this year his mother and others at home should talk to him in a one-to-one relation. Visits from the health visitor are invaluable, as she can ensure that adequate toys and picture books are available in the child's home and she can get the parents to appreciate the value of reading to their child. She can demonstrate to the mother how best to use the materials available to stimulate the child's language development. As speech is learnt mainly from adults, attendance at nursery school is unlikely to help speech development as such, though this may well help where a child's social competence is poor. This is particularly so in areas where there is much child minding, as minders will not often be aware of the need for particular kinds of stimuli and play at various stages in a child's development. Unfortunately, the provision of nursery classes in such areas is likely to be in inverse proportion to the need.

Where there is any question of mental backwardness, referral to an assessment centre is indicated and if the disability is confirmed, the GP may have to help the parents develop a realistic attitude to their child's potential. While maintaining his independent position, he will need to appear to be on their side if conflicts with the authorities arise and he must be prepared to listen to their worries, discuss their problems and act on their behalf when this is necessary.

SPEECH PROBLEMS

Where problems of speech predominate, considerable benefit will derive from treatment by a speech therapist, to whom the GP can refer a child direct. The therapist will be able to concentrate on particular aspects of the child's difficulties, such as auditory inattention or articulation defects, and she will be able to follow progress by means of standard measures such as the Reynell Language Development Scales.

Research studies on intervention programmes for pre-school children have shown that the large majority with delayed language development make accelerated progress in both receptive and expressive aspects of language. These programmes may be either in a language clinic where parents and child are seen regularly by a speech therapist for ongoing advice on how to help the child's language, or in a language class which the child attends daily and which is under the direction of a qualified teacher. Similar progress has been obtained with a program for pre-school children organised by the local primary school and administered by mothers at home. For four months, the mothers spent 30 minutes a day following a programme of general vocabulary, stimulating an understanding of time space and size relationships and reading selected books.

Most children with language difficulties do not show abnormalities in social and emotional development, and language retardation does not itself lead directly to emotional and behavioural problems. It may, however, lead to such problems through the effects of communication difficulties in social relationships, and through educational failure. When children first start at school, some five per cent speak so poorly that they are unable to make themselves understood by strangers, and one per cent are seriously retarded in their production of spoken language. At the age of seven, over ten per cent of children have an appreciable degree of speech impairment, while between one and two per cent have marked speech defect. The commonest type of defect is stuttering, and though gradual improvement often takes place, this does not always happen.

Some children pass through a period between the ages of 2½ and five years when their speech is not fluent. It is not known whether this 'non-fluency' is part of normal speech and language development or whether it is a preliminary stage in the development of stutter. Children with a family history of stutter and who are poor or late talkers are five times more likely to develop stutter than other children. In such children, parent counselling may help to prevent its development. Advice to parents should be directed towards modifying situations of communicative stress, reducing adverse reactions, and encouraging the child to enjoy talking.

In the older child, the speech therapist's analysis of the specific patterns of stutter and the child's attitude to his speech will lead to a two-dimensional approach in treatment. Specific techniques are used to increase fluency by, for example, syllable-timed speech and continuous attempts are made during treatment to reduce stress and modify the resulting symptoms. Attendance weekly at a speech therapy clinic is often inadequate and more intensive daily treatment may be needed. Group therapy is often used in children over the age of nine and in adolescents.

Specific learning disorders are amongst the commonest problems in schoolchildren, and though primarily they may be the concern of teacher or school psychologist, family doctors have an important role to play. The doctor must try to establish why a particular child has a learning difficulty; pre- and perinatal factors such as smoking during pregnancy, malnutrition or physical abuse may have played a part in the aetiology. Certainly, if special neurological examinations of children with learning disabilities are carried out, many are found to have significantly more minor neurological signs than control children. Although these signs become less obvious or disappear by about the age of 11, younger children show lags or deficits at the highest levels of central nervous functioning such as fine co-ordination.

READING RETARDATION

Although learning disabilities may show themselves in disorders of listening, thinking, talking, writing, spelling or arithmetic, low achievement is most frequent with reading ability. Over the country as a whole, about 10 per cent of all primary schoolchildren are backward readers, but in some areas as many as 30 per cent have not started to read by the age of six and a half. The controversy continues between the neurologists, who lay claim to a specific syndrome of dyslexia due to neurological abnormality, and the educational psychologists, who regard backward readers as only quantitatively different from good readers, their achievement being at one end of a continuum covering the entire range of reading abilities from fluency to severe difficulty.

Nevertheless, although reading ability follows a generally normal distribution with over-achievement and under-achievement occurring with roughly the same frequency, there is a significant departure from normality at the extreme lower end of the curve such that gross under-achievement in reading occurs at well above the expected frequency. This suggests that there is a group of children with specific reading retardation which is not explicable simply in terms of the bottom of a continuum and it is to this small group of children that the term dyslexia should be confined.

Full investigation by an educational psychologist will include tests of sensory and motor function, intelligence, reading and spelling, speech and language function, visuoperceptual function, laterality and right/left confusion. All may be within normal limits, and the reading age', may rectify itself as time goes on. However, some dyslexic children have language disorders, reading difficulty, which may have presented itself only as a delay in comparison with the standard of 'normal', showing great difficulty in putting names to objects and in recognising sounds or visual patterns. Some are handicapped by articulation defects and lack of coordination in their speech and handwriting, while others have normal speech, but a perceptual disorder makes them unable to discriminate between letters and unable to associate these with sounds.

Recent experimental results are compatible with the view that in backward readers there is a developmental lag in their visual information processing. This has led to the introduction of a test of visual sequencing for preschool children which may be used as a screening test to identify potential backward readers.

The exact part played by left-handedness, ambidexterity, and left/right cerebral dominance has not yet been clearly determined but the presence of clumsiness in such things as skipping, kicking, throwing and catching indicates a central nervous system not sufficiently organised to cope with our man-made technology of language, based as it is on skills, order and rules. Thus reading retardation may result from any one of several clusters of deficiencies in brain function, and those various defects may, themselves, each have multiple causes.

Reading retardation is strongly associated with antisocial or conduct disorder and with emotional disturbance. A vicious circle may be set up because the child, particularly the intelligent one who fails in reading, has to face negative responses to his failure and becomes discouraged, miserable and lacking in confidence, whilst these very symptoms produce low motivation for achievement and lead to continuation of the reading difficulty. Although a severe emotional upset, such as separation of parents, will obviously affect school performance, more often than not behaviour difficulties are due to failure at school. Under-achievers appear to have had in their past no more anxiety or stress than other children.

FAMILY INFLUENCES

The home environment is of crucial importance as a formative and continuing influence in a child's attainment and there is undoubted value in parents talking intelligently to their children, reading stories to them and participating alongside schools in teaching to read. However, there is a virtual absence of preparental training, such as making older pupils aware of young children's linguistic and cognitive development, or making language development a matter of concern to expectant parents in antenatal clinics. Schools do not lend books to parents of preschool children to encourage them to recognise the value of preschool reading, and home visiting schemes by teachers to aid parents of preschool children do not exist.

Within the family, a number of conditions might produce resistance to learning to read and to blocking of the capacity to learn. These include indifference of parents to the child's welfare, and hostility as shown by scolding, ridicule and encouragement of sibling rivalry. Overprotectiveness and overanxiety on the part of a parent and disturbed parental relationships are other factors. If it is not recognised that failure is due to a specific learning disorder, it may be thought that the child is not really trying or is lazy or naughty. He may actually have been trying harder than average and when success eludes him, be falsely accused and punished. It is often the mother who realises that the child is not getting a fair deal, not only at school but frequently from an authoritarian father. If she fails to get the help she knows is needed for her child, she is likely to become emotionally disturbed. Mothers of backward readers exhibit more neuroticism than normal, and while little is known about paternal influences, fathers of young children with language development lag seem to have less than average verbal interaction with their children.

The alert general practitioner may well be the first to become aware of a possible learning problem, as many of the children are brought to him by a parent because of symptoms such as headache, abdominal pain, nervousness, restlessness and poor concentration. Other children may have behavioural disturbances such as rebelliousness, destructiveness or withdrawal. The doctor may know the adverse home and school conditions which are playing a part in the particular child's problem, and with the aid of social worker or health visitor he may be able to help to resolve the child's difficulties, in which the whole family is usually involved. The educational problem itself may remain covert if the doctor does not consult with the child's head teacher, and ideally co-operation between the two is needed to decide on the provision of special help such as opportunity class or remedial teaching. Often those children most in need of assistance are those least likely to get it, and the family doctor can play an important role on a child's behalf by acting as co-ordinator and mobilising medical, educational and psychosocial specialists. General practitioners need to become increasingly involved in children's educational problems.

FURTHER READING

Cooper, J., Moodley, M. & Reynell, J. (1978) *Helping Language Development: A Developmental Programme For Children With Early Language Handicaps*. London: Edward Arnold.

Crystal, D. (1980) *Introduction to Language Pathology*. London: Edward Arnold.

Francis-Williams, J. (1974) *Children with Specific Learning Difficulties*, 2nd edn. Oxford: Pergamon Press.

Gregory, H. (ed) (1979) *Controversies About Stuttering Therapy*. University Park Press.

Morley, M.E. (1981) *The Development and Disorders of Speech in Childhood*, 4th edn. Edinburgh: Churchill Livingstone.

Rutter, M. & Martin, J.A.M. (eds) (1972) *The Child with Delayed Speech*. London: Heinemann.

Vernon, M.D. (1971) *Reading and its Difficulties. A Psychological Study*. Cambridge University Press.

48

The care of immigrant children

Margaret Pollak

WHO ARE THE IMMIGRANTS?

Britain long ago ceased to be populated by a homogeneous cultural group. It is, therefore, important for all doctors – but, perhaps, particularly for primary care doctors – to have information and knowledge of the ethnic groups who make up some of the patient population of this country.

It is only since the end of World War II that immigration by a variety of ethnic groups, some of whom have a black skin, has taken place in any numbers. The great majority of the immigrants have come from the New Commonwealth countries and Pakistan (NCWP). The NCWP is defined as consisting of: India, Pakistan, Bangladesh, the West Indies, the African continent and others which include Cyprus and Malta.

SIZE AND ORIGIN

In 1971 it was estimated that NCWP immigrants constituted 2.5 per cent of the population of Great Britain (1 371 000 people). In the same year there were 111 000 immigrants from Poland, and 109 000 from Italy. By 1977 the NCWP population had grown to 1 846 000– 3.4 per cent of the total population and an increase of 30 per cent.

During this period (1971–77) the increase in the NCWP population has not been uniform amongst the different groups of which it is composed. For example, there has been a 20 per cent increase in the numbers of people who originated in Pakistan, Asians from East Africa and Africans from Africa whilst the increase in the West Indian group has been only ten per cent, although they are still the largest single group in the NCWP. During the same period of time, other groups in the NCWP – mainly from Hong Kong and countries of the Mediterranean – have grown from 203 000 to 274 000, an increase of 35 per cent. In 1977 it is estimated that there were approximately 140 000 people of mixed descent living in UK, many of whom are immigrants.

The ways in which the different groups have increased have been different. The West Indian population, reflecting their earlier immigration compared with some other groups, has increased its numbers mainly by births in the UK whilst most of the other groups have increased by a rise in immigration numbers.

CHILDREN

In 1977 approximately 40 per cent of the NCWP population living in GB was made up of people who had been born in this country so that most of them are children. Figure 48.1 shows the age and sex structure of NCWP immigrants in 1976. For example, males under the age of 16 years made up 25.3 per cent of the population. It is seen therefore, that the majority of NCWP immigrants are young compared with the general population (Table 48.1).

The percentages of all live births to mothers from the NCWP increased from 5.3 per cent in 1971 to 6.6 per cent in 1976. (Table 48.2). It will be noticed, however, that there has been a substantial fall in the numbers of births to West Indian mothers, little change in the numbers born to mothers from Pakistan and Bangladesh and an increase in live births to African mothers.

Figure 48.2 illustrates the differences in birth order and marital status of children and parents from the indigenous population, West Indian and Indian Subcontinent immigrants and illustrates the social and family differences which occur in the different groups.

The GB population of wholly NCWP ethnic origin is projected to increase in the decade 1976–86 by between 35 and 50 per cent.

BACKGROUND AND CULTURE

There is an unfortunate tendency for some in the host country to think of all immigrants as 'foreigners'. They are, of course, made up of many different peoples with their own distinct backgrounds. Some come from ethnic

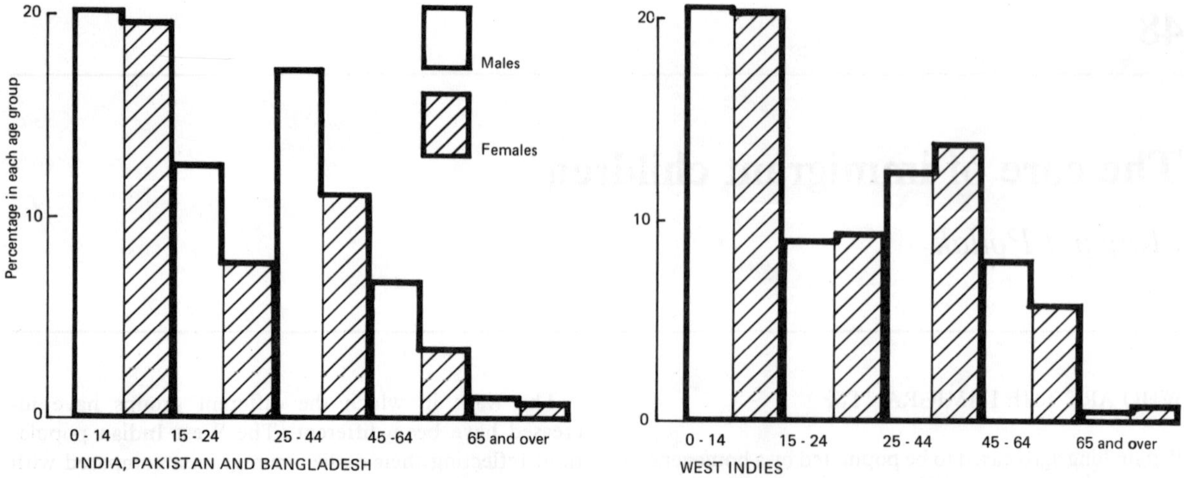

Fig. 48.1 Great Britain: Age and sex structure of populations originating from India, Pakistan, and Bangladesh, and from the West Indies, 1976. Source: Office of population censuses and surveys

Table 48.1 Population of New Commonwealth and Pakistani ethnic origin: age structure. *Source: Office of Population Censuses and Surveys*

	1971	*1976*	*1971*	*1976*
	(thousands)		*(percentages)*	
Males				
0– 4	110	122	*8.0*	*6.9*
5–14	177	227	*12.9*	*12.8*
15–24	123	195	*9.0*	*11.0*
25–44	252	276	*18.4*	*15.6*
45–64	74	119	*5.4*	*6.7*
65+	8	16	*0.6*	*0.9*
Total	744	955	*54.3*	*53.9*
Females				
0– 4	107	114	*7.8*	*6.4*
5–14	165	221	*12.0*	*12.5*
15–24	110	158	*8.0*	*8.9*
25–44	187	233	*13.6*	*13.2*
45–64	48	74	*3.5*	*4.2*
65+	10	16	*0.7*	*0.9*
Total	627	816	*45.7*	*46.1*
Total population	1371	1771	*100*	*100*

groups with long and proud traditions of culture and art. For the family doctor meeting them in the consulting room it is helpful to know something of these traditions because they may explain aspects of their family life and structure, attitudes to the English way of life and some child rearing practices.

For the West Indian immigrant there is no past history of settled family life, early marriage nor husbands involved in child rearing. There is a long tradition of working mothers. This is a matriarchal society. It is, therefore, not surprising to find a great many one parent families amongst the West Indian children living here. These children, too, have many stepfathers and step-siblings living in their family unit (Pless and Hood, 1967; Pollak, 1979). The West Indian immigrant, as indeed those born here, intends to stay in this country. He is not dreaming of returning to the Caribbean and needs very much to integrate into our way of life. In some ways, compared with other groups of NCWP immigrants, the West Indians do not find the British way of life too strange and, in particular, they are eager to participate in the educational system and happy to accept Caucasian pre-school care. The majority of West Indian immigrants are in social classes IV and V even when they may have qualifications for different types of employment. There is some suggestion that their family life is beginning to change. They have increasingly taken to marriage at an earlier age than in the West Indies (Fitzherbert, 1967) and, as seen by Table 48.1 they are having fewer babies. There is evidence that they are practising family planning and contraception (Pollak, 1979).

Asian children, on the other hand, are living in a tightly knit family structure. Father is very much the head of the household, and the mother plays a more subsidiary role compared with the West Indian structure. Many Asian marriages are arranged and parents exert considerable pressure on the young not to marry outside the culture. A dowry system is still in operation for many and young married couples continue to live with their parents who exert influence on them. In general, the Asian immigrant feels less certain that he is here for good. Many do, but have a dream of returning to the land of their birth 'one day'.

Particularly in the case of Muslims, a husband prefers his wife to be looked after by a woman doctor during

Table 48.2 Live births: by country of birth of mother. *Source: Office of Population Censuses and Surveys, General Register Office for Scotland*

	Number (thousands)				Percentage of all live births			
	1971	*1974*	*1975*	*1976*	*1971*	*1974*	*1975*	*1976*
Area/country of birth of mother:								
New Commonwealth and Pakistan:								
India, Pakistan, Bangladesh	22.1	20.6	20.4	22.2	*2.6*	*2.9*	*3.0*	*3.4*
West Indies[1]	12.6	8.2	7.7	7.2	*1.4*	*1.2*	*1.2*	*1.1*
African continent[2]	5.1	6.0	6.5	6.9	*0.6*	*0.8*	*1.0*	*1.1*
Other[3]	6.2	6.5	6.6	6.8	*0.7*	*0.9*	*1.0*	*1.0*
Total	46.0	41.2	41.3	43.1	*5.3*	*5.8*	*6.2*	*6.6*
Irish Republic[4]	22.5	15.2	13.4	11.9	*2.6*	*2.1*	*2.0*	*1.8*
Australia, Canada, New Zealand	2.7	2.6	2.4	2.3	*0.3*	*0.4*	*0.4*	*0.4*
EEC[5] (excluding UK and Irish Republic) } Other foreign (excluding Pakistan)	20.6	6.4	5.9	5.6 }	*2.4*	*0.9*	*0.9*	*0.9*
		11.7	11.8	12.2		*1.6*	*1.8*	*1.9*
Total with mother born outside UK	91.8	77.1	74.7	75.1	*10.6*	*10.9*	*11.1*	*11.6*
United Kingdom[6]	773.3	631.6	595.7	573.4	*88.9*	*89.0*	*88.7*	*88.3*
Not stated	4.8	1.3	1.0	0.7	*0.6*	*0.2*	*0.1*	*0.1*
Total births	869.9	710.0	671.4	649.2	*100.0*	*100.0*	*100.0*	*100.0*

[1]Including Guyana, and Belize (formerly British Honduras)
[2]African Commonwealth countries (including Rhodesia)
[3]Mainly Malta, Gibraltar, Cyprus, and Hong Kong
[4]Including Ireland, part not stated
[5]Figures for the EEC are not available prior to 1973
[6] Including Isle of Man and Channel Islands

her pregnancy. Wives are more likely than West Indian mothers to stay at home. They often speak little English, and Lobo (1978) points out that many, particularly from Pakistan and Bangladesh, are illiterate. Because of their poor English, the husband or children usually accompany mothers to the surgery to act as interpreters. It is not unusual to discuss an Asian mother's menstrual irregularities (about which she tends to be excessively concerned) with her through the interpretations of her small son! In the case of Asian women who do go out to work they usually prefer to have Asian child minders and go to some lengths to find them. As seen by Table 48.1 there has been little change in family size over the last few years and there is no evidence that the Asian family life is likely to change in the future.

African children find themselves in a somewhat different family unit. Their parents are usually married, they often come from the same village in Africa and sometimes from the same tribe. They have usually married before coming to Britain. Although they speak to each other in their dialect their groundwork in the English language is good. They are more likely to have come from a wealthy and cultivated home than other NCWP groups. The father is often a student or undergoing training in England whilst the wife works, often in a menial job. These African families see themselves as re-

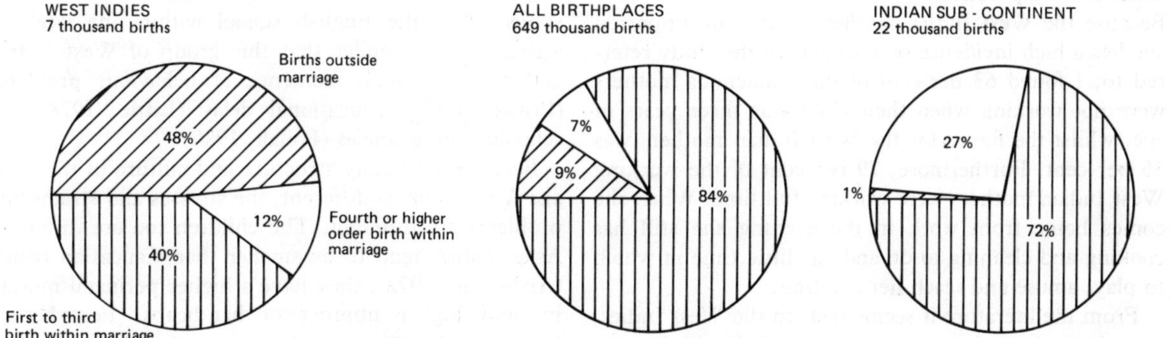

Fig. 48.2 Births in Great Britain: by birth-place of mother, 1976. Source: Office of population censuses and surveys

turning to their native land once the father has qualified. Many African parents foster their children, with Caucasians for preference. The foster parents often live at some distance away from the parents so that the children see the latter infrequently. The families have holidays back to Africa and sometimes the children are sent back without the parents for these trips.

In order to provide good care for immigrant children these family patterns are important since they have consequences for the children involved.

Feeding

Although in their own countries breast feeding is the rule, it is unfortunate that bottle feeding is one of the English habits which immigrant mothers have copied. Goel et al.(1978) have shown that, although the rate was not as high as that of the native born Scottish mothers, Asian, African and Chinese mothers of babies living in Glasgow had a high rate of bottle feeding. Lobo (1978) quotes interesting figures for the incidence of gastroenteritis in Luton amongst immigrant children, the incidence exactly following the incidence of bottle feeding. He finds a higher level of breast feeding amongst West Indian mothers compared with other mothers from NCWP countries. In a study of three year old children (Pollak, 1972) I found that 57.3 per cent of the West Indian children had been fed by a mixture of breast and bottle, bottle during day and breast at night. With the early return to work after delivery which characterises the West Indian mother it is not surprising to find the babies are often weaned earlier than is thought wise.

On the other hand, Goel *et al* (1978) and Lobo (1978) both report on the late weaning of Asian and West Indian babies. In my study (Pollak, 1972) I found that 50 per cent of the West Indian three year olds were still having at least one bottle per day but this was in addition to a satisfactory solid diet. Davis *et al* (1960) and Stroud (1965) report on the high level of iron deficiency anaemia amongst immigrant children which they associate with late weaning.

Child rearing practices

Because the West Indian mother is often unsupported she has a high incidence of working. In the study referred to, I found 63 per cent of the indigenous mothers were not working when their child was three years of age, whilst the figure for the West Indian mothers was 36 per cent. Furthermore, 79 per cent of the working West Indian mothers were working full time. When she comes home from work in the evening she still has cooking and cleaning to do and has little time in which to play, amuse and teach her children.

From the literature it seems that, in the West Indies, grannies and aunties play an important part in the care of children whilst their mothers are at work. Figure 48.1 illustrates the youth of the West Indian immigrants and this implies that there are few grandparents. When the children in my survey were seen at nine years of age (Pollak, 1979), 74 per cent of the West Indian children had no grandparents in England whom they could visit. The figures for the English and Cypriot nine year-olds were 5 per cent and 33 per cent respectively.

These facts have considerable consequences for the children because West Indian mothers, in particular, need to find pre-school care. In working class inner city areas, nurseries, playgroups and official minders are less available than for the professional classes (Social Trends, 1979) and West Indian mothers often have to resort to unofficial minders who are both easier to find and cheaper to pay. In my survey, 71 per cent of the West Indian three-year-olds were cared for by 'unofficial' sources whilst only 42 per cent of Cypriot children and 18 per cent of the indigenous children were so placed.

Illegitimacy is no stigma in West Indian culture and stepsiblings are the rule. In the same way there is a long tradition of fostering and informal adoption in the West Indies with mothers not feeling guilty if someone else brings up their children (Patterson, 1967). This pattern is reflected in the high numbers of West Indian children who are taken into care (Lobo, 1978).

A special feature of West Indian childhood which is, fortunately, becoming less frequent, is the sending by a mother or father for an 'outside' child who was left behind in the West Indies when the parent emigrated to the UK. These children were often left in the care of a grandparent or aunt. Later when the relative became ill or died and/or the parent was in better circumstances the fare to Britain was sent to these children. It is difficult to imagine the culture shock which such children undergo. Leaving 'home' in sunny Jamaica and flying to grey London might be bad enough in itself. But they meet a mother whom they have not seen for several years, probably a new stepfather and certainly new siblings and stepsiblings. They cannot begin to know what type of reception they will receive. To my own knowledge several children arriving in this way have been subjected to the English school within one week of arrival. Small wonder that this group of West Indian children have high incidence of behaviour problems (Prince, 1967), educational delay (Little, 1978) and schoolgirl pregnancies (Pollak, 1980).

Because the family structure and culture in the average Asian home is different, the stresses and strains and problems are different. The children too are different. Asian babies tend to be smaller than Caucasian babies (Arthurton, 1972), they have a higher perinatal mortality and higher number of handicaps (Fernyhough, 1979), the latter said to be due to the intermarriages. Father is the disciplinarian in the Asian home and obedience is expected and enforced. Asian children have problems with their diets, their fastings, their clothes and their hair styles.

Muslim children, living in a traditional household, will not be allowed to eat pork, and, in addition, any meat which they consume has to have been slaughtered by a special butcher. They have a real problem with school meals. Many Hindu families are vegetarian and if they do allow the children to eat meat, beef is forbidden. During the Ramadan fasting, which lasts for a month, no food is eaten between sunrise and sunset. Some children, doing a day's schooling, find this debilitating (Lobo, 1978). Lobo also mentions that there is the need to learn to use knife and fork at school since much Asian food is eaten with the fingers and/or a spoon only.

Clothes are a problem for Muslim girls. They often wear a special trouser suit which is frowned upon by schools. They are also required to have their limbs covered so that swimming suits and sports shorts are forbidden. Sikhs must wear the turban. Younger boys must not have their hair cut and this is arranged on the top of the head in a topknot which is sometimes covered by a small cloth. Such Sikh boys resent the teasing which may ensue. Both West Indian and African children – of both sexes – sometimes have their hair arranged in sections with very elaborate plaits. Some writers have described the breaking and dystrophy of hair following this style. Alopecia has also been noted.

TWO RESEARCH STUDIES AMONGST IMMIGRANT CHILDREN (POLLAK, 1972–1979).

In 1972 all the three-year-old children who were registered with a group practice in an 'inner city' area of South London were given developmental assessments and a medical examination. Extensive information was also gathered regarding their daily lives, families, income, social class, housing, environment and child rearing practices.

163 children were examined. 75 children had been born to English–born parents, 75 to West Indian born parents and the rest to 'other' groups which consisted of mainly Cypriot children and some from mixed marriages.

No difference was found in the motor development of the three groups but the West Indian children were found to have statistically significantly lower levels in personal/social, language and adaptive (non-verbal performance) development compared with the two other groups – all measured by recognised paediatric developmental tests (Table 48.3).

There was no difference between the three groups in heights, weights and serious medical conditions, although the three groups did have different patterns of illness. All the children were living in the same underprivileged area of London, often in the same streets and sometimes in the same multi-occupied house. There was no significant difference in the social class status nor income of the three groups.

The West Indian children were disadvantaged compared with the indigenous group, being in poorer housing and in their mothers working more often and longer hours. However, the third group were also disadvantaged in these respects yet were not showing the same lower developmental pattern. The ways in which the two immigrant groups differed from each other was in their family lives and daily routine. The second immigrant group came from tightly knit families, they were given toys, played with, their parents were concerned with their rearing and much parent-child interaction was taking place. The West Indian children, on the other hand, had loose family ties, stepfathers, stepsibl-

Table 48.3 Mean scores and differences between the three groups on development tests

	Adaptive development	*Language development*	*Personal social development*	*Motor development*
Mean score				
Group England	10.32	12.04	8.92	13.27
Group West Indian	3.48	3.85	6.97	12.91
Group 'Other'	9.15	10.77	8.77	12.54
't' test				
Group Eng. v Group W.I.	H.S. $p<0.001$	H.S. $p<0.01$	H.S. $p<0.001$	N.S.
Group Eng v Group 'Other'	N.S.	N.S.	N.S.	N.S.
Group W.I v Group 'Other'	H.S. $p<0.001$	H.S. $p<0.001$	H.S. $p<0.001$	N.S.

H.S. = highly significantly different
N.S. = not significantly different

ings and one parent families. They had few or no toys, play was meagre, outings rare. There was a paucity of mother-child interaction and a high level of unofficial child minding with frequent change of minder.

It was felt that this study had produced enough environmental evidence to explain the lower developmental scores. It drew attention to the importance of family life and home care in child development and highlighted the disadvantage which was suffered by the West Indian children.

The second study is a follow up of the same children at age nine. 85 per cent of the original children were traced and seen. The children were seen at school and undertook a verbal IQ, a reading and comprehension test and a test of spatial ability. The children completed a questionaire about themselves, their families, home and school. They described their wishes, hopes and fears and a great deal of information was gleaned about their life experiences. Their parents were asked questions about housing, local play facilities, schools, and their own involvement with their children. School teachers were asked to place the children on a scale both for behaviour and school achievement.

The differences in development which were noted at three years of age remain in the older children. The West Indian children had lower reading skills, lower IQs and lower spatial skills compared with the two other groups (Table 48.4).

The disadvantages which had been noted at three for the West Indian children were even more apparent at nine years of age.

The English and Group 'Other' families had improved financially, they had improved the quality of their housing and had moved to more salubrious districts. Although some West Indian families had also improved in these ways, the improvements were at a significantly lower level. The quality of life experienced by the children marked the greatest differences between the groups. The majority of English and 'Other' children had had many interesting and stimulating life experiences and adventures most of which they had encountered within the love and security of their family setting. The West Indian children were now gravely disadvantaged both in the home, due to lack of parental involvement and learning experiences and in society where their unfamilarity with events was harmful to their full integration. It was felt that schools could, however, have an important and beneficial role in helping the children to overcome some of these problems.

ILLNESSES AND DISEASES

Illnesses confined to immigrants

There are, in fact, very few illnesses and diseases which are confined to immigrants, although they do suffer

Table 48.4 Results of tests of three groups of children at nine years of age

	Group Eng.	*Group W.I.*	*Group 'Other'*	*p/x²*
I.Q. test				
Mean score	101.3	84.3	103.3	
Eng. v W.I.				$p < 0.001$
Eng. v 'Other'				N.S.
W.I. v 'Other'				$p < 0.001$
Mean number of mistakes in Reading test	11.41	20.46	10.25	
Eng. v W.I.				$p < 0.001$
Eng. v 'Other'				N.S.
W.I. v 'Other'				$p < 0.02$
Non-readers	8 (1.3%)	21(31.8%)	0(0%)	$p < 0.001$
Mean no. of questions answered correctly	5.5	4.3	5.75	
Eng. v W.I.				$p < 0.001$
Eng. v 'Other'				N.S.
W.I. v 'Others'				$p < 0.01$.
Visual perception test				
Mean no. of mistakes	4.8	7.4	4.5	
Eng. v W.I.				$p < 0.02$
Eng. v 'Other'				N.S.
W.I. v 'Other'				$p < 0.05$

more often than the host population from many diseases. Illnesses which are confined to immigrants are related to a coloured skin and affect the negro rather than all immigrants.

The pigmented, black skin appears thicker than the white skin as all those who are used to taking blood samples will be well aware. Such a skin is particularly liable to keloid formation and I have seen a particularly distressing keloid in a small girl who was scarred following burns to arms and legs.

Mongolian spots are important to recognise. They are bluish black pigmented areas often over the sacrum and buttocks in negro children. They can also occur in half caste babies. Most marked at birth, they gradually fade. I was once called by a social worker to visit a baby whom she suspected had suffered child abuse. She knew that the mother was Caucasian but did not know that the father was African. The apparent bruises were Mongolian spots.

The deeply pigmented skin seems especially susceptible to depigmentation and this of course is more obvious. It can be seen after infections of the skin and may follow tinea versicolor, vitiligo and even carbuncles. Yaws, which is not entirely confined to negros, is a tropical spirochaetal infection which causes papules on the face and extremities which may ulcerate. However, it is more common in this country to see secondary Yaws and this presents as nodules or crusted granulomatous lesions, often on the legs.

The haemoglobinopathies are diseases which are special to many immigrants. They are genetically determined and have a recessive carrier state. Married carriers have a one in four chance of an affected child. There are no reliable figures for the incidence in this country but there is no evidence that it is likely to be different from other countries. (Thalassaemia trait occurs in 15 to 20 per cent of Cypriots and 5 to 10 per cent of Southern Italians. Sickle cell trait occurs in 20 to 40 per cent of Africans and approximately 10 per cent of West Indians).

Sickle cell disease is seen in East and West Africans, West Indians and some Arabs; an abnormal and immature type of haemoglobin is inherited. This abnormal haemoglobin interferes with the oxygenation of blood and the abnormal 'sickle' cells are less sturdy than normal red cells and have a tendency to clump together. The symptoms are often due to embolic phenomena. Sickle cell disease causes a chronic, haemolytic anaemia, bone and joint pains, abdominal pains and sickle cell crises. Quite apart from the disease itself, its sequelae are important. The children are likely to have stunted growth. The skull and cheek bones often show bossing, giving a characteristic facies. They have a shortened life span and sometimes have a permanent or intermittent jaundice. They are more susceptible to infections of all kinds but particularly meningitis and pneumonia (Muller). The known association of sickle cell anaemia and G6PD deficiency is important to bear in mind because of the drug and food induced haemolysis which it may produce.

Thalassaemia major is found amongst Cypriots - both Greek and Turkish, Italians, some Asians and Chinese. In this condition the fetal haemoglobin is not replaced by Hb A, with maturity, but continues as an inherited condition. The abnormal red cells are more fragile and their circulation time is shorter than normal. Affected children are usually pale, suffer from tiredness and lethargy and have poor school records. Growth is often stunted, they also suffer from bossing and acquire a sallow yellow complexion. Life expectancy is shortened. Splenomegaly and hepatomegaly are usually present and often lymphadenitis. The children suffer from PUOs. X-ray appearances show rarefaction of the long bones and the skull has a characteristic appearance of 'hair standing on end'. The children require frequent transfusions and hospital admissions. Lately a pump, which operates only at night, offers hope of replacing transfusions in the future.

Doctors may want to consider their views on the screening and counselling of the carriers and sufferers (and parents) on their lists. The pros and cons of screening have never been successfully resolved, some finding the practice discriminatory. However, theoretically at least, the diseases could be eradicated if carriers never mated with carriers. The possibility of amniocentesis followed by termination of affected cases is, perhaps a further argument for a screening plan.

Older textbooks give grave prognoses for both sickle cell disease and thalassaemia major but with more experience and modern improvements in treatment the outlook for these children is improving and early, vigorous and effective treatment is avoiding the stunted growth and, hopefully, the shorter life span.

Infections from abroad

All the following infections have been described as being seen in immigrants in this country: Typhoid, malaria, amoebic dysentry, leprosy, leishmaniasis, trypanosomiasis. Many types of worms – hookworm, flat worms, round worms, liver and lung flukes are also described. In many years of giving primary medical care to many immigrants I have only ever encountered the hook worm (ankylostomiasis) in two West Indian child patients. The whole family was later found to be infected. Another interesting case in an adult Nigerian male was leprosy which was diagnosed from a lesion on the ear. It was thought that the patient had acquired the disease in childhood.

Conditions which are unusual in Great Britain but which have been noted as more common in immigrants

Lupus erythematosis is said to be more common in negro immigrants. There were six cases of sarcoidosis amongst West Indian patients in my London practice; all occurring in adults.

The evidence regarding tuberculosis is conflicting. There is general agreement that it is most common in the Asian immigrant (Lobo, 1979; Arthurton, 1972; Walters, 1965) but what is not agreed is the incidence amongst West Indians. Lobo considers it to be uncommon but Stroud (1965) believes it to be common. Our experience in London SW4 is that it occurs but rarely in the West Indian. However Walters (1965) mentions an acute caseous broncho-pneumonia to which negro immigrants appear especially prone. The infection is usually mycobacterium but bovine types may be found in new immigrants from India.

In children the presentation and sites may be unusual with fever, wasting, polyadenitis, peritonitis, osteomyelitis and meningitis. A clear X-ray of chest does not exclude tuberculosis and a Tuberclin test and isolation by culture are always advisable. Several writers have recommended a chest X-ray and BCG for all new Asian immigrants on entry to the UK.

Although one or two small outbreaks of rickets have been described (Arneil, 1963) it could be claimed, with justification that rickets had disappeared in the UK until the arrival of Asian immigrants. At the present time, rickets presents in three age groups of Asian children; two- to four- year-olds, adolescents and young women. Initially it was found in younger babies but as so many Asian mothers now bottle feed their babies with dried milk which has an added Vitamin D supplement, rickets is tending to occur later, after the babies have been weaned on to cow's milk, which is not supplemented, and the initial stores of the vitamin become used up.

In adolescence, both diet and lack of sunshine have been blamed. The wholemeal flour, from which chappatis etc. are made, contains phytic acid which combines and is excreted with calcium. Several writers (Dunnigan, 1972; Ford, 1977) have made a plea for the fortification of wholemeal flour with Vitamin D for Asian communities. I have seen a case of rickets in a young Asian mother who was the only member of the household to eat a traditional diet, none of the other members of the family - all of whom were eating English type of food - being affected. Lack of sunlight on the skin has been blamed for rickets occurring in older children. Girls and young women are expected to keep limbs and bodies covered, they have no tradition of sunbathing and often keep indoors for much of the day. Since they come from a warmer clime, there is no tradition of Asian mothers putting their babies outside in prams and when they do go out they are usually wrapped up in many clothes. Florid rickets is usually easy to diagnose, the bony swellings around the epiphyses, the bowing of legs due to softening are confirmed by radiological appearances of generalised osteoporesis and wide metaphyses. A raised phosphatase and lowered calcium and phosphorus confirm the diagnosis. In sub-clinical cases, however, the diagnosis is more difficult, especially as the calcium and phosphate levels may be within normal limits.

Lobo (1978) has described a survey of three year olds in Luton in which 12.8 per cent of the Asian children were found to have a raised lead level and 14.9 per cent had an iron deficiency anaemia. None of the matched Caucasian controls had a raised lead level. The use of Surma – an eye cosmetic containing lead sulphide – is cited as aetiology in some cases, the lead being absorbed through the lacrimal ducts. (The original eye make-up used in Kashmir did not contain lead). Dr Lobo puts forward the interesting theory that, because of the low mineral-calcium and iron content of the Asian diet, the children are unable to excrete the normal amounts of environmental lead which are easily dealt with by the English children living in the same district. Pica was, not surprisingly, found to be a common occurrence, in these children.

Common general practice diseases to which immigrant children are especially prone

A group practice in London SW4 in which I worked has a 24.4 per cent immigrant population and kept a disease register of the common illnesses of the practice. From this register it is apparent that the immigrant children had the following conditions in excess of expectation from their proportion in the practice: hay fever, asthma (West Indians only), infantile eczema (West Indians), otitis media (West Indians), nocturnal enuresis (West Indians), URTI (Asian and Cypriot), chilblains, iron-deficiency anaemia (West Indian and Asian), burns and accidents (West Indian), language delay (West Indian), withdrawn behaviour (West Indian), mumps (Asian) and rubella.

Several other authors (Lobo, 1978; Pollak, 1972; Arthurton, 1972) have remarked upon the apparent increased susceptibility of West Indian children to eczema and asthma. It will be interesting to note whether these conditions lessen as the immigrants become more used to the British atmosphere. The same point could apply to hay fever and chilblains.

One could speculate whether there is any connection between the higher incidence of otitis media and the reported larger number of West Indian children in schools for the deaf (Department of Education and Science, 1974).

Not all workers have confirmed the common finding of

nocturnal enuresis in West Indian children. In a recent survey, Earls and Richman, (1980) studying the prevalence of behaviour problems in three year old children of West Indian born parents found no significant increase compared with the children of British born parent controls.

In the survey of three year olds (Pollak, 1972), 85 per cent of the West Indian homes were heated entirely by paraffin stoves (figures for the English and 'Other' were 6.3 per cent and 4.6 per cent respectively). These are notoriously dangerous objects and cause many fires and burns.

Behaviour and psychiatric problems, so common amongst children are also common amongst immigrant children. Whether they are more common or not is a matter of conjecture. Rutter (1976) found a high level of conduct disorder in West Indian girls and boys but concludes that the West Indian children do not, overall, have an increased rate of psychiatric disorder. Rack (1978) finds a high level of stress symptoms amongst Asian teenage girls. Lobo (1978) also mentions the school children and young adolescents of West Indian and Asian parents as being especially liable to stress. Withdrawn behaviour has also been well described by Prince (1967). The survey by Earls and Richman (1980), already referred to compared the prevalence of behaviour problems of West Indian three-year-olds and British born three-year-olds. They found very few significant differences in rates or patterns of presentation between the two groups.

Conditions which occur with less frequency amongst immigrants

Information is scarce. From the disease register of the practice the conditions applying to children were: exchange transfusion of rhesus incompatibility (this has also been noted by Arthurton, 1972); diabetes in childhood (West Indian, African and Asian); appendicitis (West Indian).

Miles (1965), stating that acute appendicitis is undoubtedly far less common in non-European races also mentions that vomiting is a much less common symptom in non-Europeans. I think I would agree with this. I also believe that headache as a symptom in immigrant children is less common.

SPECIAL PROBLEMS IN THE CARE OF IMMIGRANT CHILDREN

Immigrant children and their parents present with special problems which because they affect their future welfare and happiness and also because some of them may be avoidable, need thought and consideration.

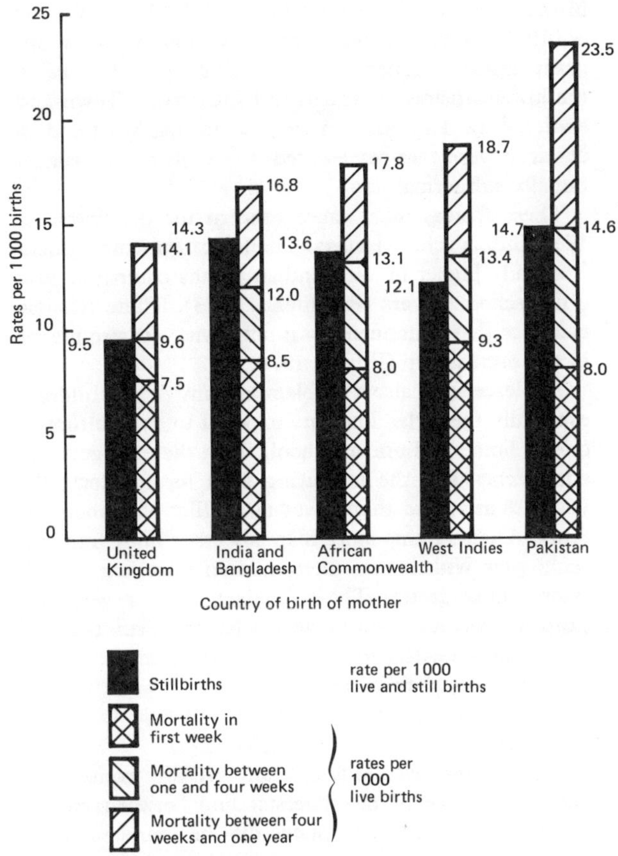

Fig. 48.3 England and Wales stillbirth and mortality rates in the first year of life 1975–1977, by country of birth of mother. Source: Studies in medical and population subjects, 41. HMSO, 1980

Perinatal problems

The high rate of stillbirths, congenital malformations and infant mortality noted in Asian babies must give rise to concern (Fig. 48.3). Poor antenatal care, poor diet and intermarriages have all been cited as aetiology. Late booking for antenatal care, often after 20 weeks gestation, is another factor stressed recently (Simpson and Walker,1980).

A particular feature of the statistics shown in Figure 48.3 is the high mortality after the first week of life, when the babies have left the maternity hospitals for their own homes. General practitioners and health visitors are therefore closely involved in the struggle to improve these figures. In the case of babies of mothers born in Pakistan, the death rate at this period is running at over twice the level for babies of mothers born in the UK.

School children and adolescents

The lower educational achievements of the West Indian children which my studies revealed have been confirmed by several other studies (ILEA, 1973; Yule *et al*, 1975). Several other studies have found that immigrant children, especially West Indians, tend to be in the lower streams in schools (NFER survey; Townsend *et al*, 1972). Townsend in 1971 noted that West Indian children were over-represented in schools for the educationally subnormal.

These factors must cause concern for the future of West Indian school leavers. The level of unemployment is already higher in West Indian youths compared with other school leavers (Richmond, 1973). There is some evidence that delinquency – if not crime – is also higher in the same group (Rutter, 1976).

Adolescence is also a problem to many Asian children, especially the girls. They are exposed to two cultures – one at home and one at school. With the emergence of adolescence and the increasing need for freedom, the young Asians find themselves in conflict with their parents. Asian parents more than any other immigrant parents view with horror their children marrying outside their ethnic group. These children have a very real problem which is difficult to resolve and even the conflict itself is hurtful to them, brought up as they are to love and obey their parents.

Attitudes

The poor language skills of many NCWP women is a potential source of misunderstanding between patient and doctor. Rack (1978) states that he found interpreters unsatisfactory. If one cannot converse with the patient about basic symptoms how can one ever hope to discuss the more subtle aspects of, for example, the mother/child relationship?

It is also useful to know that both Asian and West Indian patients find the presentation of emotional or psychiatric symptoms very difficult. Rack goes so far as to state that Asian patients only consult their GPs for physical symptoms. I have not found this to be the case but I do believe that they usually put anxiety or depressive symptoms into physical terms ('I have low feelings, Doc') or bizarre, multiple aches and burning sensations. This also applies to parents giving a history for their children.

USE OF HEALTH CARE SERVICES

How do immigrants use the NHS? The evidence is somewhat conflicting. Pinsent (1963), writing about the West Indians in Birmingham using their general practitioner service, found that they consulted at least as often as their Caucasian counterparts. Our experience in London SW4 was similar, consultations being slightly in excess but requests for visits less. Rack (1979) believes that Asians consult their GP only for physical symptoms. He further states that in Bradford where Asians make up ten per cent of the population they account for only four per cent of the hospital referrals. Arthurton (1972) on the other hand, found no significant difference between the English and Asian population in new paediatric (medical) referrals in 1969.

Low compliance and high defaulter rates have been noted in both Asian and West Indian patients. Language difficulties of understanding; change of address; poor motivation have been blamed as reasons, whilst in the case of Asians, the need for follow-up is questioned when a father may have to take time off work in order to bring the patient.

Both Asian and West Indian families have traditions of consulting 'private' doctors, herbalists and special 'healers'. It is always worthwhile asking a direct question on this score because one may be unaware of drugs which are being taken unless one does so. In South London, some doctors have thriving smalltime private practices because West Indian patients sometimes think that they get better treatment and care when they pay for it. I believe that this applies especially to children, particularly when they are handicapped.

IMMIGRANT FAMILIES FROM EUROPE

During the last war large numbers of soldiers, prisoners of war and displaced persons from Europe reached Britain, and many have settled here, often being joined by wives from their country of origin. I have had little personal experience of such families in my practice, but Dr Cyril Hart has kindly supplied information from his own practice near Peterborough, which contained over 1000 patients in this category in the late 1950s, and still numbers several hundreds. Most of these are of Polish and other Middle European extraction, but many have come from Northern Italy.

There have of course been problems of adaptation, but the overall picture is an optimistic one. The great majority have coped well with the disruption in their lives, and have settled successfully. Their children were nearly all born in Britain, and almost without exception have integrated well. Most are now virtually indistinguishable from children born of native British parents. Nearly all of the immigrant European parents remain devout Catholics, and most retain links with their homelands. The general living standards of these familes are if anything above average, and their standards of housekeeping are also high. Squalor is rare. Parents are industrious, families are close-knit, and illegitimacy is low. The family size approximates to that of the indigenous population. As might be expected, few medical problems of ethnic origin have been encountered in second generation children from these families, and still less in the third generation now being born. Such differences as still exist are subtle, and now of minor significance in medical terms.

SUMMARY

Family doctors and the primary care team cannot cure or even help all the ills to which immigrant children under their care are subject. But they can understand their special problems and offer compassionate advice and help. There is a very special need to help parents to ensure that their children achieve their full potential. They are the citizens of tomorrow and need to be educated, trained and equipped to be happy and useful members of a multiracial society. An editorial in the *General Practitioner*, February 16th, 1973, stated 'The coloured family is accepted by medicine, as it ought to be by the whole of our society, as different, equal and deserving of the best.' I hope it is true.

REFERENCES

Arneil, G.C. & Crosby, J.C. (1963) Infantile rickets returns to Glasgow. *Lancet*, **2**, 423.

Arthurton, M.W. (1972) Immigrant children and the day-to-day work of a paediatrician. *Archives of Disease in Childhood*, **47**, 251, 126-130.

Davis, L.R., Martin, R.H. & Sarkany, I. (1960) Iron deficient anaemia in European and West Indian infants in London. *British Medical Journal*, **2**, 1426.

Dunnigan, M.G. *et al* (1972) Biochemical response of late rickets and osteomalacia to a chapatti-free diet. *British Medical Journal*, **2**, 1132.

Earls, F. & Richman, N.(1980) The prevalence of behaviour problems in three-year-old children of West Indian-born parents. *Journal of Child Psychology and Psychiatry*, **21**, 99–117.

Fernyhough, D. (1979) Culture colours diagnosis. *British Medicine*, 6 – 8.

Fitzherbert, K. (1967) West Indian children in London. Occas. papers on social administration. No. 19.

Ford, J.A. et al (1977) Treatment of severe Asian rickets with Vitamin D fortified chapatti flour. *Archives of Disease in Childhood*, **9**, 743.

Goel, K.M., House, F. & Shanks, R.A. (1978) Infant feeding practices amongst immigrants in Glasgow. *British Medical Journal*, **2**, 1181–1183.

Inner London Education Authority (1973) Literacy Survey. 1971 follow-up, preliminary report. ILEA document.

Little, A.N. (1978). Educational policies for multi-racial areas. *Goldsmiths' College Inaugural Lecture*. University of London.

Lobo, E. de H. (1978). Children of Immigrants to Britain. Their health and social problems. Hodder and Stoughton.

Miles, R.P.M. (1965) Surgical diseases of immigrants. *Postgraduate Medical Journal*, **41**, 589–598.

Muller, A. Personal communication.

Patterson, S. (1963) Dark Strangers. London: Tavistock Press.

Pless, I.B. & Hood, C. (1967). West Indian one year olds. *Lancet*. 1373–76.

Pollak, M. (1972). Today's three-year-olds in London. Heinemann SIMP.

Pollak, M. (1979) Nine Years Old. M.T.P. Press. Lancaster.

Prince, G.S. (1967). Mental health problems in pre-school West Indian children. *Mat Child Care*, **3**, 483–486.

Pinsent, R.J.F.H. (1963) Morbidity in an immigrant population. *Lancet*, **i**, 437–438.

Rack, P. (1978). Immigrant children and the health service. *National Association for Maternal and Child Welfare. 65th Annual Conference Report.*

Richmond, A.H. (1973) Migration and Race relations in an English City. *A Study in Bristol.* Oxford University Press, (for institute of Race Relations).

Rutter, M. (1976). Cycles of Disadvantage. London: Heinemann.

Simpson, Hazel & Walker G. (1980) When do pregnant women attend for antenatal care? *British Medical Journal*, **2**, 104–107.

Social Trends. (1979). H.M.S.O.

Stroud, C.E. (1965) The New Environment. *Postgraduate Medical Journal*, **41**, 599–602.

Townsend, H.E.R. (1971). Immigrant pupils in England. *NFER*.

Townsend, H.E.R. (1972). Organisation in multiracial schools. *NFER*.

Walters, J.H. (1965) Infections of immigrants. *Postgraduate Medical Journal*, **41**, 584–588.

Yule, W., Berger, M., Rutter, M. & Yule, B. (1975) Children of West Indian immigrants. II Intellectual performance and reading attainment. *Journal of Child Psychology and Psychiatry*, *16*, 1–18.

49

Children with alcoholic parents

Rodney Wilkins (Ben-Dov)

'Behold, thou shalt conceive, and bear a son; and now drink no wine or strong drink.' Judges 13, 7.

The 'skid-row' alcoholic who heats gramophone records or shoe polish to extract alcohol represents only about five per cent of the alcoholic population. As general practitioners, we are far more likely to encounter a married alcoholic with children living at home. The challenge we face is to detect the alcoholic at an early stage, before the marriage breaks up. However, unfortunately, alcoholics see us more often than we see them. Failure can lead to emotional crippling of the children who may become the alcoholics of tomorrow. This essay focuses on the effects of an alcoholic parent on the children and the role of the general practitioner and the health team in identifying and managing the children who are 'the principals in a hidden tragedy. Often they remain pathetically invisible to the professional treating the alcoholic' (Bosma, 1972).

In an average general practice of 2500 patients, the GP will probably be aware of a handful of alcoholics, but a further 30 or so may be unrecognized (Wilkins, 1974). The concept of preventive medicine demands that we search out these hidden alcoholics in an attempt to reduce the damaging effects of this family illness on the patient, spouse and children.

THE FETAL ALCOHOL SYNDROME

The most frequent known teratogenic cause of mental deficiency in the Western world has been stated to be alcohol (Clarren and Smith, 1978). Over 300 cases of the fetal alcohol syndrome have now been reported since it was initially described by Lemoine (1968) and Ulleland *et al* (1970), and defined by Jones and Smith (1973). The most consistent features are: prenatal growth deficiency (expressed in length more than weight), post-natal growth deficiency (leading to failure to thrive), developmental delay and or mental deficiency, fine motor dysfunction, microcephaly, and short palpebral fissures. Found characteristically in the full-blown syndrome is a hypoplastic upper lip and a flattened elongated philtrum with thin narrow vermilion lip borders producing a facial appearance considered as specific as that of Down's Syndrome. Other abnormalities sometimes found include cardiac septal defects, abnormal dermatoglyphics, ptosis, strabismus, cleft palate, minor ear and limb defects and naevi. Recently, Warren and Rosett (1978) have reviewed the literature and suggested a link between maternal alcohol abuse and minimal brain dysfunction.

The National Institute on Alcohol Abuse and Alcoholism, under the auspices of the United States Department of Health, Education and Welfare, in 1977 issued a 'health caution' suggesting that drinking more than six hard drinks a day (or three ounces of absolute alcohol) by a pregnant woman constitutes a risk to the fetus. It is generally accepted that antenatal counselling and even better, prenatal counselling could considerably reduce the incidence of the fetal alcohol syndrome although probably few would suggest an abortion to a pregnant alcoholic (Erb and Anderson, 1978; Turner, 1978).

THE STRESSES IN AN ALCOHOLIC FAMILY

'The alcoholic is anaesthetised by the alcohol, but the family is not and suffers the pain,' the wife of an alcoholic patient of mine once told me. It would be surprising if most children reared in a home environment where one parent was an alcoholic did not exhibit some ill-effects. In the ideal situation, the child is secure in a cocoon of love and affection from both parents. He learns to expect consistent attitudes and behaviour from his mother and father. At school he is free from anxieties about what he might expect when he returns home. Contrast this with the family where the father is an alcoholic. Often drunk, he may be violent (verbally or physically) to his wife and children. Sober, he seeks to regain affection.

Four factors have been described which may harm the emotional development of the child (Clinebell, 1968). Firstly, confusion is likely because of the reversal or distortion of the parents role causing difficulty in achieving a strong sense of sexual identity. Secondly, there may be an inconsistent, unpredictable relationship with the alcoholic parent. Thirdly, the *non*-alcoholic parent is also often disturbed and therefore inadequate in the parent role. Finally, increased social isolation of the family interferes with peer relationships and with emotional support from the extended family.

Orford (1979) points out that there is a correlation between childhood problems and violence in the family which may be because violence is associated with the severity of the drinking problem. He substantiates the work of Cork (1969) who noted that children of an alcoholic parent found it difficult to make friends. Apart from the unwillingness of the alcoholic parent to have other children around, the children themselves were unwilling to invite a friend home.

The son of an alcoholic father may have feelings of helplessness and develop fear, hatred and revenge fantasies towards his father (Cover, 1968). Later he may feel guilty and fear retaliation for his thoughts. Such anxiety-producing feelings can cause difficulties with authority figures in adult life. Because the father's behaviour is so inconsistent, a son may become overdependent on his mother. His feelings and thoughts about both parents become confused and ambivalent, resulting in his turning against them. The son may also come to blame his mother for his father's drinking, thereby associating masculine independence with drunkenness. The son often has difficulty with his own masculine role and may overidentify with his mother. Homosexuality may result (Fox, 1963). Sons of alcoholics may appear to be quiet and acquiescent but have strong inner feelings of anger and rebellion (Aronson and Gilbert, 1963). They are more likely to become alcoholics than the sons of non-alcoholics (Nylander, 1960; Drew, Moon and Buchanan, 1974; Aitken, 1978).

The daughter of an alcoholic father may hate and fear him and side with her mother, or conversely, continue to love him desperately and blame her mother for his drinking. Each time he drinks, she may feel a deep personal rejection. She may also confuse independence with drunkenness. The daughter is sometimes the object of seductive behaviour from her father. In one study, the daughters of alcoholic fathers tended to be self-defeating, vulnerable, pessimistic, withdrawn, and fluctuating in their moods (Cover, 1971).

The wife of an alcoholic is no passive participant in the family dynamics. Faced with a husband who has abdicated his role as husband and father, she has to take control and organise those family affairs normally undertaken by the man. Preoccupied with the drink problem, she cannot give the necessary motherly love and attention to her children. Her normal emotions are perverted by anger and frustration with her husband often combined paradoxically with a desire to mother and protect him (Kogan and Jackson, 1965). 'The alcoholic builds up resentment and anger, brick by brick, and even love cannot penetrate the wall' it was once graphically described to me. The response of the wife is not uniform, and Whalen (1953) has described four personality types commonly observed. There is 'Suffering Susan' who needs to feel miserable, 'Controlling Catherine' who chooses a husband she can dominate, 'Wavering Winifred' who needs a husband to feel dependent on her but sometimes finds the strain unbearable, and 'Punitive Polly' whose neurotic needs are fulfilled by punishing her husband.

The classic paper of Jackson (1954) outlined seven successive stages through which she considered that families passed in making an adjustment to the crisis of alcoholism in the family. However, Orford (1979) suggests that there are two major phases in the reaction of the family to the alcoholic husband. Family recognition of the problem, first attempts by wives to control drinking, social isolation of the family and transfer of part of the husband's family role to the wife generally occur at an earlier stage than fearful reactions on the part of the wife, her feelings of hopelessness about being able to cope with the problem, decline or ceasing of marital sexual behaviour, and the seeking of outside help.

The mother who is herself an alcoholic is clearly likely to have a disastrous effect on the physical and mental development of her children. While drinking, she neglects her children. When the father adopts the mother role, she may become jealous and spiteful, competing with the child for the father's attention. When sober, she compensates with an excess of loving and mothering (Fox, 1963).

Children at risk

'The alcoholic has the illness and the family has the spots.' Can we make use of the 'spots'? I believe that it is possible to identify certain at risk factors, including some specifically relating to children which are valuable clues for identifying an alcoholic family (Wilkins, 1974). The social worker, health visitor (Wilkins, 1972) and community nurse (Wilkins, 1973) can be valuable allies in this detection process. They may have the opportunity to establish a relationship with the family which can allow the wife to talk about her own alcoholism, or the problems created by her alcoholic husband. A study by Abbott (1970), a health visitor attached to a Cardiff general practice, showed the importance of a high index of suspicion. Home visits because of absence from school, faulty personal hygeine discovered at school inspections, indifferent scholastic attainments in a child who should do better, and the keeping of an older child at home to look after younger members should lead to taking a careful alcoholic history.

Other important 'at risk' factors include repeated hospitalization, often for non-organic reasons (Nylander, 1960). There may be history of stealing, running away from home, and other antisocial acts (Glatt, 1958; Jenkins, 1968). There is considerable evidence that children of alcoholic parents are prone to anxiety, depression, attempted suicide, temper tantrums, destructive behaviour, hyperactivity, and aggressive behaviour (e.g. Roe, 1944; Kearney and Taylor, 1969; Orford, 1979). Psychosomatic illnesses such as asthma may be found. I have identified three alcoholic fathers by taking a history from the mothers of children with nocturnal enuresis. Finally, there is conflicting evidence that alcoholics are likely to batter their children (see Ch. 16).

MANAGEMENT

Identification does not automatically lead to treatment and recovery; there has to be acceptance of the diagnosis and willingness to be helped. However, even if the alcoholic and spouse are not yet prepared to accept advice, we can offer guidance to the children. The general practitioner, and the health team, if interested and knowledgeable, can discuss and explain the disease concept of alcoholism. There may be a branch of Alateen in your area (UK office: St Giles Centre, Camberwell Church Street, London SE5 8RB; 01-703 0397). This is a fellowship for the sons and daughters, aged 12–20 years, of alcoholics, and has principles similar to Alcoholics Anonymous and Al-anon (for the spouse of the alcoholic). These groups meet regularly to discuss their worries, exchange experiences, encourage one another, learn effective ways to cope with their problems, and help each other to understand about alcoholism. Amongst the principles that Alateen teach are that compulsive drinking is a disease, that the sick parent's loss of dignity should not be regarded with contempt but with compassion, that some measure of emotional detachment must be acquired in order to cope with the situation, and that it is stupid and self-defeating to resort to acts of reprisal or rebellion from which they alone will suffer the consequences. Alateen produces some excellent literature which is well worth reading.

Occasionally, it may be necessary to recommend the separation of the children from the alcoholic parent if he or she cannot or will not respond to treatment.

The return to sobriety of the alcoholic does not signal the end of all problems. The reversion to normal parental roles can produce tensions in itself, non-alcoholism stresses of the marriage may be revealed, and there is always risk of relapses.

CONCLUSIONS

Recognition of the children of alcoholics is important for two reasons. Firstly, we may abort any physical or emotional pathology and allow the child to develop normal relationships. Secondly, we may be practising preventive medicine for the next generation. Children of alcoholic parents are six times more likely to become alcoholics themselves compared with children of non-alcoholic parents (Glatt, 1975). They may marry alcoholics and produce another generation of alcoholics. They are more likely as adults to have personality difficulties, marital problems, and be inadequate parents because of their own lack of satisfactory parent models.

It must be emphasized that *early* identification is vital. Alcoholism is a progressive, insidious disease. The time to detect the alcoholic is *before* he gets married and has children.

REFERENCES

Abbott, M. (1970) Attitudes to drinking and admitted alcohol consumption in an area of mixed private and municipal housing in Cardiff. *The Journal of Alcoholism*, **5**, 96.

Aitken, P.P. (1978) *Ten to Fourteen-year-olds and Alcohol*. A developmental study in the Central Region of Scotland, Vol. III. Edinburgh: HMSO.

Aronson, H. & Gilbert, A. (1963) Preadolescent sons of male alcoholics. *Archives of General Psychiatry*, **8**, 235–241.

Bosma, W.G.H. (1972) Children of alcoholics – a hidden tragedy. *Maryland State Medical Journal*, **21**, 34–36.

Clark, B. (1969) *Health Visitor*, **42**, 451.

Clarren, S.T.C. & Smith, D.W. (1978) The Fetal Alcohol Syndrome. *New England Journal of Medicine*, **298 (19)**, 1063–1067.

Clinebell, H.J. (1968) Pastoral counselling of the alcoholic and his family. In *Alcoholism, The Total Treatment Approach*, p. 189. Ed. by R.J. Cantanzaro. Illinois: Charles C. Thomas.

Cork, R.M. (1969) The forgotten children; a study of children with alcoholic parents. Toronto: Addiction Research Foundation.

Cover, J.M. (1968) Personality correlates and antecedents of drinking patterns in adult males. *Journal of Consulting and Clinical Psychology*, **32**, 2.

Cover, J.M. (1971) Personality antecedents and correlates of drinking in women. *Journal of Consulting and Clinical Psychology*, **36**, 61.

Drew, L.R.H., Moon, J.R. & Buchanan, F.H. (1974) *Alcoholism. A Handbook*. London: Heinemann.

Erb, L.E. & Anderson B.D. (1978) The Fetal Alcohol Syndrome. *Clinical Pediatrics*, **17**(8), 644–649.

Fox, R. (1963) *The Effect of Alcoholism on Children*. New York: The National Council on Alcoholism.

Glatt, M.M. (1958) Alcoholism, crime and juvenile delinquency. *British Journal of Delinquency*, **9**, 84.

Glatt, M.M. (1975) *Alcoholism – a Social Disease*, **3rd edn.** London: English Universities Press.

Jenkins, R.L. (1968) The varieties of children's behaviour problems and family dynamics. *American Journal of Psychiatry*, **124**, (10), 134.
Jones, K.L. & Smith, D.W. (1973) Recognition of the fetal alcohol syndrome in early infancy. *Lancet*, **2**, 999–1001.
Kearney, T.R. & Taylor, C. (1969) Emotionally disturbed adolescents with alcoholic parents. *Acta Paedopsychiatrica* (Basel), **36**, 215.
Kogan, K.L. & Jackson, J.K. (1965) Stress personality and emotional disturbances in wives of alcoholics. *Quarterly Journal of Studies on Alcohol*, **26**, 486.
Lemoine, P., Harousseau, H., Borteyru, J.P. and Menuet, J.C. (1968) Les infants de parents alcooliques: anomalies observées a propos de 127 cas. *Quest Medicale*, **25**, 476–482.
Nylander, I. (1960) Children of alcoholic fathers. *Acta Paediatrica Scandinavica*, **49** (Suppl. 121), 1–134.
Orford, J. (1979) Alcohol and the Family. In Grant, M. & Gwinner, P. (eds) *Alcoholism in Perspective*, Ch. 8. London: Croom Helme.
Roe, A. (1944) The adult adjustment of children of alcoholic parents raised in foster-homes. *Quarterly Journal of Studies on Alcohol*, **5**, 378.
Turner, G. (1978) The Fetal Alcohol Syndrome. *Medical Journal of Australia*, **1**, 18–19.
Ulleland, C., Wennberg, P.R., Igo, R.P. & Smith, N.J. (1970) The offspring of alcoholic mothers. *Paediatric Research*, **4**, 474.
Warren, K.R. & Rosett, H.L. (1978) Fetal Alcohol Sydrome. *Alcohol Health and Research World*, **2**, (4), 2–12.
Whalen, T. (1953) Wives of alcoholics. Four types observed in a family service agency. *Quarterly Journal of Studies on Alcohol*, **14**, 632.
Wilkins, R.H. (1972) The Health Visitor and the Alcoholic. *Journal of Alcoholism*, **7**, 92.
Wilkins, R.H. (1973) The Community Nurse and the Alcoholic. *Nursing Times*, **69**, 1071–1072.
Wilkins, R.H. (1974) *The Hidden Alcoholic in General Practice*. London: Elek Science.

50

The handicapped child at home

Teresa Wilkinson

The child who is born with, or acquires a handicap, mental, physical or emotional, starts out in life with the scales weighted heavily against him. It is, however, most important to remember at all times that he is first and foremost a child, and is just as much dependent on his family and home to provide a stable supportive and stimulating environment in which he can grow to exploit his full potential, as is the normal child.

Any baby needs to be handled, cuddled and loved; any small child needs to play, to explore, to test his abilities and understand his limitations; any adolescent needs to assert his independence and identify his own personality. Within the boundaries set by their bodies or by their intellectual limitations, handicapped children need to do all these things, and to take part in normal family relationships, to fight with their brothers and sisters, love their mothers, rebel against their fathers and learn to enjoy the rough and tumble of life with the rest of us.

Thus, however severe the disability, almost all handicapped children are better cared for at home if this is at all possible. If their needs for specialised education demand that they should be placed in residential schools, then they need to spend many weekends and holidays at home so that the family ties are not broken.

Any family which contains a handicapped member is subject to extra stress. Most parents of a handicapped child are troubled by guilt, almost always irrational and unfounded, but no less a potent source of emotional trouble for that. Normal sibling rivalries and tensions are heightened by the presence of a child who either gets more attention than the others or holds the family back from outings and holidays.

Any general practitioner is aware of the pressures that normal family life exerts on its members. He understands the mechanisms by which marital or personality problems in the parents may be presented in other ways by the family, such as recurrent minor illness or inappropriate behaviour in the children. When dealing with a family which contains a handicapped child the doctor must always remember that this is an ordinary family with an unusual problem, and that its members function in the same way as the rest of the community. In other words, depressions, anxiety states, enuresis and temper tantrums abound in our society, and when encountered in the family with a handicapped child should be dealt with in the normal way and not be laid at his door.

In many ways the severely handicapped child is often almost removed from the general practitioner's care by a proliferation of specialists, recurrent hospital visits, operations, specialised education, physiotherapy, occupational therapy and the rest. It is very important however that the family doctor should make an effort to be aware of what is going on in relation to his patient's medical treatment and education, or else he may not be in a position properly to understand the pressures on the family or the parents' worries. Any parent of a handicapped child needs to be able to relate to one doctor out of the multiplicity that he will see over the years. This doctor need not be the 'conductor of the orchestra' but must be available to explain the nature and implications of operations, the significance of investigations and the rationale of treatments. Often this role is undertaken by a hospital consultant, a health visitor or a social worker, but if the general practitioner has the confidence of the family, and is seen to be aware of developments and concerned about them, he is in the best position to explain medical and surgical crises as they come and go, to listen to worries small and large and to give an informed opinion when decisions have to be made which will affect the child and the family.

The importance of this function cannot be overemphasised, as various studies have shown that the tensions in families with this problem are exacerbated by a lack of understanding of the nature of the medical condition and its prognosis, and by the bewilderment induced by the multiplicity of agencies which may be approached for help.

Most families with a handicapped child need help with specific problems from time to time. Nursery places for the handicapped child or for normal siblings, wheel chairs, walking aids, structural alterations to the home such as ramps and hand rails, financial assistance, holidays, transport etc. Fortunately the reorganised local authority social services are to combine the variety of agencies into one comprehensive organisation, but patients are still confused and often do not benefit from help which is available as they remain unaware of it.

The local social services department remains the first avenue to be explored when any need arises as if there is no help available from an official source, they are usually in a position to know which voluntary agencies exist or are active locally. It is important that the family should be helped by an imaginative and interested approach to forsee difficulties before they become acute, and to solve problems as they arise, so that tensions are kept to a minimum.

There are many societies and voluntary organisations which exist to support and help patients suffering from specific conditions or with specific needs. Children suffering from blindness, deafness, cerebral palsy, spina bifida, and mongolism have different needs and different problems. Their families are stressed in different ways by different tensions and the emotional support and concrete help which they may gain from membership or association with a society composed of others in the same position is enormous. There are various booklets available, such as the excellent *Handbook for Parents with a Handicapped Child*, which give details of the societies and agencies which exist, and explain their functions and activities.

The main benefit of such societies is that they provide an opportunity for parents to get together with others who have experienced the same difficulties, depressions and exasperations. They can often be helped a great deal by learning to talk to others about their hidden fears, guilt, frustrations and anger when they understand that other parents have felt the same. A doctor may be sympathetic, understanding and supportive if a mother admits guiltily to occasional feelings of disgust, irritation or rejection towards her mentally handicapped child, but if she can relate her feelings and difficulties to another mother in the way that most parents discuss teething, nappy rashes and feeding problems, she is more likely to be able to see her troubles and her achievements in a true perspective.

Parent associations also serve a useful function in that they may develop into pressure groups which campaign for improved services, promote public interest and improve general understanding of handicaps.

The aim of education and medical treatment of any handicapped child is that he should be helped to exploit his full potential and become as free, independent and useful a member of the community as he is able. This means that the child must be as well equipped as possible to face the challenge of living in a society composed of people without handicaps, and this is the point at which many parents need help. The line between overprotection and rejection in parenting a handicapped child is much more difficult to draw but needs attention, as on this to a large extent depends the child's attitude to his own disability.

How much more difficult it is for a mother to hear her disabled child jeered at by the neighbourhood children as a cripple than to hear insults hurled at her normal child. How much more difficult to judge the moment when her backward child is competent to walk in the street and visit friends alone. These are the problems of which the general practitioner should be constantly aware, and should make every effort to work out with the parents.

Many families contain and care for a handicapped child without guilt or bitterness and find it an enriching and rewarding experience for all the members. Their doctor's function is to be available at all times as a source of technical information, an imaginative lead into organisations which can provide practical help and friendships, and an understanding observer of the child's development and of the relationships within the family. The key is to remember always that the handicapped child is an individual, a member of a family, a part of the community, with hopes, fears and aspirations, rights and responsibilities, just like the rest of us.

FURTHER READING

Barnitt, R.E. (1971) Aids for the multi-handicapped child. *Physiotherapy*, September, 418–424.

Burton, L. (1973) *The Family Life of Sick Children*. London: Routledge & Kegan Paul.

Central Council for the Disabled (1975) *Holidays for the Physically Handicapped*. Booklet, 40 p, obtainable from W.H.Smith & Son. Revised annually.

Cummings, P. (1973) *Education and the Severely Handicapped Child*. National Society for Mentally Handicapped Children.

Finnie, N.R. (1974) *Handling the Young Cerebral Palsied Child at Home*, 2nd edn. London: Heinemann.

Hannam, C. (1975) *Parents and Mentally Handicapped Children*. Harmondsworth: Penguin.

Hewett, S., Newson, J. & Newson, E.(1970) *The Family with the Handicapped Child*. London: George Allen.

Parfit, J. (1972) *Services for the Young Handicapped Child*. London: National Children's Bureau.

Stone, J. & Taylor, F.(1974) *Handbook for Parents with a Handicapped Child*, 2nd edn.London: Home and Social Council. Case Publications, 17 Jackson Lane, Billericay, Essex.

Younghusband, E. *et al* (1970) *Living with Handicaps*. London: National Children's Bureau.

Wilkes, J. & Wilkes, E. (1974) *Bernard: Bringing Up our Mongol Son*. London: Routledge & Kegan Paul.

Woodburn, M. (1975) *Social Implications of Spina Bifida*. Windsor: National Foundation for Educational Research.

51

Death in childhood

Christopher Elliott Binns

INTRODUCTION

A hundred years ago death amongst children in this country was commonplace and a mother who could say she had 'successfully reared all her family' had reason to be proud. Nowadays, due largely to the decreased mortality from infective illness, childhood death is uncommon after the perinatal period, and a rarity after the age of one year. This is illustrated in Table 51.1 which shows the incidence of death from general causes, and Table 51.2 which refers to certain illnesses particularly relevant to this chapter.

Death, when it does occur, is nearly always in hospital because a general practitioner will arrange the admission of a child who is ill enough to be in danger of death and failure to do so would be considered a serious error. Only unexpected or sudden deaths normally occur at home, such as deaths from fulminating respiratory infections, trauma or cot deaths. None of these imply care during terminal illness, so even an established family doctor may never have experienced the problems of looking after a dying child in the home. He may, in fact, tend to lose contact with a child who suffers from a long term fatal illness such as leukaemia because the family bypass their own doctor and look to the hospital for help, the general practitioner merely receiving information by letter. This is an undesirable state of affairs and he should have some general system of care in readiness to ensure he is fulfilling his role as a family doctor.

This plan should cover the period from the first suspicion of a fatal illness until a year or so after the child's death when the mourning process is complete and should include the child itself, the parents, siblings, relatives and friends. It should be a team plan since the doctor should work in co-operation with the hospital staff, his practice nurse and health visitor, and others ready to give help, especially ministers of religion, as well as those mentioned above who are personally involved in the tragedy. Terminal care should be looked upon as part of a much wider field of family care, although it must never be forgotten that the primary object is to help the child die in peace and comfort.

It is logical to suppose that the best place for a child to die is in his own bed at home, surrounded by familiar objects and toys, and cared for by his mother and father. It is because childhood death, unlike death in old people, is unacceptable that both doctor and parents

Table 51.1 Deaths per 100 000 population. Major causes by age and sex, Great Britain. Source: HMSO annual abstracts of statistics. Crown Copyright

Cause of death	*Males* 1950–3 average	*Males* 1961	*Males* 1974	*Females* 1950–3 average	*Females* 1961	*Females* 1974
Ages under 1 year						
Infective diseases	249	75	67	199	71	51
Pneumonia	527	320	149	416	254	108
Congenital anomalies	460	460	403	430	455	401
All causes	3293	2450	1883	2554	1920	1419
Ages 1–14 years						
Infective diseases	15	4	3	14	3	2
Cancer (inc. leukaemia)	8	8	6	7	7	5
Pneumonia	7	6	3	7	5	3
Accidents	24	21	15	12	10	9
All causes	85	62	45	67	44	34

Table 51.2 Death rates from selected causes per million population. England and Wales, 1978. Source: OPCS Mortality Statistics Series DH3 No 5 1980. Crown Copyright

		Ages (years)						
Causes	*0–1*	*0–1*	*1–2*	*2–3*	*3–4*	*4–5*	*5–9*	*10–14*
All causes	M	4513	293	165	151	130	628	619
	F	3368	238	137	124	108	417	421
All congenital disorders	M	1081	79	31	22	18	63	54
	F	952	58	31	24	12	64	63
Spina bifida	M	164	3	1	2	3	4	6
	F	249	3	–	–	1	9	9
All respiratory disorders	M	547	52	23	17	10	38	36
	F	390	59	22	14	9	37	32
Infective and parasitic	M	170	24	10	9	6	27	9
	F	125	14	15	2	5	18	18
All neoplasms	M	26	19	24	22	30	151	130
	F	16	19	11	20	24	93	84
Diseases of lymphocytic and haemopoeitic systems (mostly leukaemia)	M	6	6	8	9	14	87	70
	F	7	8	4	11	12	32	47

Deaths from accidents are analysed in Tables 24.1–4 and deaths from congenital heart disease in Table 35.2

will feel that life should be preserved as long as possible and this usually requires treatment and nursing procedures that cannot easily be carried out in the home. The parents may feel more confident if the child is in hospital because professional help is always at hand when suffering occurs and watching their child die is more tolerable in the impersonal hospital situation. As one mother put it, 'I could not bear to think of us watching her body being taken away from the house. If she dies in hospital we can at least leave her there and come home to mourn.' There is also a fear that the siblings will react badly to death in the home.

The child's own views are difficult to ascertain but those with long term illness have become used to hospital. They accept admission as the normal procedure when they have a relapse and, especially if the parents are near, suffer no special anxiety. Fortunately childrens' wards are now organised so that the mother or father can sleep in the same room as the child.

Thus the present climate of opinion is against terminal care in the home, but many paediatricians and family doctors are wondering whether this is in fact in the best interests of the child and parents. There may well be a return to the old ideal of the child dying peacefully at home.

MEDICAL AND NURSING CARE

On the technical side the nursing of the dying child is unlikely to present many problems which cannot be managed at home once active treatment has been abandoned. This is because the child is light in weight and can be moved easily. Bedsores do not commonly occur unless the child is immobile for a long time, as in spastic conditions or prolonged unconsciousness following head injury, when hospital treatment is usually necessary anyway. Incontinence is easy to manage with the use of draw-sheets and incontinence pads and the child can be sat on a pot or commode until late in the illness. If the child is wasted an underlying synthetic sheepskin is a comfort and is washable.

Discomfort of any kind must be controlled effectively. Antiemetics may help when vomiting causes distress, but our information on their use in children is not very great, so that caution is needed. Mild pain can be treated with aspirin or paracetamol but the doctor should not hesitate to use strong analgesics when necessary. Of these diamorphine is the most effective but because it is unpleasant to take by mouth a suitable vehicle must be found, the parent knowing best the child's taste. A satisfactory alternative is tincture of opium in chlorpromazine syrup. Cocaine is undesirable in children.

If sedation alone is required diazepam, chlorpromazine or promethazine (Phenergan) are useful, but diazepam does not suit all children. Treatment of this sort should only be given if there is an indication, since many children will die peacefully without sedation or analgesia and it is incorrect to suppress the process of dying, which may be meaningful to the parents and perhaps the child himself. In conditions such as leukaemia and respiratory failure which may lead to a distressing death, diamorphine should be given in large doses, if necessary by injection.

By the terminal stage unessential treatment and investigations will have been stopped but an explanation must be given to the child, otherwise he may feel abandoned. He may be told he is being given a rest from them for the time being.

Nursing will be shared between the practice nurse and the parents and other relatives or friends. The nurse should train the parents to help with general care. This will be a great comfort to them because they know they are helping the child in a practical way. If the parents are unable to co-operate, hospital admission is indicated. The nurse should visit frequently, perhaps two or three times a day in the final phase, to give the parents moral support. During this period the practice nurse will be able to form a close relationship with the parents and child which will prove invaluable later. Being experienced she is unlikely to suffer severely from grief herself, as sometimes happens with junior nurses in a paediatric ward. Also she will accept the inevitability of death without feelings of guilt or frustration.

The doctor may find he has little practical help to offer and be tempted to visit infrequently. If he does this he is failing in his obligation because his interest and compassion are of great importance, to the parents in particular. A brief daily visit is suggested in the final days. In the bedroom the child should be the centre of attention. If the doctor is uncertain what to say he may find it helpful to sit on the side of the bed and show an interest in the child's toys. This is a good way of starting a converstaion. He should not spend his time talking across the bed to the parents, but should give them a chance to express their grief and anxiety in another room.

He should, if possible, arrange to be available when death occurs, during the night or when he is off duty, and should attend as soon as possible. His presence will be a great help to the parents and he should sit and drink a cup of tea with them even if he can find no words to comfort them.

THE CHILD'S ATTITUDE TO DEATH

Parents and attendants sometimes wonder if the child realises he is dying, or indeed if he should be made aware of his condition, either directly or in a roundabout way. Many studies of children's awareness of death have been carried out.

Under the age of three a child cannot conceive 'non-existence' and his anxieties are in relation to separation from his parents who, for this reason, should always be present or near at hand in the terminal phase of illness.

Between the ages of three and six the child develops curiosity about death, for example in relatives and pet animals, but has little fear of death as such. He may consider illness or separation is symbolic of punishment and it should be made clear to him that this is not so.

At about the age of six he will begin to fear death. He will tend to personify it and think in terms of ghosts, skeletons, being shut up in a black box and other images related to books, television and adult conversations. His attitude can be compared to the magical approach of primitive cultures and the attendants should be aware of this symbolic form of thinking. It is at about the age of ten that he will begin to understand the permanence of death and consider the matter logically.

The above account is only a rough guide since some quite young children have remarkable perceptiveness while teenagers may show an immature attitude to death.

At some time the doctor should discuss with the parents and practice nurse what they should say if the child does talk about the prospect of death. It is important not to brush aside the question, which will make the child anxious and suspicious, and he should be allowed to express his ideas, but if possible in general terms. In this way fanciful terrors may be dispelled. If the child does ask the direct question 'Am I going to die?' it is tempting to reply 'Of course not', but this may not convince older children. For them it may be better to explain that the illness is sometimes fatal and that is why they are having treatment. The matter is more complex in so-called 'doomed families' when a series of siblings die from inherited disease and the child is all too well aware of the outcome.

In practice the matter seldom arises and the doctor is advised to leave well alone unless the child develops severe anxiety or apathy for which a reason must be sought.

The child's main reaction will be towards his disablement, treatment and parental separation rather than the fear of death. Some children resist treatment, especially injections, and become aggressive, while others become oversubmissive and apathetic. The first reaction, which is more common in boys, may lead to undesirable and destructive habits with a demanding and aggressive attitude which may sadden and shock the parents. The second may lead to a depressive state in which the child gives up and loses contact with those around him or regresses to an infantile state. This can be equally upsetting.

It should be the aim of the doctor to prevent either of these extreme reactions. If the problem is a long term one it is sensible for the paediatrician and family doctor to meet the parents together in the early stages of the illness. It must be explained to them that the best service they can give the child is to encourage him to lead as normal a life as possible. He should not be spoilt and should carry on with schooling, even if it be limited. By nature all children strive and the parents should ensure that he has something to strive for, but it must be within his capabilities. As the illness progresses his attainments will become less, but his interests must be maintained and he must be encouraged to do what he can in the terminal phase.

PARENTAL ATTITUDES

Grief is a complex subject and only a parent who has lost a child can fully appreciate the nature of the tragedy. It is customary to think of the mother as the chief mourner with the father giving her support but in fact each parent is likely to suffer similar grief and they should support each other. Grief is something which must be lived through and it is harmful to suppress it. In our culture, ritual expression is usually limited to the funeral ceremony and parents are not encouraged to show extravagant sorrow.

There is usually a double bereavement, first when the parent is told the child has a fatal illness and second when death takes place. The interval between the two may be months or years and the mourning process may be almost completed by the time the child dies. Parents will sometimes lose contact with the child because they symbolically consider him already dead and experienced ward-sisters may remark that the predominant feeling at the time of death may be one of relief.

The reaction of the parents depends on their personalities, culture, religion and social class. A West Indian mother, for example, will show a very different pattern from a middle class English father although their problem is the same.

When parents are told their child has a fatal illness the initial reaction is often shock and disbelief, and this feeling may be prolonged so that they insist on a second opinion or seek help from faith healers. This attitude should not be scorned since the parents have the right to any help they can get, but they should be dissuaded from spending a lot of money on projects which will lead to disappointment.

Once reality is accepted they may ask many questions. Why has this happened to us? Is it our fault? Is the illness inherited? All these questions must be answered truthfully, patiently and often repeatedly, so that the parents have a good understanding of the situation long before the terminal phase is reached.

Sometimes one or both parents may show marked aggression towards the family doctor, the hospital, God or some object whom they feel must take the blame for the intolerable situation. Occasionally the aggression is directed at the child itself. Aggression of this sort is often a symptom of guilt, which should, if possible, be uncovered. It may be that the parent has been antagonistic to the child in the past, or did not wish him to be born in the first place.

When the parents accept the situation they will best help themselves by concentrating on the care of the child. They should become involved as much as possible both in and out of the hospital, and in the terminal stages, should be encouraged to do as much of the nursing as practicable. They may have episodes of despair and resentment and the doctor should encourage them to express their grief in words. In the later stages of the illness they may become tired, especially if they have disturbed nights, and the doctor must ensure they have some rest and relaxation. This may be difficult if the child is overdependent and unable to accept adult substitutes. The father may need help in organising his work although he will probably receive cooperation if it is known that a sick child is involved.

As the child's condition becomes hopeless the doctor should increase not decrease his attentions. After death he should visit the parents within a few days, and if he is able to attend the funeral it will make a lasting impression. There is some danger of the parents being inundated with sympathy at first and later neglected, so the practice team should discuss who should be responsible for the long term follow-up. Often the nurse is the most suitable person, having been most involved, but the health visitor or social worker may be preferred.

The parents will find comfort in being congratulated on the way they have looked after the child, and it is often helpful to explain that death is sometimes preferable to prolonged illness. For a time the parents will idealise the memory of the child and the doctor should accept this. Gradually their attitude will become more realistic and at the end of about a year their lives should have returned to normal although they will continue to be sad at times, especially at anniversaries.

Excess mourning should not be taken as a measure of the fondness of the parent for the child but as an indication of unstable relationships. A basically happy family will recover more quickly than one troubled with antagonism and guilt. It requires fine judgment by the doctor to decide when mourning is abnormal, in which case he should consider antidepressant therapy or psychiatric help.

A note of the child's death should be made in the parent's records for the benefit of future partners, because the mourning process may recur years later in some apparently unimportant circumstance such as the death of a distant relative.

SUDDEN DEATH

When death is sudden the grieving process is accentuated. The parents have no opportunity for preparation and may have strong feelings of guilt, especially if death is due to trauma which might have been preventable, such as accidents on the road or in the home, or in cot deaths. The latter is now responsible for half the deaths between the ages of one month and one year, thus posing a serious problem. The cause of sudden infant death syndrome (SIDS) is largely a matter of conjecture in spite of recent intensive investigation although contributory factors have been identified. Typically it occurs in families of class 4 or 5, often with the mother of young age but with several children born in rapid succession. It is commoner in winter or spring and also at weekends or bank holidays when the parents wake up late and find the child dead. Until recently it was thought to be associated with excessive salt in artificial feeds but now it is equally common in breast fed babies. A three year multicentre study has shown that 50 per cent of SIDS babies have had warning symptoms as compared with 26 per cent controls These however are usually mild, the most significant being drowsiness, excessive or irritable crying and refusal of feeds. Since these symptoms herald many trivial and non-fatal illnesses the parents do not think it necessary to call the doctor and the doctor, if called, would probably find no indication for hospital admission. He should however be on guard with at-risk babies especially those with a history of 'near miss' cot death.

Why do babies sometimes die in their sleep? In some cases autopsy shows evidence of acute illness, usually respiratory. In others there is nothing to show. Studies of 'near misses' have demonstrated cardiac arrythmias on 24 hour tapes but these occur in normal babies so that evidence is not conclusive. Apnoeic attacks of up to twenty seconds are also fairly common in young babies and it may be that some SIDS babies just stop breathing due to some fault in the respiratory centre, perhaps as a result of viral illness. Attention has recently been drawn to the effects of overheating. Many mothers tend to wrap up a feverish child rather than cool him down and there is some post-mortem evidence that heat exhaustion may occur in a swaddled baby with a high temperature. The matter is still undecided and this is reflected in the fact that coroners now accept a diagnosis of Cause Unknown on death certificates, whereas previously it was usual to write Suffocation on the false assumption that the baby had been asphyxiated by his pillow or 'overlayed' by his mother.

Parents react with shock and grief to a cot death. It is difficult to satisfy them with a vague diagnosis and they may feel antagonistic towards the doctor or guilty because they should have realised the child was ill. Other adverse factors are shock at finding the child dead and the need to involve the coroner, although this is necessary to prevent gossip as well as certify the cause of death.

Patient discussion is needed and the best person to undertake this may be a parent who has undergone a similar experience. A service of this kind is provied by The Foundation for the Study of Infant Deaths (see Appendix, pp. 395–6) and in some areas there are local organisations.

The emotional needs of parents at the time of stillbirth or neonatal death are comparable to SIDS although grief is not usually so prolonged because they have not had the opportunity to know the baby as a person.

It is now recommended that the mother of a stillborn child should be encouraged to see the body if she so wishes. There should be opportunity for sympathetic discussion and The Health Education Council have produced a helpful booklet. The best comfort to the mother is often another pregnancy but when this does not occur grief may be extended and feelings of guilt become ingrained.

CARE OF SIBLINGS

The death of a brother or sister may cause serious and long lasting disturbance in a child's life, although by and large children are more resilient than adults. The distress may stem more from the change of attitude of their parents and the general upheaval than from the actual death. It is therefore important for the doctor to give the parents advice at the onset of the illness about the care of the siblings.

The attitude of children to death has already been discussed. If a child should ask if his brother or sister is going to die the parents should not brush aside the question but should give an answer which is optimistic, except when the end is near. It must be remembered that remarks may be repeated to the ill child and siblings are quite capable of saying 'Didn't they tell you you are going to die?' In the case of sudden death the parents must seek a way of breaking the news to the siblings with complete honesty. It is idle to pretend the dead child will come back again.

The parents will tend to neglect the siblings in favour of the patient and this may lead to attention-seeking behaviour, aggression, regression to infantile behaviour and poor school reports. Boys in particular may become antisocial. Older children should be encouraged to help with the care of the sick child, but younger children cannot understand this and are concerned only with the loss of parental attention to themselves. A sympathetic relative or friend will be invaluable in filling this gap.

There is some danger of older girls being put in a position of running the home while the mother is involved with the sick child. The parents must be prepared to give praise and even reward and not take the help for granted. Finally the parents must accept that the siblings may show aggression towards the sick child who has ousted them, or appear apathetic about the whole matter. A child who shows more interest in his favourite television programme than the funeral is not necessarily showing abnormal behaviour.

HELP FROM OTHER SOURCES

In a situation such as the death of a child the extended family comes into its own, and it may only be with the help and sympathy of relatives that the child can be nursed at home. Neighbours also are invaluable, although the situation is now so unusual that there may be a feeling of embarrassment in the community, of a kind which would not have occurred fifty years ago.

The role of ministers of religion is of the utmost importance. In days gone by a priest would automatically be involved, but with the present secular trend this is no longer so. If the family is of religious bent they will, themselves, contact a priest who may be their chief source of support and understanding, and the doctor should accept this and be prepared to play a secondary role. The priest and doctor should never be at cross purposes and they should, if possible, discuss the matter at the onset of the illness. Even if the family are not concerned with religion the doctor should, at some time, mention the matter and without forcing the issue, suggest they seek help in that direction. The death of a child is such a tragedy that it cannot be seen in limited medical terms, and a sincere and sensible priest will help anyone in distress.

The doctor may call on various organisations such as the Parents Association, Society of Compassionate Friends, Royal Red Cross Society, National Society of Cancer Relief and the Marie Curie Memorial Foundation. He can obtain advice on where to seek help from the Social Services Department or the Citizen's Advice Bureau, but if a health visitor is attached to the practice she may make the necessary arrangements. Most families, however, receive adequate support from relatives and friends, so outside help is not needed.

SUMMARY

A family doctor will rarely be responsible for the care of a child dying at home, but when the situation does occur his worth will be tested to the full. He may feel helpless himself but must realise his interest and compassion are of enormous value. He must work in co-operation with the child, the parents and friends, and his own staff to ensure that the child dies in peace and comfort and that grief is kept within reasonable bounds. Or as Hippocrates wrote some 2400 years ago, 'The art of medicine consists of three things, the disease, the patient, and the physician. The physician is the servant of the art and the patient should combat the disease along with the physician . . . The physician must not only do what is right himself but also guide the patients, attendants and friends . . . Where there is love of man there is also love of the art'.

ACKNOWLEDGEMENT

The author wishes to acknowledge his debt to the parents, medical staff and others who have given him advice, and in particular Dr T. Wynne Williams, Sister Cecily Carter and the Rev. Leslie Turner.

FURTHER READING

Benfield, D.G. *et al* (1978) Grief response of parents to neonatal death and parent participation in deciding care. *Pediatrics*, **62**, 171–7.

BMJ Editorial (1980) Sudden infant death syndrome and ventilatory control. *British Medical Journal*, **2**, 337.

Branson, H.K. (1972) The dying child and his family. *Bedside Nurse*, **5**, 11–15.

Burton, L. (1974) *Care of the Child Facing Death*. London: Routledge & Kegan Paul.

Chapman, J.A. & Goodall, J. (1979) Dying children need help too. *British Medical Journal*, **1**, 593–594.

Cornwell, J. *et al* (1977) Family response to loss of a child by sudden infant death syndrome. *Medical Journal of Australia*, **1(18)**, 656–8.

Guntheroth, W.G. (1977) Sudden infant death syndrome (crib death). *American Heart Journal*, **93**, 784–93.

Lascari, A.D. (1978) The dying child and the family. *Journal of Family Practice*, **6**, 1279–86.

Limerick, Countess of (1974) SIDS. In Camps, F.E. (ed.) *International Symposium, Canadian Foundation for the Study of Infant Deaths*.

Limerick, Countess of, *et al* (1978) Support for families bereaved by cot death; joint voluntary and professional view. *British Medical Journal*, **1**, 1527–9.

Lowenberg, J.S. (1970) The coping behaviours of fatally ill adolescents and their parents. *Nursing Forum*, **9**, 269–287.

Olmsted, R.W. (1970) Care of the child with a fatal illness. *Journal of Pediatrics*, **76**, 814.

Preston, K.O. (1971) Nursing children with cancer. *Nursing Times*, **67**, 467–469.
Roberts Jaequeline, Lynch Margaret & Golding Jean (1980) Postneonatal mortality in children from abusing families. *British Medical Journal*, **2**, 102–103.
Stanton, A.N. *et al* (1978) Terminal symptoms in children dying suddenly and unexpectedly at home. Preliminary report of the DHSS multicentre study of postneonatal mortality. *British Medical Journal*, **2**, 1249–51.
Tietz, W. *et al*. (1977) Family sequelae after a child's death due to cancer. *American Journal of Psychotherapy*, **31**, 417–25.

Appendix: Voluntary organisations for child care

Cyril Hart

VOLUNTARY ORGANISATIONS FOR CHILD CARE

This list is corrected as far as possible up to November, 1980, but does not claim to be exhaustive. Adoption Societies are omitted, as they are listed in *The General Practitioner's Year Book* (Winthrop), and in the *Social Services Year Book*. There is also a list in *Adopting a Child*, 1980 edition, published by the Association of British Adoption and Fostering Agencies, 4 Southampton Row, London WC1B 4AA, tel. 01-242-8951. Two special adoption organisations are Parents for Children, 222 Camden High Street, London NW1, tel. 01-485-7526, which is concerned with the adoption of handicapped children within 100 miles of London; and Parent to Parent Information Advisory Service, 26 Belsize Grove, London NW3, tel. 01-722-5328, which publishes a newsletter about children in the care of local authorities who are available for adoption.

Local organisations are also omitted; information about these is best sought from your local library or social services department. Research foundations are listed in the annual reports of the National Fund for Research into Crippling Diseases, by Action Research for the Crippled Child. A general directory of voluntary social services is published by the National Council of Social Service, and many voluntary organisations are listed in the *Social Services Year Book*.

Many of these organisations have been badly hit by inflation, and are finding it difficult to maintain the range and quality of their activities. This is a great misfortune for child care in Britain today, and practitioners are urged to encourage their patients to give every possible support to these voluntary bodies.

Alateen
St Giles Centre, Camberwell Church Street, London SE5 8RB
Tel. 01 703 0397

A fellowship for the children of alcoholics. See further, p. 382.

The Association for Children with Learning Disabilities
7 Hampton Road, Folly Hill, Farnham, Surrey

Founded in 1976 to help children of average or above average intelligence who have learning difficulties.

The Association for Research into Restricted Growth
Charles Pocock, 4 Laburnum Avenue, Wickford, Essex

Promotes studies of dwarfism; encourages self help; information on clothing, aid, and mobility. Social events organised. Bimonthly magazine.

The Association for Spina Bifida and Hydrocephalus
Tavistock House North, Tavistock Square London, WC1H 9HJ
Tel. 01 388 1382

Founded in 1966, with the twin objectives of supporting families and aiding research. Eighty eight local associations cover England, Wales and Northern Ireland, with affiliated associations in Scotland and Jersey. Provides a specialised social worker service for some counties, and deals with personal problems nationwide. Maintains an appliance officer, and officer for education, training, and employment. Publishes informative booklets for parents, and a bimonthly journal called '*Link*'.

The British Association for the Hard of Hearing
16 Park St, Windsor, Berks SL4 1LU
Tel. 01 731 2034

The British Association for the Retarded
17 Penbridge Square, London W2 EP

Founded in 1977. Represents and protects the interests of the mentally retarded of all ages. Mainly educational. Course and seminars for professionals. Publishes journal called *Retardation*.

The British Deaf Association
38 Victoria Palace, Carlisle CA1 1HU
Tel. 0228 20188/9

Founded in 1899 for the profoundly deaf of all ages. Help with sign language and other communication skills. Educational activities include school leaver courses.

The British Diabetic Association
10 Queen Anne Street, London W1M OBD
Tel. 01 323 1531

Founded in 1934. A national association for all diabetics, including children. Free advisory service. Holidays and hostels for diabetic children. While on holiday, their diabetic state is stabilised as far as possible, and they are taught principles of dieting and treatment. The association organises conferences and supports research. Catalogue of wide range of publications available. Issues a journal called *Balance*, and an annual report. See further, page 306.

The British Dyslexia Association
4 Hobbart Place, London SW1

Founded in 1972 to co-ordinate interdisciplinary studies – medical, psychological and educational. This work is now based at the Dyslexia Institute, 133 Gresham Rd, Staines TW18 2AJ. Also brings together regional associations for parents and interested professional workers, already established throughout Britain. 34 local branches. The Dyslexia and Learning Disability Centre at 18 Park Square East, London N.W.1, offers help with diagnosis and tuition.

The British Epilepsy Association
Crowthorne House, New Wokingham Road, Wokingham, Berks RG11 3AY
Tel. 03446 3122

Founded in 1950. A national organisation, with regional offices in London, Leeds, Birmingham and Belfast. Activities include education – courses, lectures, literature, films – for lay and professional groups, including general practitioners. Mounts an Action for Epilepsy campaign, with 100 local groups. Sponsors research, largely in special schools for children with epilepsy. Organises parents support groups, and a Family Advice Centre. A Children's Holiday Unit runs annual holidays and periods of temporary care for children with epilepsy. Advice Bureau. Career Assessment Unit. Publishes annual symposium of articles on epilepsy by lay and medical workers, and also a magazine and newsletter. Other activities described in annual report. See further, page 320.

The British Nutrition Foundation
15 Belgrave Sq., London SW1X 8PS
Tel. 01 235 4904

Founded in 1967. Provides information on nutrition of the mother, infant, and child. Seminars for health care and education professionals. Wide range of publications.

The British Red Cross Society
9 Grosvenor Crescent, London, SW1X 7EJ
Tel. 01 235 5454

Founded in 1870. Adult courses concerned with child care include: First Aid, Nursing, Maternal and Child Health, Welfare (with special attention to needs of multi-handicapped children and social support services). Courses for junior members include Infant and Child Care, Health and Hygiene, and Accident Prevention. The juniors also run schemes to help parents to have a break from continuous strain of caring for the handicapped child. Adult services include a school for 50 handicapped children in Cambridgeshire, and a toy library.

The British Rheumatism and Arthritis Association
6 Grosvenor Crescent, London SW1X 7ER
Tel. 01 235 0902

Founded in 1947. A national association. 150 local branches. Most of its work is done with adults, but it does provide some literature on rheumatism in childhood, and organises holidays for children with rheumatism. Publishes annual report, and a quarterly magazine.

The Brittle Bones Society
Sec. Mrs. M. Grant, 63 Byron Crescent, Dundee DD3 6SS
Tel. 0382 87130
Southern rep: Mrs J. Morrow, 38 Hartford Road, Borehamwood, Herts.

About 1250 people in Britain are affected. The Society encourages research, refers members for genetic counselling, and through its 'Magpie Appeal' helps children with equipment, treatments, and holidays.

Buckets & Spades
20 Mersham Drive, Kingsbury, London N.W.9
Tel. 01 204 7414

A Jewish short-term home for mentally handicapped children of all religions, St Leonards on Sea, Sussex. No fee charged to parents, but any donation gratefully received.

The Central Council for the Disabled
34 Eccleston Square, London SW1V 1PE
Tel. 01 834 0747/8

Founded in 1919. A national co-ordinating body of voluntary organisations for physically disabled of all ages. Concentrates on housing, holidays, access to public buildings and facilities and monitoring legislation. Information bureau, and monthly bulletin.

The Cheshire Foundation Homes for the Sick
7 Market Mews, London W1Y 8HP
Tel. 01 499 2665

The first home was founded in 1948. There are now over 60 within the UK, and about the same number overseas. Most are for adults, but there is one in Surrey for 16 physically handicapped children, and three homes in Dorset and Cheshire cater for a total of 74 mentally handicapped children. Publications include a quarterly magazine, the 'Cheshire Smile', and books and films.

The Chest Heart and Stroke Association
Tavistock House North, Tavistock Square, London WC1H 9JE.
Tel. 01 387 3012/4

A national association for those of all ages with heart, arterial and chest diseases. Maintains a Children's Chest Circle for parents of children with asthma, bronchitis, and heart disease. Counselling and welfare services. Conferences and research. Publications include booklets for parents, and a quarterly magazine called *Hope*.

The Child Poverty Action Group
1 Macklin Street, Drury Lane, London WC2B 5NH
Tel. 01 242 3225 and 01 242 9149

Founded in 1965 as a vigorous pressure group to bring public attention to the needs of the poor. Wide range of pamphlets, and a quarterly journal.

The Church of England Children's Society
Old Town Hall, Kennington Road, London SE11 4QD
Tel. 01 735 2441

Founded in 1881. Works throughout England and Wales. Runs 67 residential and day-care establishments. Employs 85 social workers. Works with 1500 families on a preventive basis. Has 400 children in its own foster homes, and places about 500 children each year for adoption – half of them children with special needs. Maintains assessment centre at Balham, London. Most of the society's work is with normal children experiencing social deprivation, but some mentally and physically handicapped children are cared for, in eight homes and hostels. Issues a leaflet, *The work of the Children's Society.*

The Coeliac Society
P.O. Box 181, London NW2 2QY

Founded in 1968 to further the interests of patients with coeliac disease and to encourage research and the dissemination of information on the condition. 50 local groups have been formed. Publications include a film, a taped lecture, a newsletter, a list of gluten free foods, a booklet entitled 'The Coeliac Condition', and a comprehensive guide entitled *The Coeliac Handbook*.

Cruse, The National Organisation for the Widowed and Their Children
Cruse House, 126 Sheen Road, Richmond, Surrey TW9 1UR
Tel. 01 940 4818/9047

A counselling service with 35 branches in Britain. Monthly magazine and wide range of literature.

The Cystic Fibrosis Research Trust
5 Blyth Road, Bromley, Kent BR1 3RS
Tel. 01 464 7211/2

Founded in 1964. Finances 35 major research projects. Help and advice for parents through more than 260 local branches in Britain. Publishes a quarterly magazine, *C.F. News*, and a set of education literature for parents.

The Disabled Living Foundation
346 Kensington High Street, London W14 8NS
Tel. 01 602 2491

Founded in 1970, for research into the home problems of the disabled of all ages. Provides an information service and issues a valuable series of handbooks and pamphlets.

Dr. Barnardo's
Tanners Lane, Barkingside, Ilford, Essex 1G6 1QG
Tel. 01 550 8822

Founded in 1866. A large interdenominational Christian organistaion, active throughout the United Kingdom, also in Kenya, Australia, and New Zealand. Covers the whole range of voluntary child care. Responsible for 1200 children in 'ordinary' residential care (many from broken homes), or physically handicapped, or those who are emotionally disturbed or maladjusted, and 1000 children in 22 day care centres. Also helps 4000 children annually through its Family Care Service. Arranges adoptions, foster homes, holidays and accommodation for families with single parents. Advice on social services. Work is concentrated increasingly in the big cities and conurbations. Publications include an informative *Annual Review*.

Downs Babies Association
Quinborne Centre, Ridgacre Road, Quinton, Birmingham B32 2TW
Tel. 021 427 1374

Founded in 1970. Provides an advisory service for the parents of children with Down's syndrome (mongolism) and supports research into their care and education.

Tha Family Fund
See Joseph Rowntree Memorial Trust.

The Family Welfare Association
501 Kingsland Road, Dalston, London E8 4AU
Tel. 01 254 6251–4

Provides an information service concerning resources and administration of charities.

The Foundation for the Study of Infant Deaths
23 St. Peters Square, London W6 9NW
Tel. 01 748 7768

Help for those suffering from grief. Telephone Samaritan-type service for grieving parents in cases of 'cot deaths'. See further, page 390.

The Friends of the Centre for Spastic Children
Godfrey House, 63 Cheyne Walk, London SW3 5NA
Tel. 01 352 6740

Founded in 1954. A small day and residential centre for the assessment, treatment, and education of children with cerebral palsy. Children are referred from all over Britain, and from abroad. Training courses for professional workers in the management of cerebral palsy. Issues pamphlets on teaching the handicapped to feed and dress, and an annual report.

Gingerbread
35 Wellington Street, London W.C.2
Tel. 01 240 0953

A nationally organised self-help association, founded in 1970, to promote interests of one parent families. Over 400 local branches; social activities for parents and children. Holidays; information service. Publications include monthly magazine, *Ginger*.

The Haemophilia Society
P.O. Box 19, 16 Trinity Street, London SE1 1DE
Tel. 01 407 1010

Founded in 1950 for haemophiliacs of all ages. There are about 5000 sufferers in Britain, half of them members of the society. 24 groups meet throughout the country for mutual support. Research and holiday funds. Literature includes pamphlets and a news bulletin.

The Invalid Children's Aid association
126 Buckingham Palace Road, London SW1W 9SB
Tel. 01 730 9891

Founded in 1888. London-based, but covers also the Home Counties, with affiliated societies in Manchester and Norwich; recently has opened a school in Nottinghamshire. Primarily for helping the handicapped child at home, using a team of 22 case workers. Has a special interest in dyslexia, and maintains three schools for this, also two schools for boys with asthma. Organises conferences and conducts research. Publishes an annual report.

The Joseph Rowntree Memorial Trust
Beverley House, Shipton Road, York Y03 6RB
Tel. 0904 29241

This trust administers the Family Fund, established in 1973 to help financially families of severely handicapped children. The money is provided by the Government, but the fund is administered independently by the Trust.

Kids Centre
Easton Maudit, Northants NN9 7NR
Tel. 0933 663474

Holidays and short-term care for mentally and physically handicapped, and socially deprived children aged 4–14. Escort service to and from St. Pancras Station.

The Lady Hoare Trust for Thalidomide and other Physically Disabled Children
7 North Street, Midhurst, W. Sussex.
Tel. 073081 3696

Founded in 1961. Comprehensive help for families. Has its own team of 27 social workers. Has 600 children under care. Specialises in development of powered limbs.

The Leukaemia Society
c/o Mrs Williams, 45 Craigmoor Ave., Queen's Park, Bournemouth
Tel 0202 37459

Founded in 1967 by a small nucleus of parents. Leukaemia is diagnosed in 5000 adults and 500 children in Britain annually. Membership now extended to adult sufferers and their husbands or wives. Mainly for contacts between members of affected families. Helps financially and with holidays, transport, home nursing, and baby sitters. Publishes a booklet and a newsletter.

The Malcolm Sargent Cancer Fund for Children
6 Sydney street, London SW3 6PP.

Financial and other help for families of children with malignancies. Application to the fund should be made by a social worker.

MIND (The National Association for Mental Health)
22 Harley Street, London W1N 2ED
Tel. 01 637 0741

Formed in 1946 by the amalgamation of the Central Association for Mental Welfare, the Child Guidance Council, and the National Council for Mental Hygiene, Name changed to MIND in 1973. Promotes mental health, and helps the mentally handicapped, maladjusted, and emotionally disturbed of all ages. Coordinates activities of over 100 local associations. Homes and schools for disturbed children. Maintains an active lobby. Education and information service. Publishes *Mind Out*, a bimonthly magazine. Mail order and bookshop – Bookstall Services Ltd., 169 Malden Road, London NW5.

The Muscular Dystrophy Group of Great Britain
Nattrass House, 35 Macaulay Road, London SW4 OQP
Tel. 01 720 8055

Founded in 1959. Supports research and maintains its own laboratories at Newcastle upon Tyne. Welfare work through 300 local branches. Information for parents. Telephone enquiry service. Films. Publishes annual report, and wide range of literature including books.

The National Association for Deaf/Blind and Rubella Handicapped
Gen. Sec., Suffolk House, 10 The Butts, Coventry

Founded in 1955 by parents for mutual support and to act as a pressure group. Now a national organisation with eight regional groups. General information and help to parents, including weekend courses. Activities now extended to the deaf/blind of all ages. Publishes a newsletter.

The National Association for Mental Health
See under **MIND**

The National Association for Welfare of Children in Hospital
7 Exton Street, London SE1 8VE
Tel. 01 261 1738

Founded in 1961 to encourage regular contact between hospitals and parents of child patients. Paradoxically, it is also very concerned with the quality of home care services, and liaison with general practitioners. Coordinates the work of 65 local branches. Information and baby-sitting services for parents. Promotes research, conferences, and publications, including a newsletter.

The National Childbirth Trust
9 Queensborough Terrace London, W2
Tel. 01 229 9319

The Breast Feeding Promotion Group supplies lecturers for lay audiences on breast feeding and produces books and leaflets.

National Children's Bureau
8 Wakeley Street, Islington, London EC1V 7QE
Tel. 01 278 9441–7

Founded in 1963 to improve communications between organisations professionally or administratively concerned with the well-being of children. Individual membership also available. A link between education, medicine, and social work, and between statutory and voluntary bodies. Evaluates existing services, encourages new developments, contributes new knowledge, acts as information centre. Numerous research projects. Organises conferences covering the whole area of child care. Professional staff over 60 strong. Maintains Children's Centre at headquarters. Responsible for National Child Development Study (1958 cohort). Wide range of informative publications and films. Annual review.

National Children's Home
85 Highbury Park, London N5 1UD.
Tel. 01 226 2033

A large organisation with eight regional offices, main ly concerned with residential care, but activities include fostering, adoption, care of physically handicapped and educationally retarded, fieldwork service, and family centres.

National Council for One Parent Families
255 Kentish Town Road, London NW5 2LX
Tel. 01 267 1361

Founded in 1918, reorganised in 1973. Social workers help over 10 000 parents and individual children a year. Information service. Monitors legislation. Range of publications. Annual report.

The National Council of Social Service
26 Bedford Square, London WC1B 3HU
Tel. 01 636 4066

Founded in 1919. A co-ordinating body, to help voluntary social organisations and to prevent duplication of effort. Not directly concerned with child care, but maintains a useful information and publications section, and publishes a directory of voluntary social services.

The National Council of Voluntary Child Care Organisations
85 Highbury Park, London N5 1UD
Tel. 01 226 6592

Founded in 1943 as an association of children's homes, but membership now open to all voluntary child care organisations. Mainly a co-ordinating body. Monitors legislation, and acts as a consultative and advisory body. Maintains a list of member organisations.

National Deaf Children's Society
31 Gloucester Place, London W1H 4EA
Tel. 01 486 3251/2

Founded in 1944, enlarged in 1958 for parents and professional workers. Regional organisations throughout the UK Research committee. Casework, courses, and information. Publishes a range of booklets, a yearbook, and a quarterly magazine called *Talk*.

National Eczema Society
27 Doyle Gardens, London NW1D 3DB

Founded in 1975 for children and adults suffering from eczema. 38 local self-help branches. Magazine called *Exchange*.

The National Society for Autistic Children
1a Golders Green Road, London NW11 8EA
Tel. 01 458 4375

Founded in 1962. Provides day and residential centres for the care and education of autistic children. 30 affiliated regional societies. Advisory service for parents; information service for professionally interested people. Promotes research and publishes and distributes literature on management and education of the autistic child. There are at least 5000 children with this condition in England and Wales.

The National Society for Brain Damaged Children
The National Centre, 85 Homer Road, Solihull, Warwicks.
Tel. 021 705 5377

Founded in 1972. A small organisation started by parents and friends, with some medical members, to make the Doman Delacato method of treatment available in Britain. Referrals by doctors for evaluation and instruction at the National Centre.

The National Society for Mentally Handicapped Children
117–123 Golden Lane, London EC1Y ORT
Tel. 01 229 8941

Founded in 1946. Covers the UK, except for Scotland. Range of activities includes advisory service for professional workers and parents, holidays, residential care in three homes, welfare and counselling via 430 local societies, a trusteeship scheme for orphaned mentally handicapped children, publicity, provision for leisure activities. Residential school for profoundly handicapped children, with research data being collected by the University of Bristol. Full range of publications including books and pamphlets for professional workers and parents, two journals, and an annual report.

The National Society for Phenylketonuria and Allied Disorders
Hon. Sec. B. Talbot, 26 Towngate Grove, Mirfield, Yorks.
Tel. 0924 492873

Founded in 1973 for the medical, educational and social welfare of PKU patients and their families. Advice on diets for children. Conferences. Quarterly magazine called *News and Views*.

The National Society for the Prevention of Cruelty to Children
1 Riding House Street, London W1P 8AA
Tel. 01 580 8812

Founded in 1884. Covers the UK, except for Scotland. Annual case-load over 80 000 children, covered by a reduced inspectorate of 220 social workers, whose names and addresses are listed in the *Social Services Year Book*. Maintains a national advisory centre and seven regional treatment units for the battered child, and a national registry of child abuse cases. Offers advice and support for the whole family. Runs over 70 community and therapeutic playgroups for deprived preschool children. NSPCC Research Papers are obtained from its information service at headquarters.

Norwood, The Welfare Organisation for Jewish Children
315/317 Ballards Lane, London N12 8LH
Tel. 01 446 4271

Complete family casework service with financial and other forms of support.

The Partially Sighted Society
40 Wordsworth Street, Hove, E.Sussex BN3 5BH
Tel. 0273 736053

Founded in 1973 as a pressure group of parents of partially sighted children. Now caters nationally for the partially sighted of all ages. Advisory service on all problems encountered by the partially sighted. Design of aids and equipment, particularly large print books. Local groups. Magazine called *Oculus*. Range of low-cost booklets.

Pre-School Playgroups Association
Alford House, Aveline Street, London SE11 5DH

Founded in 1961. 13 000 groups cater for approximately 500 000 children throughout Britain. Informative magazines entitled *Contact* and *Under 5*, with sensible articles on child health and development and handicap.

The Psoriasis Association
7 Milton Street, Northampton NN2 7JG
Tel. 0604 711129

Founded in 1968. A national organisation with 4000 members in 55 branches for all sufferers from or interested in psoriasis, including children. Supports research. Educational and social activities; pressure group. Journal *Beyond the Ointment* thrice yearly.

Riding for the Disabled Association
National Equestrian Centre, Kenilworth, Warwickshire CV8 2LR
Tel. Coventry 27192

Founded in 1960. Provides safe and free riding for disabled of all ages, organised by 400 groups nationwide. The riders are of all ages, but four-fifths of them are under 18. Their disabilities are almost evenly divided between mental and physical handicap, sometimes quite severe. Trekking and riding holidays are also arranged. Publishes a directory of groups, and an informative annual report.

The Royal National Institute for the Blind
224 Great Portland Street, London W1N 6AA
Tel. 01 388 1266

Founded in 1868. Covers the whole of the UK, concerned with the whole range of care for the blind and partially sighted of all ages. Special provisions for those with additional handicaps, particularly the deaf-blind. Maintains homes and schools. Produces books and trains readers in Braille. Talking book service. Promotes research. Monitors legislation. Advisory service for parents. Family case-work. Information service for professional enquirers. Wide range of literature available.

The Royal National Institute for the Deaf
105 Gower Street, London WC1E 6AH
Tel. 01 387 8033

Founded in 1911. Wide range of services for deaf and hard-of-hearing of all ages. Social casework. Provides special aids, including a children's hearing-aid harness. Maintains Larchmoor School at Slough for maladjusted deaf and partially hearing children. Comprehensive library and information service. Maintains register of British organisations in the field of deafness. Publications include journals and annual report.

The Royal Scottish Society for the Prevention of Cruelty to Children
16 Melville Street, Edinburgh EH3 7PB
Tel. 031 225 5377/2912

Run on similar lines to the NSPCC. Names and addresses of local officers are listed in the *Social Services Year Book.*

The Royal Society for the Prevention of Accidents
Cannon House, The Priory, Queensway, Birmingham B4 6BS

18 000 Tufty Clubs throughout the country teach children aged three to eight years the principles of home, road, and water safety.

The Salvation Army
International Headquarters, 101 Queen Victoria Street, London EC4P 4EP
Tel. 01 236 7020
Scottish Headquarters, Houldsworth Street, Glasgow G3 8DU
Tel. 041 221 3378

Founded in 1865; work with young people officially established in 1880. An evangelical Christian organisation, whose work with children is particularly concerned with those suffering from various forms of neglect and deprivation. Maintains 17 homes for 445 children in the UK. Publishes a directory of its social services in the British Isles and Eire.

The Save the Children Fund
157 Clapham Road, London SW9 OPT
Tel. 01 582 1414

Founded in 1919. A large independent voluntary organisation, working internationally in the field of child care. In 1974 about one quarter of its total expenditure was for projects within the UK. Runs homes, clubs and playgroups, with emphasis on deprived children rather than the handicapped. Play advisers visit children in hospital. Its versatility enables concentration of effort where the need is greatest; in recent years there has been considerable expansion of activities in Northern Ireland.

The Scottish Council for Spastics
22 Corstorphine Road, Edinburgh EH12 6HP
Tel. 031 337 2804/2616

Founded in 1946 for spastics of all ages. Maintains three special schools for 190 pupils. Physiotherapists visit homes and schools. Team of ten social workers. Speech and occupational therapy. Day centres, and a nursery unit. Publishes annual report.

The Scottish Federation for the Welfare of the Blind
39 St. Andrew's Street, Dundee, Scotland
Tel. 0382 27101

Founded in 1917. The federation of voluntary organisations and local authorities concerned with the welfare of the blind in Scotland. Activities include coordination of work of individual societies, provision of information, summer school for teachers, examination of legislation. Maintains list of useful addresses.

The Scottish Society for the Mentally Handicapped
69 West Regent Street, Glasgow G2 2AN
Tel. 041 331 1551

Founded in 1954. Aims, objects and activities similar to those of the National Society. Sixty two branches provide a meeting point for parents. Day care centres for preschool and severely handciapped children. Two short-stay homes for the care of such children while their families have a break, or in emergencies. Caravan holidays for the families. Research, books, films and a quarterly newsletter.

The Scottish Spina Bifida Association
190 Queensferry Road, Edinburgh EH4 2BW

Similar objectives and activities to the London-based association, with which it is affiliated. Publishes two booklets on spina bifida.

The Shaftesbury Society
112 Regency Street, Westminster, London SW1P 4AX
Tel. 01 834 2656

Founded in 1844. An interdenominational Christian society, mainly for London and the Home Counties, but recently extending its activities to the North of England. Maintains five residential schools for 237 severely handicapped children, mainly with spinal disorders, muscular dystrophy, and cerebral palsy. Provides holidays for nearly 500 handicapped and disadvantaged children annually. Other activities described in annual report.

The Society of Compassionate Friends
25 Kingsdown Parade, Bristol BS6 5UE
Tel. Bristol 47316

A small organisation whose National Secretary, Mrs C. Mann, lives at the above address. Help and comfort for parents grieving the loss of their child.

The Spastics Society
12 Park Crescent, London W1N 4EQ
Tel. 01 636 5020
Family Services and Assessment Centre, 16 Fitzroy Square, London W1P 5HQ
Tel. 01 387 9571.

Founded in 1952. Covers England and Wales. A comprehensive service for spastics of all ages includes family support and advice from a team of social workers, grants for special needs, holidays, assessment, education, and research. Maintains altogether 60 establishments throughout Britain, including eight special schools for over 530 children, with an additional four affiliated schools for a further 230 children. Short term care for 43 children at four centres during family crises and holidays. The residential assessment centres in London and Pendlebury are particularly valuable, providing reports for general practitioners. 180 local branches. The society maintains a library and information centre for professional workers, and a wide range of films and publications, including a valuable Guide to Services, and the periodicals *Spastic News* (monthly) and *Special Education* (quarterly) and an annual report. Recently the society has promoted an active 'save a baby' campaign to reduce the incidence of births of spastic babies.

The Thomas Coram Foundation for Children.
40 Brunswick Square, London WC1N 1AZ
Tel. 01 278 2424

Founded in 1739 as the Foundling Hospital, Hatton Gardens. A small voluntary organisation for child care, probably the oldest in England. Activities now include counselling, adoption, fostering, a day service for local preschool children, a toy library, study days and conferences for those concerned with child care, provision of accomodation for child welfare organisations, and the Thomas Coram Research Unit in child development. Publishes an annual report.

The Trust Fund for Training of Handicapped Children in Arts and Crafts
8 Claremont Road, Wallasey, Merseyside L45 6UE

Set up in 1978 by the association of Mouth and Foot Painting Artists, – to promote the art education of handicapped children. Practical and financial help to individuals and groups.

Multiple choice questions

Constructed by Ian Stanley

The following multiple-choice questions consist of an initial statement (or stem) followed by a number of completions (or items) identified by the letters A, B, C, D, E. In each question any number of items may be true or false.

— To assess your knowledge of the factual content of this book attempt to identify every item as true or false.

— An answer key is provided after the questions.

— It is the convention with this type of question that a mark be deducted from your score for each item incorrectly identified.

1. In considering perinatal mortality it is correct to say that:

A. the rate of improvement in the U.K. over the last 10 years is similar to that of Scandinavian countries.

B. neonatal mortality rate measures deaths in the first month of life per 1000 live births.

C. World-wide, deaths in the first week exceed those in the whole of the first year of life.

D. in the U.K. in the last 10 years least improvement has occurred in the crude perinatal mortality rate.

E. post neonatal mortality rates in the U.K. are comparable with those of Scandinavia and Holland.

2. Of young people in care it is true to say that:

A. social services may take a child into care only after a court order has been obtained.

B. parental rights may be assumed by the local authority despite the wishes of the parents once care has continued for 3 months.

C. they must be under 18 years of age.

D. after 6 months in care the parents may be required to give 28 days notice of their intention to remove the child.

E. some will have been removed from home because they have committed a criminal offence.

3. Adoption:

A. may, exceptionally, be undertaken by a single person rather than a married couple.

B. will be formalised in an adoption order only after the child has lived with the adoptive parents for 6 months.

C. applications to a court will be followed by the appointment of a guardian ad litem.

D. requires the permission of both natural parents when the child is illegitimate.

E. is irrevocable once the adoption order is finalised.

4. The training of a health visitor:

A. lasts one year.

B. requires the participant to be a state certified midwife.

C. takes place in a teaching hospital.

D. includes a 3 month period supervising a case load of 100 families.

E. does not include specific training in geriatrics.

5. Social workers:

A. are now attached to about 40 per cent of group practices in the U.K.

B. regard preventive work as their major priority in child welfare.

C. are usually not involved in field conferences.

D. are employed by the Area Health Authority.

E. generally see themselves as replacing voluntary welfare services.

6. Perinatal deaths:

A. are most often due to congenital anomalies.

B. show wide regional variation in incidence in the U.K.

C. are twice as common in social class V as in social class I.

D. are unrelated to the marital status of the mother.

E. are more common in the children of immigrant mothers than in the children of non-immigrants.

7. Smoking in pregnancy is known to increase the risk to the infant of:

A. dysmaturity.

B. perinatal death.

C. a wide range of congenital malformations.

D. neural tube defects.

E. cleft lip and palate.

8. The following maternal conditions are associated with increased risk to the offspring:

A. herpes genitalis.

B. toxoplasmosis.

C. alcohol abuse.

D. treatment with long-acting sulphonamides.

E. D/D genotype.

9. Maternal serum alpha-feto protein levels:

A. are highest at the end of the first trimester of a normal pregnancy.

B. are usually measured between 16 and 18 weeks gestation.

C. are likely to be raised in about 1 per cent of pregnancies.

D. are an appropriate screening test only in those with a family history of neural tube defect.

E. are raised in the presence of intrauterine death of a normal fetus.

10. The fetal heart rate:

A. varies by as much as 15 beats/min in a normal pregnancy.

B. shows persistent acceleration if sparine is administered to the mother.

C. shows 'type I' dips of less than 20 beats/min in normal pregnancy.

D. shows loss of beat-to-beat variation if diazepam is given to the mother.

E. shows 'type II' dips as a response to hypoxia.

11. In considering contraindications to the immunisation of children it is true to say that:

A. Schick testing is a prerequisite to diphtheria immunisation in children over the age of 10 years.

B. allowance should be made for prematurity in the timing of the initial dose of an immunisation programme.

C. the DHSS recommend complete recovery from a respiratory infection before pertussis vaccine is given.

D. any previous evidence of penicillin sensitivity is an absolute contraindication to oral polio vaccine.

E. a strong family history of convulsions is an absolute contraindication to measles vaccination.

12. Routine surveillance of children in the pre-school years:

A. is carried out in practice-based child care clinics in 80 per cent of U.K. general practices.

B. will be facilitated by 'year-books' derived from an age-sex register.

C. will involve a work load of about 500 children in a practice of list size 10 000.

D. is likely to result in a decline of 5–10 per cent in overall practice work load.

E. does not include the monitoring of weight gain in children over one year of age.

13. Ill-treated children ('battered babies'):

A. are more often the first or last born child.

B. are seen equally in all social classes.

C. are more often of low birth weight.

D. are more often adopted children.

E. often have a ruptured frenulum of the tongue.

14. In otitis media:

A. requiring antibiotics, ampicillin is preferable to penicillin V in the child over 5 years of age.

B. vomiting is a recognised presentation of the acute form in infancy.

C. with signs of glue ear, spontaneous resolution is unlikely.

D. of the chronic serous form, the insertion of grommets will preclude swimming.

E. in children most acute perforations heal rapidly.

15. In the diagnosis and management of respiratory tract infection in childhood it is correct to say that:

A. indrawing of the alae nasi is characteristic of nasal obstruction due to upper respiratory tract infection.

B. acute epiglottitis is commonest in the first year of life.

C. a previous history of otitis media is a recognised indication for the prescription of antibiotics in coryza.

D. para-influenza viruses have a special propensity for causing croup.

E. characteristically bronchiolitis is accompanied by high fever.

16. In influenzal infection in childhood:

A. pain on eye movement is a well recognised symptom.

B. the clinical attack rate is likely to be only half of the true attack rate.

C. influenza A is twice as common as influenza B as a cause of school epidemics.

D. acute polyneuritis is a recognised complication of influenza B infection in those over the age of ten years.

E. an increased incidence of streptococcal infection is a recognised sequel.

17. In the differential diagnosis of the acute exanthemata of childhood:

A. babies born to mothers who have been actively immunised against measles in childhood, inherit substantial passive immunity.

B. the incubation period of measles is 14 days.

C. desquamation is not seen following the rash of measles.

D. many types of virus infection mimic rubella.

E. second attacks of chicken pox in childhood do not occur.

18. In Scarlet fever:

A. a throat infection by an erythrogenic strain of streptococcus is a prerequisite.

B. typically the rash begins on the neck.

C. erythema maginatum is a recognised sequel.

D. pre-school children are seldom affected.

E. characteristically desquamation spares the hands and feet.

19. Infection by herpes simplex virus:

A. is the commonest identified cause of conjunctivitis in infants in the U.K.

B. has an incidence related to social class.

C. is a recognised cause of gingivostomatitis.

D. is a recognised cause of napkin rash.

E. due to HSV2 is a recognised cause of perinatal death.

20. The following statements about viral infections in childhood are correct:

A. mumps is infectious for one week before and two weeks after the onset of glandular swelling.

B. a common complication of glandular fever in childhood is a coexistent streptococcal throat infection.

C. hepatitis A infection has a peak incidence in springtime.

D. rotavirus infections are uncommon after the age of 6 years.

E. rotavirus infections cause upper respiratory tract signs in the early stages.

21. In the differential diagnosis of the acute abdomen in childhood:

A. foetor oris is a recognised sign of acute appendicitis.

B. an inflamed retrocaecal appendix will be accompanied by tenderness on rectal examination.

C. constipation is usual in mesenteric adenitis.

D. intussusception is twice as common in girls as in boys.

E. characteristically a sausage-shaped swelling is found in intussusception.

22. Of accidents and poisoning in childhood it is true to say that:

A. they are now the commonest cause of death.

B. tricyclic antidepressants are now the commonest cause of death from medicinal substances.

C. tetanus is a recognised risk to injured children aged 9–12 years who have had full routine immunisation.

D. poisoning is a recognised form of child abuse.

E. the rate of accidental death in the U.K. is the lowest of 27 European countries.

23. The Moro reflex:

A. if unilateral suggests a fractured clavicle on the immobile side.

B. is elicited by sharp lowering of the head 2–3 inches from the horizontal plane.

C. is depressed or abolished by sedative drugs.

D. is increased in the presence of brain damage.

E. consists of a symmetrical embracing movement.

24. Neonatal convulsions:

A. are effectively controlled by rectal diazepam.

B. occurring at the end of the first week in breast fed babies suggest hypocalcaemia.

C. occurring 48 hours or more after birth are a recognised sign of meningitis.

D. due to hypoglycaemia are more common in the baby 'light for dates'.

E. usually conform to the classical grand mal pattern.

25. In assessing maturity of the newborn it is correct to say that:

A. the term premature has now been abandoned.

B. ten per cent of normal infants are 'light for dates'.

C. pre-term infants are of 28–36 weeks gestation.

D. dysmature infants may be 'heavy for dates'.

E. a post term infant with birth weight between 10th and 90th percentile may be 'normal for dates'.

26. Recognised causes of a 'light for dates' infant include:

A. increased maternal urinary oestriol excretion during pregnancy.

B. toxoplasmosis.

C. maternal cigarette smoking.

D. maternal diabetes mellitus.

E. social class.

27. In breast feeding:

A. the let-down reflex is inhibited by emotional tension.

B. the rooting reflex is not essential.

C. prior induction of labour is associated with a high rate of successful breast feeding.

D. stilboestrol (5 mg a day for 1–2 days) is a safe and effective remedy for severe breast engorgement.

E. the requirements of the infant for iron are adequately provided for.

28. Threadworms:

A. are most common in pre-school children.

B. are more common in girls than in boys.

C. are readily diagnosed by inspection of the faeces for adult worms.

D. produce ova which when shed remain viable for up to 3 weeks.

E. treated with piperazine will usually result in the patient being constipated for a day or two.

29. Head lice:

A. are a recognised cause of enlarged occipital lymph nodes.

B. are typically very numerous in the scalp of an infested child.

C. are reliably killed by gamma benzene hexachloride.

D. in a child are an indication for treatment of the whole family.

E. treated with malathion will need the subsequent removal of nits with a Sacher comb.

30. The following statements about childhood skin conditions are correct:

A. guttate psoriasis is a recognised sequel to an upper respiratory tract infection.

B. the herald patch of pityriasis rosea shows characteristic collarette scales.

C. granuloma annulare requires no treatment.

D. pseudominia is an early sign of atopic eczema.

E. plantar warts are no longer infectious after one week's treatment with nightly soaks in 3 per cent formalin solution.

31. Of the orthopaedic disorders of childhood it is correct to say that:

A. chondromalacia patellae typically causes pain on climbing stairs.

B. a permanently enlarged tibial tubercle may result from Osgood-Schlatters disease.

C. slipped upper femoral epiphysis is commonest in thin underweight boys between 12 and 15 years of age.

D. knock-knee is usually a normal variant which corrects itself by the age of seven years.

E. flat foot may be the result of femoral or tibial torsion.

32. Urinary infection in childhood:

A. has an incidence related to social class.

B. is associated with enuresis more commonly in girls than in boys.

C. where associated with vesicoureteric reflux is likely to be a famililal problem.

D. is due to E coli more commonly in boys than in girls.

E. is not accompanied by pyuria in about one case in three.

33. Anaemia in childhood:

A. is a characteristic feature of Henoch-Schonlein purpura.

B. due to folic acid deficiency is a recognised complication of fibrocystic disease.

C. is a typical presenting feature of leukaemia.

D. due to spherocytosis is invariably accompanied by a high reticulocyte count.

E. is a characteristic finding in sickle-cell trait.

34. Dental caries:

A. affects 97% of children in the U.K. by the age of 15 years.

B. progresses faster in permanent teeth than in primary teeth.

C. is as effectively prevented by fluoride toothpaste as by fluoridation of drinking water.

D. is a recognised hazard of long term medicinal syrups.

E. is defined as rampant where the primary dentition is affected before eruption.

35. In the aetiology and management of asthma in childhood:

A. atopy is defined as a constitutional liability to develop type I hypersensitivity.

B. monozygotic twins show complete concordance for asthma.

C. the extrinsic type is less amenable to treatment than the intrinsic type.

D. cycling is a form of exercise less likely to provoke asthma than running or jumping.

E. corticosteroid aerosols are seldom effective as initial treatment.

36. Deafness in childhood:

A. is suggested by excessive monotonous crying by an infant.

B. when unilateral and mild (20 to 30 db evenly distributed over speech frequencies) will cause some difficulty in speech discrimination.

C. is of little importance to the development of the child during the first year of life.

D. is present to some extent in 20% of primary school entrants.

E. is readily excluded in infants and toddlers by the use of a pure-tone audiometer.

37. In childhood, visual disorders:

A. due to refractive errors are well established by school entry.

B. due to hypermetropia predispose to squint.

C. of colour perception are twice as common in males as in females.

D. due to alternating squint will not be detected by the cover test.

E. due to vertical squint are typically accompanied by head tilt.

38. Epilepsy in childhood:

A. causing status epilepticus is most commonly due to the abrupt withdrawal of anticonvulsant therapy.

B. of the Rolandic type characteristically improves in the second decade of life.

C. of the petit mal type usually ceases in adolescence.

D. with incomplete seizure control is an absolute contraindication to swimming.

E. provoked by television viewing is best managed without anticonvulsant drugs.

39. The following disorders may be reliably predicted in the offspring following examination of the amniotic fluid:

A. galactosaemia.

B. Down's syndrome due to translocation.

C. Nieman Pick's disease.

D. club foot.

E. respiratory distress syndrome.

40. Immigrant children in the U.K.:

A. are more commonly bottle-fed than the children of British mothers.

B. of West Indian ancestory are over represented among those taken into care.

C. are commonly found to be harbouring hookworm (ankylostoma).

D. of Asian origin tend to develop signs of rickets before weaning.

E. of West Indian parents have an increased liability to develop atopic conditions.

MCQ ANSWER KEY

Q	1	2	3	4	5	6	7	8	9	10
A	T	F	T	T	F	T	T	T	T	T
B	T	F	F	F	T	T	T	T	T	T
C	T	T	T	F	F	T	F	T	T	T
D	F	T	F	T	F	F	F	T	F	T
E	F	T	T	F	F	T	T	F	T	T

Q	11	12	13	14	15	16	17	18	19	20
A	T	F	T	F	F	T	F	F	T	T
B	T	T	F	T	F	T	F	F	T	T
C	T	T	T	F	T	T	F	T	T	F
D	F	T	F	T	T	F	T	T	T	T
E	F	F	T	T	F	T	T	F	T	T

Q	21	22	23	24	25	26	27	28	29	30
A	T	T	T	T	T	F	T	F	T	T
B	F	T	T	F	T	T	F	T	F	T
C	F	T	T	T	T	T	F	F	F	T
D	F	T	F	T	T	F	T	T	T	F
E	F	T	T	F	T	T	F	F	F	T

Q	31	32	33	34	35	36	37	38	39	40
A	T	F	F	T	T	T	F	T	T	F
B	T	T	T	F	F	T	T	T	T	T
C	F	T	T	F	F	F	F	T	T	F
D	T	F	F	T	T	T	F	F	T	F
E	T	T	F	F	T	F	T	T	T	T

Index

abdomen, acute, 174–80
abdominal distension, 230
  pain, 47
abortion, 79, 126
  following amniocentesis, 80
  habitual, 77
  missed, 81
  selective, 72
abruptio placentae, 79, *and see* placenta
absence seizures, 312
accessibility, 122
accident and emergency departments, 105, 109, 121
accidents, 14, 181–191, 353, 376, 386
  home, 181–2, 349
  prevention, 127–8, 188–9, 394
  proneness, 47
  road, 181–2, 349
acetazolamide, 319
achondroplasia, 76
acidosis, 315, *and see* ketoacidosis, lactic acidosis
acne vulgaris, 218
Actifed, 134
activity centres, 32
Acts of Parliament, *see*
  Affiliation Proceedings Act 1957
  Bail Act 1976
  Births and Deaths Registration Act 1926
  Child Care Act 1980
  Children Act 1975
  Children and Young Persons Acts 1933, 1969
  Consumer Protection Acts 1961, 1978
  Domestic Proceedings and Magistrates' Courts Act 1979
  Education Act 1944
  Employment of Children Act 1973
  Explosives (Age of Purchasing) Act 1929
  Family Law Reform Act 1969
  Guardianship Acts 1971 to 1973
  Health Services and Public Health Act 1968
  Hypnotism Act 1952
  Indecency with Children Act 1960
  Infant Life (Preservation) Act 1929
  Law Reform (Miscellaneous Provisions) (Scotland) Act 1968
  Legitimacy Act 1959
  Maternity and Child Welfare Act 1918
  Matrimonial Causes Act 1973
  Mental Health Act 1959
  Nurseries and Child Minders Act 1948
  Sexual Offences Act 1956
  Tatooing of Minors Act 1969
  Vaccine Damage Payments Act 1979
adhesions, abdominal, 177
adenitis, *see* lymphadenitis
adenoidal hypertrophy, 132, 134, 136–7
adenoidectomy, 133, 135–6
adenotonsillectomy, 46, 137, *and see* tonsillectomy
adenoviruses, 140, 144, 148, 171, 175
admission
  children's home, 123
  hospital, 11, 20, 23, 25, 58, 123, 125, 157, 184
Admune, 149
adolescence, 378
adoption orders, 29, 38–9
  societies, 37–8, 393
adrenalin, 95, 281–2
adrenoreceptor stimulants, 291–2
affiliation orders, 38
Affiliation Proceedings Act 1957, 38
Africa, 244, 375
  Central, 213
  East, 369, 375
  West, 375
African Commonwealth, 377
age-sex register, 20–2, 45, 53, 55, 58, 105–7
agranulocytosis, 318
Aicardi syndrome, 313
airflow obstruction, 141–2, 284–7, 290–4, 311
airway, 186, 188, 199
alarm bed, 359
albinism, 331
albuminuric purpura, 248
alcohol, 128–30, 183
  legislation, 34
  maternal, 77, *and see* fetal alcohol syndrome
alcoholism, 310, 380–2
Alcopar, 214
alkaline phosphatase, 81
alkalosis, 276, 312
allergic purpura, 247–8
allergy, 14, 94, 136, 283, 285–6, 288, 349
  milk, 60
alphafetoprotein, 81–3
allopurinol, 276–7
alopecia, 262, 373
amantadine, 149
ambidexterity, 367
amelogenesis imperfecta, 251
America, North, 214, 278
  South, 213, *and see* USA
aminophylline, 291–2, 295
aminotransferase, 164
amitryptyline, 359
amnesia, retrograde, 312
amniotic fluid, bilirubin, 81
  creatinine, 81
  estimation, 80–1
  lecethin-sphingomyelin ratio, 81
  urea, 81
amniocentesis, 80–3, 203, 339, 375
amoebic dysentery, 375
amoxycillin, 50, 144, 233, 259
amphetamine, 359
ampicillin, 82, 133, 135, 144, 153, 162, 170, 199, 206, 256, 258–259, 262
amputation, digits, 86
  fingertips, 185
anaemia, 14, 60, 79, 133, 181
  aplastic, 236, 245, 247
  dyshaemopoeitic, 238
  folic acid deficiency, 239–40
  haemolytic, 238, 243–4, 375
  hypochromic, 278
  hypoplastic, 238
  in leukaemia, 240–1
  iron deficiency, 238–9, 372, 376
  macrocytic, 236, 240
  megaloblastic, 239, 265, 318
  microcytic, 236
  normochromic, 288
  nutritional, 238, *and see* blood
analgesics, 88–9, 167, 184, 206, 244, 258
anaphylactoid purpura, 247–8, 279
ancillary staff, *see* practice
androgenic steroids, 77
anencephaly, 73–4, 76, 81, 334
angina, 275

angiocardiography, 274
angioma, 225
ankylosing spondylitis, 280–1
Ankylostoma duodenale, 213–4, 375
anorexia, 133, 354
anoxia, 73, 195, 198, 309, 311, 315
antenatal care, 8, 58–9, 67–8, 72–83, 87, 234, 334
  clinics, 42, 79, 82–3
ante partum haemorrhage, *see* haemorrhage
antibiotics, 45, 49–50, 94, 98, 132–5, 140–1, 143, 153, 155, 161–2, 167, 170–1, 199, 206, 222, 228, 233–4, 241, 244, 248, 256–7, 258, 274, 277, 279, 292–3, 310
anticholinergic drugs, 143, 290
anticoagulants, 77
anticonvulsants, 94, 236, 239, 255, 311, 315–9
antidepressants, 359, 384
  tricyclic, 47, 187, 258, 359
antidiarrhoeals, 258
antiemetics, 387
antigenic drift, 146
  shift, 146
antihistamines, 134, 136, 164, 220, 258, 262, 279, 304
antimalarials, 280
antinuclear factor, 280, 282
antistreptolysin O titre, 247, 278, 280
antithyroid drugs, 77
anxiety, 106, 333, 352, 354, 367, 378, 380–2, 384
aortic aneurysm, 174
  regurgitation, 256
  stenosis, 268–9, 272–3
  valve replacement, 273
Apgar score, 88, 195, 334
aphonia, 186
apnoeia, 310, 350, 390
appendicitis, 147, 175, 212, 351, 377
  acute, 152, 174, 176–7
appointments, 22–3
Arabia 374–5, *and see* Saudi Arabia
area health authority *see* local authority
arithmetic attainment, 351–2
arthralgia, 153
arthritis, 278, 394
  rheumatoid, 278
  suppurative, 228, 278, 280
  tuberculous, 278, 280, *and see* haemophilia
arthropathy, influenzal, 147
Arthus reaction, 96
artificial respiration, 186
  rupture of membranes, 86
Ascaris lumbricoides, 212–3
Aschoff nodes, 278
Asia, South East, 213
Asian communities, 68, 269–72, 375–8
aspariginase, 241
asphyxia, 142, 185, 305, 350
  neonatal, 196
aspirin, 34, 149, 151, 187, 246, 259, 262, 278, 387
  poisoning, 188

assessment centres, 365
asthma, 14, 17, 23, 25, 46, 95, 138, 141–4, 147–8, 219, 283–96, 316, 349, 376, 395–6
astigmatism, 327–8
ataxia, 167, 262, 318
atelectasis, 79
atopy, 287–8
atrial septal defect, 256, 268–9, 272
at risk registers, 35, 56, 122, 124–5, 177, 322, 332, 390
atropine methonitrate, 143
attachment schemes, 57
attendance centres, 31–2
audit, peer, 24–6
audiometry, 22, 56, 116–7, 132–3, 135, 267, 323–5
aureomycin, 134
  ointment, 219, 222
Australia, 4
autism, 365, 397–8
automatism, 310
autoimmune diabetes, 299
azathioprine, 282
azotaemia, 248

baby sitters, 34
bacterial endocarditis, 247, 273
bacteriological specimens, 132
bacteriuria, 46, 230–1
Bail Act 1976, 31
balanitis, 300
Balham, London, 395
Bangladesh, 369–71, 377
barbiturates, 187, 259, 317–8
Batley, Yorkshire, 68
battered babies, *see* child abuse
BCG, *see* tuberculosis immunisation
Beconase spray, 136
bedsores, 387
bedwetting, *see* enuresis
begging, 34
behaviour disorders, 14, 30, 32, 60, 352, 354–60, 377, 382
behavioural development, 113
Belfast, 396
Belgium, 4, 17–18
Belize, 371
belladonna, 359
benzoic acid, 287
benzyl benzoate, 216
bephenium hydroxynaphthoate, 214
bereavement, *see* mourning
Berkshire, 8, 58, 83
bicuspid aortic valve, 256, 272–3
biguanidines, 301
bilirubin, 260 *and see* plasma
binding over, 32
biparietal skull diameter, 81, 203
Birmingham, 96, 159, 167, 213, 378, 394
birth certificate, 38–40
  complications, 20
  trauma, 73, 86–90, 198
  weight, 7, 197–8, *and see* low birth weight

Births and Deaths Registration Act 1926, 39
Blalock shunt, 256, 267, 273
bleeding time, 247
blindness, 385, 397, *and see* visual disorders
blood blast cells, 241
  culture, 228
  disorders, 234–249
  dyscrasias, 318
  eosinophilia, 211, 214
  factor VIII, 245–6
    IX, 245–6
  granulocytes, 236
  group, ABO, 79
  grouping, 82
  haematocrit, 237–8
  haemoglobin, 236–9, 245
  leucocytes, 136, 236
  lymphocytes, 236
  MCH, 237–9
  MCHC, 237, 239
  MCV, 237, 239
  neutropaenia, 241
  normal values, 237
  occult, faecal, 238
  platelets, 239–41, 247, 279
  red cell count, 237–8
    fragility, 244
  reticulocytes, 237
    response, 240
  reticulocytosis, 343
  sickle cell disease, 238–9, 244–5, 281, 375
    trait, 244
  spherocytosis, 238, 243–4
  sugar, 209, 305
  thalassaemia, 238, 243–5, 375
    trait, 375
  thrombocytopaenia, 241, *and see* platelets
  transfusion, 33, 183, 241, 244–5, 375
    exchange, 377
    incompatible, 79
  volume, 236, *and see* haemoglobin, plasma, serum
boils, 218
bonding, 59, 65
bone marrow depression, 265
  examination, 240
  in leukaemia, 240–1
  transplant, 241
Bordetella pertussis, 139–40, 143
Borstals, 31–3
bottle feeding *see* feeding
bow legs, 226
boxing, 191
brachial plexus injury, 86
Bradford, 8, 378
braille, 399
brain damage, 350, *and see* birth trauma
brandy, 127
breast engorgement, 206
breath holding attacks, 355–6
breathing exercises, 137
breech delivery, 79, 81, 89, 225, 348
Briggs report, 57

Bristol, 191, 398
British births survey, 202
British Honduras, 371
bronchiectasis, 140, 143, 284, 289, 291–2
bronchiolitis, 14, 141, 143–4, 287
bronchitis, 14, 46, 138–142, 147–9, 277, 283–96, 349–50, 395
bronchodilators, 258, 288–90, 293–7
  aerosols, 286, 291
bronchopneumonia, 143, 274, 309, 376
bronchospasm, 46, 213, 270, 286, *and see* asthma, wheezy bronchitis
brucellosis, 148
bruises, 121
Buckinghamshire, 7–8, 57
Bulgaria, 4
bullying, 360
buphthalmos, 330–1
burns, 34, 120–1, 174, 183–4, 243, 376
Buscopan, 359
Byelorussia, 14

Caesarian section, 79, 87, 158
calamine lotion, 155, 220
Calderdale, 8
calories, 351
Cambridgeshire, 394
Canada, 19
cancer, 14, 386–7, 396
  cervical, 333
candida albicans, 220
caput succedaneum, 86
carbamazepine, 262, 316, 318
carbaryl, 215
carbohydrate metabolism, 317
  in diabetes, 301
carbon dioxide, snow and slush, 220–1
  monoxide, *see* poisoning
carboxyhaemoglobin, 76
carbuncles, 218, 375
card reader, 53
cardiac, *see* heart
cardiomegaly, 278
cardiopulmonary bypass, 269, 273
cardiotocography, 81, 87–8
Cardiff, 381
care order, 31–2, 64
  proceedings, 30, 33, 35–6
caries, dental, 254–5
Carylderm, 215
case conferences, 35, 67, 124
Castellani's paint, 221
casualty officers, 183
cataracts, 329, 331
  congenital, 78, 327, 330
  diabetic, 305
catarrh, 45, 136–7, 152
Catford, London, 70
catheterisation, 232
cauterisation, 232
cellulitis, 218, 257
Cendehill strain of rubella virus, 99
central nervous system congenital disorders, 73
  diseases, 14
  in leukaemia, 241
  malformations, 74, 82–3
cephalexin, 259
cephalhaematoma, 86
cephaloridine, 256, 274
cephalosporins, 156
cereals, 59
cerebral calcification, 78
  dysfunction, 308
  dysrhythmia, 313
  oedema, 87, 199
  palsy, 86–7, 109, 321–2, 336, 350, 365, 385, 396, 400, *and see* spasticity
  tumour, 331
cerebrovascular accidents, 79
cervical dilatation in labour, 88–9
Channel Islands, 371, *and see* Jersey
chappatis, 376
Cheshire, 394
chicken pox, *see* varicella
chilblains, 376
child abuse, 27, 29, 33–5, 38, 49, 56, 61, 67, 85, 105, 109, 120–6, 188, 310, 331, 349, 366, 382, 398–9
  register, 35
Child Care Act 1980, 36
child destruction, 33
  development clinics, 48, 330, 354
  guidance, 116, 396
  health clinics, 23, 26, 60, 72, 101–110, 323, 352
  minders, 37, 365
  morbidity rates, 27
  mortality rates, 12–13, 27
  proof containers, 34, 187, 263
  psychiatry, 23–6, 102, 116–9
Children Act 1975, 37–8
Children and Young Persons Act 1933, 33–5
  1969, 30, 35
Children Committee, 8, 12, 16, 99, 109, 202
children of the family, 39
children's homes, 35–6
China, 214, 272, 275
chiropody, 116, 129, 348
Chlamydia psittaci, 139
choking, 184
cholecystitis, 174–5, 179
cholestasis, 163
cholesteatoma, 134
chondromalacia retropatellae, 226
chorea, Huntingdon's, 310
  rheumatic, 279
chorioretinitis, 78
chloral, 357
chloramphenicol, 199, 236, 238, 262
chlorhexidine, 136
chlorpheniramine, 136
chlorpromazine, 243, 337
chlorthiazole, 276
Chlostridium welchii, 243
Christmas disease, 245–6
chromosome anomalies, 76–7, 81, 268–9
circulatory defects, congenital, 73
claw foot, 227
cleft palate, 76, 194, 196, 316, 334, 380
cling film, 184
clinical trials, 49–50
clonazepam, 317
clotting factors, 316
  mechanism, 77
cloxacillin, *see* flucloxacillin
club foot, 80, 217
clubbing of fingers, 273
clumsiness, 101, 350
coagulation time, 247
coal tar, 219, 223
coarctation of aorta, 256, 268–70, 272–3, 316
cocaine, 387
coeliac disease, 239, 395
coloboma, 330
colour blindness, 329
Coltapaste, 219
coma, 167
Committee on Safety of Medicines, 95
common cold, *see* coryza
communication, 106, 130
  disorders, 365–7
  practice, 122–3
  problems, 48
  skills, 112
community child health services, 33, 328
  handicap team, 349
  physician, 26, 102–3, 107, 113, 125, 156, 215, 320, 323
  and see local authority
complement fixation, 139, 143
compliance, parental, 9
computers, 20, 23, 53–6
conditional discharge, 31–2
confidentiality, 34, 54, 124
congenital deafness, 322–3
  defects, 14, 20, 72–3, 76, 78, 87, 194, 202
    viral, 78
  dislocation of hip, 196, 225, 333–4, 338
  heart disease, 14, 72–3, 78, 148, 199, 267–78, 334
conjunctival pallor, 238
conjunctivitis, 14, 151–2
  herpetic, 158–9
constipation, 14, 174, 176–8, 351, 354–5
Consumer Protection Act 1961, 34
  1978, 189
conurbations, 25, 73
convulsions, 12, 78, 101, 143, 147, 167, 171, 198–9, 212, 230, 308–11
  febrile, 48, 149, 151, 312–5, 319
  jacknife, 312
  neonatal, 94
  vaccine, 97–8
Cooley's anaemia, 244
coordination, 112
coronary heart disease, 209
  thrombosis, 275
corticosteroids, 95, 153, 208, 241, 247–8, 258, 278–82, 286, 290–3, 295, 330, *and see* hydrocortisone, prednisolone
coryza, 140–2, 153

cot death, 27, *and see* death
cotrimoxazole, 50, 233, 263
cough, 132, 142
  in influenza, 147
  linctuses, 258
  paroxysmal, 143
  persistent, 140
  suppressants, 142, 261
County Court, 39
Court Report, 34, 17–8, 20, 26–7, 41–2, 44–5, 49, 58, 92, 101–2, 106, 109, 111, 115, 119
Courts, *see* County, Crown, High, Juvenile, Magistrates, Sheriff
Coxa vara, 226
Coxsackie B virus, 154, 165–6, 168, 269, 299
craniopharyngioma, 329
cretinism, 198, 238
cri du chat syndrome, 269
cricothyroidotomy, 184
criminal law, 30–5
  proceedings, 31
  responsibility, 30–1
cromoglycate, sodium, 136, 290, 293–5
croup, 140–2
Crown Court, 30–3
cryoprecipitate, 246
crystalluria, 319
sulthiame, 318
curly fingers, 228
Cushingoid facies, 265, 280
custodianship order, 38–9
cyanocobalamine, *see* vitamin B12
cyanosis, 140, 142, 184, 186, 230, 275, 277
  central, 196
  in neonates, 198–9
cyanotic attacks, 79
  heart disease, 203, 264–71, 273
cyclophosphamide, 262
Cypriots, Greek, 375
  Turkish, 375
Cyprus, 37, 369, 371–2
cystic fibrosis, 161, 284–5, 289, 349, 395
cystitis, 231, 234
cystoscopy, 233
cytomegalic inclusion disease, 82, 198
cytomegalovirus, 78, 161, 309
cytotoxic drugs, 77, 95, 236, 241, 249, 262
Czechoslovakia, 9

dander, 288
day nurseries, 37, 384
DCH examination, 44, 115
DDT, 215
deafness, 78, 106, 109–110, 112, 117, 129–134, 137, 322–6, 333–4, 349, 365, 385, 393, 398–9
  congenital, 350
  following mumps, 160
  nerve, 323
death, 10, 183–4, 353, 356, 386–91, 395–6
  accidental, 181–2
  register, 20
  see also cot death, mortality
Debendox, 77
decongestants, nasal, 142
defibrillation, 274
dehydration, 12, 170, 174, 197, 207, 310
  neonatal, 198
delinquency, 352, 364
  in immigrants, 378
delirium, 313
dendritic ulcers, 158
Denmark, 4–6, 17–8, 316
dental care, 129
  caries, 252–4, 349
  defects, 250–1
  development, 250–2
  discolouration, 251
  extraction, 274
  hypocalcification, 251
  hypomineralisation, 251
  hypoplasia, 251
  malocclusion, 253
  and see teeth
dentition, 251–3
depression, 106, 378, 382, 384
  post influenzal, 147
  puerperal, 120
deprivation, 121, 129
deputising services, 9–12, 25
Derbac, 215–6
dermatomyositis, 281
desensitisation, 136, 390
desquamation in scarlet fever, 155
detention centres, 31–2
  order, 31
developmental assessment, 42, 117, 267
  milestones, 252
  paediatrician, 324–5
  surveillance, 11, 20, 27, 48, 53, 60, 92, 101, 107, 111, 115, 349, 363, 373
    first year, 105–110
    pre-school, 111–113
    and see screening
  warning signals, 334
dexamethazone, 316
dextropropoxyphene, 246
dextrose, 171, 305
Dextrostix, 304, 365
DF 118, 246
diabetes mellitus, 14, 16, 73, 79, 83, 148, 164, 202, 208, 246, 299–306, 309, 316–7, 333, 349, 369, 377, 393–4
  following mumps, 160
diamorphine, *see* heroin
diaphragmatic hernia, 270
diarrhoea, 12, 14, 49, 94, 170–1, 174, 357
Diastix, 304
diazepam, 88–9, 180, 197, 199, 259–60, 315, 317, 358–9, 387
dichloralphenazone, 357
Dickens, Charles, 6, 9, 12, 18
digestive disorders, congenital, 73
digoxin, 259–60, 273–4, 276–7, 279
dihydrocodein, 246
dimethyl sulphoxide, 159
dioctyl sodium sulphosuccinate, 358
Dioralyte, 171
diphenoxylate, *see* Lomotil
diphtheria, 14, 34, 91, 93, 135
  immunisation, 94–7
  toxoid, 241
dipslides, 46–7, 233
disability, *see* handicap
discotheques, 313, 326
disinfectants, 151
disodium cromoglycate, *see* cromoglycate
disproportion, 73, 79
disseminated lupus erythematosus, 282
district nurse, *see* nurse
diuretics, 277, 279
diverticula, vesical, 233
diving, 133–4, 189
divorce, 39
dog bites, 190
Doloxene, 246
Domestic Proceedings and Magistrates' Courts Act 1978, 38
domiciliary confinement, 9, 79–80, 89–90
Dorset, 394
Down's syndrome, 73, 76–7, 82–3, 196, 240, 255, 257, 268, 330–1, 334, 339, 380, 385, 395
drooling, 252, 311
drowning, 181, 185
drowsiness, 12
drug absorption, 259
  abuse, 128, 131
  compliance, 263
  distribution, 259
  dosage, 261, 276
  excretion, 260–1
  in pregnancy, 56
  metabolism, 259–60, 315
ductus arteriosus, 316
Dulcolax suppositories, 178
dummies, 252
duodenal ulcer, 355
dwarfism, 231
dysentery, 168
dyslexia, 366, 394, 396
dysmaturity, 76, 87, 89, 202, 309, 334
dysphagia, 238
dystonia, 262
dysuria, 231–2

ear, nose and throat disorders, 117, 132–137
  syringing, 134–5, *and see* deafness
earache, 133–4
earrings, 189
East Anglia, 7, 13, 74, 213
East Midlands, 7
ecchymoses, 246–7
Echo viruses, 154, 165–8
eclampsia, 79
ectopic pregnancy, 174
  ureteric orifice, 233

eczema, 14, 95, 158–9, 218, 276, 397
  atopic, 219, 222
  infantile, 219
  nummular, 222–3
  of pinna, 134
  seborrhoeic, 219
  vaccination, 155
Edinburgh, 213
Education Act 1944, 117
education welfare officer, 23, 36
educational psychology, 60, 116–8, 325, 366
  retardation, 35, 397
    of immigrants, 378
  strain, 260–1
  subnormality, 114, 118
Eire, *see* Ireland, South
Eisenmenger syndrome, 256
electrocardiograph, 199, 278
electrochleograph, 325
electroencephalograph 311, 314, 320, 356
  changes in encephalitis, 152
  recording, 312–3
emergency admissions, *see* admissions
  care, 25
emotional crises, 125–6
  deprivation, 105, 121
  development, 117
  disorders, 120, 396–7
emphysema, 277
Employment Medical Adviser, 329
employment of children, 36–7
emulsifying ointment, 219
empyema, 141, 144, 292
encephalitis, 98, 309, 322, 337
  herpetic, 158–9
  measles, 152–3
  mumps, 160
  rubella, 153
  varicella, 154
  viral, 15–17
encopresis, 47, 355, 357–8
endocardial fibroelastosis, 274
endocarditis, 256, 273–4
endotracheal intubation, 195
England, 3–7, 9, 11–13, 38, 54, 64, 72–5, 78–80, 96, 98, 109, 117, 146–7, 151–4, 157, 162–3, 165–7, 181, 186–7, 214, 250, 252–3, 269, 347–9, 351, 371–2, 374, 377, 393, 395, 398
  Eastern, 7
  Northern, 7, 12–13, 74
  North Western, 7, 73–4
  South Eastern, 7
  South Western, 7, 13, 74
enteric fever, 148
Enterobius vermicularis, *see* threadworms
enterovirus infection, 94, 97, 167
enteroviruses, 140, 165, 168, *and see* Echo virus, Coxsackie virus
Entonox 89, 184
enuresis, 47, 67, 231, 234, 300, 349–50, 352, 354, 358–9, 384
  nocturnal, 376–7, 382
environmental health officer, 61
enzyme defects, 77
  induction, 260
enzymes, liver, 315, *and see* alkaline phosphatase, glucoronyl transferase, glucose-6-phosphate dehydrogenase, and transaminases
eosinophilia, 211, *and see* blood
Epanutin, *see* phenytoin
ependyoma, 312
ephedrine, 359
epidemiology, 23–4, 26–7, 46, 83, 127, 139, 333, 337, 349
  accidents, 181–2
  asthma, 284, 286–7
  congenital heart disease, 267–8
  dental disease, 250
  diabetes mellitus, 299–300
  epilepsy, 308–9
  gastroenteritis, 171
  gingivitis, 255
  infective hepatitis, 162–3
  influenza, 146–7
  poisoning, 186–7
  scabies, 216
  skin disorders, 208
  threadworms, 211–2
  urinary infection, 230
  visual disorders, 331
epidermolysis bullosa dystrophia, 251
epididymo orchitis, 179
epiglottitis, acute, 140, 142, 184
epilepsy, 14, 78, 86, 120, 192, 214, 254–5, 308–320, 331, 359, 394
  flicker, 319
  focal, 318
  grand mal, 199, 310–2, 318–9
  Jacksonian, 311
  myoclonic, 313–4, 318–9
  petit mal, 23, 312, 318–9
  psychomotor, 311–2
  reflex, 314
  Rolandic, 311
  television, 314
  temporal lobe, 311–2, 318, 320
  uncinate, 311–2
epiloia, 308, 310
epiphyses, damage, 182
  distal femoral, 81, 203
  in rickets, 374
  knee, 226
  premature fusion, 280
  slipped, 280
  union, 280
  upper tibial, 203
episiotomy, 88, 90
episode rates, 20
epistaxis, 134
Epstein Barr virus, 156–7, 161, 165, 175
erythema annulare, 280
  infectiosum, 156
  nodosum, 278
  multiforme, 278
erythrogenesis, 243, 245, *and see* blood
erythromycin, 135, 143–4, 156, 250, 256, 259, 278–80
Escherichia coli, 168, 176, 230, 233, 309
ethics, 45, 54
ethnic groups, 68, 238
  variations, 48
ethosuximide, 263, 318–9
Eumydrin, 179
Europe, 4, 17–19, 72, 78, 278
  East, 4–5, 19
  Economic Community, 371
  North 6–7, 212
  West, 4–5, 18–19
eustachian obstruction, 132–4
exanthemata, acute, 151–7, 166–7
Exeter Computer Project, 54–5
exomphalos, 83
expectorants, 142, 258
Explosives (Age of Purchasing) Act 1976, 34
external cephalic version, 79
eye, congenital disorders, 73
  contact, 197
  injuries, 187, *and see* visual disorders

facial asymmetry, 275
Fallot's tetralogy, 256, 268–70, 273, 276
familial acholuric jaundice, 243
family breakdown, 30, 64
  care, 336–7
  counselling, 32
  disorder, 47–8
    in alcoholism, 381
  law, 37–40
  planning, 59, 127, 348
Family Doctor booklets, 128–9
Family Fund, 396
Family Law Reform Act 1969, 34, 38
Far East, 238, 244
fat atrophy, insulin, 303
fara beans, 243
febrile convulsions, *see* convulsions
feeding, 107, 129, 197–8, 254, 373, 376
  advice, 106
  artificial, 310
  baby foods, 59
  bottle, 58, 108, 170, 372, 376
    sterilisation, 171
  breast, 58–60, 106, 128, 287
  demand, 207
  infant, 59–60, 195, 205–6, 238
  overfeeding, 208
  problems, 47, 335–6, 362
  prop, 59
femoral pulses, 196, 271
ferrous sulphate, 239, *and see* iron
fertility, 79
fetal alcohol syndrome, 77, 380
  blood, acid-base balance, 81
  growth retardation, 81
  heart rate, 81, 87–9
  maturity tests, 80–1
  scalp blood sampling, 86–8
fetus, 72–83
fetor, 174
fibrocystic disease, 239
fines, 32
finger clubbing, 271
  sucking, 228

Finland, 3
fireworks, 189
  legislation, 34
first aid, 127, 130, 394, *and see* drowning
fish bones, 135
fissure sealants, 254–4
fits, *see* convulsions
flat foot, 227
flea powder, 220
floppy valve syndrome, 271
flucloxacillin, 199, 259
flukes, liver, 375
fluoride, 127, 207, 253–5
Fluvirin, 149
flying squad, 80, 89
folate deficiency, 316
folic acid, 205, 238–40, 244–5
  antagonists, 239
  metabolism, 236
fontanelle depression, 171
foot care, *see* chiropody
forceps delivery, 87–90
foreign body in ear, 132–3
  in larynx, 142, 184–5
  in nose, 133, 185
  in throat, 135
formalin, 221
Fortral, 246
foster homes, 37, 395
  parents, 29, 36–7, 39, 397
fractures, 120, 182, 184
  clavicle, 86
  elbow, 184
  greenstick, 183
  humerus, 87
  skull, 87, 184
fragilitas ossium, 183
France, 3–4, 17–19, 348
frenulum, ruptured, 120
Friars Balsam, 206, 220
frusamide, 276
Fuchs-Rosenthal counting chamber, 232
fucidic acid, 134
fungal infections, respiratory, 139
  skin, 218

G6PD deficiency, 375
galactosaemia, 77, 81, 330
galactose-7-phosphate uridylyl transferase, 77
gallstones, 179, 243
gamma benzene hexachloride, 215–6
gastroenteritis, 157, 168–72, 177–8, 206–7, 300, 310, 372
Gateshead, 11
General Household Surveys, 15, 17
general practitioner obstetric units, 9
  paediatrician, 17, 111
genetic counselling, 82, 244–5, 330
genitalia, neonatal, 196
genitourinary defects, congenital, 73
  system, 14
gentamycin, 260
gentian violet, 221
genu valgum, 226
Germany, East, 41
  West, 4, 17–19
gestational age estimation, 203
Gibraltar, 371
gingival hyperplasia, 252, 318
gingivitis, 255
  in leukaemia, 241
gingivostomatitis, 157–9
Glamorgan, 181
glandular fever, 38, 99, 133, 136, 153, 157, 160–2, 175
Glasgow, 15–16, 105, 372
glaucoma, congenital, 330–1
glossitis, atrophic, 238
Glucagon, 305
Glucocheck, 304
glucoronyl transferase, 260
glucose-6-phosphate dehydrogenase, 343
glucose tolerance test, 79
glue ear, 134–5, 323
glycosuria, 147, 304–5
gonococcus, 199
gout, 280
  iatrogenic, 276
grand mal, *see* epilepsy
grandparents, 37
granuloma annulare, 222
grasp reflex, 196–7
Greece, 4, 244
griseofulvin, 316
grommets, 134
growth, 101, 236, 239, 349–61, 375, 380
  charts, 24, 102–3, 113, 203, 208, 351
  hormones, 113, 208
  retardation, 271, 280–1, 393
  uterine, 202, 350
guardian, 29, 35, 39
  ad litem, 38–9
Guardianship Acts 1971 to 1973, 39
Guedet airway, 183
Guthrie test, 59, 77, 82
Guyana, 371

haemagglutinisation inhibition test for rubella, 154
haemarthrosis, 246, 280
haematocrit, 238
haematoma, 183, 252
haematuria, 231, 248, 279
haemoglobin, 82, 236–7, 244
  A, 375
  estimation, 133
  F, 244
  fetal, 236–7, 375
  in diabetes, 304
haemoglobinopathies, 243–6, 375
haemolysis, 240
haemolytic anaemia, congenital, 79
haemolytic disease of newborn, 73, 78, 81, 239, 343
haemolytic disorders, 238
haemophilia, 183, 190, 238, 245, 247, 278, 396
  arthritis, 281
Haemophilis influenzae, 133, 139, 140, 142, 153, 165, 243, 289
haemopoeitic system, 236
haemoptysis, 213
haemorrhage, 186, 239
  antepartum, 79, 83, 87, 333
  cerebral, 316
  chronic, 238
  fetomaternal, 79
  gastrointestinal, 236, 279
  in leukaemia, 241–1
  intra-articular, 236, 281
  purpuric, 238, 248
  retinal, 331
  scurvy, 238
  spontaneous, 316
haemorrhagic disease of newborn, 73, 198
haemosiderosis, 243
hallucinations, 313
hallux rigidus, 227
  valgus, 227
handicap, 14, 16, 20, 48, 57, 60, 64, 67, 105, 108, 115, 118, 127, 277, 304–5, 308, 320, 349–50, 356, 372, 378, 394–5, 400
  clinical care, 333–9
  deafness, 323–6
  definition, 333, 349
  mental, 83, 101, 331
  register, 67
  visual, 327–32
hare lip, 76, 194, 334
Harrington squares, 220
hay fever, 14, 46, 95, 136, 288, 294, 349, 376
HBAg, 164
head banging, 212
  circumference of neonates, 197
  injury, 184, 310
headache, 133, 367, 377
  in glandular fever, 161
  tension, 354
Heaf test, *see* tuberculin test
health centres, 47, 102, 106, 128, 343
  education, 20, 22–3, 47, 57, 61–2, 101, 103, 107–8, 127–9
    officers, 128
  expenditure statistics, 17–19
Health Education Council, 128–9, 189–190, 214
Health Services and Public Health Act 1968, 156
health visitors, 10, 12, 20, 22–4, 26–7, 43, 47–8, 55, 57–60, 65, 68–9, 77, 92–3, 101–3, 105–8, 111–2, 115–7, 122–3, 125–6, 127–8, 162, 164–5, 183, 194–5, 206–7, 215, 267, 280, 306, 323–5, 327–8, 344, 348, 354, 357–8, 365, 377, 381, 386, 391
hearing, *see* deafness, audiometry
heart arrhythmias, 310
  block, 310
    congenital, 274
  catheterisation, 274
  disorders, 349, 395
  failure, 270, 277
  massage, 184–5

murmurs, 196, 238, 269–70
septal defects in alcoholism, 380
sounds, 270–1
and see congenital and rheumatic heart disease
heat exhaustion, 390
height charts *see* growth
Heimlich manoeuvre, 184
helmets, safety, 189–90
hemiplegia, infantile, 311
Henoch Schonlein purpura, 247–8, 279
hepatitis serum, 162
viral, 157, 161–4
hepatomegaly, 163, 214, 238, 270, 300, 375
in leukaemia, 240
hepatosplenomegaly, 78
hernia diaphragmatic, 199
inguinal, 177, 179
strangulated, 175
heroin, 73, 387–8
linctus, 276
herpes genitalis, 78, 158
simplex, 157–9, 165, 168, 222
zoster, 154, 158–9, 165
virus, 167
Herpid, 159
Hess tourniquet test, 238, 247–8, 279
hexosaminidase A, 77
High Court, 38–9
Hindus, 373
hip disorders, 225–6, *and see* congenital dislocation of hip
Hirschsprung's disease, 170
hirsutes, 318
hoarseness, 184
Hodgkin's disease, 95, 247–9
home care team sister, 16
delivery, *see* hospital confinement
environment, 87
nursing, 127, 133, *and see* nurse
safety, 58, 61, 129, 190
visits, 20, 23
homicide, 31, 35
homosexuality, 29, 381
holidays, 385
for diabetics, 306
for handicapped, 275, 277
Holland, 4–6, 9, 17–19
Hong Kong, 369, 371
hook foot, 227
hookworms, 170, 213–4, 238, 375
hormone pregnancy tests, 77
hormones *see* growth human/placental lactogen, Oestriol, oestrogens, plasma
horse riding, 189
hospital care, 27–6
and domiciliary care, 16–17
Houghton Committee, 38
house dust mite, 136, 142, 288–9, 294
housing, 73, 125, 350, 352, 365, 373
density, 12
departments, 61
human biology, 127
immunoglobulin, measles, 98
lymphocytic antigen, 299
Humberside, 8, *and see* Yorkshire
Humotet, 186
Hungary, 4
Huntington's chorea, 310
hydramnios, 73, 79
hydrocephalus, 73, 78, 331, 334, 393
hydrocortisone, 226, 292–3
cream, 134
hydrops foetalis, 79
hypnotics, 357
Hypnotism Act 1952, 34
hypocalcaemia, 198–9, 207
hypochondriasis, 352
Hypocount, 304
hypogonadism, 331
hypoglycaemia, 77, 79, 101, 198–9, 300–1, 303–6, 309
hypopituitarism, 252
hyposensitisation, 290, 294
hypotension, 186
hypothermia, 10, 59, 89, 185, 188–9, 197, 199
hypothyroidism, 113, 252, 284
hypotonia, neonatal, 89
hypoxia, 73, 86–9, 101, 142–3, 184, 292, 322
hypsarrhythmia, 313
hysterotomy, 79

iceberg, illness, 15
Iceland, 4
ichthyol, 219–20, 223
Ichthyopaste, 219
icterus gravis neonatorum, 79
IDU, 159
IgA deficiency, 137, 164
IgE, 290
antibody, 285
IgM antibody
to rotavirus, 167
to rubella, 154
in virus hepatitis, 164
illegitimacy, 9, 20, 29, 38, 58, 75–6, 378
imipramine, 359
impetigo, 14, 61, 116, 215, 218, 222
immaturity, 73, 191
immigrants, 68, 75, 91, 93, 99, 102, 211, 351, 369–379
Asian, 228
Indian, 209
Pakistani, 209
immunisation, 9, 20, 22–5, 48–9, 59–60, 91–9, 101, 105–7, 112–3, 116–7, 127–8, 287, 313, 338, 348
in leukaemia, 241
programmes, 42, 93–5
rate, 103
reactions, 97
records, 55–6
see also diphtheria, influenza, measles, mumps, pertussis, poliomyelitis, rubella, tetanus, tuberculosis
immunoglobulins, 139, 156
herpes zoster, 241
measles, 153
rubella, 154
tetanus, 186
varicella, 155
see also IgA, IgE, IgM
immunological deficiency, 94–5, 99, 139, 154
mechanisms, 285
immunosuppression, 158–9, 241
immunosuppressive drugs, 282
incest, 34–5
incontinence pads, 387
incubators, 199
indecency, 31, 35
Indecency with Children Act 1960, 34
India, 244, 313, 369–72, 376–7
induction of labour, 79, 81–2, 205
Infant Life (Preservation) Act 1929, 33
infant mortality, 3–7, 9–11, 353
rate, 105, 109, 154, 347, 377
total wastage, 5
welfare clinics, *see* child health clinics
infanticide, 33
infectious mononucleosis, *see* glandular fever
influenza, 140, 144, 146–50, 214, 269
immunisation, 149, 241
surveillance, 146
viruses, 140, 144, 146–7
Influvac, 149
infundibular resection, 272
ingrowing toenails, 227
inhalation, steam, 142
inner city problems, 20, 25
Inner London Education Authority, 30
insect bites, 155, 174
insomnia, *see* sleep disorders
insulin, 79, 246, 260, 299, 301–5
Intal, *see* cromoglycate, sodium
intercostal recession, 199
interferon, 139
intermediate treatment, 32
intestinal infections, 14
obstruction, 177–8, 198
intrapartum care, 8
intrauterine death, 74
intravenous pyelogram, 233
intussusception, 174–5, 177–8, 248, 279
ipecacuanha syrup, 190

Jacksonian epilepsy, 311
Jamaica, 372
Japan, 3, 17–18
jaundice, 77, 199, 230
acholuric, 243
in infective hepatitis, 164
neonatal, 198–9
Jersey, 393, *and see* Channel Islands
Jews, 243
Julius Caesar, 308
Juvenile Courts, 30, 32, 35–6
juvenile offenders, 30–5
Jobson-Horne probe, 135
joint ankylosis, 280
contractures, 280

kaolin, 49, 171
Kenya, 395
keratitis, herpetiform, 158
kernicterus, 77, 310

Kernig sign, 166
ketoacidosis, 300–1, 303, 305
ketogenic diets, 316
ketones, 87
Ketrax, 212, 214
Keystone apparatus, 328
Kirklees, 8
Klebsiella pneumoniae, 140
Klinefelter's syndrome, 76
knee disorders, 226
koilonychia, 238
Koplik spots, 152–3
kyphosis, 224–5, 244

labour, prolonged, 88–9
lacrimation, 330
lactation, 33, 206, *and see* feeding, breast
lactic acid, 254
 acidosis, 301
lactulose, 358
Ladies Sanitary Reform Association, 57
language development, 25
 problems in immigrants, 378
lanoxin, 276, *and see* digoxin
lanugo hair, 203
laparotomy, 177
large babies, 79
laryngitis, 147, 152
laryngotracheitis, acute, 142, *and see* croup
Lassars paste, 219–20
Laurence Moon Biedle syndrome, 331
Law Commission, 29
Law Reform, (Miscellaneous Provisions) (Scotland) Act 1968, 38
lead lotion, 219–20
 poisoning, 236, 300
learning disorders, 365–7, 393
Leeds, 8, 394
left handedness, 367
Legitimacy Act 1959, *and see* illegitimacy
leishmaniasis, 375
Lennox syndrome, 313
leprosy, 375
lethargy, neonatal, 198
letters, hospital, 24
leucopaenia, 318
leukaemia, 95, 136, 161, 238–42, 247, 278, 280–1, 333, 349, 386–7, 396
 acute myeloblastic, 240, 242, 283
  lymphatic, 240–2
 chronic myelocytic, 240
  lymphocytic, 240
 gingivitis in, 255
 radiation, 77
levallorphan, 88
levamizole, 212, 214
lice, *see* louse
light for dates infants, 202, 309
 sensitivity, 318
limp, 226–7
lincomycin, 259
linctuses, 142, 153
liquor, 74
 meconium stained, 81, 87–9
Listeria monocytogenes, 309
Little's area, 136
Liverpool, 181, 213
Livingstone New Town, 49
local authority, 29–33, 35–6
 education, 30, 36
 health, 92–3, 102, 128, 323
 homes, 31
 see also child health clinics, community child health services, social services
Lomotil, 171, 187
 poisoning, 190
London, 47, 213, 336, 347–8, 376, 378, 393–4, 396
 boroughs, 30, 214
 East, 46
 South, 373
 South East, 67
 and see Inner London Education Authority, metropolitan districts
Lorexane, 215–6
Lothian region, 49
louse, body, 215
 head, 61, 129, 202–4, 214–5
 pubic, 215
low birth weight, 7, 78, 83, 101, 322, 327, 349–50
Lucosade, 301
lumbar puncture, 160, 165, 167, 242, 310
lung abscess, 140, 144
lupus erythematosis, 376
Luton, 372
lymphadenitis, 280, 375
 axillary, 90, 175
 cervical, 135–6, 175, 225
 in glandular fever, 161
 inguinal, 175
 mediastinal, 152
 mesenteric, 161, 175–6
 occipital, 215
 regional, 257
lymphadenoma, 161
lymphadenopathy, 78

macrophages, 139
Magistrates' Court, 30–1, 39
magnesium deficiency, 309
majority, age of, 29
malabsorption, folic acid, 239
 iron, 239
 syndrome, 349
maladjustment, 30, 118, 335, 395–6
 index, 337–8
malaria, 109, 148, 243–4, 375
Malathion, 215–6
malnutrition, 209, 331, 366, *and see* nutrition
malpresentation, 73, 79, 88
Malta, 369, 371
Manchester, 396
manual rotation, 87
manualism, 325
Marfan's syndrome, 269, 271
marital dysharmony, 125–6, 194, 338, 356
marriage breakdown, 64
 of minors, 39
Marsh, Geoffrey, 75
Masse cream, 206
mastoiditis, 132
masturbation, 310
maternal age, 9–11
 deprivation, 109
 parity, 9–11, *and see* multiparity
Maternity and Child Welfare Act 1918, 101
maternity unit, general practitioner, 58–9
 hospital, 58–9
Matrimonial Causes Act 1973, 34
matrimonial proceedings, 39
maturity, fetal, 202–4
measles, 34, 49, 78, 151–3, 160, 165, 241, 283, 331, 334, 338
 immunisation, 91, 94, 97–9, 108, 153
Meckel's diverticulum, 177, 238
meconium, 81, 89, *and see* liquor
Medic-alert bracelets, 190
Mediterranean, 213, 238, 243–4
Melbourne, 168
membranes, artificial rupture, 88
memory, computer, 53
meningeal infiltration in leukaemia, 240–1
meningism, influenzal, 147
meningitis, 157, 198–90, 280, 309, 322, 331, 375–6
 bacterial, 165
 enteroviral, 157
 haemophilus influenzae, 165
 in glandular fever, 161
 meningococcal, 165–7
 mumps, 160
 traumatic, 184
 viral, 165–7
meningococcal infection, 157, 165–7, 248–9
meningococcus, 247
meningoencephalitis, rheumatic, 279
mental cruelty, 34
 disorders, 14, 36
 handicap, 101, 395
 retardation, 78, 83, 86–7, 238, 313, 325, 327, 331, 349–50, 352, 365, 380, 393, 396, 398
Mental Health Act 1959, 35
menthol and eucalyptus inhalation, 142
meprobamate, 82
merbendazole, 213
Mersey, 13, 74
mesenteric adenitis, *see* lymphadenitis
mesenteric artery occlusion, 174
mesial temporal sclerosis, 313
metabolic disorders, 77, 81, 101, 313
metatarsus primus varus, 227
metformin, 301
methaemoglobinaemia, 243
methadone linctus, 276
methotroxate, 339, 341
methyl nitrite, 179
 xanthine, 290
metoclopromide, 262
metropolitan districts, 30, 214
MFV-Ject, 149

microangiography, 300
microcephaly, 78, 380
micturating cystogram, 231, 233
middle ear infection, *see* otitis media
Middle East, 213, 238, 244
Midlands, West, 13
midwife, 20, 26–7, 43, 57–8, 61, 80, 89–90, 106, 128, 194–5, 206
migraine, 14, 97, 310, 354–5
abdominal, 179–80
milk, allergy to
formulae, 197–8
national dried, 47
supplements, iron, 207, 238
fluoride, 207
vitamin C, 207
vitamin D, 207
and see feeding
ministers of religion, 391
Mini-Wright peak flow meter, 286
minors, treatment of, 34
Mintezol, 212–3
mitral regurgitation, 256, 272
Mogadon, 357
molluscum contagiosum, 222
Mongolian spots, 275
Monglism, *see* Down's syndrome
monilial infection, 262
Monospot slide agglutination test, 162
monosulfiram, 216
moral danger, 35
morbidity, postneonatal, 10
rates, 12–17
register, 20
seasonal, 11, 13, 20
surveys, 14–15
and see National Morbidity Survey
Moro reflex, 196–7
morphine, 273, 276, 387
mortality rates, child, 12–13
infant, 12–13, 27
neonatal, 5, 8, 72, 79
perinatal, 5–6, 8, 72–6, 82–3, 202, 349, 353, 372
postneonatal, 7, 9–11, 349
regional, 12–13
and see total infant wastage
mothercraft, 58–9, 61
motor development, 373
dysfunction, 380
moulding, 196
mourning, 335, 386, 389, 400
mouth breathing, 134
MRCGP examination, 42, 44
mucopolysaccharidoses, 81, 182, 309
mucus extractor, 195
multigravidae, 80, 88
multiparity, 79, 203
multiple sclerosis, 152
mumps, 78, 157, 159–61, 166–7, 299, 334, 376
immunisation, 160–1
Murphy's sign, 179
muscle relaxation, 203
tone, 203
muscular dystrophy, 396–7, 400
musculoskeletal defects, congenital, 73
Muslims, 370–1, 373
marriages, 68
Mustard operation, 273
mustine hydrochloride, 249
Mycobacterium tuberculosis, 376
Mycoplasma pneumoniae, 139–41, 144
myocardial depression, fetal, 88
myocarditis, 79
mumps, 160
rheumatic, 278
myopia, 328, 331
myxovirus parotidis, 157–9, 165

naevus, 380
cavernous, 221
spider, 221–2
nalidixic acid, 234
napkin, 58
rash, 107, 170, 219–20, 358
herpetic, 158
narcotics, 78
nasal discharge, 142
obstruction, 142, 194
Naseptrin cream, 136
nasopharyngitis, 14
National Child Health Computer System, 54
national dried milk, 47
National Morbidity Survey, 13
Necator americanus, 213–4
negroes, 243–4, 375–6
neomycin, 49, 98–9, 134, 136
neonatal care, 58, 194–201
examination, 194–6
and see mortality
nephrectomy, 231
nephritis, 282
in scarlet fever, 155
purpuric, 248
neuropathy, diabetic, 305
nephrotic syndrome, 318
Netherlands, *see* Holland
neural tube defects, 72, 76, 81, 83, 166, 339
neuritis, peripheral, 153
neuropathy, diabetic, 305
neurotoxin, 143
neurotropic viruses, 157
newborn, *see* neonates
Newcastle upon Tyne, 27, 47, 203, 347, 350, 396–7
New Commonwealth, 75, 369–72
Newsom Committee, 350
New Zealand, 4, 49, 395
Niemann Pick's disease, 77
Nigeria, 109, 375
night blindness, 331
night dresses, 34
Nightingale, Florence, 57
nightmares, 212, 357
nipples, cracked, 206
shields, 206
nocturia, 231–2
non-accidental injury, *see* child abuse
non-attenders, 27
Normax, 358
Northamptonshire, 8
Norwalk viruses, 169–70
Norway, 4, 6, 17–18
Norwich, 396
NSPCC, 35, 58, 121–3, 125
nurse, district, 20, 61, 115, 183, 277, 280, 300, 381, 388
practice, 20, 22, 68, 92, 102–3, 128, 162, 164, 183, 234, 386
school, 23–4, 26–7, 48, 60, 116–7, 328–9
Nurseries and Child Minders Act 1948, 37
nursery school, 365
nutrition, 76, 101, 107, 151, 205–9, 350–1, 394
nystagmus, 318, 331

obesity, 47, 103, 113, 127, 129, 198, 206, 208–9
obsessiveness, 352
occupational therapy, 384, 399
oesophageal varicies, 258
oestriol, 81–2
oestrogens, 81, 203
oligohydramnios, 196
oliguria, 171
olive oil, 134
onchocerciasis, 331
Oncovin, 249
one parent families, 396–7
ophthalmia neonatorium, 14, 199
opiates, 187
opium, tincture, 381
optic atrophy, 331
oralism, 325
orbiviruses, 168
orciprenaline, 292
orchitis, mumps, 160
organochlorine insecticides, 215
organogenesis, 77
organophosphate insecticides, 215
ornithosis, 139
orthopaedic disorders, 224–8
orthoptists, 116, 328
Ortolani's test, 225
ossification centres, 81, 203
osteochondritis, 280
navicular, 227
patellar, 226
tibial tubercle, 226
ostodystrophy, 252
osteogenesis imperfecta, 251, 394
osteomalacia, 316
osteomyelitis, 228, 280, 376
osteoporosis, 280–1, 376
otitis externa, 46, 132–4
media, 40, 98, 133–4, 138, 140, 142, 147, 149, 153, 170, 313, 323, 349–50, 376
actue, 14, 50, 132–3, 135
recurrent, 133, 136
secretory, 133, 136
ototoxicity, 77
ovarian cyst, 174
overcrowding, 349, 351, 365
over protection, 129, 305, 367
Oxford region, 7–8, 13, 74
oxygen, 89, 143, 211, 244, 273, 277, 327
fetal, 76

Paddington, 68
paediatric psychiatry, *see* child psychiatry
paediatricians, 22–6
Pakistan, 75, 369–71, 377
Palmer automatic injector, 305
pancreatitis, 174
  mumps, 160
papilloedema, 312
paracetamol, 34, 179, 246, 252, 259
paraffin stoves, 377
para influenza, 159
  viruses, 140, 142
paraldehyde, 317
paralytic ileus, 175
paraplegia, 350
parasites, intestinal, 211–4
parasitic diseases, 14
parental attitudes, 305–6
  compliance, 105
  consent, 33–4
  deprivation, 120
  rights, 36
  and see overprotection
parentcraft classes, 58 *and see* mothercraft
parents, 12, 15, 20, 23–4, 47–8, 63, 194, 204, 331, 336, 348, 354–5, 360, 362–3, 367, 372–3
  alcoholic, 380–2
  and terminal care, 386–91
  groups, 306
  immigrant, 378
  of handicapped, 335, 384–5
paronychia, 222
parotid duct, 159
  gland, 159–60
  pain, 132
parotitis, suppurative, 160
paroxysmal supraventricular tachycardia, 256, 270, 272, 274
  vertigo, 310
partially sighted, *see* visual defects
patent ductus arteriosus, 78, 256, 268–73
patients' associations, 112, 128
Paul Bunnell test, 135, 160, 162
peak expiratory flow, 286, 290–1, 293, 295
  meter, 46, 291
pediculosis humanis capitis, 214, 222
  corporis, 215
Pel-Ebstein fever, 249
pelvic abnormality, 73
pemphigus, 216
Pendlebury, 400
penicillin, 94, 135, 144, 166–7, 195, 243, 258, 262, 274, 278–9
  benzyl, 135
  G, 256–7
  phenoxymethyl, 133, 135, 162
  prophylactic, 137
  rash, 95
  V, 153, 156, 162, 256–7
penicillamine, 280
pentazocine, 246
peptic ulcer, perforation, 174
percussion, 293
pericarditis, 278, 280, 282
pericolic abscess, 174
peridontal disease, 355
perinatal care, 8 *and see* mortality
peripheral neuropathy, 147
peritonitis, 176–7, 282, 376
permissiveness, 354
Perthe's disease, 226
pertussis, 34, 48–9, 108, 139, 140, 143, 287, 310
  immunisation, 48–9, 91, 94–7, 143, 166
  notification, 96
pes cavus, 227
petechiae, 164, 166, 238, 240, 246–8
  in glandular fever, 161
Peterborough, 378
pethidine, 78, 88
pethilorfan, 88
petit mal, *see* epilepsy
petrol agar, 358
Peyer's patches, 179
pharyngitis, 14, 135–6, 140, 175
phenacetin, 243, 280
Phenergan, *see* promethazine
phenformin, 301
phenobarbitone, 143, 260, 262, 313, 318, 320
phenothiazines, 187
phenyl alanine hydroxylase, 77
phenyl butazone, 238, 280
phenyl ketonuria, 77, 113, 283, 309–10, 333, 398
phenytoin, 235–6, 238–9, 255, 260, 262, 316–8, 320
phimosis, 333
Phthirus pubis, 215
photophobia, 151, 166
photosensitivity in epilepsy, 309
physical fitness, 129
physiotherapy, 44, 46, 58, 118, 142, 183, 280–1, 293, 384, 399
phytate intake, 209
phytic acid, 376
pica, 236, 376
picornavirus, 162
Pierre Robin syndrome, 196
pigeon toes, 225
pigmentation, 375
pinhole meatus, 233
piperazine phosphate, 212–3
pityriasis rosea, 222–3
placenta, disorders, 73
  failure, 81
  function, 203, 333
  infarction, 73, 203
  insufficiency, 309
  lactogen in human serum, 81
  praevia, 73
  retained, 79
  transmission, 77
plasma albumen, 77
  bilirubin, 77
  fibrinogen, 246
  half life concentration, 316
  non esterified fatty acids, 208
  oestriol, 81
  phosphorus, 207
  proteins, 246
  sodium, 310
play groups, 37, 61, 356, 398
pleural effusion, 180
pleurisy, 144, 147, 282
pleurodynia, 166
Plowden Committee, 27
pneumonia, 14, 46, 139–41, 144, 147, 149, 153, 275, 300, 349–50, 353, 375, 386
  aspiration, 311
  influenzal, 148
pneumonitis, 152, 280
  haemorrhagic, 213
pneumothorax, 140, 270
podophyllin, 220–1
poikilocytosis, 239
poison centres, 190
poisoning, 14, 47, 127, 181–90, 264, 254
  aspirin, 188
  carbon monoxide, 187
  drugs, 129
  iron, 188
Poland, 369, 378
police, 35, 125, 183, 189
poliomyelitis, 14, 34, 78, 103, 141, 278
  immunisation, 91, 93–4, 97–8, 241
poliovirus, 165
pollen hypersensitivity, 288, 294
polyadenitis, 376
polyarteritis nodosa, 281
polyarthritis, 282
  rheumatic, 280
polycythaemia, 270, 273, 276–7
polydactyly, 316, 331
polydipsia, 231
polymyxin, 98–9
polyneuritis, influenzal, 148
polyuria, 231
Pony Club, 189
Posalfillin, 221
positive discrimination, 19, 27–8
postmaturity, 203
postnasal drip, 132, 142
postnatal care, 8, 158
  visits, 108
post neonatal mortality, *see* mortality
post-term infants, 202
postural defects, 112, 117
  drainage, 293
potassium chloride, 171
  supplements, 277
poverty, 64, 120, 125, 346–53, 395
  definition, 346–7
practice premises, 2–3
  receptionist, 12, 128
  records, 111-3
  secretary, 107
  staff, 111
  treatment room, 47
  and see health visitor, midwife, nurse
precipitate labour, 79
prednisolone, 247, 262, 292–4, 319
prednisone, 160
pre-eclampsia, 79, 83, 202–3
pregnancy, multiple, 73, 79, 83
  termination, 80–3, 98, 338–9, 375
    in rubella, 154
premature labour, 80, 350
  rupture of membranes, 73

prematurity, 60–1, 65, 78–9, 86–7, 89, 95, 97, 202
prepuce, retraction, 194
pre-school surveillance, 48
prescribing, 45, 50, 259–265
  antibiotics, 141
pre-term infants, 202
primary care team, 12, 14, 16–7, 19–20, 22–6, 59, 63, 69, 106, 115, 119, 128, 267, 335, 344, 379, 381
primidone, 236, 316, 318
primigravidae, 58, 80, 88, 93
Prioderm, 215–6
Prior, Matthew, 264
Pripsen, 212–3
prison, 31, 33
Probanithine, 359
probation officer, 31–2, 35, 61
problem orientated records, 20
procaine amide, 274
processor, computer, 53
prochlorperazine, 262
progressive systemic sclerosis, *see* scleroderma
prolapsed intervertebral disc, 225
promazine, 89
promethazine, 155, 387
pronunciation, 112
propanolol, 273–4, 276
propantheline, 359
proteinuria, 234
Proteus, 233
pruritis, 218
  ani, 212
  vulvae, 300
pseudamina, 272
pseudoephedrine, 134
Pseudomonas pyocyanea (aeruginosa), 140, 333
psoriasis, 218, 220, 223, 398
psychological problems, 47
psychologists, 22
psychometric assessment, 320
psychosis, 120, 333
psychotherapy, 86, 120
psychotropic drugs, 47
ptosis, congenital, 330
puberty, 77, 180, 316
Public Health (Infectious Diseases) Regulations 1968, 156
pulled elbow, 228
pulmonary blood flow, 270
  hypertension, 270
  oedema, 270
  stenosis, 256, 268–9, 272
pulp death, 257
punishment, 363
purpura, 238, 240, 246–8
  after rubella, 153
  Henoch Schonlein, 178–9
  influenzal, 147
  in meningococcal infection, 166
  non-thrombocytopaenic, 247–8
  thrombocytopaenic, 78, 245, 247
  toxic, 245
pyelitis, 175, 309, 313
pyelonephritis, 234
  acute, 230–1
  chronic, 231, 233–4
pyloric stenosis, 179
pyridoxine, *see* vitamine B6

quadriplegia, 350
Quellada, 215–6
questionnaires, 48
quinsey, 135, 137, 147

rabies, 166
radiation, 78, 80
radioactive iodine, 77
radiography, 144
radiotherapy in leukaemia, 241
Ramadan, 373
random case analysis, 44
rape, 31
reading attainment, 351
  difficulty, 101, 330
  retardation, 352, 366–7
records, 45, 53, 58, 60, 124
  antenatal, 80
  child health, 23–4
  immunisation
  local authority, 101
  practice, 106–7
  school medical, 117
Red Cross escorts, 61
Reed-Sternberg cells, 248–9
reflex, glabellar, 203
  let down, 205
  Moro, 312
  neck righting, 203
  pupil, 203
  rooting, 196–7
Reflo test, 304
refraction, 350
regional adviser, 43
regional mortality, *see* mortality
Registrar of Births and Deaths, 39–40
Registrar General, 39
registration, births, 39
  partially sighted, 332
  stillbirths, 39
rehabilitation, 320
reimplantation of ureters, 231
relaxation classes, 58, 61, 128
renal abnormalities, 196
  colic, 231
  dialysis, 234
  failure, 234
  osteodystrophy, 231
  glucose threshold, 79
reovirus, 168
research, 45–50
residential care, 32–3
respiratory defects, congenital, 73
  depression, 88–9
  disorders, 14, 41, 45–6, 138–45, 349, 387
  distress, 12
    syndrome, 81–2, 199, 270
  failure, 317, 387
  function tests, 46
  infection, 10, 46, 49–50, 97, 157, 176, 238, 376
  rate, 196
  syncytial virus, 140, 143, 148, 287
restlessness, 142
resuscitation, 195
reticulocytosis, *see* blood
retinal dystrophy, 329, 331
  haemorrhage, 331
  microaneurysm, 300
retinitis pigmentosa, 331
retinoblastoma, 214, 329, 331
retinopathy, 78, 185
  diabetic, 301, 305
retrograde amnesia, 310–1
  pyelogram, 235
retrolental fibroplasia, 331
Reynel language development scales, 366
rhesus factor, 78–9
  incompatibility, 238, 310, 322, 377
  haemolytic disease, *see* blood
rheumatic fever, 135, 278–9, 338
  heart disease, 278
  nodules, 200–1
rheumatism, 14, 278–81, 394
rheumatoid arthritis, 279–80
rhinitis, allergic, 141
  perennial, 132, 136
  see also hay fever
rhinoviruses, 140, 142, 289
Rhodesia, 371
Rhondda, 76
Ribena, 301
rickets, 14, 183, 209, 228, 316, 376
riding for the disabled, 398
rifampicin, 362
ringworm, 116, 222–3
river blindness, 331
Rochester, Kent, 32
Romania, 4
roseola infantum, 151, 156
ROSPA, 189
rotahaler, 295
rotaviruses, 157, 168–70
Rotersept spray, 206
round shoulders, 227
roundworms, 212–4, 375
Rovsing's sign, 177
rubella, 34, 49, 55, 78, 82–3, 136, 151, 153–6, 196, 203, 251, 269, 309, 322, 324, 330–1, 376, 397
  congenital, 154, 198, 203
  immunisation, 49, 55, 91, 98–9, 129, 160
rugby football, 189
rural areas, 73, 80

Sacker comb, 215
salbutamol, 143, 292, 295, *and see* Ventolin
salicylates, 246, 248, 259, 278–80
salicylic acid, 219
salivary calculus, 160
  duct, 160
  glands, 159–60
Salmonella sonnei, 168
sarcoidosis, 283, 376

Sarcoptes scabei, 215–6
Saudi Arabia 244, *and see* Arabia
scabies, 61, 116, 130, 215–6, 222
scalds, 121
Scandinavia, 350
scarf sign, 203
scarlet fever, 135, 140, 151, 155–6
school attendance, 23, 349
legislation, 36
dentist, 116
health service, 23, 26, 55, 92–3, 115–9, 132
meals, 347, 362
medical examination, 105
officer, 115, 117–9, 146, 149, 189, 215, 326
phobia, 359–60
reports, 31, 320
teacher, 23, 61, 116–7, 154, 189, 222, 230, 330, 353, 362, 399
welfare officer, 61
and see nurse
schools, residential, 67, 144–5, 149, 155
for deafness, 325, 376
for handicapped, 118, 334, 336
for spastics, 400
for visual defects, 330
Schwartz strain of measles virus, 98
scleroderma, 281
scoliosis, 224–5
Scotland, 6–7, 10, 13, 33–4, 49, 54, 166, 187, 347, 351–2, 372, 397–9
screening, 23–5, 47, 83, 101, 103, 108, 113, 116–7, 128, 132, 375
bacteriuria, 234
congenital heart disease, 267
deafness, 322, 324
phenylketonuria, 333
programmes, 14
urine, 231, 233
visual defects, 328–9
and see developmental surveillance
scurvy, 238, 247
sealants, fissure, 254
seborrhoeic dermatitis, 218
secondary care, 19–20, 22–6
sedatives, 84, 256, 387
self help, 129
senna, 214
sense organs, diseases, 14
septicaemia, coliform, 230
in leukaemia, 241
meningococcal, 166, 247–8
serum alkaline phosphatase, 81
alphafetoprotein, 81–3
aminotransferase, 164
amitryptyline, 359
anticonvulsant levels, 316
bilirubin, 243
calcium, 376
folate, 240
lead, 376
SGOT, 162
SGPT, 162
phosphatase, 376
phosphorus, 376
and see plasma
sex education, 127, 129
sexual maturation, 208
Sexual Offences Act 1956, 34, 39
shaking injuries, 126, 185, 310
Sheffield, 11, 47
Sheldon Committee, 119
Sheriff Court, 33
Shetland Isles, 49
shigellae, 168
shire counties, 30
Short, Renee, 8
sickle cell disease and trait, *see* blood
sign language, 325
Sikhs, 273
silicone barrier cream, 220
sinusitis, 135, 138, 142, 147
skate board injury, 189
skeletal defects, 117, *and see* orthopaedic disorders
skin disorders, 14, 218–223
pigmentation, 375
skull biparietal diameter, 203
bossing, 243–5, 375
slapped cheek disease, 156
sleep disorders, 47, 64, 106–8, 113, 122, 142, 219, 252, 354, 356–7
Slough, 399
small for dates, *see* dysmaturity
smallpox, 14, 34, 76, 78, 91, 155, 165
immunisation, 241
smoking, 46, 58, 80, 127–9, 151, 306, 348–9, 366
Snellen's test types, 327–8
snuffles, 106
social class, 9–13, 16, 20, 73–5, 87, 101, 105, 161, 181, 189, 205, 256, 299, 347–52, 370, 373
social services departments, 30–1, 39, 58, 63–69, 127, 185, 277, 332, 335, 397
voluntary, 129, 335
social worker, 22–4, 27, 31–2, 35, 37, 47, 61, 63–69, 123, 125–6, 325, 330, 344, 358, 375, 381, 399–400
socio-economic variation, 7
sodium bicarbonate, 171, 222
ion, 243
sonicaid amplifier, 87–8
Sparine, *see* promazine
spasticity, *see* cerebral palsy
special care baby unit, 194, 199, 204
speech development, 58, 60, 112, 117, 325
disorders, 101, 119, 350, 365–6
therapy, 23, 116, 118, 324, 366, 399
spermatic cord, torsion, 179
spherocytosis, *see* blood
sphingomyelinase, 77
spina bifida, 73, 76, 81, 225, 334, 359, 385, 387, 393, 399
spinal disorders, 400
injury, 86, 186
splenectomy, 243, 245, 247
splenomegaly, 238, 243, 245, 247, 249, 274, 279, 375
in glandular fever, 161
in leukaemia, 240
splints, 184
Spock, Benjamin, 65, 354
spoiling, 362–4
sprains, 182
Sprengl's shoulder, 227
squatting attacks, 271, 273
squint, 25, 60, 106, 109, 112, 117, 327–9, 331, 333, 350, 380
staphylococcus, 199, 228
albus, 233
aureus, 233
pneumoniae, 148
pyogenes, 139–40, 153–4, 222
statistics, 41, 74–7
status epilepticus, 259, 311, 313, 317, 319
step parents, 29, 39
stercobilin, 243
Steristrip, 186
sternomastoid tumour, 223
steroid aerosols, 293–5
metabolism, 316
therapy, 155
topical, 219–20
and see corticosteroids, prednisolone
stilboestrol, 82, 206
stillbirth, 5, 39, 72–6, 79, 390
rate, 7, 348, 377
register, 70
Still's disease, 279–80
Stockton, 75
stomatitis, 147
strabismus, *see* squint
strangury, 331
strawberry tongue, 55
streptococcus, 243
beta haemolytic, 135, 139–40, 148, 154–5, 222, 247, 278–9
faecalis, 333
mutans, 253
pneumoniae, 139–40, 144, 153
streptococcal throat infection, 161
streptomycin, 77, 256, 260
stridor, 141–2, 184
Stuart's medium, 132
stutter, 366
Stycar hearing tests, 109, 112, 132, 324
vision tests, 109, 112, 327–8
subacute sclerosing panencephalitis, 313
subaortic stenosis, 256
subdural haematoma, 120–1, 185, 310
suckling, 206, 252
sudden infant death syndrome, 390
sugar, 59, 254–5
suicide, 126
attempted, 382
Suleo, 215
sulphonamides, 77, 137, 233, 238, 243, 262, 310
sulphur dioxide, 287
sulthiome, 316, 318, 320
summary proceedings, 30
supervision order, 32
supplementary benefit, 351
suprapubic aspiration, 232
suturing of lacerations, 187
surveillance, *see* developmental surveillance
Sweden, 3–4, 6, 9, 17–19, 189

sweets, 127, 129, 187, 208, 253, 301
swimming, 133–4, 185, 315
Switzerland, 4–5, 7, 18–19
Sydenham's chorea, 279
syndactyly, 316
synovitis, 280
syntocin, 84
syphilis, congenital, 78, 203

tachycardia, neonatal, 84
talipes equinovarus, 76, 196, 227, 334
tartrazine, 287
Tatooing of Minors Act 1969, 34
Tay Sachs disease, 77, 310
teenage mothers, 75
teeth, 14, 77, 129, 133, 209, 212, 239, 250–7
teething, 158, 252, 385
television, 314–5
temper tantrums, 67, 355
temporomandibular joint, 132
Ten Day Rule, 78
tendo achilles, shortening, 227
tendon sheath infections, 228
tetanus, 34, 182, 186–7, 190
  immunisation, 93–7
  toxoid, 186, 241
tetany, 389
Tetmosol, 216
tetracyclines, 77, 251, 258–9, 262, 278
tetralogy of Fallot, *see* Fallot's tetralogy
Tetretol, 262
teratogenesis, 77, 380
  drugs, 316
  smoking, 76
terbutaline, 292
Terman Merrill intelligence test, 320
terminal care, 386–8
termination, *see* pregnancy
testicular biopsy, 241
testis, ectopic, 175
  torsion, 175, 179
thalassaemia, *see* blood
thalidomide, 77, 333, 349, 396
Thames regions, 13, 74
theophylline, *see* aminophylline
thiabendazole, 212–4
threadworms, 175, 178, 211–2
throat infections, 132
thrombocytopaenia, 94, 99, 319, 340–1
thrush, 139, 158
  diarrhoea, 170
  in leukaemia, 241
thymus-derived lymphocytes, 241
thyroid disorders, 77
thyrotoxicosis, 79
thyroxin, 238
tinea versicolor, 375
tobacco legislation, 34
Todd's palsy, 311
Tofranil, 359
toilet, neonatal, 197
  training, 60
tonic-clonic movements, 310, 319
tonsillectomy, 135–7, *and see* adenotonsillectomy
tonsillitis, 14, 23, 133, 135–6, 138, 140, 147, 155, 158, 160–1, 174, 176, 195, 313
toothache, 127
tooth buds, 250
tooth pastes, 254
torticollis, 223
total infant wastage, 5
tower blocks, 351
toxaemia, 73, 333
toxicity, 141–2, 188
Toxocara canis and catis, 214
toxoplasmosis, 78, 82, 161, 198, 203, 309
toy libraries, 60, 400
toys, 374
trachoma, 331
tranquillisers, 256
transaminases, 81, 163
transfusion, *see* blood
translocation mongols, 76, 82
transposition of the great arteries, 256, 268–9, 273
Trent region, 13, 74
trichloracetic acid, 221–2
trichloryl, 357
Trichuris trichiuria, 213
Triclofos syrup, 319, 357
tricuspid regurgitation, 72
trigeminal ganglion, 158
trigger finger and thumb, 228
trismus, 159
trivia, 109
Trollope, Anthony, 205
troxidone, 318
truancy, 36, 352, *and see* School phobia
trypanosomiasis, 375
tryptizole, 359
tuberculin test, 94, 376
tuberculosis, 14, 34, 79, 136, 166, 275, 278, 283, 376
  bovine, 376
  immunisation, 91, 94, 99, 376
  spinal, 228
  urinary tract, 231
tuberose sclerosis, 308, 310
Tunbridge Wells Committee, 120
Turner's syndrome, 76–7, 240, 268–9
twin pregnancy, 81
Twist, Oliver, 6, 9, 12, 18
typhoid, 375

ultrasound, 79–80, 82, 180, 203
umbilical artery, single, 269
  blood vessels, 334
  cord, 73, 197–8
    prolapse, 87
    sepsis, 309
unconsciousness, 183–4, 356
unemployment, immigrants, 378
United Kingdom, 4–7, 9, 12, 17–19, 41, 45, 72–5, 95, 99, 103, 105, 108–9, 123, 153, 159–62, 169, 190, 205, 209, 308, 319, 331–3, 369–71, 376–7, 394–5
unmarried mothers, *see* illegitimacy
uraemia, 264
ureteric calculus, 174
  transplantation, 234
ureterocoele, 333
urinalysis
urinary incontinence, 243
  tract infection, 23, 46–7, 50, 60, 230–4, 238
urine bacteria, 231–4
  bile, 238
  culture, 117
  leucocytes, 232
  microscopy, 232–4
  oestriol, 81–2
  pus, 234
  protein, 234
  specimens, collection, 232
  tests, 79, 82, 232
  urobilinogen, 164, 238, 243
urobilin, 243
urticaria, 147, 218, 262
  papular, 220, 222
uterine rupture, 79
uteroplacental function tests, 81–2
  insufficiency, 87
USA, 17–19, 139, 161, 169, 189, 206, 231, 350, 380
USSR, 4

vaccination, *see* immunisation
Vaccine Damage Payments Act 1979, 34
vaccinia, 159, 165
vagina, adenocarcinoma, 77
Valium, *see* diazepam
valproate, sodium, 316, 319
valproic acid, 315
valvulotomy, 272–3
vancomycin, 256
Van den Bergh reaction, 243
Vanquin, 212
varicella, 78, 154–5, 165, 241
variola, *see* smallpox
vasectomy, 10
vasovagal attacks, 310–1
ventricular septal defect, 268–70, 272–3
Vermox, 212–3
vernix caseosa, 88
verrucae, *see* warts
vesico-ureteric reflex, 231, 233–4
Vincents infection, 158
vincristine, 241, 249, 262
vioform, 134
violence, 14, 381
viprinium embonate, 212
viruses, diagnostic tests, 139
  hepatitis, 78
  of love, 158
  replication, 158
  respiratory, 46
visceral larva migrans, 214
vision defects, 78, 116–8, 327–32, 349–50, 398
vitamins, 60, 348
  B6, 310
  B12, 238, 240, 283
  C complex, 238–40
  D, 209, 228, 316, 375
  K, 316
  supplements, 60, 205

vitiligo, 375
vocabulary, 12
vocational training, 25–6, 42–3, 45, 49, 67–69, 102, 129
Volkmann's contracture, 183
voluntary organisations, 128–9, 393–400
vomiting, 12, 14, 174
  cyclical, 355
Von Willebrand's disease, 245, 247
vulvovaginitis, herpetic, 158

Wales, 3–7, 9, 11–13, 38, 54, 64, 75–6, 78–80, 96, 98, 117, 146–7, 151–2, 157, 162–3, 165, 167, 181, 186–7, 250, 253, 269, 347–8, 351–2, 377, 393, 395, 398
Waller's shells, 206
wardship, 39–40
Warnock Committee, 117–8
warts, 14, 218, 220–1
  plantar, 116, 185, 221
Waterson's shunt, 256
wax, 134
weaning, 60, 108, 129, 206, 372, 384
welfare, *see* social services
weighing, 107–8, 209
weight charts, 113
  loss, 230–1
  record, 23
Weil's disease, 164
Wessex, 7, 13, 74
West Indians, 68, 213, 351, 363–6, 372–4, 376–7
West Midlands, 7, 74
West's syndrome, 312
wheezy bronchitis, 46, 140–1, 143, 284–5, 287–9, 293, 295
whipworms, 213
Whitfield's ointment, 223
whitlows, herpetic, 158
whooping cough, *see* pertussis
window sign, 203
winter vomiting disease, 169
Wood's light, 223
worms, 375
Wright peak flow meter, 286
wry neck, 223

yaws, 375
yeast infection, *see* thrush
yolk sac, 82
Yorkshire, 7–8, 13, 74
youth employment officer, 326
  organisations, 129

zinc oxide, 219–20, 223